Seminars in Child and Adolescent Psychiatry

College Seminars Series

For details of available and forthcoming books in the College Seminars Series please visit:
www.cambridge.org/series/college-seminars-series/

Seminars in Child and Adolescent Psychiatry

Third Edition

Edited by
Shermin Imran
Greater Manchester NHS Foundation Trust

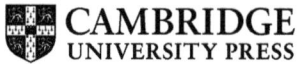

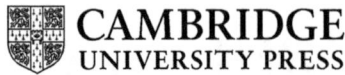
CAMBRIDGE
UNIVERSITY PRESS

Shaftesbury Road, Cambridge CB2 8EA, United Kingdom

One Liberty Plaza, 20th Floor, New York, NY 10006, USA

477 Williamstown Road, Port Melbourne, VIC 3207, Australia

314–321, 3rd Floor, Plot 3, Splendor Forum, Jasola District Centre,
New Delhi – 110025, India

103 Penang Road, #05–06/07, Visioncrest Commercial, Singapore 238467

Cambridge University Press is part of Cambridge University Press & Assessment,
a department of the University of Cambridge.

We share the University's mission to contribute to society through the pursuit of
education, learning and research at the highest international levels of excellence.

www.cambridge.org
Information on this title: www.cambridge.org/9781009114233

DOI: 10.1017/9781009110266

© The Royal College of Psychiatrists 1993, 2005, 2026

This publication is in copyright. Subject to statutory exception and to the provisions
of relevant collective licensing agreements, no reproduction of any part may take
place without the written permission of Cambridge University Press & Assessment.

When citing this work, please include a reference to the DOI 10.1017/9781009110266

First published 1993
Second edition 2005
Third edition 2026

A catalogue record for this publication is available from the British Library

A Cataloging-in-Publication data record for this book is available from the Library of Congress

ISBN 978-1-009-11423-3 Paperback

Cambridge University Press & Assessment has no responsibility for the persistence
or accuracy of URLs for external or third-party internet websites referred to in this
publication and does not guarantee that any content on such websites is, or will remain,
accurate or appropriate.

For EU product safety concerns, contact us at Calle de José Abascal, 56, 1°, 28003 Madrid, Spain, or email
eugpsr@cambridge.org

....

Every effort has been made in preparing this book to provide accurate and up-to-date information
that is in accord with accepted standards and practice at the time of publication. Although case histories
are drawn from actual cases, every effort has been made to disguise the identities of the individuals
involved. Nevertheless, the authors, editors, and publishers can make no warranties that the information
contained herein is totally free from error, not least because clinical standards are constantly changing
through research and regulation. The authors, editors, and publishers therefore disclaim all liability
for direct or consequential damages resulting from the use of material contained in this book. Readers
are strongly advised to pay careful attention to information provided by the manufacturer of any drugs
or equipment that they plan to use.

Contents

List of Contributors vii
List of Abbreviations xi

1 **Children's Mental Health Services in Context** 1
Prathiba Chitsabesan, Paula Lavis and Guy Northover

2 **Normal Childhood Development: Theories and Influence** 19
Reshmi Nijjar and Dushyanthan Mahadevan

3 **Risk Factors for Childhood Psychopathology** 34
Joanne L. Doherty and Alka S. Ahuja MBE

4 **Infant Mental Health** 49
Zoë Davidson and Anne McFadyen

5 **Classification and Epidemiology** 67
Josephine Holland, Kapil Sayal and Elena Garralda

6 **Law in Relation to Children and Young People** 81
Tina Irani, John O'Brien and Shermin Imran

7 **What Does a Good Assessment in Children and Adolescents Look Like?** 96
Kishan Sharma[†] and Rachel Elvins

8 **Neurodevelopmental Disorders in Children and Young People** 113
Catherine J. Gregory, Hannah Slevin and Shruti Garg

9 **Intellectual Disabilities in Children and Young People** 130
Mark Lovell and Ashley Liew

10 **Antisocial Behaviours in Young People** 144
Paul A. Tiffin and Oliver O'Mara

11 **Attachment, Anxiety Disorders and Experience of Trauma in Children and Adolescents** 161
Emma Williams and Bridie Gallagher

12 **Self-Harm and Suicide in Young People** 176
Mindy Reeves, Eleni Frisira and David Kingsley

13 **Mood Disorders in Young People** 190
Amy McCulloch, Stephen Connery Adams, Aditya Sharma and Bernadka Dubicka

14 **Psychosis in Children and Adolescents** 219
Sofia Manolesou and Marinos Kyriakopoulos

15 **Substance Misuse in Young People** 231
Paul McArdle and Eilish Gilvarry

16 **Evolving Perspectives on Eating Disorders: From Diagnosis to Digital Therapies** 244
Cecily M. Donnelly and Dasha Nicholls

17 **Benefits and Risks of the Digital World** 264
Alka S. Ahuja MBE and Gemma Johns

18 **Bodily Distress Disorder and Dissociative Disorders** 278
Charlotte Ulrikka Rask and Karen Hansen Kallesøe

19 **Psychosocial Approaches in CAMHS** 296
Shaziyah Afzal, Samantha Todd and Paul Wallis

20 **Gender Diversity and Mental Health in Young People** 313
Akhgar Ghassabian, Melissa Santos and Tonya White

21 **Mental Health Prevention in Services for Children** 323
Carmen Chan, Matthew Lister and Nick Hindley

22 **Moving from Models of Liaison Psychiatry to Psychological Medicine: New Approaches** 339
Isabel Paz, Kate Green, Harriet Stewart, Karen Steinhardt and Mina Fazel

23 **Forensic Mental Health Services for Young People** 353
Oliver White

Index 363

Contributors

Shaziyah Afzal
Systemic Psychotherapist, Greater Manchester Mental Health NHS Foundation Trust, UK

Alka S. Ahuja MBE
Consultant Child & Adolescent Psychiatrist, Aneurin Bevan University Health Board; National Clinical Lead, TEC Cymru, UK; Visiting Professor, University of South Wales and Honorary Professor Cardiff University, UK; Chair of Wales Devolved Council, Royal College of Psychiatrists, UK

Carmen Chan
Consultant Clinical Psychologist and Clinical Lead; Horizon (Oxfordshire CAMHS), Oxfordshire Outreach Team and Oxfordshire CAMHS trauma pathway, UK

Prathiba Chitsabesan
Consultant Child and Adolescent Psychiatrist, Pennine Care NHS Foundation Trust; Visiting Professor, University College London and Manchester Metropolitan University, UK

Stephen Connery Adams
Consultant Child and Adolescent Psychiatrist, Manchester University NHS Foundation Trust, UK.

Zoë Davidson
Consultant in Infant Mental Health Psychiatry, NHS Lanarkshire and Glasgow Infant and Family Team, NSPCC, UK

Joanne L. Doherty
Consultant Child and Adolescent Psychiatrist, Cardiff and Vale University Health Board; Honorary Senior Research Fellow, Cardiff University, UK

Cecily M. Donnelly
Honorary Research Associate, Division of Psychiatry, Imperial College London, UK

Bernadka Dubicka
Consultant Child and Adolescent Psychiatrist Greater Manchester Mental Health NHS Foundation Trust; Professor of Child and Adolescent Psychiatry HYMS University of York; honorary consultant Pennine Care NHS Foundation Trust; honorary MAHSC Professor University of Manchester; Editor-in-Chief *Child and Adolescent Mental Health*, UK

Rachel Elvins
FRCPsych, MD, Consultant Child and Adolescent Psychiatrist, Manchester University NHS Foundation Trust, UK

Mina Fazel
Consultant in Child and Adolescent Psychiatry and Professor of Adolescent Psychiatry, Department of Psychiatry, University of Oxford, Oxford, UK

Eleni Frisira
Academic Clinical Fellow in Child and Adolescent Psychiatry, University of Nottingham, UK

Bridie Gallagher
Consultant Clinical Psychologist, Strategic Lead for Wigan and Bolton Intensive Support Team, Greater Manchester Mental Health GMMH NHS Trust, UK

Shruti Garg
Division of Psychology, Communication and Human Neuroscience, School of Health Sciences, University of Manchester, Manchester, UK; Royal Manchester

Children's Hospital, Manchester University NHS Foundation Trust, Manchester, UK

Elena Garralda
Emeritus Professor in Child and Adolescent Psychiatry, Imperial College London, UK

Akhgar Ghassabian
Departments of Pediatrics and Population Health, New York University Grossman School of Medicine, NY, USA

Eilish Gilvarry
Consultant Psychiatrist Newcastle Addictions Service Cumbria, Northumberland, Tyne and Wear NHS Foundation Trust; Honorary Professor University of Newcastle, UK

Kate Green
Principal Clinical Psychologist, Department of Children's Psychological Medicine, The Oxford Psychological Medicine Centre, Oxford University Hospitals NHSFT, Oxford, UK

Catherine J. Gregory
Division of Psychology, Communication and Human Neuroscience, School of Health Sciences, University of Manchester, Manchester, UK

Karen Hansen Kallesøe
Department of Child and Adolescent Psychiatry, Aarhus University Hospital Psychiatry, Denmark; Department of Clinical Medicine, Aarhus University, Denmark

Nick Hindley
Consultant Child and Adolescent Psychiatrist, Forensic CAMHS and Link Teams; Lead Named Doctor for Children's Safeguarding, Oxford Health NHS Foundation Trust; Honorary Senior Lecturer, University of Oxford, UK

Josephine Holland
Clinical Assistant Professor in Child and Adolescent Psychiatry, University of Nottingham, UK

Shermin Imran
Consultant Child and Adolescent Psychiatrist Forensic CAMHS, Gardener Unit, Greater Manchester Mental Health NHS Foundation Trust, UK; Vice Chair CAP faculty, Royal College of Psychiatrists, UK

Tina Irani
Austen House, Southern Health NHS Foundation Trust, Southampton, Hampshire, UK

Gemma Johns
Head of Research, TEC Cymru, UK

David Kingsley
Consultant Child and Adolescent Psychiatrist and Clinical Director CAMHS, Priory Healthcare, UK

Marinos Kyriakopoulos
South London and Maudsley NHS Foundation Trust, London, UK; National and Kapodistrian University of Athens, Athens, Greece; Institute of Psychiatry, Psychology and Neuroscience, King's College London, London, UK

Paula Lavis
Policy Manager, NHS Confederation, UK

Ashley Liew
Consultant Paediatric Neuropsychiatrist, South London and Maudsley NHS Foundation Trust, UK

Matthew Lister
Head of Psychological Therapies for Oxfordshire CAMHS; Consultant Clinical Psychologist, Oxford Health NHS Foundation Trust, UK

Mark Lovell
Consultant Child and Adolescent
Intellectual Disability Psychiatrist, Tees Esk
and Wear Valleys NHS Foundation
Trust, UK

Dushyanthan Mahadevan
Consultant in Child & Adolescent
Psychiatry, East Lancashire Hospitals NHS
Trust, UK; Deputy MRCPsych Course
Director, Health Education England North
West, UK

Sofia Manolesou
South London and Maudsley NHS
Foundation Trust, London, UK; National
and Kapodistrian University of Athens,
Athens, Greece

Paul McArdle
Child and Adolescent Psychiatrist and Lead
Consultant for Child and Adolescent
Mental Health Service, Northumberland,
Cumbria, UK; Northumberland, Tyne and
Wear NHS Foundation Trust, UK;
Honorary Senior Lecturer Newcastle
University, UK

Amy McCulloch
Psychiatrist Manchester University NHS
Foundation Trust and Clinical Research
Fellow University of Manchester, UK

Anne McFadyen
Infant Mental Health Clinical Advisor,
Scottish Government, UK

Dasha Nicholls
Professor of Child and Adolescent Psychiatry,
Imperial College London; Honorary
Consultant Child and Adolescent
Psychiatrist, Central and North West London
NHS Foundation Trust, UK; National
Specialist Advisor on Eating Disorders, NHS
England, UK; Clinical & Strategic Director,
National Audits & Research, CCQI, Royal
College of Psychiatrists, UK

Reshmi Nijjar
Specialty Doctor in Child & Adolescent
Psychiatry, East Lancashire Hospitals NHS
Trust, UK

Guy Northover
Consultant Child and Adolescent
Psychiatrist, Lead Clinical Director and
Chief Clinical Information Officer,
Berkshire NHS Foundation Trust, UK;
Chair of the Child and Adolescent
Psychiatry Faculty, Royal College of
Psychiatrists, UK

John O'Brien
Ardenleigh, Birmingham and Solihull
Mental Health NHS Foundation Trust,
Birmingham, UK

Oliver O'Mara
Tees, Esk and Wear Valleys NHS
Foundation Trust, UK

Isabel Paz
Consultant in Child and Adolescent
Psychiatry, Department of Children's
Psychological Medicine, The Oxford
Psychological Medicine Centre, Oxford
University Hospitals NHSFT,
Oxford, UK

Charlotte Ulrikka Rask
Department of Child and Adolescent
Psychiatry, Aarhus University Hospital
Psychiatry, Denmark; Department of
Clinical Medicine, Aarhus University,
Denmark

Mindy Reeves
Forensic Child and Adolescent Psychiatrist,
Greater Manchester Mental Health NHS
Foundation Trust, UK

Melissa Santos
Department of Pediatrics, University of
Connecticut School of Medicine,
CT, USA

Kapil Sayal
Professor of Child and Adolescent Psychiatry, Institute of Mental Health, School of Medicine, University of Nottingham, UK

Aditya Sharma
Consultant Psychiatrist and Lead National Adolescent Bipolar Service, Northumberland Tyne and Wear NHS Foundation Trust, UK; Senior Lecturer in Child and Adolescent Psychiatry, Newcastle University, UK

Kishan Sharma[†]
MBBS, MRCPsych, Consultant Child and Adolescent Psychiatrist and Honorary Clinical Lecturer, Manchester University NHS Foundation Trust, UK

Hannah Slevin
Specialist Trainee in Child and Adolescent Psychiatry, Manchester University NHS Foundation Trust and Clinical Research Fellow, University of Manchester, UK

Karen Steinhardt
Consultant Clinical Psychologist, Department of Children's Psychological Medicine, The Oxford Psychological Medicine Centre, Oxford University Hospitals NHSFT, Oxford, UK

Harriet Stewart
Consultant in Child and Adolescent Psychiatry, Department of Children's Psychological Medicine, The Oxford Psychological Medicine Centre, Oxford University Hospitals NHSFT, Oxford, UK

Paul A. Tiffin
University of York, UK; Hull York Medical School, UK; Tees, Esk and Wear Valleys NHS Foundation Trust, UK

Samantha Todd
Consultant Clinical Psychologist, Manchester University NHS Foundation Trust, UK

Paul Wallis
Consultant Clinical Psychologist, Director of Psychological Services CAMHS, Manchester University NHS Foundation Trust, UK

Oliver White
Consultant Child and Adolescent Forensic Psychiatrist, Oxford Health NHS Foundation Trust, UK

Tonya White
Chief of Section on Social and Cognitive Developmental Neuroscience, National Institute of Mental Health, Bethesda, MD, USA

Emma Williams
Lead Clinical Psychologist for Inpatient CAMHS, Greater Manchester Mental Health NHS Foundation Trust, UK

Abbreviations

AAP	American Academy of Pediatrics
ABAS	Adaptive Behaviour Assessment System
AC	Approved Clinician
ACE	Adverse Childhood Experiences
aCGH	array comparative genomic hybridisation
ACT	Acceptance and Commitment Therapy
ADHD	Attention Deficit Hyperactivity Disorder
ADI-R	Autism Diagnostic Interview Revised
ADOS/ADOS-2	Autism Diagnostic Observation Schedule
AFP-AN	adolescent-focused psychotherapy for AN
AMBIT	Adolescent Mentalization-Based Integrative Therapy
AMHP	Approved Mental Health Practitioner
AN	Anorexia Nervosa
ANTD	antenatal depression
APSD	Antisocial Process Screening Device
ARFID	Avoidant Restrictive Food Intake Disorder
ARMS	At Risk Mental State
ASD	Autism Spectrum Disorder
BA	Behavioural activation
BAS	British Ability Scales
BCE	benevolent childhood experiences
BD	bipolar disorder
BDD	Bodily Distress Disorder & body dysmorphic disorder
BDI	Beck Depression Inventory
BED	Binge Eating Disorder
BMI	Body Mass Index
BN	Bulimia Nervosa
BPD	borderline personality disorder
BPI	brief psychosocial intervention
CAMHS	Child and Adolescent Mental Health Services
CAPA	Child and Adolescent psychiatric assessment
CAPT	Child and Adolescent Psychotherapists
CBCL-PBD	Child Behaviour Checklist-Pediatric Bipolar Disorder
CBT	Cognitive Behaviour Therapy
CBT-ED	Cognitive Behavioural Therapy for Eating Disorders
CCG	clinical commissioning groups
CD	conduct disorder
CDDG	Clinical Descriptions and Diagnostic Guidelines
CDOP	Child Death Overview Panels
CDR	child death review
CFF-CBT	child and family-focused cognitive-behavioural therapy
CFT	compassion-focused therapy
CHDS	Christchurch Health and Development Study

CHR-P	Clinical/Ultra High Risk for Psychosis
CI	confidence interval
CJS	criminal justice system
CMRS-P	Child Mania Rating Scale-Parent version
CMV	cytomegalovirus
CNVs	copy number variants
COSLA	Convention of Scottish Local Authorities
COSP	Circle of Security Parenting
CPM	Children's Psychological Medicine
CPP	Child–Parent Psychotherapy
CPS	Crown Prosecution Service
C-PTSD	Complex Post-Traumatic Stress Disorder
CRT	cognitive remediation therapy
CYP	children and young people
CYPMH	children and young people's mental health
DAWBA	Development and Well-Being Assessment
DBT	Dialectical Behaviour Therapy / for self-harm
DBT-A	Dialectical Behaviour Therapy for Adolescents
DCD	Developmental Coordination Disorder
DD	Dissociative Disorders
DEB	disordered eating behaviour
DISC	Diagnostic Interview for Children
DM	diabetes mellitus
DMDD	disruptive mood dysregulation disorder
DNSD	dissociative neurological symptom disorder
DoLS	Deprivation of Liberty Safeguards
DPs	deviant peers
DSED	Disinhibited Social Engagement Disorder
DSM-5	Diagnostic and Statistical Manual of Mental Disorders (5th Edition)
DTO	detention and training orders
DUP	duration of untreated psychosis
DUST	Drug Use Screening Tool
ED	eating disorders
EDE-Q	Eating Disorders Examination – Questionnaire
EEG	electro-encephalography
EIP	Early Intervention in Psychosis (Services)
EMCDDA	European Monitoring Centre for Drugs and Drug Addiction
EMDR	Eye Movement Desensitisation Re-processing
EOP	early-onset psychosis
EPO	Emergency Protection Order
EQ5DY	Health-Related Quality of Life Instrument for Children and Adolescents
ERP	Exposure Response Prevention
FACE-CARAS	Functional Analysis in Care Environments-Child and Adolescent Risk-Assessment Suite
FFT	Functional Family Therapy
FFT-EOY	Family Focused Treatment for Early Onset Mood and Psychotic Disorders in Youth

FIM	Future in Mind
FNP	Family Nurse Partnership
FOMO	fear of missing out
FSH	Follicle Stimulating Hormone
FSS	functional somatic syndromes
FT-AN	Family Therapy for Anorexia Nervosa
FYFVMH	Five Year Forward View for Mental Health
GBDS	Global Burden of Disease Study
GDPR	General Data Protection Regulation
GMC	General Medical Council
GWAS	genome-wide association studies
HIV	human immunodeficiency virus
HoNOSCA	Health of the Nation Outcome Scales for Children and Adolescents
HSE	Health Survey for England
IAPT	Improving Access to Psychological Therapy
IBT	internet-based technology
ICBs	Integrated Care Boards
ICD/DSM	International Classification of Diseases Diagnostic and the Statistical Manual of Mental Disorders
ICD-11	International Classification of Diseases (11th Edition)
ICP	Integrated Care Partnerships
ICS	integrated care systems
ICU	Inventory of Callous-Unemotional Traits
ID	Intellectual Disabilities
IED	intermittent explosive disorder
IMH	Infant Mental Health
IPCC	inferior parietal cortex convexity
IPT	Interpersonal Psychotherapy
IPT-A	Interpersonal psychotherapy for depressed adolescents
IQ	Intelligence Quotient
J-SOAP-II	The Juvenile Sex Offender Assessment Protocol-II
KBIT	Kaufman Brief Intelligence Test
K-SADS	Kiddie Schedule for Affective Disorders and Schizophrenia
LGBT	lesbian, gay, bisexual and transgender
LGBTQ	lesbian, gay, bisexual, trans and queer
LH	luteinising hormone
LPS	Liberty Protection Safeguards
LSU	low secure unit
LTP	Long Term Plan
MBT	Mindfulness-Based Therapies
MBT-A	mentalisation-based treatment for adolescents
MCA	Mental Capacity Act 2005
MCAST	Manchester Child Attachment Story Task
MDD	Major Depressive Disorder
MDT	multidisciplinary team
MEED	Medical Emergencies in Eating Disorders
MFQ	Moods and Feelings Questionnaire

MSU	medium secure unit
MHCYP	Mental Health of Children and Young People
MHRA	Medicines and Healthcare products Regulatory Agency
MHST	Mental Health Support Teams
MIPO	Manchester Inventory for Playground Observation
MoJ	Ministry of Justice
MST	Multisystemic Therapy
MUS	medically unexplained symptoms
NBAS	Brazelton Neonatal Behavioural Assessment Scale
NBO	Newborn Behavioural Observation
NCISH	National Confidential Inquiry into Suicide and Homicide by People with Mental Illness
NCMD	National Child Mortality Database
NCS-A	National Comorbidity Study – Adolescent Supplement
ND	neurobehavioral disinhibition
NDDs	neurodevelopmental disorders
NDST	non-directive supportive therapy
NES	non-epileptic seizures
NG	naso-gastric
NHS	National Health Service
NICE	National Institute for Health and Care Excellence UK
NSSI	non-suicidal self-injury
NVR	non-violent resistance
OBP	offspring of bipolar parents
OCD	obsessive-compulsive disorder
OCEAN	Openness, Conscientiousness, Extraversion, Agreeableness and Neuroticism
OCPD	obsessive-compulsive personality disorder
ODD	Oppositional Defiant Disorder
ONS	Office of National Statistics
OR	odds ratio
OSFED	Other Specified Feeding and Eating Disorders
OT	Occupational Therapy
PACT	Preschool Autism Communication Treatment
PANDAS	paediatric autoimmune neuropsychiatric disorders
PCL-YV	Psychopathy Checklist-Youth Version
PDA	Pathological Demand Avoidance
PICU	Psychiatric Intensive Care Units
PMIS	paediatric multisystem inflammatory syndrome
PNTD	postnatal depression
PPS	persistent physical symptoms
PR	parental responsibility
PREM	patient reported experience measures
PROM	patient-reported outcome measures
PRS	polygenic risk score
PTSD	Post-Traumatic Stress Disorder
P-YMRS	Young Mania Rating Scale-Parent version

QT	Quick Test
RAD	Reactive Attachment Disorder
RC	Responsible Clinician
RCADS	revised child anxiety and depression scale
RCT	Randomised Controlled Trials
RDoC	Research Domain Criteria
RHSE	relationships and sex education and health education
RO-DBT	radically open DBT
ROM	Routine Outcome Measures
SAL	speech and language assessments
SAVRY	Structured Assessment of Violence Risk in Youth
SBMT	school-based mindfulness training
SCAS	Spence Children's Anxiety scale
SCH	secure children's homes
SCQ	Social Communication Questionnaire
SDI	Socio-Demographic-Index
SDQ	Strengths and Difficulties Questionnaire
SEND	Special Educational Needs and Disability
SGA	Second Generation Antipsychotics
SLE	systemic lupus erythematosus
SNP	single nucleotide polymorphisms
SNRI	Serotonin-Norepinephrine Reuptake Inhibitor
SNV	single nucleotide variants
SOAD	Second Opinion Appointed Doctor
SOC	Standards of Care
SRS	Social Responsiveness Scale
SSRI	Selective Serotonin Reuptake Inhibitor
START:AV	Short-Term Assessment of Risk and Treatability: Adolescent Version
STC	secure training centres
STP	Sustainability and Transformation Partnership
SUD	substance use disorder
TADS	Treatment for Adolescents with Depression Study
TIA	Trauma-Informed Approaches
TORDIA	Treatment of Resistant Depression in Adolescents
TRD	treatment resistant depression
VCSE	Voluntary Community and Social Enterprise
VIG	Video Interaction Guidance
WAIS	Wechsler Adult Intelligence Scale
WHO	World Health Organisation
WIAT	Wechsler Individual Attainment Test
WISC	Wechsler Intelligence Scale for Children
WISC-V	Wechsler Intelligence Scale for Children-Fifth Edition
WNV	Wechsler Nonverbal Scale of Ability
WPATH	World Professional Association for Transgender Health
WPPSI	Wechsler Preschool and Primary Scale of Intelligence
YOI	young offender institutions
YP	young person

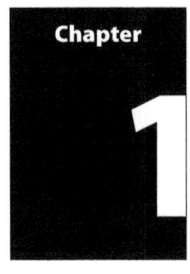

Chapter 1

Children's Mental Health Services in Context

Prathiba Chitsabesan, Paula Lavis and Guy Northover

Introduction

Children and young people's mental health services (sometimes called CAMHS: Child and Adolescent Mental Health Services) refers to a range of services that provide assessment and treatment to children and young people (CYP) who are experiencing mental health needs. Following the Health and Social Care Act (2012) [1], the government has increased its focus on mental health services, and has now committed to providing 'parity of esteem' for mental and physical health services. Parity of esteem means that mental health is valued as much as physical health including equal access to care and allocation of resources proportionate to need.

Health care is devolved, so all the home nations will have their own mental health policies. This chapter will explore the different policy frameworks but will go into more detail concerning policy in England and look at the changes to the National Health Service (NHS) and how the system works.

Epidemiology

In the UK, mental health disorders are the leading cause of child disability [2]. The prevalence of mental ill-health in CYP in England has increased steadily over the last 30 years. By 2017, a large national survey using the Development and Well-Being Assessment (DAWBA), indicated that 12.8% of 5–19-year-olds met the criteria for a mental health disorder, with higher rates for older adolescents [3].

When comparing between ethnic groups, surveys indicate that prevalence rates of mental health difficulties is higher for white children than children from ethnic minority backgrounds [3]. However, limitations of existing surveys include poor sampling of those from different ethnic minority communities in population level surveys.

The Covid-19 pandemic has affected all of us in one way or the other. CYP have been disproportionately adversely affected, as they have had to adapt to extraordinary changes to the world around them. National surveys in England using the Strengths and Difficulties Questionnaire, found an increase in rates of probable mental health disorder in young people 6 to 16 years of age from 11.6% (2017) [3] to 16.4% (2020) [4] and subsequently 17.4% (2021) [5]. By 2023 20.3% of 8- to 16-year-olds and 23.3% of 17- to 19-year-olds were found to have a probable mental health disorder (2023) [6]. Of concern is the rising prevalence rates of mental health conditions in adolescent girls (2023) [6].

Children and young people with a probable mental disorder were more likely to also have a parent experiencing a higher level of psychological distress and to report poor family connectedness and functioning [3] (see Chapter 5 – Classification and Epidemiology for more information). However, considerable differences were observed between individuals, and most children remained mentally well.

The prevalence of self-harm and suicide in young people of 10–24 years of age had been on the increase before the pandemic struck. In England, the National Child Mortality Database Programme was established in 2018 to collate and analyse data on all children in England, who die before their 18th birthday. The data are collated from the 58 regional Child Death Overview Panels across England who provide a multi-agency joint response as part of the child death review process. A report from the National Child Mortality Database found that 108 young people (under 18 years) had died by likely suicide over a 12-month period (April 2019–March 2020) [7]. As for adults, causes of suicide are multifactorial. Common themes identified in deaths by suicide in CYP[7] include family factors such as parental mental illness, abuse and neglect, loss and bereavement, bullying, suicide-related internet use, problems at school, physical health needs, alcohol and drug use, mental health and neurodevelopmental needs and risk-taking behaviours including self-harm.

Health Inequalities

Health inequalities are unfair and avoidable differences in health across the population, and between different groups within society [8]. Health inequalities can contribute to young people experiencing higher rates of mental health needs, as well as poorer access, experience and outcomes from services.

The poorest young people are more likely to experience mental health problems than the wealthiest [4]. Young people and adults who identify as LGBT experience higher rates of poor mental health while those with intellectual disabilities have poorer mental health than their non-disabled peers [9]. Additionally, young people and adults from ethnic minority communities are less likely to be able to access services that could help to prevent any mental health problems from escalating [9,10].

Research also suggests individuals with neurodevelopmental disorders such as autism will experience severe health inequalities compared to their neurotypical peers: average life expectancy among those with autism is 25 years shorter [11]. The annual cost of failing to adequately support autistic people in the UK is estimated to be at least £32 billion – more than heart disease, cancer and strokes combined [12]. The NHS Long Term Plan (LTP) (2019) made a commitment to reduce waiting times for assessment for young people with autism and to improve post-diagnostic support [10].

In addition, there are inequalities in the provision of CAMHS. A report by the Children's Commissioner found that areas higher in deprivation were more likely to have longer waiting times, lower spend per child and a greater need for mental health services [13].

The pandemic is likely to have long-term economic and social effects. There are concerns about widening health inequalities with studies suggesting that CYP with special educational needs and those living in disadvantaged families were more likely to have higher and persistent rates of mental health needs [3,5,6].

Children and Young People's Mental Health Policy

Wales

The mental health strategy in Wales covers all ages and is wide ranging [14]. In relation to CYP, the strategy will be delivered in accordance with the Welsh Government's due regard to duty as part of the Rights of the Children and Young People's (Wales) Measure 2011 [15]. A new 10-year mental health strategy is currently being developed.

Wales has been working to improve mental health support in schools for a considerable time; since 2013, local authorities have been required to secure provision of an independent counselling service for secondary age children and those in year 6 in primary schools [16].

The Together for Mental Health Delivery plan 2019–22 was reviewed in response to Covid-19 and includes several priority areas for CYP including improving access to mental health and well-being support in schools and improving young people's mental health and crisis services and psychological therapies [17].

Scotland

The Scottish government published their all age, Mental Health and Wellbeing Strategy in 2023 [18], which includes 10 core principles. These include being outcome focused, trauma informed and trauma responsive, based on the whole person and on a no wrong door approach and it is informed by people with lived experience. It is based on a life stage approach and focuses on prevention, early detection, recovery and treatment of mental illness and poor mental well-being, minimising risk factors and enhancing protective factors and providing support at important stages of life, which include infant and early years, and children, young people and families.

The Children and Young People's Mental Health Taskforce report from 2019 [19] was commissioned by the Scottish government and Convention of Scottish Local Authorities and looked at how CYPMH should be organised, commissioned and provided in order to make it easier for CYP to access help and support when it is needed. It sets out 13 wide-ranging recommendations for how to do this and focuses on both preventative approaches and specialist mental health services.

Scotland also has a perinatal and infant mental health programme board delivery plan 2019–20 [20], which has four key areas: improve capacity, increase the number of staff, invite more voices including people with lived experience such as parents and carers, and develop infant mental health networks and services.

Northern Ireland

Northern Ireland published its mental health strategy in 2021 [21] that sets the direction for mental health services over the next decade. It is a wide-ranging strategy and covers prevention through to specialist services, is aimed at all ages, covers workforce issues and links with the suicide prevention strategy.

The strategy includes several actions to improve prevention and early intervention, but also to improve access and the quality of CAMHS, which includes services for infants and better transitions between child and adult mental health services.

Northern Ireland also has an infant mental framework, which was published in 2016 [22]. It has three key priorities: promote the evidence around infant mental health; ensure frontline staff have the necessary knowledge and skills around infant mental health; and service development.

England

The current transformation work in England started with Future in Mind (FIM), which was published in 2015 [23]. One of the key proposals in FIM to help implementation was the development of transformation plans, where clinical commissioning groups (CCGs) work in partnership with local authorities, public health, education, youth justice and the voluntary sector to develop local plans.

The previous government published a new Special Educational Needs and Disability (SEND) and Alternative Provision Improvement Plan in 2023 to address the significant concerns raised about the SEND system. A road map was published to set out the various actions, which include establishing statutory SEND and alternative provision partnerships. However, given the change of government it is unclear to what extent this new policy will continue [24].

The Five Year Forward View for Mental Health (FYFVMH) was published in 2016 [25]. It covered all ages and set out several measurable commitments including improving access to mental health support and the roll-out of eating disorder and crisis care services. (The FYFVMH is detailed in various sections in the chapter.)

The government set out plans to further improve CYPMH provision in 2017, in the Transforming CYP Mental Health Provision Green Paper [26]. This included setting up Mental Health Support Teams in schools, that would be able to provide evidence-based psychological therapies to young people with mild to moderate mental health issues as well as the training of designated senior leads in schools, who will lead on whole school approach to mental health in schools. While significant progress has been made, further funding is required to roll out these services nationally.

The NHS LTP was published in 2019 and put forward a plan for the next 10 years but, in reality, only had funding for the next 5 [10]. There was a ring-fenced local investment fund for mental health as a whole, worth £2.3 billion per year by 2023/24. There were several commitments for mental health, which built on the progress made in the FYFVMH [25]. For CYP these include commitment to improve the number of young people accessing NHS funded mental health support, but a crucial difference was to improve support for young people aged 0–25 working across key stakeholders.

Also relevant to CYPMH were the proposals to transform perinatal mental health services. These included the development of specialist community perinatal mental health services, improving access for women with moderate to severe perinatal mental health difficulties including building new mother and baby units, enabling their partners to have an assessment of their mental health and developing maternity outreach clinics across England.

There is also a drive to reduce the reliance on using inpatient beds, reducing inappropriate out-of-area placements and improving community mental health provision. This is for people with mental health problems, including young people, but also for people with learning disabilities and autistic people. Transforming Care was published in 2012, following the Winterbourne View Hospital expose of abuse of patients with learning disabilities and/or autism [27]. The commitment was that following a review, everyone who was deemed inappropriately placed in hospital should be moved to community-based support. This commitment was also included in the LTP [10], the Mental Health Act reforms [28] and the Autism Strategy [29]. The new Mental Health Bill is currently passing through parliament and will have an increased focus on patient advocacy and choice and ensuring care is provided in the least restrictive environment.

Concerns have been raised about health and social care staff's knowledge and training with regard to working with people with a learning disability and autistic people. The Oliver McGowan mandatory training is looking to address this by providing appropriate training for all staff [30].

A new government 10-year health plan to include mental health is due to be published in 2025. This will build on the findings of an independent investigation into the NHS in England and is likely to focus on a move away from hospital to community care, prevention and the role of various digital therapies and technologies to support care.

Changes to NHS Structures in England

Integrated Care Systems and Provider Collaboratives

England has been moving to a system that enables various organisations to work together more effectively for several years building from Sustainability and Transformation Partnership, which was first announced in December 2015.

Sustainability and Transformation Partnerships subsequently developed into integrated care systems (ICSs) that encourage closer partnerships between NHS organisations, local authorities and others to take collective responsibility for planning services across their local population. Changes to the Health and Care Act (2022) [31] have put ICSs on a statutory footing and replaced CCGs. There are 42 ICSs across England supported by seven regional teams, covering populations of around 500,000 to 3 million people. Through the development of Integrated Care Boards (ICBs) and Integrated Care Partnerships, ICSs must achieve four key aims: improving outcomes in population health and health care, tackling inequalities in outcomes, experience and access, enhancing productivity and value for money and helping the NHS to support broader social and economic development. Provider collaboratives are partnership arrangements involving at least two trusts working at scale across multiple places to reduce unwarranted variation and inequalities in health outcomes [32].

New models of care pilots (now referred to as provider collaboratives) covered CYPMH inpatient services. There were six pilots across England and the aim was to improve outcomes for young people in inpatient mental health services. These pilots focused on CYP who are treated outside of their area, often long distances from their home, by providing appropriate support locally, closer to their homes where possible. An economic evaluation of these pilots found that by investing in local services, each of the sites had achieved reductions in overall spending at the same time as a significant expansion of community-based care with comprehensive offers of 24-hour availability of highly skilled teams and innovative models of support [33]. Transformation of specialised children's mental health services and delegation to ICBs supports delivery of care closer to home in less restrictive environments.

There have also been recent changes to primary care, with the setting up of primary care networks, which are groups of local GP practices [34]. Primary care already provides mental health support, and the aim is to increase this with the development of the mental health practitioner roles. The community mental health transformation work is to support the integration of primary and secondary care by delivering mental health services through new integrated neighbourhood hubs [35].

Referral and Access

Investment in mental health care for CYP has been underfunded for many years. In the FYFVMH [25], the UK government set a target for England that 35% of CYP with mental health needs should access services by 2021, based on the 2004 prevalence data. This was from a low baseline of only 25% of young people accessing mental health services in 2016.

Against the 2023 prevalence estimate, 48% of CYP with a mental health condition had contact from mental health services [36]. While access to children's mental health services has improved with more CYP accessing support, the treatment gap has also contributed to longer waiting times for support.

The Office of the Children's Commissioner (2021) assessed the provision of NHS children's mental health services and found that there were enormous levels of variation between different local areas in expenditure and waiting times for services [13]. Those with the best outcomes typically spend more than average per person.

The NHS LTP sought to address this disparity by investing in CAMHS at a rate faster than both overall NHS funding and total mental health spending. The NHS LTP aimed that by 2023/24, at least an additional 345,000 CYP aged 0–25 would be able to access support [10].

Under proposals set out in the 2017 Green Paper on Transforming Children and Young People's Mental Health, the government committed to trialling a four-week waiting time for access to specialist NHS CAMHS [26]. Further work is progressing to develop all-age standards across mental health services for both those requiring routine care as well as an urgent or emergency response (clinically led review of standards).

Service Delivery

The prevalence of mental health difficulties in CYP has risen significantly over the last 30 years in the UK and, consequently, mental health services aimed at supporting CYP have also changed.

It is now well established that mental health is an integral part of CYP's general health and well-being, and therefore CYPMH provision needs to be embedded in a wide range of services for young people. This includes universal health promotion and prevention programmes to services provided in education and community settings, including targeted provision for vulnerable groups of young people such as those in local authority care or in contact with the criminal justice system.

Universal services (services available to everybody, such as children's centres/family hubs, schools, colleges, primary care and youth centres) can be important in preventing mental health problems. Schools and colleges are an existing universal system to support prevention and early identification and support for mental well-being and mental health needs. A whole school approach refers to a universal, school-wide and multi-component approach to the promotion of well-being and mental health among the whole school community: children, young people, families and staff. In England all schools will be required to teach pupils about maintaining mental well-being through the new relationships and sex education and health education curriculum. Local authorities play an important role, in part through their statutory duties relating to public health, in promoting children's and families' physical and mental well-being.

The NHS LTP (2019) committed to providing services in an integrated and holistic way, working across agencies and settings and across physical and mental health care [10]. However, differences in language and culture between the wider systems (health, education, social care), as well as within systems (adult versus child and adolescent services), can make systems working difficult and co-ordinating service delivery challenging.

Values-based practice, working in partnership with evidence-based practice, can help to provide the skills and other resources needed to support balanced decision-making between stakeholders, within a framework of shared values. While all stakeholders have a shared values base for promoting good outcomes for CYPMH, they have different perspectives on what matters or is important in achieving those perspectives. Unaddressed, such differences can lead to barriers to providing joined-up care. However, when acknowledged, it is possible to develop a framework of shared values within which balanced decisions can be made in partnership.

Co-production acknowledges that people with 'lived experience' of a particular condition or services are often best placed to advise on what support and services will make a positive difference to their lives. Done well, co-production helps to ground discussions in reality and to maintain a person-centred perspective. It is part of a range of approaches that includes citizen involvement, participation, engagement and consultation. Co-production should be at the heart of developing any local offer and should start from the earliest stages of service design, development and evaluation. There is no single, universal model of co-production, and the way in which it is done is specific to the task, context and the people involved. It requires thinking about people (service users, carers and staff), power, partnerships and resources differently.

The Amplified programme (Young Minds) was funded by NHS England and NHS Improvement to support and build participation in every part of the CYPMH system [37]. As part of the Amplified project, a number of participation toolkits were created that combine learning from the project and best practice guidance, with the aim of supporting the development of participation practices within organisations.

Approaches to Service Delivery

The most well-known framework describing CAMHS was a model dividing service provision into four tiers. This model helped differentiate between the different forms of services that might be available to children and young people. However, more recent models focus on the needs of children and young people and include a systems-wide framework in considering how support can be delivered by a range of different practitioners and agencies, including the role of parents and carers.

Data and Quality Improvement

Data has become integral to how we now practice health care in the UK: health data can be used to benefit individuals, public health, and medical research and development. Digitisation and health information technology have expanded both the ability to collect data and to use it. Our use of electronic health records, electronic prescribing, patient portals and shared care records has enabled enhanced access to patient information to drive patient care.

The uses of health data are classified as either primary or secondary. Primary use data or data for 'individual care' is when health data is used to deliver health care to the individual from whom it was collected. Secondary use data, or data for 'Improving health, care and services through research and planning' is when health data is used outside of health care delivery for that individual [38].

Patient data, when used for purposes beyond an individual's care, for example understanding the health needs of a population, provision of operational and clinical assurance and for audit/research is known as 'secondary use' – secondary to the original reason for collection. Outcome measures may also be used as secondary data to determine service effectiveness or service improvement. In addition to the improvement of client outcomes, collecting ongoing progress data can also facilitate quality enhancement at multiple levels within organisations [39].

Routine Outcome Measures capture information from the clinician's perspective and may be based on investigations or a functional assessment. Patient-reported outcome measures (PROMs) capture information from the client's perspective. Patient-reported experience measures provide vital information on the experience of care.

PROMs assess patients' experiences of their symptoms, their functional status and their health-related quality of life and when collected across a patient treatment journey, can provide information on the effectiveness of the treatment for the individual patient and guide the therapeutic sessions. When using outcome measures it is imperative to ensure that the measure is validated for the intended use. The CYP-IAPT project has identified and validated the use of a range of outcome measures which cover the vast majority of presentations to CAMHS.

The process of collecting outcome data drives improvement in local services without any other change in the clinical model [40]. Using outcome data has been consistently found to reduce deterioration and improve outcomes [41]. Despite this evidence and drive, there are concerns that primary data in the form of outcome measures still remains underutilised by clinicians and services within child and adolescent mental health.

It is increasingly possible to compare services through national benchmarking, as championed by NHS Benchmarking with their CYPMH data collection covering service modes, access, activity, workforce and finance [42]. Such comparison can identify variations in care. Getting It Right First Time is a national initiative using national and local data to identify unwarranted variations in care, and through the use of clinical leadership allowing services to understand the underlying cause of this variation and support the development of quality improvement plans to reduce it [43]. A GIRFT programme for CYP's inpatient and crisis services identified a significant variation in most data metrics and clinical delivery of care, resulting in a significant variation in the length of admissions. A lack of robust outcome monitoring was also highlighted. The report identified a need for a whole pathway approach to crisis care, ensuring a seamless transition between services without the need for reformulation of the young person's needs. There is a need to improve the quantity and quality of data collection and ensure that it is used in both strategic planning of services and everyday clinical work.

Secondary use of data has led to numerous positive benefits for patients. However, such benefits can come with concerns about the risk of privacy breaches. The General Data Protection Regulation (GDPR) provides a set of data protection rules, which enhance how people can access information about themselves, and places limits on what organisations can do with personal data. Explicit consent under the GDPR is distinct from implied consent for sharing for direct care purposes under the common law duty of confidentiality.

Quality improvement in health care is based on a principle of organisations and staff continuously striving to improve how they work. There is no single definition, but can be understood as 'quality improvement is about giving the people closest to issues affecting care quality the time, permission, skills and resources they need to solve them. It involves a systematic and coordinated approach to solving a problem using specific methods and tools with the aim of bringing about a measurable improvement' (Health Foundation) [44].

There is no single quality improvement methodology that is recommended for mental health; however, all of them have a strong emphasis on co-production and service user involvement. Techniques that have been applied in health care can all be adapted for use in mental health settings.

Quality improvement projects typically involve simple changes in staff behaviour and interactions. Generally, the interventions selected involve relatively minor practice modifications with minimal associated patient safety risk. Using quality improvement at scale also improves the experience of staff delivering care as well as driving efficiencies [45].

Integrated and Holistic Models

Integrated care is about delivering health care in a coordinated and unified way where the different social, psychological and medical needs of a person are met together rather than separately, and where organisations work in partnership. Integrated services can reduce confusion, repetition, delay and duplication in service delivery.

The physical and mental health of a child or young person are not distinct entities that can be treated separately. Children with a long-term physical condition are at increased risk of a mental health condition [4].

The Mental Health Foundation have identified a number of factors for effective integrated care for those with mental health problems that include: (1) information-sharing systems; (2) shared protocols setting out the responsibilities of each; (3) joint funding and commissioning; (4) co-located services; (5) multidisciplinary teams [46]. The report stressed the need to refrain from thinking of physical and mental health separately and to consider the wider determinants of health. Having the *'right people with the right skills and attitudes'* was also seen to be an important requirement for the successful integration of physical and mental health care.

Developing and supporting integrated and multi-agency services requires commitment and leadership across the relevant agencies. The government has recognised the effectiveness of integrated working. The Department of Health and Social Care white paper (2021) *Integrations and Innovation: Working Together to Improve Health and Social Care Outcomes For All* aims to build on the innovations that have been seen through the Covid pandemic, improving services at a time when the pressure on them has been the highest [47].

Trauma-Informed Approaches

Trauma-Informed Approaches (TIAs) are based on the understanding that many CYP in contact with services have experienced adversity and trauma and may consequently find it difficult to develop trusting relationships with staff providing care, and to feel safe within services [48]. TIAs are informed by neuroscience, psychology and social science as well as attachment and trauma theories, and give central prominence to the complex and pervasive impact that adversity and trauma have on a person's world-view and interrelationships.

Within TIAs the basic safety of environments is prioritised (physical, psychological, social and moral). Training, reflective practice (including clinical supervision) and support for staff are seen as essential to help them recognise and focus on the impact of trauma on CYP and their support systems. TIAs incorporate key trauma principles and practices across the whole organisational and system cultures.

AMBIT [49], MAC-UK's 'integrate' model [50], Trauma Recovery Model and Enhanced Case Management [51] are promising examples of trauma-informed approaches introduced in the UK.

Thrive

Thrive aims to replace the tiered model with a conceptualisation of a whole system approach. The Thrive categories are needs-based groupings [40]. The Thrive framework conceptualises five needs-based groupings for young people with mental health difficulties and their families: thriving, getting advice, getting help, getting more help and getting risk support. Each of the five groupings is distinct in terms of the needs and/or choices of the individuals within each group, skill mix required to meet these needs, dominant metaphor used to describe needs (well-being, ill health, support), resources required to meet the needs and/or choices of people in that group. The groups are not distinguished by severity of need or type of problem. Rather, groupings are primarily organised around different supportive activities provided by CYPMH services in response to mental health needs and influenced by client choice.

0-25 Services

The majority of CYPMH services have been commissioned to provide services for young people 5 to 18 years of age. However, this underestimates the importance of early years provision and transition from 18 years.

Supporting Children in the Early Years

The early years play a large role in determining mental health through childhood and beyond. In the early years, infants make emotional attachments and form relationships that lay the foundation for future mental health. The positive mental health and well-being of children and their parents during the first few months and years of a child's life enable their future health and attainment. There is good evidence for a range of interventions that can promote mental health and well-being. Policy initiatives focusing on supporting parents, and particularly mothers with mental health needs and infant mental health, are increasingly common [10,25]. Targeted support for vulnerable parents, such as the Family Nurse Partnership programme and positive parenting programmes, can also improve outcomes for this group (see Chapter 4 – Infant Mental Health).

The government has recognised the pivotal importance of this time, most recently in its Early Years Healthy Development Review Report [52], supported with additional funding. Specifically, investment in health visiting, expansion of parent–infant mental health teams and investment in a national network of family hubs.

Transition and Support for Adolescent and Young Adults

It is well recognised that transition to adult mental health services can be challenging with many young adults failing to access services. Centre for Mental Health's Missed Opportunities report [53] articulates the prepandemic issues faced by people aged 16–25. Just 22.7% of 16-24-year-olds with symptoms of common mental health problems were receiving treatment. The likelihood of a mental health difficulty increases with age. The pandemic has had a significant impact on the life chances of young people, and the long-term changes to income, employment and housing will impact their mental health.

The NHS LTP [10] aimed to create a comprehensive mental health offer for people aged 0–25, working in partnership across services and agencies. NICE transition guidance [54] emphasises the need for transition to be multiagency and to involve service users in the design and development of services.

Early support hubs are recommended in Future in Mind (Department of Health & NHS England 2015) [23] and described as an effective delivery mechanism of mental health care and support for young people in the community in less stigmatising and more accessible settings. Previous evidence from the UK, Australia, Denmark and Ireland also indicates that early support hubs are able to attract young people who are less likely to engage with NHS mental health support [55]. A hallmark of the hubs is that they develop and respond to specific local need and are often a partnership between voluntary, community and social enterprises and health care services. Expanding provision of hubs (young futures hubs) are a commitment from government with a plan for further pilot and evaluation.

Eating Disorder Services

Eating disorders are serious, potentially life-threatening conditions that affect a person's emotional and physical health. Eating disorders commonly start in childhood and adolescence but affect people of all ages, genders and sexual orientation. Studies put the prevalence rates of lifetime eating disorders at 8.4% for girls/women (peak onset is often in adolescence) and 2.2% for boys/men [56]. However, rates of eating disorders were found to have increased significantly for young people 17–19 years of age to 12.5% by 2023 [6]. Anorexia nervosa has the highest mortality rate of any psychiatric disorder, from medical complications associated with the illness as well as suicide. Evidence highlights the importance of early intervention as soon as eating disorder is suspected, to prevent development of entrenched, long-term illness [57].

In response, 70 community eating disorder services were developed across the England to deliver NICE evidence-based treatment as part of the FYFVMH Programme [25]. This was supported by whole team training and increasing access to IAPT training programmes for family and Cognitive Behavioural Therapy interventions. The access and waiting time standards set a target that 95% of CYP with an eating disorder should access treatment within 1 week for urgent cases and 4 weeks for routine cases [58].

NHS England guidance on eating disorders in CYP outlined a whole pathway approach from prevention and early identification with GPs, and schools to intensive outreach, ward admission or home treatment when required [58,59]. The revised guidance from NHS England also considers support for the increasing number of CYP presenting with disordered eating and ARFID (Avoidant Restrictive Food Intake Disorder).

Early Intervention Psychosis Services

Psychosis is a severe mental illness associated with significant impairment in social functioning and shorter life expectancy. A long duration of untreated psychosis is associated with poorer personal recovery, increased service use and poorer economic outcomes in both the short and long term [60].

Early Intervention in Psychosis consists of multidisciplinary teams set up to seek, identify and reduce treatment delays at the onset of psychosis and promote recovery by reducing the probability of relapse following a first episode of psychosis [61]. Timely access to specialist treatment is shown to have a significant long-term impact on the lives of individuals with psychosis and their families.

All CYP, aged 14 and above, experiencing their first episode of psychosis should receive a comprehensive package of NICE concordant care within 2 weeks of referral to a specialist service [61]. A specialist service includes any team that is identified as delivering a component of the locality's specialist early intervention psychosis response, which must be comprehensive across the full 14–65 years age range. The updated plan includes sections for CYP and those with At Risk Mental States (ARMS). The overall aim of ARMS provision is to delay or prevent the onset of severe mental health problems, including psychosis and also to support a reduction in the Duration of Untreated Psychosis (DUP).

Looked-After Children

The challenges faced by looked-after children are widely recognised as impacting on their mental health. The importance of supporting positive relationships in the young person's care network and placement stability is well recognised [62]. Mental health services for children in care support young people in the care system, recognising that the impact of childhood trauma or neglect may present as pervasive difficulties that occur throughout the lives of young people, rather than diagnosable mental health problems.

Services for looked-after young people are overseen by social care, but many integrate mental health provision, through either systemic or psychology practitioners, to provide either direct input, consultation to social workers or training and advice to carers. To ensure that looked-after children are not disadvantaged by potential placement changes or more frequent moves, teams to support them often integrate education and physical health offers that wrap around the young person to ensure there is the same level of consistent oversight that would be expected of young people with a more stable caring relationship [62].

It is also recognised that higher levels of placement breakdown or change are associated with poorer outcomes against a wide variety of metrics, hence support is designed to scaffold placements (either family or residential homes) to maintain placements.

Crisis Services and Home Treatment Teams

A mental health crisis is a situation that the person or anyone else believes requires immediate support, assistance and care from an urgent and emergency mental health service.

A functioning crisis response unit is an essential part of mental health care. The NHS LTP aimed to have comprehensive crisis services available by 2024 [10]. The crisis offer should have the following four functions: (1) A single point of access, including through 111, to crisis support, advice and triage; (2) Crisis assessment within the emergency department and in community settings; (3) Crisis assessment and brief response within the emergency department and in community settings, with CYP offered brief interventions; and (4) Intensive home treatment services aimed at CYP who might otherwise require inpatient care, or intensive support that exceeds the normal capability of a generic CAMHS community team.

It is imperative that appropriate crisis response services are operational. Their absence has resulted in some CYP being sent far from home for treatment and/or placed in adult wards that are inappropriate for their age groups. The mobilisation of all age crisis helplines 24/7 by local mental health trusts is an integral part of the crisis care pathway.

Trials of community-based treatments for young people, both in the UK and abroad, have reported good clinical outcomes [63]. Although there is some variation in the results from randomised controlled trials, overall, the findings indicate that these outcomes are comparable to those of inpatient treatment [64,65]. There is also some evidence that the clinical improvements associated with intensive community treatments are equally stable at follow-up as those associated with inpatient treatment, although further research is needed to establish this more firmly [66].

Workforce Development

Transforming the mental health workforce is fundamental to creating sufficient capacity to deliver accessible, quality services and good outcomes for CYP. Stepping Forward to 2020/2021 [67] outlined the mental health workforce plan for England to support delivery of the Five Year Forward View for Mental Health [25]. The report highlighted the importance of addressing retention of staff as well as recruitment, recognising the importance of supporting staff mental health and well-being. The report also identified the need to develop new roles such as Child Well-Being Practitioners as well as a wider roll of recently developed roles, such as advanced practitioners, physician associates, non-medical prescribers, nursing associates and allied health professionals, including pharmacists. The NHS Long Term Workforce Plan (2023) sets out a comprehensive workforce plan to meet the needs of a changing population, including the expansion of psychiatrists, mental health nurses and psychological professionals [68].

Developing integrated care models means building flexible teams working across organisational boundaries and ensuring they have the full range of skills and expertise to respond to service user needs in different settings.

Professionals supporting children with mental health needs may work in a variety of different settings and come from a variety of different backgrounds. Therefore, consideration needs to be given to the training of the wider workforce within communities as well as those working in specialist mental health settings. Staff working in front line community services should also have access to regular supervision and consultation to support provision of effective services. Maintaining staff well-being is also crucial for sustaining the growth of the workforce, as poor well-being can culminate in problems with the retention of staff.

The children and young people's IAPT (Improving Access to Psychological Therapy) programme provides an important opportunity for training the workforce. It seeks to combine evidence-based practice with user involvement and outcome evaluation to embed best practice in child mental health. It includes 5 key principles underlying transformation: participation, increasing mental health awareness and reducing stigma, improving access and engagement, delivering evidence-based therapy and demonstrating outcomes and accountability through data collection.

Summary

In recent years, there has been an unprecedented focus on mental health within the NHS, providing greater transparency regarding the needs of CYP, as well as the commissioning and service delivery required to meet those needs. A third of all mental health problems have been established by the age of 14, rising to almost two-thirds by age 24 [69]. It is likely that the Covid-19 pandemic has further broadened income gaps between households, putting more CYP at risk [6].

Important principles in delivering effective CYPMH services include the need to: build resilience, consider prevention and early intervention, as well as developing a clear joined-up approach linking services through care pathways. Delivering evidence-based interventions for young people with mental health needs requires a sustainable, well-supported workforce with the relevant skills and competencies working across the full system.

New models of care can stimulate effective collaboration between commissioners and providers to develop integrated, accessible services for all. Expanding access to digital services can enable more people to receive effective care and provide greater accessibility and choice. A system-wide focus on quality improvement can support staff and patients to improve care through effective use of data, with support from professional networks. All new models must be developed in partnership with experts-by-experience, carers and community and voluntary organisations. Systemic investment in services and the staff who provide them is needed to meet the ambitions set by governments.

References

1. UK Parliament. *Health and Social Care Act.* 2012. Available from: https://www.legislation.gov.uk/ukpga/2012/7/contents (accessed 3 April 2025).
2. World Health Organisation. *Global Health Estimates: Leading Causes of DALYs.* World Health Organisation, 2020. Available from: https://www.who.int/data/gho/data/themes/mortality-and-global-health-estimates/global-health-estimates-leading-causes-of-dalys (accessed 7 April 2025).
3. NHS Digital. *Mental Health of Children and Young People in England 2017: Summary of Key Findings.* London: NHS Digital, 2018. Available from: https://digital.nhs.uk/data-and-information/publications/statistical/mental-health-of-children-and-young-people-in-england/2017/2017 (accessed 23 September 2024).
4. NHS Digital. *Mental Health of Children and Young People in England 2020: Wave 1 Follow Up to the 2017 Survey.* London: NHS Digital, 2020. Available from: https://digital.nhs.uk/data-and-information/publications/statistical/mental-health-of-children-and-young-people-in-england/2020-wave-1-follow-up (accessed 23 September 2024).
5. NHS Digital. *Mental Health of Children and Young People in England 2021: Wave 2 Follow Up to the 2017 Survey.* London: NHS Digital, 2021. Available from: https://digital.nhs.uk/data-and-information/publications/statistical/mental-health-of-children-and-young-people-in-england/2021-follow-up-to-the-2017-survey (accessed 23 September 2024).
6. NHS Digital. *Mental Health of Children and Young People in England, 2023: Wave 3 Follow Up to the 2017 Survey.* London: NHS Digital, 2023. Available from: https://digital.nhs.uk/data-and-information/publications/statistical/mental-health-of-children-and-young-people-in-england/2023-wave-4-follow-up (accessed 23 September 2024).
7. National Child Mortality Database Programme Thematic Report. *Suicide in Children and Young People.* Bristol: National Child Mortality Database, 2021. Available from: www.ncmd.info/publications/child-suicide-report/ (accessed 23 September 2024).
8. NHS England. *Core20PLUS5 – An Approach to Reducing Health Inequalities for Children and Young People.* NHS England, 2021. Available from: www.england.nhs.uk/about/equality/equality-hub/national-healthcare-inequalities-improvement-programme/core20plus5/core20plus5-cyp/ (accessed 23 September 2024).
9. NHS England *Advancing Mental Health Equalities Strategy.* NHS England, 2020. Available from: www.england.nhs.uk/publication/advancing-mental-health-equalities-strategy/ (accessed 23 September 2024).
10. NHS England. *NHS Long Term Plan.* NHS England, August 2019. Available from: www.england.nhs.uk/publication/the-nhs-long-term-plan/ (accessed 3 April 2025).
11. Hirvikoski T, Mittendorfer-Rutz E, Boman M, Larsson H, Lichtenstein P, Bölte S. Premature Mortality in Autism Spectrum Disorder. Br J Psychiatry. 2016 Mar; 208(3):232–38. https://doi.org/10.1192/bjp.bp.114.160192. Epub 2015 Nov 5. PMID: 26541693.
12. Buescher AV, Cidav Z, Knapp M, Mandell DS. Costs of Autism Spectrum Disorders in the United Kingdom and the United States. JAMA Pediatr. 2014 Aug;168(8):721–28. https://doi.org/10.1001/jamapediatrics.2014.210. PMID: 24911948.

13. The Children's Commissioner. *The State of Children's Mental Health Services 2020/2021*. The Children's Commission, January 2021). Available from: https://assets.childrenscommissioner.gov.uk/wpuploads/2021/01/cco-the-state-of-childrens-mental-health-services-2020-21.pdf (accessed 3 April 2025).
14. Welsh Government. *Together for Mental Health: Our Mental Health Strategy*. Welsh Government, 2012. Available from: https://www.gov.wales/together-mental-health-our-mental-health-strategy (accessed 3 April 2025).
15. Welsh Government. *Rights of Children and Young Persons (Wales) Measure 2011*. Welsh Government, 2011. Available from: https://law.gov.wales/rights-children-and-young-persons-wales-measure-2011 (accessed 3 April 2025).
16. Welsh Government. *School and Community-Based Counselling Operating Toolkit (revised 2020). WG37758 Counselling Toolkit for Schools*. Welsh Government, 2020. Available from: www.gov.wales/school-and-community-based-counselling-operating-toolkit (accessed 3 April 2025).
17. Welsh Government. *Review of the Together for Mental Health: Delivery Plan 2019–2022 in Response to Covid-19*. Welsh Government, 2021. Available from: www.gov.wales/sites/default/files/publications/2021-11/review-of-together-for-mental-health-the-plan-for-2019-to-2022-in-response-to-covid-19_1.pdf (accessed 3 April 2025).
18. Scottish Government. *Mental Health and Wellbeing Strategy*. Scottish Government, 2023. Available from: www.gov.scot/publications/mental-health-wellbeing-strategy/ (accessed 3 April 2025).
19. Scottish Government. *Children and Young People's Mental Health Taskforce: recommendations*. Scottish Government, 2019. Available from: www.gov.scot/publications/children-young-peoples-mental-health-task-force-recommendations/ (accessed 3 April 2025).
20. Scottish Government. *Perinatal and Infant Mental Health Programme Board 2020–2021: Delivery Plan*. Scottish Government, 2020. Available from: www.gov.scot/publications/perinatal-infant-mental-health-programme-board-2020-2021-delivery-plan/ (accessed 3 April 2025).
21. Department of Health. *Mental Health Strategy 2021–2031*. Northern Ireland Government, 2021. Available from: www.health-ni.gov.uk/publications/mental-health-strategy-2021-2031 (accessed 3 April 2025).
22. Public Health Agency. *Infant Mental Health Framework for Northern Ireland*. HSC Public Health Agency, 2016. Available from: www.publichealth.hscni.net/publications/infant-mental-health-framework-northern-ireland (accessed 3 April 2025).
23. Department of Health & NHS England. *Future in Mind. Improving Mental Health Services for Young People*. Department of Health & NHS England, 2015. Available from: https://assets.publishing.service.gov.uk/government/uploads/system/uploads/attachment_data/file/414024/Childrens_Mental_Health.pdf (accessed 3 April 2025).
24. HM Government. *Special Educational Needs and Disabilities (SEND) and Alternative Provision (AP) Improvement Plan*. HM Government, 2023. Available from: www.gov.uk/government/publications/send-and-alternative-provision-improvement-plan (accessed 3 April 2025).
25. NHS England. *Five Year Forward View for Mental Health*. NHS England, 2016. Available from: www.england.nhs.uk/publication/the-five-year-forward-view-for-mental-health/ (accessed 3 April 2025).
26. Department of Health & Department for Education. *Transforming Children and Young People's Mental Health Provision*. Department of Health & Department for Education, 2017. Available from: www.gov.uk/government/consultations/transforming-children-and-young-peoples-mental-health-provision-a-green-paper (accessed 3 April 2025).
27. Department of Health. *Transforming Care: A National Response to Winterbourne View Hospital*. Department of Health, 2012. Available from: www.gov.uk/government/publications/winterbourne-view-hospital-de

28. Department of Health and Social Care. *Reforming the Mental Health Act*. Department of Health and Social Care, 2021. Available from: www.gov.uk/government/consultations/reforming-the-mental-health-act (accessed 3 April 2025).

29. Department for Education & Department of Health and Social Care. *The National Strategy for Autistic Children, Young People and Adults: 2021 to 2026*. Department for Education & Department of Health and Social Care, 2021. Available from: www.gov.uk/government/publications/national-strategy-for-autistic-children-young-people-and-adults-2021-to-2026 (accessed 3 April 2025).

30. NHS England. The Oliver McGowan Mandatory Training on Learning Disability and Autism. Workforce, training and education. NHS England, 2024. Available from: www.hee.nhs.uk/our-work/learning-disability/current-projects/oliver-mcgowan-mandatory-training-learning-disability-autism (accessed 3 April 2025).

31. UK Parliament. *Health and Care Act*. UK Parliament, 2022. Available from: www.legislation.gov.uk/ukpga/2022/31/enacted (accessed 3 April 2025).

32. NHS England. *Working Together at Scale: Guidance on Provider Collaboratives*. NHS England, 2021. Available from: www.england.nhs.uk/wp-content/uploads/2021/06/B0754-working-together-at-scale-guidance-on-provider-collaboratives.pdf (accessed 23 September 2024).

33. O'Shea N. *Bringing Care Back Home*. London: Centre for Mental Health, 2020. Available from: www.centreformentalhealth.org.uk/wp-content/uploads/2020/03/CentreforMH_BringingCareBackHome_0.pdf (accessed 24 March 2025).

34. NHS England. *Primary Care Networks*. www.england.nhs.uk/primary-care/primary-care-networks/ (accessed 23 September 2024).

35. NHS England. *Next Steps for Integrating Primary Care*. NHS England, 2022. Available from: www.england.nhs.uk/wp-content/uploads/2022/05/next-steps-for-integrating-primary-care-fuller-stocktake-report.pdf (accessed 23 September 2024).

36. The Children's Commissioner. *The State of Children's Mental Health Services 2022–2023*. Available from: www.childrenscommissioner.gov.uk/resource/childrens-mental-health-services-2022-23/ (accessed 3 April 2025).

37. Young Minds. Amplified. Available from: www.youngminds.org.uk/professional/consultancy-and-service-design/case-studies/amplified/ (accessed 23 September 2024).

38. Safran C, Bloomrosen M, Hammond WE, et al. Toward a National Framework for the Secondary Use of Health Data: An American Medical Informatics Association White Paper. JAMA. 2007; 14(1):1–9.

39. Chorpita BF, Bernstein A, Daleiden EL. Research Network on Youth Mental Health. Driving with Roadmaps and Dashboards: Using Information Resources to Structure the Decision Models in Service organizations. Adm Policy Ment Health. 2008; **35**(1–2):114–23.

40. Wolpert M, Harris R, Jones M, et al. Thrive – The AFC-Tavistock Model for CAMHS. London: Anna Freud Centre and the Tavistock and Portman NHS Foundation Trust, 2014.

41. Bickman L, Kelley SD, Breda C, De Andrade ARV, Riemer M. Effects of Routine Feedback to Clinicians on Mental Health Outcomes of Youths: Results of a Randomized Trial. Psychiatr Serv. 2011; 62(12):1423–29.

42. NHS Benchmarking International Benchmarking – NHS Benchmarking Network. Available from: www.nhsbenchmarking.nhs.uk/ (accessed 8 October 2024).

43. NHS England. *Getting it Right First Time*. Available from: www.gettingitrightfirsttime.co.uk/what-we-do/ (accessed 5 February 2022).

44. Health Foundation. *Quality Improvement Made Simple: What Everyone Should Know About Healthcare Quality Improvement*. London: Health Foundation, 2021.

45. Shah A, Course S. Building the Business Case for Quality Improvement: A Framework for Evaluating Return on Investment. FHJ. 2018;**5**(2):132–37.
46. Mental Health Foundation. *Crossing Boundaries Improving Integrated Care for People with Mental Health Problems.* Mental Health Foundation, 2013. Available from: https://swsenate.nhs.uk/wp-content/uploads/2014/01/4-Crossing-boundaries.pdf (accessed 3 April 2025).
47. Department of Health and Social Care. *Integrations and Innovation: Working Together to Improve Health and Social Care Outcomes for All.* Department of Health and Social Care, 2021. Available from: www.gov.uk/government/publications/working-together-to-improve-health-and-social-care-for-all (accessed 3 April 2025).
48. Sweeney A, Clement S, Beth F, Kennedy A. Trauma-Informed Mental Healthcare in the UK: What Is It and How Can We Further Its Development? MHRJ. 2016;**21**(3):174–92.
49. Anna Freud. *Adaptive Mentalization Based Integrative Treatment (AMBIT).* Available from: www.annafreud.org/clinical-support-and-services/adaptive-mentalization-based-integrative-treatment-ambit/ (accessed 23 September 2024).
50. MAC-UK. *Our Approach.* Available from: www.mac-uk.org/our-approach (accessed 23 September 2024).
51. Opinion Research Services. *Enhanced Case Management (ECM) Evaluation: Phase 1 Report.* 2023. Available from: https://assets.publishing.service.gov.uk/government/uploads/system/uploads/attachment_data/file/1151734/ECM_Evaluation_Phase_One_Report.pdf (accessed 23 September 2024).
52. Her Majesty's Government. *The Best Start for Life A Vision for the 1,001 Critical Days: The Early Years Healthy Development Review Report.* 2021. https://assets.publishing.service.gov.uk/government/uploads/system/uploads/attachment_data/file/973085/Early_Years_Report.pdf (accessed 23 September 2024).
53. Khan L. *Missed Opportunities: Children and Young People's Mental Health.* London: Centre for Mental Health, 2016. Available from: www.centreformentalhealth.org.uk/publications/missed-opportunities (accessed 23 September 2024).
54. NICE. *Transition from Children's to Adults' Services for Young People Using Health or Social Care Service.* Available from: www.nice.org.uk/guidance/ng43 (accessed 23 September 2024).
55. O'Keeffe L, O'Reilly A, O'Brien G, Buckley R, Illback R. Description and Outcome Evaluation of Jigsaw: An Emergent Irish Mental Health Early Intervention Programme for Young People. Ir J Psychol Med. 2015;**32**(1):71–77. https://doi.org/10.1017/ipm.2014.86.
56. Galmiche M, Déchelotte P, Lambert G, Tavolacci M-P. Prevalence of Eating Disorders over the 2000–2018 Period: A Systematic Literature Review. Am J Clin Nutr. 2019 May 1;**109**(5):1402–13. https://doi.org/10.1093/ajcn/nqy342.
57. NICE. *Eating Disorders: Recognition and Treatment.* 2017. Updated 2020. Available from: www.nice.org.uk/guidance/ng69 (accessed 23 September 2024).
58. NHS England. *Children and Young People's Eating Disorder Access and Waiting Time Commissioning Guide.* 2015. Available from: https://www.england.nhs.uk/wp-content/uploads/2015/07/cyp-eating-disorders-access-waiting-time-standard-comm-guid.pdf (accessed 23 September 2024).
59. NHS England. *Addendum – Inpatient and Intensive Day Care Extension to the Community Eating Disorder Guidance.* 2019. Available from: www.england.nhs.uk/publication/addendum-inpatient-and-intensive-day-care-extension-to-the-community-eating-disorder-guidance/ (accessed 23 September 2024).
60. Marshall M, Lewis S, Lockwood A, Drake R, Jones P, Croudace T. Association Between Duration of Untreated Psychosis and Outcome in Cohorts of First-Episode

Patients: A Systematic Review. Arch GenPsychiatry. 2005;**62**:975–83.

61. NHS England. *Implementing the Early Intervention in Psychosis Access and Waiting Time Standard: Guidance.* 2023. Available from: www.england.nhs.uk/wp-content/uploads/2023/03/B1954-implementing-the-early-intervention-in-psychosis-access-and-waiting-time-standard.pdf (accessed 23 September 2024).

62. NICE. *Looked-After Children and Young People.* 2021. Available from: www.nice.org.uk/guidance/ng205/resources/lookedafter-children-and-young-people-pdf-66143716414405 (accessed 23 September 2024).

63. Ougrin D, Zundel T, Corrigall R, Padmore J, Loh C. Innovations in Practice: Pilot Evaluation of the Supported Discharge Service (SDS): Clinical Outcomes and Service Use. CAMH. 2014;**19**(4):265–69.

64. Kwok KHR, Yuan SNV, Ougrin D. Alternatives to Inpatient Care for Children and Adolescents with Mental Health Disorders. CAMH. 2016;**21**(1):3–10.

65. Ougrin D, Corrigall R, Poole J, et al. Comparison of Effectiveness and Costeffectiveness of an Intensive Community Supported Discharge Service Versus Treatment as Usual for Adolescents with Psychiatric Emergencies: A Randomised Controlled Trial. Lancet Psychiatry. 2018;**5**(6):477–85.

66. Schmidt MH, Lay B, Göpel C, Naab S, Blanz B. Home Treatment for Children and Adolescents with Psychiatric Disorders. Eur Child Adolesc Psychiatry. 2006;**15**(5):265–76.

67. Health Education England. *Stepping Forward to 2020/21: The Mental Health Workforce Plan for England.* London: NHS. 2017. Available from: www.hee.nhs.uk/sites/default/files/documents/Stepping%20forward%20to%202020201%20-%20The%20mental%20health%20workforce%20plan%20for%20england.pdf (accessed 23 September 2024).

68. NHS England. *NHS Long Term Workforce Plan.* 2023. Available from: www.england.nhs.uk/publication/nhs-long-term-workforce-plan/ (accessed 23 September 2024).

69. Solmi M, Radua J, Olivola M, et al. Age at Onset of Mental Disorders Worldwide: Large-Scale Meta-analysis of 192 Epidemiological Studies. Mol Psychiatry. 2022;**27**(1):281–95. https://doi.org/10.1038/s41380-021-01161-7. Epub 2021 Jun 2. PMID: 34079068; PMCID: PMC8960395.

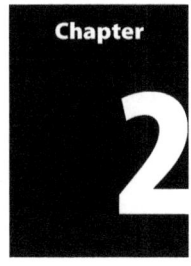

Chapter 2

Normal Childhood Development: Theories and Influence

Reshmi Nijjar and Dushyanthan Mahadevan

Introduction

A thorough and detailed understanding of normal development in childhood provides a basis upon which knowledge of children's mental health difficulties can be built. Development refers to expected patterns of change over time, beginning at conception and continuing throughout the lifespan. It is a lifelong process and encompasses different domains, including the physical, social, emotional and cognitive.

Is the way my child plays with others suggestive of autism? Could his bad dreams indicate anxiety? Does the fact she can't sit through a whole film mean she has ADHD? Only with an in-depth knowledge of what is developmentally 'normal' can we begin to elicit whether behaviours that deviate from these norms might indicate disorder. This is the basis of the developmental psychopathology that underpins the practice of child and adolescent psychiatry. What is considered 'normal' development involves a complex and continuous interplay between genetic and environmental (including socio-cultural) factors. Despite some variation, there is a consistency and reliability of functioning in children that remains steadfast from generation to generation.

This chapter briefly describes aspects of childhood development and includes an overview of some theories of development. While developmental theories may aid your academic understanding, these are most clinically useful when applied within the context of the children that you see and interact with, both personally and in your clinical practice. In order to enhance your understanding of children and young people and their development, you must be observant. It is important to consider which features of a child's presentation both conform to, and diverge from, what is expected.

In this chapter we will consider areas including the milestones of development in early childhood; attachment theory, temperament and personality; theories of emotional, cognitive and social development; and development in adolescence. There are areas of development that are not included in the scope of this chapter (e.g. the development of bowel and bladder function), and it is recommended that further reading on the vast subject of human development supplements the topics covered in this introductory chapter.

Developmental Milestones

The sequence of development is similar in all healthy children, although the exact timing for each individual child may vary. Developmental milestones represent what a healthy child can do around a particular age. Children reach various milestones relating to how they move, speak, act and learn. Reaching milestones at the typical ages given in Table 2.1

Table 2.1 Developmental milestones in early childhood

Age	Motor	Speech	Vision and hearing	Social development
4–6 weeks				Smiles at mother
6–8 weeks		Vocalises		
3 months	Prone: head held up for prolonged periods. No grasp reflex	Talks a great deal	Follows dangling toy from side to side. Turns head to sound	Squeals with pleasure appropriately Discriminates smile
5 months	Holds head steady. Goes for objects and gets them. Objects taken to mouth	Enjoys vocal play		Smiles at mirror image
6 months	Transfers objects from one hand to the other. Pulls self up to sit and sits erect with supports. Rolls over prone to supine. Palmar grasp of cube	Double syllable sounds such as 'mumum' and 'dada'	Localises sound 45 cm lateral to either ear	May show 'stranger shyness'
9–10 months	Wriggles and crawls. Sits unsupported. Picks up objects with pincer grasp	Babbles tunefully	Looks for toys dropped	Apprehensive of strangers
1 year	Stands holding furniture. Stands alone for a second or two, then collapses with a bump	Babbles 2 or 3 words repeatedly	Drops toys, and watches where they go	Cooperates with dressing, waves goodbye, understands simple commands
18 months	Can walk alone. Picks up toy without falling over. Gets up/downstairs holding onto rail. Begins to jump with both feet. Can build a tower of 3 or 4 cubes and throw a ball	'Jargon'. Many intelligible words		Demands constant mothering. Drinks from a cup with both hands. Feeds self with a spoon
2 years	Able to run. Walks up and down stairs 2 feet per step. Builds tower of 6 cubes	Joins 2–3 words in sentences		Parallel play Dry by day

Table 2.1 (cont.)

Age	Motor	Speech	Vision and hearing	Social development
3 years	Goes up stairs 1 foot per step and downstairs 2 feet per step. Copies circle, imitates cross and draws man on request. Builds tower of 9 cubes	Constantly asks questions. Speaks in sentences		Cooperative play. Undresses with assistance. Imaginary companions
4 years	Goes downstairs 1 foot per step, skips on 1 foot. Imitates gate with cubes, copies a cross	Questioning at its height. Many infantile substitutions in speech		Dresses and undresses with assistance. Attends to own toilet needs
5 years	Skips on both feet and hops. Draws a man and copies a triangle. Gives age	Fluent speech with few infantile substitutions		Dresses and undresses alone
6 years	Copies a diamond. Knows right from left and number of fingers	Fluent speech		

demonstrates that a child is developing as expected in early childhood. However, not reaching particular milestones, or reaching them much later than children of a similar age, can be an early indicator that the child may have a developmental delay.

Attachment Theory

The process of bonding between parents and infants was studied by John Bowlby, a British psychoanalyst. Through his work with hospitalised and institutionalised children, and his observations of infants separated from their caregiver, he formulated a theory of the relationship between the caregiver and parent known as 'attachment theory'.

This is based on the concept that an infant must develop a relationship with at least one primary caregiver for optimal social and emotional development to occur, and that the primary caregiver must be available and responsive to the infant's needs for the child to develop a sense of security. Bowlby believed that the quality of this early relationship has a significant psychological impact, which may continue into adult life. He believed that human infants have an innate set of behaviours that enable them to seek close physical proximity to their caregiver, improving their chances of survival. He formulated that attachment is a two-way process, in that the ability of the caregiver to recognise and respond appropriately to these behaviours contributes to their effectiveness.

The Four Attachment Styles

Mary Ainsworth [1] expanded on Bowlby's attachment theory and noted that infants use their caregivers as a secure base from which to explore. She considered how the degree of sensitivity a caregiver shows to their infant can contribute to varying styles of attachment.

Ainsworth developed the 'strange situation procedure' in order to measure the quality of infants' attachment to their caregiver. During this procedure, the baby is observed when they are separated from their caregiver, exposed to a stranger, and then reunited when their caregiver returns to the room. The behaviours observed through a one-way screen were the child's activity level, proximity and willingness to engage with a stranger, as well as distress and attempts to gain the caregiver's attention. From this, Ainsworth identified that there were three main attachment styles, which resulted from interactions with the child's caregiver early in life, and a fourth was later described.

Secure Attachment

From Ainsworth's study, 60–65% of children are securely attached. These infants appear confident that their caregiver will be present to meet their needs and will seek to interact with them when they return. The caregiver provides a secure base from which they can explore their surroundings as well as return. The caregiver can easily comfort and ease any distress the child may exhibit.

Ambivalent Attachment

Around 20% of children fall into this group. These children show high levels of distress upon separation from the caregiver initially. However, they then demonstrate a pattern of alternately seeking contact with the caregiver upon their return but then resisting or pushing away from them. They may cry wanting to be picked up, but squirm angrily and resist when they are picked up and want to get down. This style is thought to occur when the child has not been able to form a secure enough bond and feel safe enough with the caregiver to explore their environment. It has been proposed that this behaviour results from insufficient responsiveness to their needs by the attachment figure.

Avoidant Attachment

These children avoid interaction with the caregiver upon their return and may choose to ignore them entirely or show mixed attempts to interact with them. They are equally distressed at being left alone by both a stranger and their caregiver. Such children may have a caregiver who is unable to be sensitive to their needs – for example disengaged or rejecting – and who may be unavailable at times of emotional upset.

Disorganised Attachment

Work by Main and Solomon [2] identified a fourth pattern of attachment known as disorganised attachment. These children may exhibit unusual behaviours in the 'strange situation procedure', including repetitive and jerky movements, and become frozen and dissociated from their surroundings. There are high rates of maltreated children, or children of parents with severe and enduring mental illness, in this group.

Considering a child's attachment pattern can help us understand the impact of parenting on a child's development. Children who are securely attached as infants have been shown to build stronger self-esteem as they develop, with lower rates of anxiety and depressive disorders, and the ability to develop satisfying relationships with others. However, the absence of secure attachment can affect behaviour in later childhood and lead to a basic mistrust of their social world. Children who are later diagnosed with oppositional defiant disorder, conduct disorder or post-traumatic stress disorder often show insecure attachment. This may be linked to early experience of abuse, neglect or trauma.

Temperament and Personality

Temperament

Temperament involves the study of individual differences in how babies respond to physical and emotional stimulation, and the general characteristics of their mood as well as its changeability. These traits may be biologically rooted, although modified by environmental, social and cultural factors.

Alexander Thomas and Stella Chess began researching temperament in the late 1950s in the New York Longitudinal Study. They asked parents to fill in questionnaires at various intervals, beginning shortly after their baby's birth. As the children grew older, Thomas and Chess supplemented the questionnaires with interviews with teachers and tests of the children. Analysis of the results showed nine behavioural traits that provided an overall description of the child's temperament. These included rhythmicity (the predictability of activities such as eating or sleeping), activity level, approach/withdrawal (how the infant reacts to different situations), adaptability (how easily a response is modified), threshold for responsiveness (how strong a response needs to be before the infant reacts), intensity (how energetic reactions are), mood, distractibility (how easy it is to interrupt the infant's activities) and attention span (the extent to which the infant remains engaged in an activity). Further analysis allowed Thomas and Chess to propose three main categories of temperament: easy, difficult and slow to warm up [3].

Children with an 'easy' temperament were characterised as being sociable, happy in mood, adaptable and having regular biorhythms. These made up 40% of the study population. Children with a 'difficult' temperament made up approximately 10% of the study population. This category encompassed children who had opposite behaviours: being easily upset, negative responses to novel situations and a negative mood overall. 'Slow-to-warm-up' children, who accounted for approximately 15% of the study population, were characterised by gradual adaptation to novel situations through repeated contact over time.

It may be clinically helpful to consider individual approaches to each child to maximise interactions. For example, an 'easy' child may require less intervention but still has needs that must be met. A difficult child may require extra time to adapt to new situations. A 'slow-to-warm-up' child may need to be given advance warning prior to introduction of a new situation.

Thomas and Chess also developed the concept of 'goodness of fit' in order to consider how temperament can be influenced by parental expectations and behaviours. Their observation was that unrealistic parental expectations may lead to behavioural difficulties in the child. Parents may be supported to understand their child's difficulties by having insight into their specific temperament and being more in tune with their needs, and this helps to avoid 'blaming' of the child. Parents who can recognise and accept their child's temperament can encourage more effective interaction and communication.

Vulnerability and Resilience

The concepts of vulnerability and resilience are important when considering the development of temperament. Vulnerability refers to certain disadvantages a child may have. These may be innate, such as physical health difficulties, or environmental, such as poverty, malnutrition or abuse. Being able to overcome these challenges and showing the ability to adapt is considered resilience. Resilience can be attributed to certain innate factors, such as an easy temperament, intelligence or warmth; and environmental factors, which may include a supportive family and school system. Clinically, the combination of several vulnerability factors and low resilience is likely to lead to poorer outcomes, for example a child of poor physical health with a difficult temperament being raised in an unhygienic and abusive household.

Personality

Temperament is considered central to an individual's formation of their personality. Personality encompasses certain characteristics relating to how an individual thinks, feels and behaves. One influential theory of personality is the 'Big Five' theory of Paul Costa and Robert McCrae [4]. Based on repeated factor analysis of personality traits, they concluded that personality is comprised of five universal dimensions: Openness, Conscientiousness, Extroversion, Agreeableness and Neuroticism (OCEAN). There are other important theories of personality development, and this area may reward further reading.

Psychoanalytic theories relating to the development of personality are also well established. Freud stated that the personality is composed of three main structures. The id refers to the most primitive part of personality present from birth and operates on the pleasure principle. The ego operates on the reality principle. The superego holds internalised morals and standards we acquire from our parents and society. Freud believed that an imbalance between these components may lead to a maladaptive personality [5].

Emotional Development

Emotions are often divided into two general categories. There are 'basic emotions' (or primary emotions) such as interest, happiness, anger, fear, surprise, sadness and disgust. These tend to occur by the age of 6 months and can be gauged by the child's facial expression. The range of emotions that children can express broadens as they become older. Then there are 'secondary emotions', which include envy, pride, shame, guilt, doubt and embarrassment. These tend to appear towards the age of 2, as children start to develop a sense of self-awareness in line with the development of their cognitive ability. The understanding of emotions also develops through the process of social referencing, when children seek out information from others' emotional expression allowing them to interpret different situations or events.

Emotional regulation is the process by which we can control our emotional states so that we can attain goals. This process is made up of an interplay between intrinsic and extrinsic processes, including biological changes in the brain, changes in cognitive and linguistic abilities and feedback from caregivers and wider society. Infants have a very limited ability to adjust and control their emotional states, hence they rely on extrinsic factors for this process. Temperament also plays a role in children's ability to control their emotional state, which will be discussed later in this chapter. Exposure to repeated trauma in childhood is associated with disrupted ability to acquire emotional regulation skills.

The ability to understand emotions, not only in ourselves but also in other people, is known as emotional literacy. This term was coined by Claude Steiner [6] and encompasses an awareness of feelings, having a sense of empathy, managing emotions and repairing emotional difficulties. This may be seen as a skill that is variable between individuals and dependent on factors, such as temperament, developmental stage and influences from adult caregivers. It is thought that high emotional literacy may be linked with more favourable predictors for life, such as higher social competence and positive peer relationships.

Cognitive Development

Jean Piaget (1896–1980) was an influential Swiss psychologist who explored children's ability to think and reason. He sought to recognise and distinguish the ways in which a child's thought process differed from that of an adult. He believed that children seek to construct schemas, a set of concepts employed to understand or predict their environment. He believed that children could adapt to their environment through the processes of assimilation and accommodation of their current schemas.

Assimilation refers to interpreting new knowledge by integrating it into their current schemas. Accommodation conversely is the process of adjusting old schemas to fit to a new environment. Piaget proposed that our need to understand the world comes from a desire for cognitive equilibrium; a balance between what we see of the outside world and what we know. If children experience something they cannot understand, they attempt to restore equilibrium by changing their thoughts or altering the experience to change and fit into what they do know [7].

Piaget considered that the organisation of cognitive structures occurs in four stages:

(1) Sensorimotor stage (0–2 years). By encountering objects and people around them and using their senses and motor skills, children learn to distinguish between themselves and others. They achieve **object permanence**, the concept that objects continue to exist regardless of our ability to perceive them.

(2) Preoperational stage (2–7 years). Children are now familiar with the properties of objects and develop the use of symbols, particularly words, to be able to think about the world. Their understanding of how the physical world operates remains limited, and they tend to exhibit animistic thinking, attributing lifelike qualities to inanimate objects. Children in this stage remain **egocentric**, meaning they tend to think only from their own perspective.

(3) Concrete operational stage (7–12 years). Children start to use categories and classifications. They develop the ability to think logically about the physical world. They develop an understanding of concepts, such as size, distance and constancy of matter, including **conservation**. Conservation is the understanding that a quantity can remain the same despite an adjustment in its apparent size (e.g. the same volume of liquid can be present in a tall, thin glass as that in a short, wide glass).

(4) Formal operational stage (12 years onwards). By this stage, children develop skills to think logically about both concrete and abstract concepts. They can consider possibilities and **hypothesise**, developing the ability to contemplate ideas about situations they have not directly encountered, thus allowing them to appreciate the world from the point of view of others.

Language Development

There are different models to consider when thinking about the development of language. One is learning theory, which encompasses the concepts of reinforcement and punishment as proposed by Skinner [8]. He proposed that language is like other forms of behaviour acquired through operant conditioning, for example, a child learning to say a word and a parent 'rewarding' this through recognition and reinforcement. Social learning theory, as proposed by Bandura [9], suggests that children learn language through observation, picking up words they overhear.

Another is nativist theory, which is demonstrated through the work of Noam Chomsky [10]. He argued that children have innate abilities to learn language instinctively, and that aspects of learning language are biologically determined. He believed in the 'language acquisition device', which refers to the existence of a 'universal grammar' that can operate with reference to any language.

Understanding how development of language takes place is complex and involves both understanding of basic neurological functioning as well as cognitive processing. There is some evidence that language development begins before birth, as foetuses may be able to hear and recognise language from around 26 weeks gestation. Newborn babies seem to respond preferentially to their native language, which may indicate that language development has already begun before the baby is born [11]. The process of language development continues during the newborn period with intentional vocalisations, such as cooing. Cooing serves as practice for vocalisation as the infant hears their own voice and tries to repeat sounds. They can recognise their own mother's voice from birth. They express pain and hunger by crying and are also able to see and aim their gaze. They may develop different vocalisations for different emotions, including anger, content and hunger.

At about 4–6 months of age, infants begin babbling and make more elaborate vocalisations that include the sounds required for any language. They are usually able to recognise their own name at around 6 months. At around 10 months, the infant can understand more than they are able to say. They tend to use gestural language, such as pointing, to indicate their needs, and can engage in two-way play, including games such as peek-a-boo. They usually begin using their first words at about 12 or 13 months of age and may use partial words to try and convey their thoughts.

One-year-olds typically have a vocabulary of about 50 words. At 12–18 months they may be able to recognise pictures and objects. At 18–24 months they experience a 'vocabulary spurt' and begin to associate words with actions. Their grammatical understanding begins to develop, and they may start to use plurals and verb endings. By the time they become toddlers, most children have a vocabulary of about 200 words and begin putting those words together in either 2-word sentences or telegraphic speech. They may also be able to use intonation appropriately and identify rhyming words.

The acquisition of theory of mind between 3 and 5 years can enable them to take the role of another person during play. By the age of 5, usually children have mastered the basic building blocks for language including more complex grammar. The rest of childhood is spent in focusing refining language so that it can be used during increasingly complex tasks, such as reading, writing and debating. There are wide variations in the development of speech, which can be influenced by a range of genetic, auditory, environment and intellectual factors. The development of theory of mind and 'make-believe' play promotes an understanding of symbolic and abstract language.

Development of Social Competence and Morals

Kohlberg's work [12] consisted of exploring how morality develops. He believed that children develop morality through stages, and their ability to do so was dependent upon their cognitive ability. He demonstrated use of a moral judgement interview, presenting children with stories that involved conflicts between two moral values and evaluating their responses. The most famous of these is known as 'the Heinz dilemma':

> In Europe, a woman was near death from a special kind of cancer. There was one drug that the doctors thought might save her. It was a form of radium that a druggist in the same town had recently discovered. The drug was expensive to make but the druggist was charging ten times what the drug cost him to make. He paid $200 for the radium and charged $2,000 for a small dose of the drug. The sick woman's husband, Heinz, went to everyone he knew to borrow the money but he could only get together about $1,000, about half of what the drug cost. He told the druggist that his wife was dying and asked him to sell it cheaper or let him pay later. But the druggist said: 'No, I discovered the drug and I'm going to make money from it.' Heinz got desperate and broke into the man's store to steal the drug for his wife. Should the husband have done that?

Kohlberg concluded that there were three levels of moral development:

Level One – Pre-conventional Morality

The first stage is based on the concept of punishment, with children evaluating the wrongness of an action based upon the amount of damage it causes. The children base their thinking on self-interest and reward. Their answer to the Heinz dilemma would tend to be based on what would happen to the man as a result of the act, for example the man should not break into the pharmacy because the pharmacist might find him and beat him. Or they might say that the man should break in and steal the drug for his wife. Both decisions were based on what would physically happen to the man as a result of the act. This is a self-centred approach to moral decision-making.

Level Two – Conventional Morality

In this stage, children judge the morality of an act based on conformation to rules, which are seen as rigid and absolute. Their answers are also based upon what people would think of the man as a result of the act. For example, they might say he should not break in because it is against the law. The focus is on how situational outcomes impact others and contributes to the overall well-being of society. For example, they might answer that the man should steal the drug because that is what good husbands do. At this stage they acknowledge the importance of social norms or laws and want to be a good member of the group or society. A good decision is one that gains the approval of others or one that complies with the law. Older children and adolescents tend to use this reasoning.

Level Three – Post-conventional Morality

During this stage, people move beyond conforming to rules and demonstrate the ability to question rules based on their own ethical principles. They are also able to show that they can apply abstract reasoning. Not all adolescents and adults move to this stage.

Development of Peer Relationships

A child's interactions with their caregiver play a significant role in how they relate to other children, and the development of their peer relationships. Infants may show an awareness of each other by the age of 6 months, and by the end of their first year they develop the ability to respond to other infants' behaviours. Social interaction between toddlers becomes more complex and they develop the concept of turn-taking and engaging in pretend play. Dominance hierarchies develop in pre-school age groups of children.

In school-age children, there is a significant increase in the amount of time spent with peers, and groups tend to increase in size in settings that are less supervised by adults. In early adolescence, children seek peer acceptance, which is based on several different factors, some of which are not particularly rational. These may include physical attractiveness, name familiarity, sex and age. The common theme is similarity. Being accepted by other children is an important source of self-esteem for children, and peer rejection may precede later behavioural difficulties. Friendships tend to become more stable and enduring as children grow older, which correlates with how the characteristics on which the friendships are formed continue to evolve and change with time.

Play

Play is the work through which children learn about themselves, others and the world in which they live. It starts when the infant is just a few weeks old and is social, with reciprocal smiles, movements and vocalisations with the caregiver developing into play such as peek-a-boo. By the end of the first year, children are learning to clap, smile, play hide-and-seek and are seeking approval within games. Rhymes, stories, songs, dancing and make-believe play follow. As the child develops, there is increasing cooperative play with others, puzzle-solving, building and drawing (Figures 2.1 and 2.2). Play supports the positive development of relationships with peers and caregivers in early childhood, and the exploration of identity and transition to new roles in adolescence. New technologies and socio-cultural shifts can impact on the quality and availability of tools for play for children (Figure 2.3). However, play remains intertwined with language and social learning, and is essential for the development of autonomy, reciprocity, creativity and resilience in adult life.

Sleep

Newborn babies alternate frequently between sleeping and waking, with a total sleeping time of 16–17 hours per day. This develops into more structured sleep with time, usually consisting of two naps during the day and a longer sleep at night.

Sleep patterns throughout childhood are influenced by environmental factors, such as changes in routine, anxiety and parental responses to waking. By the time children are 4 years old they are able to recognise dreams and speak of them, although few can describe traumatic dreams [13]. Nightmares occur in rapid eye movement sleep. By contrast night terrors occur in deep non-rapid eye movement sleep, with children therefore not having recall of these events. Night terrors are most common in children between the ages of 3 and 8.

Sleep problems are common in adolescence, owing to marked psychological and social changes during this stage of development. Adolescents may experience altered sleep patterns due to a range of factors including changes in melatonin release, anxiety, the use of psychoactive substances (caffeine, alcohol, tobacco or drugs) or psychiatric disorder.

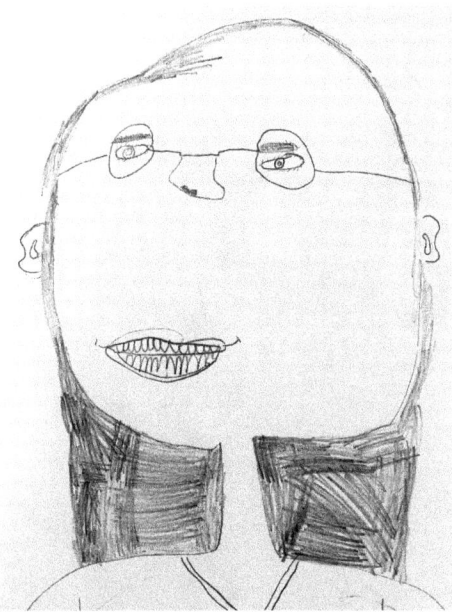

Figure 2.1 A self-portrait of a 6-year-old girl. There is detailed drawing of specific facial features (eyes, mouth) from the current perspective of the child, with some features rendered symbolically

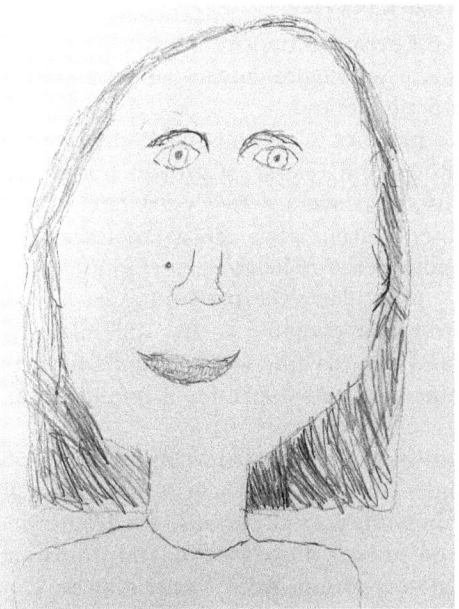

Figure 2.2 A self-portrait of a 10-year-old girl. Note the attention to the sizing and distances between features, creating a coherent (and feminine) whole

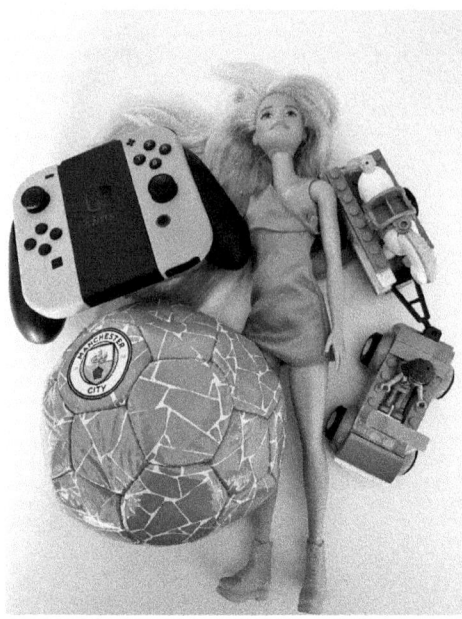

Figure 2.3 Favoured toys of girls in primary school in Lancashire in 2022. It is interesting to consider socio-cultural factors that may influence their play

Development in Adolescence

Adolescence is defined as the period of transition between childhood and adulthood. This is a crucial time in biological, psychological and social development, and an outline of some key factors linked to this period follows.

Adolescents tend to experience a 'growth spurt', defined as a rapid increase in their height and weight resulting from release of growth hormones, thyroid hormones and androgens. In males, this is on average two years later than females. The brain also undergoes extensive changes during adolescence. Adolescents often engage in increased risk-taking behaviours and experience heightened emotions during puberty. This may be since the frontal lobes – particularly the pre-frontal cortex, which are responsible for judgment, impulse control and planning – are still maturing until early adulthood. Adolescents weigh risks and rewards differently to adults, as their brain's sensitivity to the neurotransmitter dopamine peaks. As dopamine is implicated in reward circuits, rewards may outweigh the risks.

There are vital cognitive and social developments during adolescence. In this period there is development of capabilities in abstract thought. Adolescents develop the ability to imagine hypothetical situations, to debate and to consider different points of view. They tend to seek close peer relationships and become more heavily influenced by their social peer group. Adolescents may develop different interests and seek independence from attachment figures, in an important period of separation and individuation.

Puberty is a developmental period during which hormonal changes lead to physical alterations in the body. The first phase begins when Follicle-Stimulating Hormone and

Table 2.2 Tanner's five stages of puberty

Stage	Boys	Girls
1	Pre-adolescent	Pre-adolescent
2	Slight amount of pubic hair, slight enlargement of penis and scrotum	Sparse pubic hair, breasts begin to develop
3	Increased pubic hair, penis longer, testes bigger	Increased pubic hair, breasts enlarged
4	Pubic hair pattern resembles adult pattern but still sparser than in adults	Abundant pubic hair (less than in adults), nipples become more prominent
5	Adult male distribution of pubic hair, adult size testes and penis	Adult female pattern of pubic hair, breasts of mature adult

Luteinising hormone released from the pituitary gland stimulate the production of the male sex hormone testosterone in boys and the female sex hormones oestrogen and progesterone in girls. This is triggered by the hypothalamus releasing GnRH. Release of these hormones triggers the development of the primary sex characteristics, the sex organs concerned with reproduction. Secondary sexual characteristics are visible changes in the body, not directly linked to reproduction, but indicating sexual maturity. These include breast development, voice change and pubic, facial and body hair.

Tanner [14] classified the development of secondary sexual characteristics into five stages (Table 2.2).

Development of Gender Identity

Development of gender identity and sexual orientation occurs during childhood, adolescence and beyond. A brief overview of terms related to development in this area is given in this section.

'Sex' refers to the physiological differences between male, female and intersex people, including primary and secondary sex characteristics. This is determined by a combination of biological and chromosomal processes that occur prenatally and postnatally.

Gender refers to the socio-cultural and psychological differences associated with each sex. Gender identity refers to an individual's internal sense of being male, female, androgenous or non-binary. Gender is often regarded as a social construct, meaning it does not exist naturally, but is a concept created by society and is a subjective experience. From birth, children are socialised to conform to certain gender roles based on their biological sex and the gender to which they are assigned.

The term 'gender role' refers to the social construct of how men and women are expected to act, including specific attitudes and behaviours that are typically linked with each sex. During early social development, children are introduced to gender roles that are culturally specific and often stereotypically linked to their biological sex within the society they are living in. These may be subtle and vary over time. For example 'pink for girls, blue for boys' is a relatively recent construct in developed Western countries and is binary. 'Non-binary' is a construct which identifies a continuum of genders, that may evolve over time, as opposed to binary female/male gender roles.

Influences on the gender identity of children are likely to include the predominant gender roles in their socio-cultural groups; biological factors such as genetics and hormone levels; and psychological and social factors that provide constant feedback, including the influence of family, peers and media. Children will develop and explore their gender identity through observation of the gender-linked behaviours of others and subsequent experimentation.

A person's subjective experience of their gender may not correspond with the sex they were 'assigned' at birth, which may lead to distress and a desire to be of another gender. 'Transgender' is a term for persons whose gender identity, gender expression or behaviour does not conform to that typically associated with the sex to which they were assigned at birth.

An individual's sexual orientation is their emotional and sexual attraction to a particular sex or gender. Many sexual orientations are specifically defined, including heterosexuality (attraction to the opposite sex/gender), same-sex attraction (previously referred to as homosexuality), bisexuality, polysexuality or pansexuality (attraction to two, multiple or all sexes/genders, respectively) and asexuality (no sexual attraction to any sex/gender). There is no scientific consensus regarding the exact reasons why an individual holds a particular sexual orientation.

Conclusion

An understanding of normal development is key to clinical practice in child and adolescent psychiatry. A complex and fascinating interplay of biological, psychological and socio-cultural factors – involving the child, their family and the wider environment – influence development. This chapter has summarised a range of historical theories which relate to various aspects of childhood development, including attachment, temperament and theories of emotional, cognitive and social development, as well as issues related to adolescence. Many of these theories have stood the test of time and remain fundamental to achieving a holistic understanding of the patient seen in-clinic. We hope that this chapter highlights the range of domains and factors that must be considered in the assessment of childhood development.

Acknowledgements

With thanks to Dr Latha Hackett (Consultant in child and adolescent psychiatry, and MRCPsych Course Director in Health Education England North West).

References

1. Ainsworth M, Blehar M, Waters E, Wall SN. *Patterns of Attachment: A Psychological Study of the Strange Situation*. Routledge, 1978.
2. Main M, Solomon J. Discovery of an Insecure-Disorganised/Disoriented Attachment Pattern: Procedures, Findings and Implication for the Classification of Behaviours. In TB Brazelton & M Yogman (eds.), *Affective Development in Infancy*. Ablex Pub. Co, 1986, 95–124.
3. Thomas A, Chess S. *Temperament and Development*. Brunner/Mazel, 1977.
4. Costa PT, McCrae RR. *Revised NEO Personality Inventory and NEO Five-Factor Inventory*. Research Psychologists Press, 1992.
5. Freud S. *Three Essays on the Theory of Sexuality: The 1905 Edition*. Verso, 2016.

6. Steiner C, Perry P. *Achieving Emotional Literacy.* Bloomsbury, 1997.
7. Piaget J, Inhelder B, Weaver H. *Psychology of the Child.* Basic, 2000.
8. Skinner BF. *Verbal Behaviour.* Appleton Century Crofts, 1957.
9. Bandura A. *Social Foundations of Thought and Action: A Social Cognitive Theory.* Prentice Hall, 1986.
10. Chomsky N. *Aspects of the Theory of Syntax.* MIT Press, 1965.
11. Moon C, Cooper RP, Fifer WP. Two-Day-Olds Prefer Their Native Language. Infant Behav. Dev. 1993 Oct;**16**(4):495–500.
12. Kohlberg, L. Stage and Sequence: The Cognitive Developmental Approach to Socialisation. In DA Goslin (ed.), *Handbook of Socialisation Theory and Research.* Rand MacNally College Publishing Company, 1969, 347–480.
13. Terr LC. Childhood Traumas: An Outline and Overview. *American Journal of Psychiatry.* 1991 Jan;**148**:10–20.
14. Tanner JM. *Growth at Adolescence: With a General Consideration of the Effects of Hereditary and Environmental Factors upon Growth and Maturation from Birth to Maturity.* 2nd ed. Blackwell Scientific Publications, 1962.

Further Reading

Bates JE, Wachs TD. *Temperament: Individual Difference at the Interface of Biology and Behaviour.* American Psychological Association, 1994

Bowlby J. *Attachment and Loss. Vol. 2, Separation: Anxiety and Anger.* Pimlico, 1973.

Carr A. *The Handbook of Child and Adolescent Clinical Psychology: A Contextual Approach.* Taylor & Francis Ltd, 2017.

Devi L. *Child Development: An Introduction.* Institute for Sustainable Development, Lucknow, 1998.

Graham PJ, Verhulst FC, Turk J. *Child Psychiatry: A Developmental Approach.* Oxford University Press, 1999.

Salter Ainsworth, Mary D, Blehar MC, Waters E, Wall S. *Patterns of Attachment: A Psychological Study of the Strange Situation.* Erlbaum, 1978.

Paris J, Ricardo A, Rymond D. *Child Growth and Development: An Open Educational Resources Publication.* College of the Canyons, 2019.

Royal College of Psychiatrists. *TrOn – Development of Language* [Internet]. Available from: https://elearninghub.rcpsych.ac.uk/product?catalog=23_TRON_Dev_lang (cited 27 April 2022).

Royal College of Psychiatrists. *TrOn – Emotion* [Internet]. Available from: https://elearninghub.rcpsych.ac.uk/product?catalog=50_TRON_Emotion (cited 27 April 2022).

Thomas A, Chess S. The New York Longitudinal Study: From Infancy to Adult Life. In R Plomin, J Dunn (eds.), *The Study of Temperament: Changes, Continuities and Challenges.* Erlbaum, 1986, 39–52.

Chapter 3

Risk Factors for Childhood Psychopathology

Joanne L. Doherty and Alka S. Ahuja MBE

Introduction

In 2020, the Mental Health of Children and Young People in England survey found that 1:6 (16%) of children aged between five and sixteen has a probable mental illness [1]. Furthermore, research has shown that most psychiatric disorders have their origins in childhood, even if they are typically diagnosed in adulthood [2,3]. Childhood represents a critical period of physical, cognitive, psychological, behavioural and social transformation. Identifying risk and protective factors that alter the typical developmental trajectory could have long-term educational, social, societal and economic implications. This chapter will address what is meant by the term risk factor and how these can be identified, provide examples of risk factors thought to be important in child and adolescent psychiatry and conclude with some case vignettes to highlight the importance of taking a developmental biopsychosocial approach to identifying risk, considering predisposing, precipitating, perpetuating and protective factors.

Risk and Protective Factors

Epidemiological studies can tell us not only about the frequency (incidence or prevalence) of symptoms and disorders but also their associations. Through carefully designed studies of large samples of people with and without the symptoms or disorder of interest, statistical associations can be made between potential risk or protective factors and outcomes. Epidemiologists can then conduct investigations to determine whether any observed associations are likely to be causal or non-causal (artefactual) and thus identify factors that may play an important aetiological role and plan strategies for early intervention and prevention.

A risk factor is any attribute, characteristic or exposure that increases the likelihood of an individual developing a disease or injury while a protective factor reduces this likelihood. Risk and protective factors can act both directly or indirectly via intermediary factors. Table 3.1 below lists some of the terminology used in epidemiological research.

Figure 3.1 below shows examples of relationships between two variables, A and B, highlighting potential difficulties in determining whether associations are causal.

The biopsychosocial model was proposed by George Engel in 1977 to explain the complex relationships between biological, psychological and social dimensions in the development of mental illness [4]. Evidence is continuing to accumulate for both correlation and interaction between risk factors across these dimensions. Most of the risk factors identified to date do not map onto individual disorders on a 1:1 basis, nor do they act in a linear or hierarchical fashion. Rather, multiple risk factors (biological, psychological and

3 Risk Factors for Childhood Psychopathology

Table 3.1 Examples of terminology used in epidemiological research

Terminology	Example
Risk factor	If the factor of interest is present, the probability that the effect will occur is increased
Protective factor	If the factor of interest is present, the probability that the effect will occur is decreased
Sufficient cause	If the exposure is present, the outcome will occur
Necessary cause	The exposure must be present for the outcome to occur but may also be present in the absence of the outcome of interest
Directly causal	The exposure exerts its effect in the absence of intermediary factors
Indirectly causal	The exposure exerts its effects via intermediary factors
Non-causal	The association is statistically significant but no causal relationship exists e.g. other factors explain the observed association or the temporal relationship is incorrect
Reverse causality	There is an association between two variables but the direction of effect is opposite to that anticipated e.g. the hypothesised outcome causes the exposure.

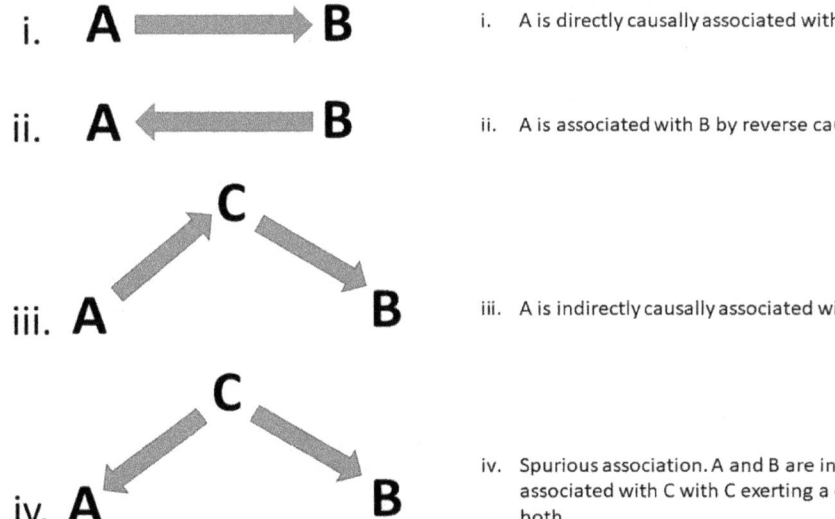

Figure 3.1 Examples of relationships between two variables

social) may act at different levels and at different stages of development. These factors may predispose an individual to one or more disorders or precipitate/perpetuate their presentation. It is likely that the number, nature, timing, severity and chronicity of risk factors influences the probability of an individual developing symptoms or disorder, as seen in Figure 3.2. In the next section, we will explore some of these risk factors in more detail.

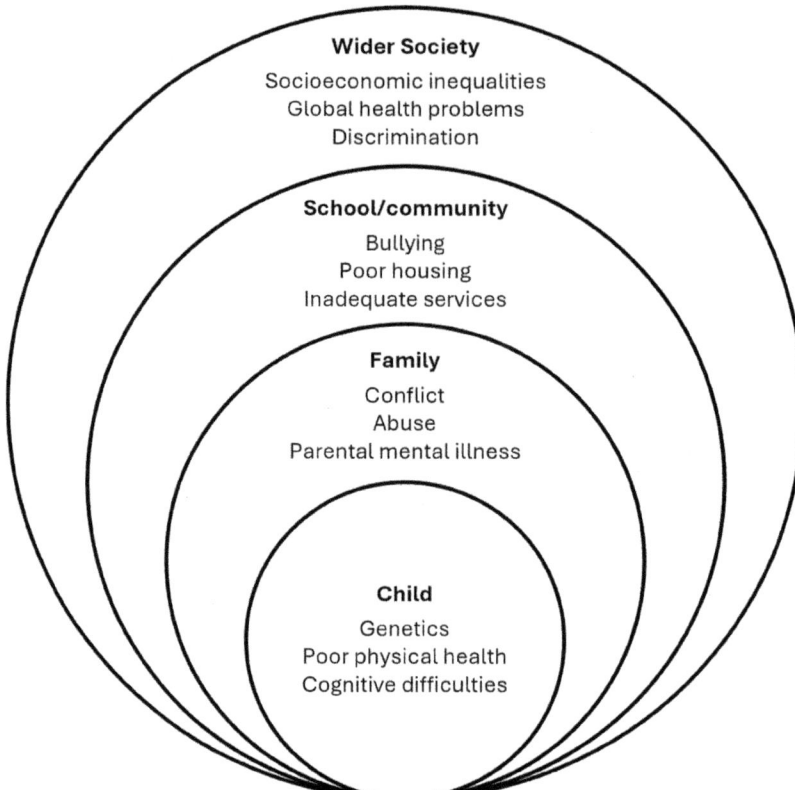

Figure 3.2 Levels at which risk factors for childhood psychopathology may exert their effects

Genetic Factors

It has long been known that psychiatric disorders tend to cluster in families. In the last two decades there have been tremendous advances in psychiatric genetics due to technological developments and collaborative working among large consortia. Evidence to date suggests that as with many other common medical conditions, the genetic architecture of psychiatric disorders is extremely complex, with no single gene being either necessary or sufficient for the clinical phenotype [5].

Heritability refers to the proportion of population variability that is attributable to inherited as opposed to environmental factors. This ranges from approximately 30% for depression to 80% for attention deficit hyperactivity disorder (ADHD) [6]. The genetic variants identified so far include small DNA sequence variants (single nucleotide variants (SNVs) and single nucleotide polymorphisms (SNPs)), submicroscopic deletions and duplications of chromosomal segments (copy number variants (CNVs)) and large chromosomal abnormalities (translocations and aneuploidies), each differing in their frequency and penetrance. Overall, these variants seem to act probabilistically and additively, such that the more variants an individual carries the higher their risk of disorder.

Many genetic variants show pleiotropy, impacting multiple phenotypic traits. For example, the 22q11.2 deletion is a CNV involving deletion of 1.5–3 million base pairs. It is rare, affecting about 1:4000 of the population. The CNV is neither necessary nor sufficient for any specific psychiatric disorder; however, 40% of carriers have autism spectrum disorder (ASD) and/or ADHD and 25% develop schizophrenia in adulthood [7]. People with the deletion may also have learning disability and a range of physical manifestations including cleft palate and structural heart defects. There are a number of different CNV syndromes that are associated with high risk of neurodevelopmental disorders and learning disability [8]. SNVs and SNPs tend to exert smaller individual effects on disorder risk than larger structural variants, but these have also been shown to cross diagnostic boundaries [9].

In recent years there has been increasing interest in gene environment interplay, with acknowledgement that genetic risks can influence environmental factors and vice versa through epigenetics. Gene environment correlation occurs when an individual's genotype (or that of their parents) influences their exposure to environmental conditions. Gene environment interaction on the other hand, occurs when the effect of a genetic risk factor is altered by the presence of an environmental risk factor. It is likely that both mechanisms play an important role in child mental health outcomes [5].

Environmental Factors

While it is clear that genetic risk factors are important in childhood psychiatric disorders, heritability estimates suggest that environmental factors must also play a crucial role. In this section, we will explore some of the associations between these factors and mental health outcomes.

Prenatal/Perinatal Factors

Obstetric complications have repeatedly been associated with psychiatric disorders, including schizophrenia, ASD and ADHD [10,11]. Determining whether these associations are causal is challenging due to the potential impact of confounding by other factors affecting foetal well-being.

Alcohol is a known teratogen that can significantly affect foetal brain development with the potential for long-term physical, cognitive and mental health consequences [12,13]. A spectrum of neuropsychiatric sequelae has been found in foetal alcohol spectrum disorders including cognitive deficits affecting learning and memory, language, visuospatial ability, attention and executive functioning. They are also associated with psychiatric co-morbidity including ADHD, depression, anxiety disorders and conduct problems [14,15].

Much less is known about the long-term mental health effects of other recreational substances during pregnancy; however, associations with cognitive function and behavioural disturbances have been reported [16]. Antenatal exposure to prescribed medications has also been associated with psychopathology. These include antibiotics [17], paracetamol [18], mood stabilisers such as sodium valproate [19,20] and antidepressants [21]. However, there are several confounding factors that could, at least in part, explain the observed relationships, for example, genetic factors, maternal infections and inflammatory disorders.

Physical Health

Physical and mental health are interrelated. Children with physical health conditions and their families are more likely than their healthy peers to have mental health problems and vice versa [22,23,24]. Furthermore, children with multimorbidity experience greater symptom severity and impairment [25]. Physical illness can impact on the physical, social and emotional well-being of children and their families and increase the risk of adverse mental health outcomes. Conversely, mental health disorders can affect physical well-being, for example, by effects on the immune system, cardiovascular function, diet and exercise [26].

Several infectious agents have direct associations with mental health problems including toxoplasmosis, syphilis, chlamydia, human immunodeficiency virus (HIV), cytomegalovirus, leptospirosis, herpes simplex, measles, malaria and streptococcus. A population-based cohort study based on registry data found that both community and hospital-treated infections were associated with higher rates of mental health problems with both dose-response and temporal relationships [27]. The observed relationships may be secondary to direct effects of the infectious agent on the brain, the resulting immune response or the effects of treatment.

In addition to the effects of the immune system in infectious diseases, there is increasing recognition of the associations between psychiatric disorders and autoimmune conditions including type 1 diabetes mellitus [28], systemic lupus erythematosus [29] and anti-NMDA receptor encephalitis [30], as well as other common inflammatory conditions such as childhood asthma [10] and eczema [11]. The relationships between autoimmune/inflammatory and psychiatric disorders could be mediated by a number of mechanisms, including but not limited to direct effects on the brain, the psychosocial impact of chronic disease and the effects of treatment.

Seizures are common in childhood, affecting about 4–5% of children [31]. Childhood epilepsy has been associated with psychiatric disorders both in childhood and in later life. There are consistently reported associations with neurodevelopmental conditions such as ASD and ADHD as well as behavioural, mood, anxiety and psychotic disorders [32,33,34,35]. The mechanisms underlying these relationships are not well understood but may be secondary to the direct effects of the seizures themselves on the brain, shared underlying pathophysiology (including genetic susceptibility) and the psychosocial consequences of living with a chronic illness. Febrile seizures on the other hand have previously been considered to be relatively benign, with no significant long-lasting sequelae. However, a study conducted in a large Danish cohort found that the risk of any psychiatric disorder was raised in those with a history of febrile seizures (hazard ratio 1.12) and that the risk increased with the number of seizure-related hospitalisations [36].

Traumatic brain injury is another important but under-recognised risk factor for neuropsychiatric problems. It has been found to be associated with ADHD [37], mood and anxiety symptoms [38]. The nature and severity of the symptoms are likely to be related to mechanism of injury and the brain regions and networks that are impacted.

Cognitive Ability

Children and adolescents with lower cognitive ability are at increased risk of psychiatric disorders compared to those of average or high IQ. For example, IQ in childhood has been found to predict adult-onset schizophrenia, depression and anxiety [39]. Over a third of children with learning disability meet criteria for a psychiatric or neurodevelopmental disorder, the most common of which is ASD. They are also at increased risk of ADHD, conduct disorder, emotional disorders, psychosis and depression [40].

There are many possible explanations for the observed associations between cognitive ability and mental health. Shared genetic contributions are one potential mechanism, with both polygenic factors and specific cognitive variants likely to play a role. For example, at least 60% of children with severe learning disability have an identifiable genetic risk variant [41]. Language ability has been shown to be associated with psychopathology, independently of IQ and to have shared polygenic risks [42,43,44]. Environmental mechanisms are also plausible. Families caring for children with a learning disability face many challenges and are more likely to experience psychosocial adversity (including financial difficulty) than other households. Parents of children with learning disability have been found to be at increased risk of depression, anxiety and emotional distress [45,46,47]. Children and young people with a learning disability may have problems developing peer relationships, accessing clubs and recreational activities and may have additional health problems like epilepsy.

Substance Use

Adolescence represents a time when peer influences gain primacy and sensation seeking may occur. Substance use disorders and mental health problems frequently co-occur. Early recreational drug use is a risk factor for later substance use disorders [48]. Adolescents with substance use disorders are three times more likely to make a suicide attempt compared to those who do not use substances, making them a particularly high-risk group [49]. The direction of effect has been the subject of much research. There is some evidence that both internalising and externalising disorders may precede substance use disorders [50,51], while cannabis use in adolescence has been associated with future psychosis [52] and earlier onset of psychosis [53]. The aetiological and neurobiological mechanisms underlying the co-occurrence of substance use disorders and psychiatric disorders have not been fully elucidated. It may be that psychiatric symptoms increase vulnerability to substance use disorders due to the reinforcing effects of particular substances. Alternatively, substance use disorders may increase the risk of mental health problems by triggering the onset of symptoms in people who may be vulnerable but who in the absence of substances would have remained well. It is also possible that there are shared/overlapping risk factors – both genetic and environmental that can help to explain the associations.

Temperament and Personality

Child temperament has been associated with a range of adverse outcomes both in childhood and in adult life. Temperament refers to early-appearing variations in emotional reactivity, which is in itself under the strong influence of genetic and environmental factors. Temperamental disposition towards experiencing negative emotions and low inhibitory control have been linked to several psychiatric disorders. For example, high negative activity has been associated with major depression [54], anxiety disorders [54] and substance abuse [55]. While depression and anxiety have been associated with low levels of extraversion [56], both of these factors are associated with substance misuse [55]. Temperament and personality factors have also been identified in patients with eating disorders. High levels of reward dependence have been found in people with anorexia nervosa and novelty-seeking in those with bulimia nervosa [57]. Patients with eating disorders report high levels of perfectionism and negative affect. Those with restricting presentations tend to score higher on measures of rigidity and obsessive-compulsiveness than those with binge-purging presentations, who score more highly on measures of extraversion and affect instability [58].

Family Factors

Healthy family relationships play an important role in child development and the risk of mental health problems. Secure attachment with a caregiver from early infancy is a key factor in social and emotional development. Consistent and sensitive caregiving results in children seeing their caregiver as a secure base from which the environment can be explored. This affects their expectations about themselves, other people and the world around them [59]. Inconsistent caregiving is associated with insecure attachment [60,61], which is in turn a risk factor for both internalising and externalising problems [62].

Maternal mental health is a robust predictor of child mental health [63,64,65]. While there has been more research into the role of mothers, fathers' mental health is also known to be important [66]. There are many potential aetiological mechanisms that could underlie the associations between parent and child mental health. These include shared vulnerabilities (e.g. inherited factors and psychosocial stressors), family separation, attachment difficulties, stigma/bullying, caring responsibilities, anxiety about each other's mental well-being and co-morbid substance abuse.

Beyond the parent–child dyad, wider family relationships are also important for children's mental well-being. Exposure to frequent, intense and poorly resolved inter-parental conflict increases a child's risk of mental health problems [67]. Sibling relationships have been less extensively researched, though there is some evidence that the quality of these relationships is associated with both internalising and externalising symptoms [68].

School and Community

The school environment is an important predictor of mental health problems in children [69]. Bullying in particular has been highlighted as a potent risk factor. Children who experience bullying are more likely to have depression and anxiety disorders, to self-harm and to have suicidal thoughts [70]. Multiple school factors have been identified as being associated with positive mental health outcomes including school connectedness, positive friendships and good pupil–teacher relationships [69,71]. Outside of the classroom setting, studies have shown that other aspects of a child's social interactions are important for mental well-being. High levels of social support, good social networks and participation in sport, clubs and organisations have been found to act as protective factors [72,73,74].

Technology and Social Media

There has been increasing interest in the mental health effects of technology and in particular online communities and social media. There is some preliminary evidence that in contrast to offline social networks, online social networks can have a negative impact on mood, self-esteem, life-satisfaction, body image and subjective emotional well-being [75]. Young people with mental health problems are more likely to use social media every day than those without a disorder. They are also more likely to feel that they compare themselves to others on social media, to have been bullied and to have bullied others [1]. There is some early evidence that social media usage is associated with eating disorder cognitions and behaviours in young adolescents [76] and with effects on the risk of deliberate self-harm, particularly in vulnerable young people [77,78]. Social media and digital platforms do also offer opportunities to increase young people's social interactions and expand supportive networks [79]. There are opportunities for professionals to engage with these platforms and increase public health messaging around mental health, improve access to services and offer online interventions [80]. This has proven to be particularly important during the Covid-19 pandemic when access to face-to-face support was very limited.

Adverse Childhood Experiences

Children with mental health problems are more likely than those without to have experienced certain types of adversity in their lives including parental separation, financial crisis, abuse and neglect. These are collectively termed 'adverse childhood experiences' (ACEs). It is thought that ACEs repeatedly activate the stress response system and impact on brain, endocrine, immune and metabolic function and development [81,82,83]. Unfortunately, ACEs are extremely common, and many children experience more than one type of ACE. A study using survey data from England and Wales found that approximately 47% of adults in Wales had suffered at least one ACE during childhood and 13% to have suffered four or more. Figures for England were lower with 44% experiencing at least one ACE and 8% experiencing four or more. ACEs have been found to act cumulatively on risk of poor outcomes. Risks of poor mental health outcomes were higher for individuals with any level of ACE and the relative risk increased with ACE level. The relative risk of having one ACE was 1.56 for depression and 1.43 for anxiety. This increased to 2.76 and 2.75, respectively, for those with four or more ACEs [83].

Migration

UNHCR data shows that children and adolescents comprise over half of the world's refugees and asylum seekers [84]. These children are at high risk of internalising disorders, with high rates of post-traumatic stress disorder (PTSD), anxiety and depression being reported [85]. Migrant and refugee children are potentially exposed to numerous stressors before, during and after migration. Cultural factors including stigma may affect health-seeking behaviour, engagement with services and adherence to treatment. Unaccompanied children are of particular concern and studies have found these children to be at higher risk of mental health problems than accompanied peers [86].

Socio-economic Inequalities

Children living in poverty in the UK are four to five times more likely to have mental health problems than children from high income families, and this gap has widened over time [87]. Families living in poverty experience many disadvantages including poor quality housing, food insecurity, lack of educational and employment opportunities, bullying and social exclusion. They are also more likely to have had ACEs.

There is a lack of high-quality research into the relationship between ethnicity and mental health in the UK. Differences in disorder prevalence have been found with girls from mixed ethnic backgrounds being at greater risk of mental health problems than white British girls [87]. Ethnic minority groups disproportionately live in substandard, overcrowded housing and experience discrimination on the basis of their race [88]. They may also face barriers in accessing mental health services [89]. The mechanisms underlying the observed associations are likely to be complex and multifactorial and show correlation/interaction with other socio-economic, cultural and educational factors.

Covid-19

The impact of the Covid-19 pandemic and the resulting policies to reduce its spread had wide-reaching effects on the mental health of young people. While the physical health consequences have not been as severe for children and adolescents as for older age groups, children have been exposed to numerous stressful experiences during this period. A systematic review concluded that school closures in particular were associated with considerable harm to children and young people's health and well-being [90]. Furthermore, children who started school during the pandemic are thought to be struggling with their personal, social and emotional development [91].

Referrals to NHS eating disorder services have almost doubled since the start of the pandemic with resulting increases in waiting times [92]. Of particular concern at this time are children with pre-existing risk factors. In a study of 142 children aged 4–8 years old who were identified as being 'at risk' by their teachers before the pandemic, Adegboye et al. [93] found a significant increase in mental health problems, particularly anxiety. They also found that financial strain indirectly predicted increases in child mental health problems through effects on parental mental health. This is an important finding as it highlights the importance of providing financial support to families in need to improve both parent and child mental health.

Case Vignettes

Salim is an 11-year-old boy who has been referred for a neurodevelopmental assessment. He has been having difficulty paying attention in class and concentrating on his work. He is unable to stay seated and has been noted to be constantly fidgeting and looking out of the window. He has also been having difficulty making friends. Salim was born at 34 weeks after a difficult pregnancy. His mother has a history of depression and has been taking antidepressants for over 10 years. Salim's father had problems in school and left without any qualifications. Salim has an 8-year-old brother who has a diagnosis of ASD.

Salim has a number of predisposing risk factors for neurodevelopmental disorders including: male gender, a positive family history, antenatal risk factors and maternal depression/antidepressant use. His symptoms may have been perpetuated by difficulties accessing adequate services and management of his symptoms or lack of social support for the family. He lives at home with his parents and brother, which may act as a protective factor.

Emily is a 15-year-old girl whose mother is worried that she has become low in mood and socially withdrawn. She is tearful most of the time, has no appetite and lacks energy. Her sleep has become increasingly erratic. She has been struggling with exam preparation and is no longer doing her usual after school activities. Her parents separated when she was 13-years-old and she does not have contact with her father. There is a history of domestic violence. Emily lives with her mother and older sister. Due to financial pressures, the family recently had to move to a new area. Since starting at her new school, Emily has experienced bullying. There is a family history of depression and anxiety with her grandmother and maternal aunt being admitted to hospital with severe depressive episodes.

Emily is predisposed to developing depression due to a family history of mood disorders and a history of multiple ACEs. Her presentation to services may have been precipitated by increased bullying at school and exam pressure. Possible perpetuating factors include ongoing conflict in the family, financial insecurity and lack of support networks in their new location.

Nia is a 13-year-old girl referred to CAMHS with disordered eating. She is known to be a high-achiever in school and played hockey and netball for her county. She found the national Covid-19 lockdowns extremely difficult and was unable to engage with online learning, falling behind in several subjects. She missed playing sport and became increasingly preoccupied with her shape and weight. Last summer, her mother lost her job and became low in mood. There were lots of arguments at home and Nia became worried that her parents might separate. At the start of the new school year, Nia's friends noticed that she had lost weight, and she received lots of compliments about this. She started to restrict her food intake and spend hours doing online exercise videos. She also spent a lot of time on social media.

Nia is noted to have been a high-achiever in her academic and sporting activities. The Covid-19 national lockdowns stopped her from being able to access face-to-face teaching, extracurricular activities and social networks. Nia's parents experienced financial stress and there was increasing conflict at home, which may have precipitated restrictive eating patterns. She may also have experienced pubertal changes, affecting her body image. This, accompanied by increasing use of social media, may have acted as a maintaining factor for her disordered eating.

Tom is an 8-year-old boy with 22q11.2 deletion syndrome. He has a mild learning disability and a diagnosis of ASD. Over the last three months, he has become increasingly anxious. His worries vary from day to day. He frequently experiences abdominal pain on school days and feels tense and anxious most of the time. He struggles to get to sleep because he worries that something bad might happen during the night. This has left his family feeling exhausted. There is no known family history of mental illness. He is an only child and lives with both parents. Recently, his father has given up his job to care for him. Tom has a history of congenital heart disease and has had to have several operations in the past. He is due to have further surgery in the next year. He has frequent infections, often resulting in hospitalisation.

Tom has a genetic disorder associated with psychiatric illness, including anxiety disorders. He also has a diagnosis of ASD, which is frequently co-morbid with anxiety. In addition, he has a complex medical history with frequent hospitalisations, which may have been traumatic for both him and his family. He has cognitive difficulties, which further predispose him to a range of mental health problems. His current symptoms may have been precipitated by concerns about further surgery, changes at home including the loss of his father's income or stressors at school. Children with genetic syndromes may not receive recognition or care for their mental health needs in as timely a fashion as their physical health needs, which may act to maintain their symptoms.

References

1. NHS Digital. *Mental Health of Children and Young People in England, 2020: Wave 1 follow up to the 2017 survey.* NHS Digital, 2020.
2. Kessler RC, Berglund P, Demler O, Jin R, Merikangas KR, Walters EE. Lifetime Prevalence and Age-of-Onset Distributions of DSM-IV Disorders in the National Comorbidity Survey Replication. Arch Gen Psychiatry. 2005 Jun;**62**(6):593–602.
3. Paus T, Keshavan M, Giedd JN. Why Do Many Psychiatric Disorders Emerge During Adolescence? Nat Rev Neurosci. 2008 Nov 12;**9**(12):947–57.
4. Engel GL. The Need for a New Medical Model: A Challenge for Biomedicine. Science. 1977 April 8;**196**(4286):129–36.
5. Laver-Bradbury C, Thompson MJJ, Gale C, Hooper CM. (eds.). *Child and Adolescent Mental Health: Theory and Practice.* 3rd ed.

CRC Press, 2021. https://doi.org/10.4324/9781003083139.

6. Pettersson E, Lichtenstein P, Larsson H, et al. Genetic Influences on Eight Psychiatric Disorders Based on Family Data of 4 408 646 Full and Half-siblings, and Genetic Data of 333 748 Cases and Controls. Psychol Med. 2019 May 1;**49**(7):1166–73.

7. Schneider M, Debbané M, Bassett AS, et al. Psychiatric Disorders from Childhood to Adulthood in 22q11.2 Deletion Syndrome: Results from the International Consortium on Brain and Behavior in 22q11.2 Deletion Syndrome. Am J Psychiatry. 2014;**171**(6):627–39.

8. Chawner SJRA, Owen MJ, Holmans P, et al. Genotype–Phenotype Associations in Children with Copy Number Variants Associated with High Neuropsychiatric Risk in the UK (IMAGINE-ID): A Case-Control Cohort Study. Lancet Psychiatry. 2019 Jun 1;**6**(6):493–505.

9. Cross-Disorder Group of the Psychiatric Genomics Consortium, Hong Lee S, Ripke S, et al. Genetic Relationship Between Five Psychiatric Disorders Estimated from Genome-Wide SNPs. Nat Genet. 2013;**45**(9):984–94.

10. Arango C, Dragioti E, Solmi M, et al. Risk and Protective Factors for Mental Disorders beyond Genetics: An Evidence-Based Atlas. World Psychiatry. 2021 Oct 1;**20**(3):417–36.

11. Kim JH, Kim JY, Lee J, et al. Environmental Risk Factors, Protective Factors, and Peripheral Biomarkers for ADHD: An Umbrella Review. Lancet Psychiatry. 2020 Nov 1;**7**(11):955–70.

12. Jones KL, Smith DW. Recognition of the Fetal Alcohol Syndrome in Early Infancy. Lancet. 1973 Nov 3;**302**(7836):999–1001.

13. Aiton N. Neglect of Fetal Alcohol Spectrum Disorder Must End. BMJ. 2021 Dec 6;**375**:n2969.

14. Mattson SN, Bernes GA, Doyle LR. Fetal Alcohol Spectrum Disorders: A Review of the Neurobehavioral Deficits Associated with Prenatal Alcohol Exposure. Alcohol Clin Exp Res. 2019 Jun 1;**43**(6):1046–62.

15. Mukherjee RAS, Cook PA, Norgate SH, Price AD. Neurodevelopmental Outcomes in Individuals with Fetal Alcohol Spectrum Disorder (FASD) with and Without Exposure to Neglect: Clinical Cohort Data from a National FASD Diagnostic Clinic. Alcohol. 2019 May 1;**76**:23–28.

16. Ross EJ, Graham DL, Money KM, Stanwood GD. Developmental Consequences of Fetal Exposure to Drugs: What We Know and What We Still Must Learn. Neuropsychopharmacology. 2015 Jan 1;**40**(1):61.

17. Lavebratt C, Yang LL, Giacobini MB, et al. Early Exposure to Antibiotic Drugs and Risk for Psychiatric Disorders: A Population-Based Study. Transl Psychiatry. 2019 Nov 26;**9**(1):317.

18. Liew Z, Ritz B, Rebordosa C, Lee PC, Olsen J. Acetaminophen Use During Pregnancy, Behavioral Problems, and Hyperkinetic Disorders. JAMA Pediatr. 2014;**168**(4):313–20.

19. Christensen J, Pedersen L, Sun Y, Dreier JW, Brikell I, Dalsgaard S. Association of Prenatal Exposure to Valproate and Other Antiepileptic Drugs with Risk for Attention-Deficit/Hyperactivity Disorder in Offspring. JAMA Netw Open. 2019 Jan 4;**2**(1):e186606.

20. Christensen J, Grnøborg TK, Srøensen MJ, et al. Prenatal Valproate Exposure and Risk of Autism Spectrum Disorders and Childhood Autism. JAMA. 2013 Apr 24;**309**(16):1696–703.

21. Liu X, Agerbo E, Ingstrup KG, et al. Antidepressant Use During Pregnancy and Psychiatric Disorders in Offspring: Danish Nationwide Register Based Cohort Study. BMJ. 2017 Sep 6;**358**:j3668.

22. Hysing M, Elgen I, Gillberg C, Lie SA, Lundervold AJ. Chronic Physical Illness and Mental Health in Children. Results from a Large-Scale Population Study. J Child Psychol Psychiatry. 2007 Aug;**48**(8):785–92.

23. Dobbie M, Mellor D. Chronic Illness and Its Impact: Considerations for Psychologists. Psychol Health Med. 2008 Oct;**13**(5):583–90.

24. Ferro MA, Lipman EL, Van Lieshout RJ, et al. Cohort Profile: Multimorbidity in Children and Youth Across the Life-course (MY LIFE) Study. J Can Acad Child Adolesc Psychiatry. 2021;30(2):104–15.

25. Merikangas KR, Calkins ME, Burstein M, et al. Comorbidity of Physical and Mental Disorders in the Neurodevelopmental Genomics Cohort Study. Pediatrics. 2015 Apr 1;135(4):e927–38.

26. Carney R, Imran S, Law H, Folstad S, Parker S. Evaluation of the Physical Health of Adolescent In-patients in Generic and Secure Services: Retrospective Case-Note Review. BJPsych Bull. 2020 Jun;44(3):95–102.

27. Köhler-Forsberg O, Petersen L, Gasse C, et al. A Nationwide Study in Denmark of the Association Between Treated Infections and the Subsequent Risk of Treated Mental Disorders in Children and Adolescents. JAMA Psychiatry. 2019 Mar 1;76(3):271–79.

28. Buchberger B, Huppertz H, Krabbe L, Lux B, Mattivi JT, Siafarikas A. Symptoms of Depression and Anxiety in Youth with Type 1 Diabetes: A Systematic Review and Meta-analysis. Psychoneuroendocrinology. 2016 Aug 1;70:70–84.

29. Quilter MC, Hiraki LT, Korczak DJ. Depressive and Anxiety Symptom Prevalence in Childhood-Onset Systemic Lupus Erythematosus: A Systematic Review. Lupus. 2019 Jun 1;28(7):878–87.

30. Kayser MS, Dalmau J. Anti-NMDA Receptor Encephalitis in Psychiatry. Curr Psychiatry Rev. 2011 Aug 29;7(3):189.

31. Friedman MJ, Sharieff GQ. Seizures in Children. Pediatr Clin North Am. 2006 Apr;53(2):257–77.

32. Bertelsen EN, Larsen JT, Petersen L, Christensen J, Dalsgaard S. Childhood Epilepsy, Febrile Seizures, and Subsequent Risk of ADHD. Pediatrics. 2016 Aug 1;138(2):20154654. https://doi.org/10.1542/peds.2015-4654. Epub 2016 Jul 13. PMID: 27412639.

33. Gaitatzis A, Trimble MR, Sander JW. The Psychiatric Comorbidity of Epilepsy. Acta Neurol Scand. 2004 Oct 1;110(4):207–20.

34. Gillberg C, Lundström S, Fernell E, Nilsson G, Neville B. Febrile Seizures and Epilepsy: Association with Autism and Other Neurodevelopmental Disorders in the Child and Adolescent Twin Study in Sweden. Pediatr Neurol. 2017 Sep 1;74:80–86.e2.

35. Vestergaard M, Pedersen CB, Christensen J, Madsen KM, Olsen J, Mortensen PB. Febrile Seizures and Risk of Schizophrenia. Schizophr Res. 2005 Mar 1;73(2–3):343–49.

36. Dreier JW, Li J, Sun Y, Christensen J. Evaluation of Long-Term Risk of Epilepsy, Psychiatric Disorders, and Mortality Among Children with Recurrent Febrile Seizures: A National Cohort Study in Denmark. JAMA Pediatr. 2019 Dec 1;173(12):1164–70.

37. Gerring JP, Brady KD, Chen A, et al. Premorbid Prevalence of ADHD and Development of Secondary ADHD After Closed Head Injury. J Am Acad Child Adolesc Psychiatry. 1998 Jun 1;37(6):647–54.

38. Max JE, Koele SL, Smith WL, et al. Psychiatric Disorders in Children and Adolescents After Severe Traumatic Brain Injury: A Controlled Study. J Am Acad Child Adolesc Psychiatry. 1998;37(8):832–40.

39. Koenen KC, Moffitt TE, Roberts AL, et al. Article Childhood IQ and Adult Mental Disorders: A Test of the Cognitive Reserve Hypothesis. Am J Psychiatry. 2009;166(1):50–57.

40. Emerson E, Hatton C. The Mental Health of Children and Adolescents with Learning Disabilities in Britain. Br J Psychiatry. 2007 Dec; 191:493–99. https://doi.org/10.1192/bjp.bp.107.038729.

41. Gilissen C, Hehir-Kwa JY, Thung DT, et al. Genome Sequencing Identifies Major Causes of Severe Intellectual Disability. Nature. 2014;511(7509):344–47.

42. Yew SGK, O'Kearney R. Emotional and Behavioural Outcomes Later in Childhood and Adolescence for Children with Specific Language Impairments: Meta-analyses of Controlled Prospective Studies. J Child Psychol Psychiatry. 2013 May;54(5):516–24.

43. Toseeb U, Oginni OA, Dale PS. Developmental Language Disorder and Psychopathology: Disentangling Shared Genetic and Environmental Influences. J Learn Disabil. 2022 May–Jun;55(3):185–99. https://doi.org/10.1177/00222194211019961.

44. Newbury DF, Gibson JL, Conti-Ramsden G, Pickles A, Durkin K, Toseeb U. Using Polygenic Profiles to Predict Variation in Language and Psychosocial Outcomes in Early and Middle Childhood. J Speech, Lang Hear Res. 2019 Aug 19;62(9):3381–96.

45. Emerson E. Mothers of Children and Adolescents with Intellectual Disability: Social and Economic Situation, Mental Health Status, and the Self-Assessed Social and Psychological Impact of the Child's Difficulties. J Intellect Disabil Res. 2003 May;47(4–5):385–99.

46. Emerson E, McCulloch A, Graham H, Blacher J, Llwellyn GM, Hatton C. Socioeconomic Circumstances and Risk of Psychiatric Disorders Among Parents of Children with Early Cognitive Delay. Am J Intellect Dev Disabil. 2010 Jan;115(1):30–42.

47. Baker K, Devine RT, Ng-Cordell E, Raymond FL, Hughes C. Childhood Intellectual Disability and Parents' Mental Health: Integrating Social, Psychological and Genetic Influences. Br J Psychiatry. 2021 Jun 1;218(6):315–22.

48. Winters KC, Tanner-Smith EE, Bresani E, Meyers K. Current Advances in the Treatment of Adolescent Drug Use. Adolesc Health Med Ther. 2014 Nov 20;5:199–210.

49. Bukstein OG, Brent OA, Perper JA, et al. Risk Factors for Completed Suicide Among Adolescents with a Lifetime History of Substance Abuse: A Case-Control Study. Acta Psychiatr Scand. 1993;88(6):403–08.

50. O'Neil KA, Conner BT, Kendall PC. Internalizing Disorders and Substance Use Disorders in Youth: Comorbidity, Risk, Temporal Order, and Implications for Intervention. Clin Psychol Rev. 2011 Feb 1;31(1):104–12.

51. Wilens TE, Martelon M, Joshi G, et al. Does ADHD Predict Substance-Use Disorders? A 10-Year Follow-Up Study of Young Adults with ADHD. J Am Acad Child Adolesc Psychiatry. 2011 Jun;50(6):543–53.

52. Arseneault L, Cannon M, Witton J, Murray RM. Causal Association Between Cannabis and Psychosis: Examination of the Evidence. Br J Psychiatry. 2004 Feb;184:110–17.

53. Large M, Sharma S, Compton MT, Slade T, Nielssen O. Cannabis Use and Earlier Onset of Psychosis: A Systematic Meta-analysis. Arch Gen Psychiatry. 2011 Jun;68(6):555–61.

54. Clark LA, Watson D. Tripartite Model of Anxiety and Depression: Psychometric Evidence and Taxonomic Implications. J Abnorm Psychol. 1991;100(3):316–36.

55. Wills TA, Windle M, Cleary SD. Temperament and Novelty Seeking in Adolescent Substance Use: Convergence of Dimensions of Temperament with Constructs from Cloninger's Theory. J Pers Soc Psychol. 1998;74(2):387–406.

56. Rettew DC, McKee L. Temperament and Its Role in Developmental Psychopathology. Harv Rev Psychiatry. 2005 Jan;13(1):14–27.

57. Bulik CM, Sullivan PF, Weltzin TE, Kaye WH. Temperament in Eating Disorders. Int J Eat Disord. 1995;17(3):251–61.

58. Vitousek K, Manke F. Personality Variables and Disorders in Anorexia Nervosa and Bulimia Nervosa. J Abnorm Psychol. 1994;103(1):137–47.

59. Bowlby, J. (1969). Attachment and Loss. Vol. 1: Attachment. Attachment and Loss. New York: Basic Books

60. Ainsworth MDS, Blehar MC, Waters E, Wall SN. *Patterns of Attachment: A Psychological Study of the Strange Situation*. 1st ed. New York: Psychology Press, 1979.

61. Main, M., Solomon, J. Procedures for Identifying Infants as Disorganized/Disoriented During the Ainsworth Strange

Situation. In MT Greenberg, D Cicchetti, EM Cummings (ed.), *Attachment in the Preschool Years: Theory, Research, and Intervention*. The University of Chicago Press, 1990, 121–60.

62. Madigan S, Brumariu LE, Villani V, Atkinson L, Lyons-Ruth K. Representational and Questionnaire Measures of Attachment: A Meta-analysis of Relations to Child Internalizing and Externalizing Problems. Psychol Bull. 2016 Apr 1;**142**(4):367–99.

63. Weissman MM, Feder A, Pilowsky DJ, et al. Depressed Mothers Coming to Primary Care: Maternal Reports of Problems with Their Children. J Affect Disord. 2004;**78**(2):93–100.

64. Tully EC, Iacono WG, McGue M. An Adoption Study of Parental Depression As an Environmental Liability for Adolescent Depression and Childhood Disruptive Disorders. Am J Psychiatry. 2008 Sep;**165**(9):1148–54.

65. Brophy S, Todd C, Rahman MA, Kennedy N, Rice F. Timing of Parental Depression on Risk of Child Depression and Poor Educational Outcomes: A Population Based Routine Data Cohort Study from Born in Wales, UK. PLoS One. 2021 Nov 1;**16**(11):e0258966.

66. Ramchandani P, Stein A, Evans J, O'Connor TG. Paternal Depression in the Postnatal Period and Child Development: A Prospective Population Study. Lancet. 2005 Jun 25;**365**(9478):2201–05.

67. Harold GT, Sellers R. Annual Research Review: Interparental Conflict and Youth Psychopathology: An Evidence Review and Practice Focused Update. J Child Psychol Psychiatry Allied Discip. 2018 Apr 1;**59**(4):374–402.

68. Buist KL, Deković M, Prinzie P. Sibling Relationship Quality and Psychopathology of Children and Adolescents: A Meta-analysis. Clin Psychol Rev. 2013 Feb 1;**33**(1):97–106.

69. Kidger J, Araya R, Donovan J, Gunnell D. The Effect of the School Environment on the Emotional Health of Adolescents: A Systematic Review. Pediatrics. 2012 May;**129**(5):925–49.

70. Arseneault L, Bowes L, Shakoor S. Bullying Victimization in Youths and Mental Health Problems: 'Much Ado About Nothing'? Psychol Med. 2010 May;**40**(5):717–29.

71. Eccles JS, Roeser RW. Schools As Developmental Contexts During Adolescence. J Res Adolesc. 2011 Mar;**21**(1):225–41.

72. Moak ZB, Agrawal A. The Association Between Perceived Interpersonal Social Support and Physical and Mental Health: Results from the National Epidemiological Survey on Alcohol and Related Conditions. J Public Health (Oxf). 2010 Jun;**32**(2):191–201.

73. Jewett R, Sabiston CM, Brunet J, O'Loughlin EK, Scarapicchia T, O'Loughlin J. School Sport Participation During Adolescence and Mental Health in Early Adulthood. J Adolesc Health. 2014 Nov 1;**55**(5):640–44.

74. Oberle E, Ji XR, Guhn M, Schonert-Reichl KA, Gadermann AM. Benefits of Extracurricular Participation in Early Adolescence: Associations with Peer Belonging and Mental Health. J Youth Adolesc. 2019 Nov 1;**48**(11):2255–70.

75. Webster D, Dunne L, Hunter R. Association Between Social Networks and Subjective Well-Being in Adolescents: A Systematic Review. Youth & Society. 2020 May 14;**53**(2):175–210. https://doi.org/10.1177/0044118X20919589.

76. Wilksch SM, O'Shea A, Ho P, Byrne S, Wade TD. The Relationship Between Social Media Use and Disordered Eating in Young Adolescents. Int J Eat Disord. 2020 Jan 1;**53**(1):96–106.

77. Dyson MP, Hartling L, Shulhan J, et al. A Systematic Review of Social Media Use to Discuss and View Deliberate Self-Harm Acts. PLoS One. 2016 May 18;**11**(5): e0155813.

78. Marchant A, Hawton K, Stewart A, et al. A Systematic Review of the Relationship Between Internet Use, Self-Harm and Suicidal Behaviour in Young People: The

79. Best P, Manktelow R, Taylor B. Online Communication, Social Media and Adolescent Wellbeing: A Systematic Narrative Review. Child Youth Serv Rev. 2014;41:27–36.

80. Robinson P, Turk D, Jilka S, Cella M. Measuring Attitudes Towards Mental Health Using Social Media: Investigating Stigma and Trivialisation. Soc Psychiatry Psychiatr Epidemiol. 2019 Jan 28;54(1):51.

81. Teicher MH, Andersen SL, Polcari A, Anderson CM, Navalta CP. Developmental Neurobiology of Childhood Stress and Trauma. Psychiatr Clin North Am. 2002;25(2):397–426.

82. Teicher MH, Samson JA, Anderson CM, Ohashi K. The Effects of Childhood Maltreatment on Brain Structure, Function and Connectivity. Nat Rev Neurosci. 2016 Sep 19;17(10):652–66.

83. Hughes K, Ford K, Bellis MA, Glendinning F, Harrison E, Passmore J. Health and Financial Costs of Adverse Childhood Experiences in 28 European Countries: A Systematic Review and Meta-analysis. Lancet Public Heal. 2021 Nov 1;6(11):e848–57.

84. UNHCR. UNHCR Global Report [Internet]. UNHCR, 2018. Available from: https://www.unhcr.org/publications/fundraising/5e4ff98f7/unhcr-global-report-2018.html (cited 26 January 2022).

85. Blackmore R, Gray KM, Boyle JA, et al. Systematic Review and Meta-analysis: The Prevalence of Mental Illness in Child and Adolescent Refugees and Asylum Seekers. J Am Acad Child Adolesc Psychiatry. 2020 Jun 1;59(6):705–14.

86. Corona Maioli S, Bhabha J, Wickramage K, et al. International Migration of Unaccompanied Minors: Trends, Health Risks, and Legal Protection. Lancet Child Adolesc Heal. 2021 Dec 1;5(12):882–95.

87. Morrison Gutman L, Joshi H, Parsonage M, Schoon I. *Children of the New Century: Mental Health Findings from the Millennium Cohort Study.* Centre for Mental Health, 2015 Nov. Available from: https://www.centreformentalhealth.org.uk/publications/children-new-century/.

88. Bignall T, Jeraj S, Helsby E, Butt J. *Racial Disparities in Mental Health: Literature and Evidence Review.* Race Equality Commission, 2019. Available from: https://raceequalityfoundation.org.uk/wp-content/uploads/2022/10/mental-health-report-v5-2.pdf (accessed 4 April 2025).

89. Memon A, Taylor K, Mohebati LM, et al. Perceived Barriers to Accessing Mental Health Services Among Black and Minority Ethnic (BME) Communities: A Qualitative Study in Southeast England. BMJ Open. 2016 Nov 1;6(11). doi.org/10.1136/bmjopen-2016-012337.

90. Viner R, Russell S, Saulle R, et al. School Closures During Social Lockdown and Mental Health, Health Behaviors, and Well-being Among Children and Adolescents During the First COVID-19 Wave: A Systematic Review. JAMA Pediatr. 2022 Apr 1;176(4):400–409.

91. Bowyer-Crane C, Bonetti S, Compton S, Nielsen D, D'apice K, Tracey L. The Impact of Covid-19 on School Starters: Interim Briefing 1: Parent and School Concerns About Children Starting School. Education Endowment Fund UK, 2021. Available from: https://files.eric.ed.gov/fulltext/ED620337.pdf.

92. Solmi F, Downs JL, Nicholls DE. COVID-19 and Eating Disorders in Young People. Lancet Child Adolesc Heal. 2021 May 1;5(5):316–18.

93. Adegboye D, Williams F, Collishaw S, et al. Understanding Why the COVID-19 Pandemic-Related Lockdown Increases Mental Health Difficulties in Vulnerable Young Children. JCPP Adv. 2021 Apr 1;1(1). https://doi.org/10.1111/jcv2.12005.

Chapter 4

Infant Mental Health

Zoë Davidson and Anne McFadyen

The Importance of Infant Mental Health

The mental health of babies and young children has been a neglected area of health care and is only now beginning to receive the wider recognition and funding that it deserves. This focus has been primarily on infancy, the period from birth to the age of 3 years, but mental health problems presenting in the preschool period have also received attention from clinicians and researchers. The Royal College of Psychiatrists has published a report, which makes the case for action with respect to the early years [1]. It highlights the need for timely evidence-based mental health care for infants experiencing serious mental health problems as well as emphasising the importance of good early years mental health for the prevention of mental health conditions across the lifespan. Significantly, the report brings into sharp focus the relevance of the early years to psychiatrists of all specialties whose patients may be parents or carers of babies and young children.

The needs and developmental tasks of babies and toddlers are distinct from those of 3- to 5-year-olds, and this has led to most definitions of 'infant' referring to the period up to the third birthday only. Some diagnostic classification systems, most notably the Diagnostic Classification of Mental Health and Developmental Disorders of Infancy and Early Childhood, DC:0-5v0.2 [2], consider this age group in its entirety.

Infant Mental Health (IMH) is the developing capacity of the child 'to experience, regulate and express emotions, form close and secure relationships, and explore the environment and learn' [3]. It concerns both 'being and becoming mentally healthy' [4].

Good IMH is nurtured when babies receive warm, predictable care, and experience positive, consistent, safe and attuned relationships with their primary caregivers. These relationships begin at conception as does the development of the baby's brain and mind. This development is influenced by both genetics and the environment.

When an attuned, safe caregiving environment is not present, babies' functioning and development is significantly affected, and they are more likely to experience mental distress and disorder.

Mental health problems in infancy are common. The prevalence is thought to be similar to that of older children, with estimates ranging from 10% to 22% [5,6,7].

Good mental health in infancy is crucial for later mental and physical health. It underpins the development of a sense of self, empathy, self-regulation, the capacity to make and sustain relationships, resilience and ultimately the likelihood of achieving your potential and having a sense of purpose and satisfaction with life.

A Healthy and Safe Start

Galloway et al [8] describe the 'key ingredients' needed 'for babies to have a healthy and safe start in life'.

A Healthy Pregnancy

Mothers' mental and physical health in pregnancy is crucially important for babies' later well-being and development. Adequate nutrition and the absence of toxins plays an important role in ensuring the healthy development of a foetus, as does the psychological well-being of their mother. Poor maternal health during pregnancy is associated with low birth weight and premature birth, postnatal depression and longer term cognitive and emotional difficulties for the child.

Alcohol use in pregnancy is associated with Fetal Alcohol Spectrum Disorder [9], while substance use impacts on development in a number of ways, and in the case of opiates may lead to Neonatal Abstinence Syndrome.

Healthy Early Relationships

Babies need their caregivers to provide sensitive, attuned and consistent care. They thrive when their caregivers have healthy relationships with one another too. An infant's brain develops through interaction with others and is particularly influenced by their relationship with their primary caregivers.

Infants need attuned caregivers, noticing and being responsive to their cues and recognising the underlying communication in their behaviour. The to-and-fro of interaction, where a caregiver notices and responds to the baby's initiations is known as 'serve and return'. Sometimes the 'ball' will be dropped and communication missed or misinterpreted, and there will be an interruption or disconnect. This is known as a 'rupture' in the relationship. It is impossible for caregivers to be attuned all the time and ruptures are a normal event. What matters most is how this rupture is repaired and how the dyad gets back on track together. 'Rupture' and 'repair' is therefore an important experience in the development of internal working models for relationships in the future.

Infants rely on caregivers to 'Be With' them through their range of feelings, showing that they've understood, are not overwhelmed and can help. Early experiences of validation and co-regulation support the capacity for self-regulation skills needed throughout the lifespan.

There are many reasons why these early relationships can be challenging, and the development of a secure relationship can be derailed. These include domestic abuse, poor mental health, life stressors, caregivers' own history of attachment relationships and childhood abuse and neglect.

Temperament, and differences in the baby's development, which may also be related to prematurity, congenital disorders, or maternal alcohol and substance use can also affect the attachment relationship.

The association between maternal mental health problems and infant development has been well made. The prevalence of depression at any time in the perinatal period is estimated to be 10–15%, while postpartum psychosis, a severe illness of rapid onset, can affect 1:500 women after birth [10]. Perinatal mental health problems can have lasting effects on the emotional, behavioural, intellectual and social development of children [10,11]. Children of mothers with mental health problems are twice as likely to develop psychiatric disorders, with poor maternal mental health/well-being at 9 months, and 3 years of age strongly associated with challenging child behaviour at age 5. Postnatal depression and other mental illness have been linked to behavioural disturbance at home, less creative play and greater levels of disturbed or disruptive behaviour at primary school, poor peer relationships, and a decrease in self-control with an increase in aggression [12]. Looking beyond what you see, and recognising behaviour as a communication of something, rather than a problem located within the child, is of course central in understanding what might be happening for these children.

While much of the research in IMH has been with mothers, Stein et al [13] have described the growing evidence that fathers' mental health is also significantly associated with child developmental outcomes.

The impact of parental functioning on an infant's development is mediated through the quality of parent–infant interaction. Generally, those working in IMH believe that parents are doing the best they can but for many, attuned parenting is difficult. A depressed parent may not tune into their baby's emotional state while someone experiencing acute psychosis may be incongruent or unpredictable in their responses. Traumatised parents may withdraw from their infants while anxious or obsessive parents can be over-organised and intrusive. Harm to the infant's mental health and development is not inevitable, however. Schore [14] notes:

> The concept of 'early experiences' connotes much more than an immature individual being a passive recipient of environmental stimulation. Rather, these events represent active transactions between the infant and the early environment.

The resilience of some babies in these situations is not yet fully understood and is multifactorial.

A Safe and Stimulating Environment

Babies need a safe and stimulating environment providing appropriate sensory, social and emotional stimulation, with the space and scaffolding to play, explore, learn and be creative.

Play is essential for brain development, and it is also an important mode of communication, in that infants and young children can show, rather than tell others about their thoughts, feelings and experiences.

Effective Care and Support for Caregivers

Parents and other primary caregivers need respectful care and timely support in addressing the problems they face, so that they have the practical and emotional resources to care for their baby. This is especially the case for parents who have mental health or substance use problems, or past experiences of poor care themselves, and for those who are facing stressors such as discrimination, poverty, housing insecurity and domestic abuse.

Integrating Models of Understanding

The burgeoning of research into child development and early relationships necessitates the development of a model of understanding that embraces many different viewpoints. Like young children who are often at the centre of a complex system of relationships, especially if deemed to be vulnerable or at risk, so too must our understanding reflect a synthesis of the complex relationships between different theoretical models.

Genetics and Epigenetics

The influence of genes on development is seen most starkly in disorders that have well-evidenced genetic transmission. Some chromosomal mutations, which affect the expression of genes, are also well recognised as having a major impact on development. Autism and ADHD, however, are neurotypes that have a strong genetic component, but are not associated with one specific gene.

Genes play an important part in all aspects of who we are from physical appearance through to temperament, but the physical, emotional and social or relational environment, has the power to affect how and when genes are expressed, known as epigenetics. This refers to:

> The capacity to change gene expression in response to environmental pressures by adding a chemical signature above the gene that determines whether or not it is expressed [11].

This is very relevant to in utero and early experiences, which influence children's developing brains and minds. Importantly these influences are potentially malleable and later experience and interventions have the potential to alter outcome. Epigenetic research may also further the understanding of resilience in infants born in adverse circumstances.

Brain Development

Berens and Nelson [15] have summarised the many research studies that have contributed to our understanding of functional brain development. This happens largely sequentially from the brainstem regulatory systems essential for life, through to emotion and memory in the limbic system right up to the development of cortical functions like empathy, decision-making, logic and reasoning. From conception onwards, experience affects the structure and function of the brain. Early relationships affect brain circuitry as neuronal pathways are laid down in response to interactions with the world.

> In the first few years of life, more than 1 million new neural connections form every second [16].

Over time the neural pathways used most are made stronger and faster with myelin formation and those not used are 'pruned back' as the brain responds and adapts to its environment.

According to Leach [17] optimal brain development in the first 1001 days (from conception to the second birthday) 'not only gives a new child the best possible start in life but also enables him or her to make the most of the lifetime which is to follow'. This is the time when the brain is growing most rapidly and is also most plastic.

> It is easier to influence the configuration of a baby's developing brain than it is to rewire parts of its circuitry in later years [9].

Optimal conditions for brain growth are achieved when a baby receives safe, attuned care with someone who can buffer the impact of stress and adversity. Some stress is normal and tolerable but high levels produce elevated levels of stress hormones such as cortisol, which can have a 'toxic' impact on brain and body [16].

Adverse Childhood Experiences

The term ACEs was used originally by Felitti et al [18] when describing the association between traumatic events in childhood and later physical and mental health. ACEs include physical and emotional abuse and neglect, and significant life events such as family breakdown or the loss of a parent. These experiences can alter brain circuitry and biochemistry and affect the immune system. We also know that children who experience poverty and other structural inequalities are more likely to experience adversities[19,20]. Marryat and Frank [21] found that 11% of children in the most deprived socio-economic group had experienced four or more adverse experiences by the age of 8 years compared to 3% overall.

The relationship between health and poverty is bidirectional. Poverty is one of the main determinants of poor physical and mental health, and its association with adversity in childhood and later outcomes is complex. Inequalities and associated discrimination and stigma, significantly affect health outcomes. Reducing inequality and adversity is therefore one of the most impactful health interventions possible.

Ethology, Psychoanalysis and Attachment Theory

Ethologists like Mead [22] studied childhood in natural situations in different cultures, but it is fair to say that in contemporary writing about child development and parenting, not enough attention has been paid to the influence of culture, race and ethnicity.

Through their exploration of the early lives of their adult and child patients in psychoanalysis, Anna Freud and Melanie Klein among others developed theories about early influences on personality development. Winnicott, who was both a psychoanalyst and paediatrician, articulated these ideas in a very accessible way.

Unlike Freud and Klein, Winnicott did not think of infants and their mothers as separate. But he did not disregard their notions of drives, which included the drive for life and integration as well as that for death and disintegration. He placed great significance on the idea that the infant and its (maternal) care comprised a single unit: 'There is no such thing as an infant' [23].

Babies need their carers to support them to develop their own identity and allow them to develop autonomy. This is seen nowhere more obviously than Winnicott's notion of the good-enough mother who can mend her failures. In order to learn to self-regulate and manage their emotions, babies do not need 'perfect' parenting. If their needs were to be met before they even sensed them or experienced the distress and frustration of not getting immediate relief, then development would halt.

Attachment theory, first proposed by Bowlby [24] and developed by Ainsworth [25] and others, not only integrated and expanded but also diverged from some key ideas from ethology and psychoanalysis. Attachment 'refers to the close bond a child has to his/her parents or carers, which serves the purpose of helping a child feel safe, and comforted when worried or anxious' [26]. Young children explore the world from a secure base and safe haven (attachment figure), and development moves forward under the influence of both a desire to be close, and a need to find out about and be stimulated by the world. Attachment is a relationship specific emotional bond, driven by the need for regulation and safety. Infants and adults alike have attachment relationships and associated emotions and behaviours that will look different across the lifespan.

Attachment behaviours can be observed at times of stress. Typical attachment behaviours for instance might include cueing needs through crying or seeking proximity. Ainsworth [25] categorised attachment behaviour patterns into secure and insecure. Insecure attachment is common (40%) and can be seen as an adaptive survival process to the type of caregiving experience. For instance, a baby whose caregiver can't cope with their crying, may develop an insecure avoidant attachment style to avoid feelings of rejection. While this may have been adaptive to their environment at that time, problems can arise when these same avoidant patterns occur in what would be safer, more responsive environments. Attachment categories are not mental disorders but a description of the relationship.

An important concept that forms part of attachment theory relates to the idea that 'each partner builds in his or her mind, working models of self and of other and of the patterns of interaction that have developed between them' [27]. This is an important link between early experience and later adaptive functioning. These models exist in a reflexive relationship with experience.

Fraiberg, a social worker and psychoanalyst, coined the phrase Infant Mental Health. Her work to integrate psychoanalysis and developmental psychology through a lens of understanding intergenerational trauma was ground-breaking and is at the heart of IMH work today. Fraiberg understood that infants exist within relationships and transactional interactions. She brought into consciousness the concept of 'Ghosts in the Nursery' [28] as well as noticing what an infant brought to the relationship and helping parents gain insight into their own and their babies' mental states.

> In every nursery there are ghosts. They are the visitors from the unremembered past of the parents, the uninvited guests at the christening. Under all favorable circumstances the unfriendly and unbidden spirits are banished from the nursery and return to their subterranean dwelling place. The baby makes his own imperative claim upon parental love and, in strict analogy with the fairy tales, the bonds of love protect the child and his parents against the intruders, the malevolent ghosts [28].

Ghosts represent the repetition of the past in the present and thus she conceptualised the unconscious re-enactment of past relational experiences disturbing the infant–parent relationship in the present.

Lieberman et al [29] introduced the idea of 'Angels in the Nursery' that she described as a positive, rich and powerful benevolent care-receiving experience from childhood, which can emerge in the current dyad, co-existing with ghosts 'in dynamic tension with each other'.

It is important to hold in mind that attachment theory was largely developed, in observing neurotypical children. Attachment behaviour in neurodivergent children may be more subtle and nuanced.

Behaviourism and Cognitive Theory

Historically, learning theory informed the understanding of human behaviour, but as Black [30] observed 'most theories tend(ed) to oversimplify'. The proposal that all human and animal behaviour is learned by conditioning has been replaced by a more complex set of ideas informed by our understanding of the infant's developing mind and relationships. The main applications of learning theory currently relate to behavioural approaches to specific anxieties or phobias, and to some parenting programmes. Cognitive theory successfully informs the management of some mental disorders in older children and adults. Therapy that links feelings and actions and challenges negative cognitions has its origin in social learning theory [31].

The Case for Infant Mental Health Services

Indisputably there are far-reaching benefits of good mental health for individual infants and their families, but it also makes sound economic sense to invest in the early years. Heckman's research on the 'economics of human flourishing' makes a convincing case for investment from conception. He argues not only that money will be saved, but that there will be return on that investment, with the earlier the investment, the bigger the return [32].

> For every $1 spent on early child development interventions, the return on investment can be as high as $13 [33].

This is supported by Segal et al [34] who said that 'the consequences of not investing in the mental health needs of children at the earliest stages of life means denying thousands of children the opportunity to reach their life potential as well as accumulating huge financial costs'. The benefits of giving babies a good start in life are seen at a societal and personal level, with potential alleviation of distress and disorder in the early years and later, and prevention of the transmission of difficulties from one generation to the next.

As stated, in the section Healthy Early Relationships, the prevalence of IMH problems is high. Infants can show joy and sadness within the first 6 months of life and so 'depressive affects also may be possible at this stage of development' [35]. Symptoms such as being subdued, withdrawn, shutdown, anxious, irritable and lacking interest can be seen in babies just as they can in older children. Infants can show many features of mental distress in their behaviour as well as physiological signs, that let you know that they are not okay.

Infants can develop safety strategies such as dissociation, avoidance and miscuing to cope with the overwhelm of early trauma and allow the mind to escape. Dissociation observed in traumatised infants presents in ways such as avoidance of eye contact, freezing or zoning out, appearing not to listen or regression. Continued trauma within the context of primary relationships floods the brain and body with fear, with no opportunity for the normative, enriching experiences necessary for all aspects of development. Resulting hypersensitive threat systems can be triggered in ways that can feel difficult or confusing for caregivers, especially when the immediate threat has been removed. This can lead to misattributions of a child's behaviour and communication. This is especially true for children in care following maltreatment. Relational and developmental trauma impacts a child's sense of self and their internal working models of relationships, long into the future. A safe and secure relationship has the power to support trauma recovery and protect the infant and their developing brain [36].

Infant Mental Health Services

There is no denying that infants experience mental health problems that can be detected early and treated with cost effective evidence-based interventions. Service provision has not grown to match this need however, although endeavours have been made across the UK in recent years to raise awareness and develop specialist IMH or infant–parent relationship teams.

Services must be designed to be infant centred. A holistic approach needs a multidisciplinary team with a shared frame of reference and vision, and a diverse range of professional perspectives. Many eyes are needed to really see babies as individuals and within key relationships and families, interacting with their wider world.

The origins of the word infant come from the Latin 'unable to speak' and so it is the responsibility of adults to notice, understand and respond to babies' communication:

> This patient, who cannot talk, has awaited articulate spokesmen [28].

The Voice of the Infant Best Practice Guidelines and Infant Pledge [37] provide invaluable advice on how to create the right *Space* to facilitate the infant's *Voice*, and ensure that their views are acted upon (*Audience* and *Influence*). Its theoretical background and development are described by McFadyen et al [38].

Specialist IMH teams will vary in composition but might include psychiatrists, psychotherapists, psychologists, social workers, early-years workers, creative therapists, health visitors, occupational therapists and speech and language therapists. They are part of a wider system of statutory (NHS, Education and Social Services) and third sector services addressing the mental health needs of young children and their families. As well as providing direct services to babies and their families, the specialist teams, 'as experts and champions', should raise awareness as well as offer 'training, consultation and/or supervision to other providers and advice to systems leaders and commissioners' [39].

Universal health services for babies are delivered by midwives, health visitors, family nurses and GPs. In Scotland health visitors have a statutory obligation to coordinate services around the child. Social workers also provide direct services to infants at risk of, or experiencing abuse or significant harm, and may identify these babies before they are born. Early years and education services also have a direct role in caring for and supporting the healthy development of children under 5 years. Many third sector services support families and may also offer specific interventions. Any one of these providers should be able to raise concerns and ask for more specialist assessment and treatment.

> Ideally services should operate a 'stepped care model' which matches families' needs with the least intensive intervention that has the best chance of achieving positive outcomes [39].

Health Boards and Trusts should have clear pathways that support referrals to the most appropriate service. Figure 4.1 is an example of such a pathway as described by the Perinatal Mental Health Network Scotland [40].

Scotland's Mental Health and Wellbeing Strategy has highlighted the relevance of mental health at every stage of development by adopting a life stage model 'delivering mental health care from preconception and the earliest years [with] opportunities to influence intergenerational health and wellbeing' [41]. One of the priorities of this strategy is to 'reduce the risk of poor mental health and well-being in adult life by promoting the importance of good relationships and trauma-informed approaches from the earliest years of life, taking account where relevant of adverse childhood experiences'. Understanding patients' early experience is important in all specialties in psychiatry, and the Royal College supports the inclusion of IMH in the training of all psychiatrists.

The Role of Infant Mental Health Psychiatrists

Psychiatry is in the unique position of holding a bio-psychosocial framework to assessment, formulation and intervention, drawing on knowledge in medicine, neuroscience, normative child development and psychological theories. A psychiatrist has skills in infant observation and the capacity to notice what is 'hidden in plain sight', for instance working to understand the complex and at times confusing strategies very young children can develop to survive early adversity and trauma. Infant psychiatrists can construct a meaningful formulation and

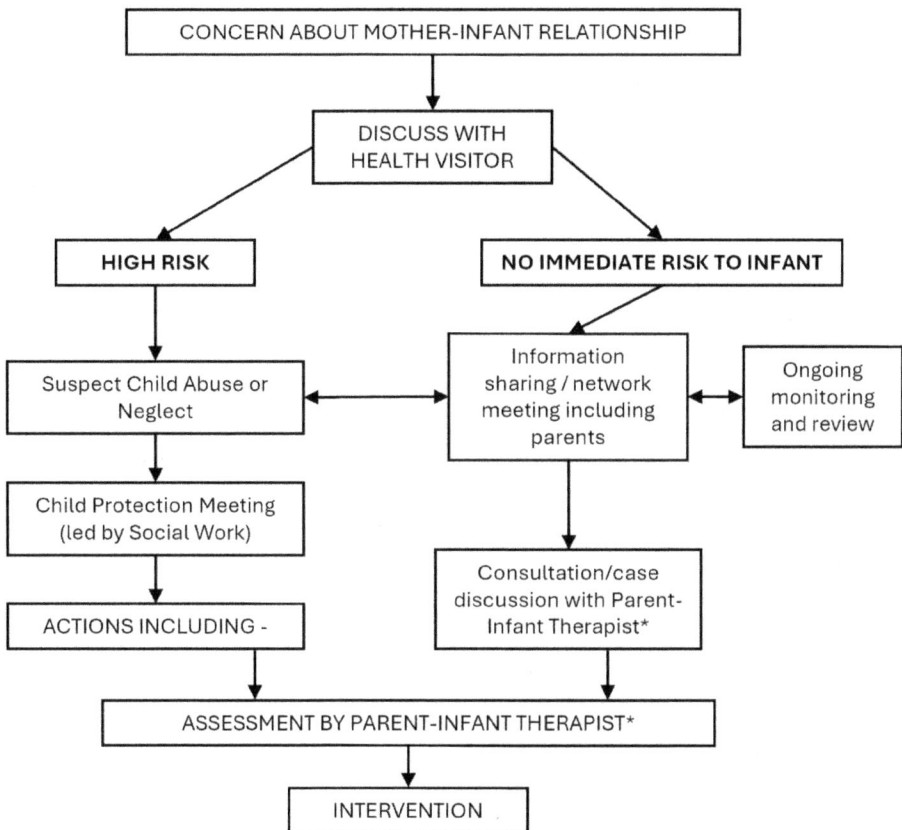

*The Parent-Infant Therapist may be a member of the perinatal mental health team or a parent-infant specialist service and may be from a range of progressions (e.g., psychiatrist, psychotherapist, psychologist, VIG practitioner).

Figure 4.1 Scottish Perinatal Mental Health Care Pathway. Published by Perinatal Mental Health Network Scotland, NHS National Services Scotland (2021).
Republished with permission

provide a range of psychological interventions and treatments. They are able to see the infant through a psychodynamic and attachment lens embedded in the experience of systems theory, cognitive/behavioural models and trauma-informed practice. Psychiatrists bring additional knowledge and expertise about neurodevelopment, general medicine and parental mental illness, as well as an understanding of intergenerational transmission and the impact of inequality.

Psychiatrists have an important role in infant advocacy and IMH awareness raising and training, as well as professional and multiagency liaison and consultation, strategic service development and clinical quality and governance. A psychiatrist also brings experience in containment and reflective practice having the capacity and relevant experience to see things from many different perspectives.

Assessment in Infant Mental Health

The Observation of Infants and Its Applications

The observation of infants and their relationships is central to a number of endeavours. These include child development and attachment research, where interactions may be coded and also supplemented by other measures such as measurement of cortisol levels or even brain scanning. The microanalysis of mother–infant interactions in the laboratory situation as described, for example by Brazelton et al [42], sought to identify the characteristics of the developing relationship. A longitudinal perspective is often included, permitting the testing of hypotheses about the link between data collected about early experience with later cognitive functioning, affect, behaviour and relationships. This kind of research exists in a recursive relationship with the development of theory, including psychoanalytic theories of personality development.

In clinical work, culturally informed observation and curiosity as to emotional, behavioural, physiological and social cues is essential when getting to know infants and their families.

Beebe [43] noted however that the therapist's attention is often exclusively on the adults in the room:

> Even in current approaches to mother-infant treatment, the infant is in danger of being the 'forgotten patient'.

Learning to notice the baby in the room and look 'in the right way' [44] is central to therapeutic work that seeks to address concerns about the infant or the relationships around them. There is a value in recording observations 'in everyday, non-theoretical language' [43] before applying a more theoretically informed lens. Observation is not just seeing; it includes awareness of other senses and importantly one's own emotions, which Miller [46] advises not to regard as 'a distraction or contaminant'.

Assessment Tools and Measures

There are many tools that supplement therapeutic and holistic infant assessment and can inform evaluation and measure change:

- The Brazelton Neonatal Behavioural Assessment Scale (NBAS) [47] (*see Intervention*).
- The Ages and Stages Questionnaire [48] is a developmental screener highlighting potential delays in development.
- Crowell Play Procedure [49] observes the child and caregiver engaging in play and completing tasks, as well as experiencing a separation and reunion designed to activate the child's attachment system in real-time. The use of video in assessment can help to slow down the clinicians' observation to see the subtleties of communication and interaction.
- Working Model of the Child Interview [49] explores caregivers' perceptions and internal representations of the child through a structured interview.
- Mothers Object Relations Scales [50] is a self-report questionnaire used to measure representations of their infant.
- Child Behaviour Checklist [51] is a caregiver rating to identify behavioural and emotional problems.

- Lanarkshire IMH Observational Indicator Set [52] is an observational tool designed to provide a lens through which to observe the mental health of infants. Indicators are organised into five areas of infant functioning/development: Relationship with Main Carer; Emotional; Cognitive; Sense of Self; and Social Interaction.

As with all assessments in infant, child and adolescent psychiatry a thorough developmental history is important too.

Mental Health Problems in Infancy: Diagnosis and Formulation

Diagnosis in Infancy Encourages Debate

The limitations of widely used ICD and DSM diagnostic categorisation prompted the formation of the DC:0–5 [2]. This attempted to use a dimensional approach to diagnosis within a developmental and relational context.

Zero to Three have produced a 'Crosswalk' [54] of diagnostic categories, comparing the DC:0–5, DSM-5 and ICD-10. This summary divides diagnostic categories into Neurodevelopmental Disorders, Sensory Processing Disorders, Anxiety Disorders, Mood Disorders, Obsessive Compulsive and Related Disorders, Sleep, Eating and Crying Disorders, Trauma, Stress and Deprivation Disorders and Relationship Disorder.

Infant psychiatric diagnosis is not common in the UK, with IMH services focussing on 'what has happened?' rather than categorising 'what is wrong with the child?'. There is a general consensus however that any diagnosis in infancy or later has to be considered meaningful and helpful before it is given, and for some families this will be the case. Additionally, diagnosis may have a place in professional communication giving a shared reference point as well as being important in research and the development of evidence-based interventions.

Features of neurodivergence can be observed in infancy and many in the field of neurodevelopment are moving away from the deficit led diagnostic models of disorder, to think about neurodiversity and different neurotypes, understanding the uniqueness and strengths of each child.

Overall, there is most value in collaborative formulation and communicating a picture of an infant's strengths and challenges, using a bio-psychosocial framework, identifying protective factors and acknowledging a shared hope between clinicians and families, for things to be better. Formulation can take many different forms but aims to meaningfully make sense of the infant as an individual existing within a dyad, within a family, within a social network and within wider society.

Infant Mental Health Intervention

Formulation informs intervention and there is a growing evidence base for effective mental health intervention in infancy. While there are differences of approach across countries and professionals taking into account cultural context, relationships remain the cornerstone to any IMH intervention. Multidisciplinary input is the rule and IMH services work closely and in collaboration with a wide range of professionals, including health, social work, education and early years, welfare and criminal justice systems and voluntary sector support services. Broadly IMH intervention includes working with the infant as an individual, strengthening the dyad/triad and family system, supporting caregivers and working with the wider professional network around a child.

Examples of common interventions in IMH service are summarised as follows:

Narrative

All infants have a right to a developmentally informed explanation of what has happened and what is happening in their lives. The concept of having a coherent narrative is important for all ages. The misperception that young children will not remember, understand or pick up on what is happening around them is harmful and we know that memory formation begins before an infant has words. Developmentally appropriate narrative therefore speaks honestly to the child's experience and prevents children from filling in the gaps in memory or explanation, often resulting in feelings of shame, guilt and self-blame.

As a specific intervention, narrative books detailing the child's journey, or life story work, is especially pertinent for care-experienced infants and young children who are often given very little information as to why they are not in their birth parents' care.

The Neonatal Behavioural Assessment Scale (NBAS)

This is a comprehensive neurobehavioral assessment available for newborn babies, which gives a strength-based, in-depth profile of an individual baby [47]. The NBAS can be used with babies from birth to 2 months, premature babies from 35 weeks gestation and developmentally delayed babies. The NBAS shows the newborn's responses to their new extra-uterine environment, contribution to the parent–infant relationship and individuality.

The NBAS's therapeutic value lies in supporting parents' observation or 'noticing' skills, and the development of an appreciation of their infant's strengths and communications.

The Newborn Behavioural Observation

This is a relationship-building tool for practitioners to share with babies under 4 months and their caregivers [55]. It is designed to support caregivers to read and understand their newborn's unique communication.

Infant–Parent Psychotherapy

In Infant–Parent Psychotherapy and Parent–Infant Psychotherapy the intervention builds on the methodology at the heart of psychoanalytic infant observation.

The differences between Infant–Parent Psychotherapy and Parent–Infant Psychotherapy are not obvious, with the preferred term appearing to be influenced by the author's position. According to Hopkins [56], 'infant-parent psychotherapy is focused, and the focus is on the development of the infant who is always in the sessions'. It is an intervention that effectively combines the use of observation and narrative, exploring as it does, the ways in which the parent's past affects the way in which they relate to the baby in the present. This approach was first described in depth by Fraiberg as described earlier.

Acquarone [57], reflecting on Parent–Infant Psychotherapy in the context of disability, considers:

> In parent–infant psychotherapy and early intervention, the baby, the parents and the therapist each have a role to play in re-wiring, re-discovering and re-developing their relationship.

Child–Parent Psychotherapy (CPP)

CPP was developed by Lieberman et al [58] and has its roots in the work of Fraiberg, drawing together psychoanalytic thinking, attachment theory and developmental psychology. CPP uses a number of intervention modalities but at its core it is a relationship-based treatment for infants and young children who have experience of trauma. The goal of CPP is the development of physical and psychological safety. CPP involves work with the caregiver individually and with the caregiver–child dyad to understand what has happened before and the impact of this trauma now on relationships and aspects of development and functioning. The foundational phase of CPP is assessment and engagement and involves a number of observations and assessment measures designed to hear and see what has happened to young children and their family in their own 'voice'. The caregiver and therapist then co-construct what is known as the 'triangle of explanation'. The triangle helps build an understanding of the child's experience, how this now affects their feelings and behaviour and how treatment in CPP might help. This is a powerful experience delivered by the caregiver to the child (or by the therapist) to 'speak the unspeakable' and acknowledge and validate the child's trauma experience. CPP understands that memory formation begins preverbally, and therefore in dyadic sessions, play is the child's language. As the child and caregiver spend time together, the therapist offers observation, curiosity and gentle explanation to give a voice to what is being played out and might be happening. Toy choice in CPP is very important with toys chosen that represent relationships, trauma, care and nurture, and which also give opportunity for regulation and normative play.

Circle of Security Parenting

The Circle of Security Parenting (COSP) programme, developed by Powell and colleagues [59], distils the key concepts of the attachment system as initially described by Bowlby [27]. It guides caregivers with an attachment 'map' to help them better understand their children's cues and needs, with the aim of improving security. The Circle illustrates a child's need for a secure base for exploration and a safe haven to return to for comfort, protection and to 'refill their emotional cup'. COSP is used individually and in groups drawing on a caregiver's capacity for self-reflection and supporting them to be 'Bigger, Stronger, Wiser and Kind' (Figure 4.2) [60].

Video Interaction Guidance

Video Interaction Guidance (VIG) is used widely to support the relationship between infant/child and caregiver, specifically focussing on attunement and parental sensitivity [61,4]. VIG draws on a wide range of theories and approaches such as attachment and mentalisation and works to promote positive intersubjective experiences. It has a sound evidence base and is also recognised by NICE [62] as an effective intervention for children and young people who are adopted from care, in care or at high risk of going into care. VIG is designed to be collaborative, starting with the development of the caregiver's 'helping question' or area that they would like to see change in. The VIG practitioner then films a period of interaction between child and caregiver and watches this back to find 'micro-moments' of attunement, following VIG principles such as being attentive, receiving initiatives, being attuned together and guiding. The VIG practitioner then shows these

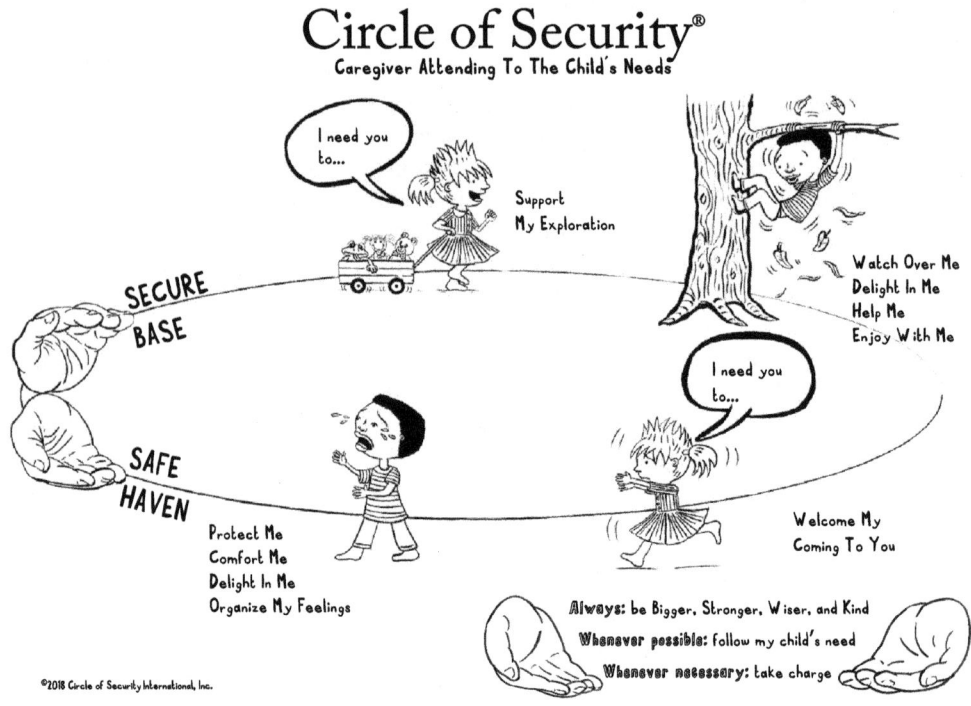

Figure 4.2 *The Circle of Security*: A visual 'map' of caregiver–child attachment. Reproduced with permission from Circle of Security International

selected video clips to the caregiver in a shared review session and encourages mentalisation with curiosity, thoughtfulness and reflection, aiming to build on strengths, that is, when you see what you're doing well, you're likely to do more of it.

The Family Nurse Partnership (FNP)

This is an evidence-based, intensive nursing home visiting programme for young parents and babies from pregnancy until the age of 2. Goals of FNP are to improve pregnancy and birth outcomes through improved prenatal health behaviours, positive, responsive caregiving and supporting the economic self-sufficiency of the family.

Other Interventions

Other commonly used interventions include individual Child Psychotherapy, Mellow Programme; Play Therapy; Watch Me Play; TripleP; Watch, Wait & Wonder; The Incredible Years; Solihull. Most are perceived as useful to families, and some require further research and evaluation.

Conclusion

Infancy is a time of great opportunity and hope. Every infant has the fundamental right to good mental health. As psychiatrists we must prioritise the care of infants if we want to see systemic change in the health and well-being of our society. Infants' minds matter.

References

1. Royal College of Psychiatrists. *Infant and Early Childhood Mental Health: The Case for Action.* College Report 238. Royal College of Psychiatrists, 2023. Available from: https://www.rcpsych.ac.uk/improving-care/campaigning-for-better-mental-health-policy/college-reports/2023-college-reports/infant-and-early-childhood-mental-health-the-case-for-action-(cr238) (accessed 4 April 2025).
2. Zero to Three. *Diagnostic Classification of Mental Health and Developmental Disorders of Infancy and Early Childhood: DC:0-5.* 2nd ed. Zerotothree, 2021.
3. Zero to Three. *Definition of Infant Mental Health.* Washington, D.C.: Zero to Three Infant Mental Health Steering Committee, 2001.
4. Hogg, S, Moody, J. *Understanding and Supporting Mental Health in Infancy – A Toolkit to Support Local Action in the UK.* UNICEF UK, 2023.
5. Egger HL, Angold A. Common Emotional and Behavioral Disorders in Preschool Children: Presentation, Nosology, and Epidemiology. JCPP. 2006;**47**:313–37. https://doi.org/10.1111/j.1469-7610.2006.01618.x.
6. Skovgaard A. Mental Health Problems and Psychopathology in Infancy and Early Childhood. An Epidemiological Study. Danish Medical Bulletin. 2010;**57**:10.
7. Wichstrøm L, Berg-Nielsen TS, Angold A, Egger HL, Solheim E, Sveen TH. Prevalence of Psychiatric Disorders in Preschoolers. JCPP. 2011;**53**:695–705. https://doi.org/10.1111/j.1469-7610.2011.02514.x.
8. Galloway S, Haynes A, Cuthbert C. *An Unfair Sentence: All Babies Count.* NSPCC, 2014.
9. SIGN 156. *Children and Young People Exposed Prenatally to Alcohol: A National Clinical Guideline.* Scottish Intercollegiate Guidelines Network, 2019. Available from: www.sign.ac.uk/media/1092/sign156.pdf.
10. Gregoire A. Antenatal and Postnatal Mental Health Problems: Prevention and Treatment. In P Leach (ed.), *Transforming Infant Wellbeing: Research, Policy and Practice for the First 1001 Critical Days.* Routledge, 2018, 89–97.
11. Balbernie R. Circuits and Circumstances: Importance of Earliest Relationships and Their Context. In P Leach (ed.), *Transforming Infant Wellbeing: Research, Policy and Practice for the First 1001 Critical Days.* Routledge, 2018, 19–27.
12. Wave/Department of Education. *Conception to Age 2 – The Age of Opportunity.* DoE, 2013. Available from: https://www.wavetrust.org/conception-to-age-2-the-age-of-opportunity (accessed 4 April 2025).
13. Stein A, Pearson R, Goodman SH, et al. Effects of Perinatal Mental Disorders on the Fetus and Child. Lancet. 2014;**384**:1800–19.
14. Schore A. The Neurobiology of Attachment and Early Personality. JOPPPAH. 2002;**16**(3):249–63.
15. Berens AE, Nelson CA. Neurobiology of Fetal and Infant Development: Implications for Infant Mental Health. In CH Zeanah Jr. (ed.), *Handbook of Infant Mental Health.* 4th ed. New York: The Guilford Press, 2019, 41–62.
16. Roehrich S. *Key Concepts: Brain Architecture.* Centre on the Developing Child Harvard University, 2020, 41–62. Available from: https://brain.harvard.edu/hbi_news/the-architecture-of-the-brain/.
17. Leach P. Fifty Years of Childhood. In P Leach (ed.), *Transforming Infant Wellbeing: Research, Policy and Practice for the First 1001 Critical Days.* Routledge, 2018, 3–10.

18. Felitti VJ, Anda RF, Nordenberg D, et al. Relationship of Childhood Abuse and Household Dysfunction to Many of the Leading Causes of Death in Adults: The Adverse Childhood Experiences (ACE) Study. AJPM. 1998;14:245–58.

19. Treanor MC. *Child poverty. Aspiring to survive*. Policy Press, 2020.

20. Shonkoff JP, Slopen N, Williams DR. Early Childhood Adversity, Toxic Stress, and the Impacts of Racism on the Foundations of Health. Annu Rev Public Health. 2021;42:115–34. Available from: www.annualreviews.org/doi/full/10.1146/annurev-publhealth-090419-101940#_i2.

21. Marryat L, Frank J. Factors Associated with Adverse Childhood Experiences in Scottish Children: A Prospective Cohort Study. BMJ. 2019. Available from: https://bmjpaedsopen.bmj.com/content/3/1/e000340.

22. Mead M. *Coming of Age in Samoa: A Psychological Study of Primitive Youth for Western Civilisation*. New York: W. Morrow & Company, 1928. Available from: https://archive.org/details/comingofageinsam00mead (accessed 4 April 2025).

23. Winnicott DW. The Theory of the Parent-Infant Relationship (1960). In DW Winnicott (ed.), *The Maturational Processes and the Facilitating Environment*. Karnac Books, 1990, 37–55.

24. Bowlby J. *Attachment and Loss: Volume 1: Attachment*. Penguin, 1969.

25. Ainsworth MD, Bell SM. Attachment, Exploration, and Separation: Illustrated by the Behavior of One-Year-Olds in a Strange Situation. Child Dev. 1970;41:49–67. https://doi.org/10.2307/1127388.

26. Fearon P. Attachment Theory: Research and Application to Practice and Policy. In P Leach (ed.), Transforming Infant Wellbeing: Research, Policy and Practice for the First 1001 Critical Days. Routledge, 2018, 28–36.

27. Bowlby J. Developmental Psychiatry Comes of Age. AJP. 1988;145:1–10.

28. Fraiberg S, Adelson E, Shapiro V. Ghosts in the Nursery: A Psychoanalytic Approach to the Problems of Impaired Infant-Mother Relationships. J Am Acad Child Psychiatry. 1975;14:387–421.

29. Lieberman AF, Padrón E, Van Horn P, Harris WW. Angels in the Nursery: The Intergenerational Transmission of Benevolent Parental Influences. Infant Ment Health J. 2005;26:504–20.

30. Black, D. Causes of Disorder, I. Theoretical Perspectives. In D Black, D Cottrell (eds.), *Seminars in Child and Adolescent Psychiatry*. Royal College of Psychiatrists, 1993, 28–38.

31. Bandura A. *Social Learning Theory*. Prentice Hall, 1977.

32. García JL, Heckman JJ, Leaf DE, Prados, MJ. The Life-Cycle Benefits of an Influential Early Childhood Program. 2016. Available from: https://heckmanequation.org/resource/research-summary-lifecycle-benefits-influential-early-childhood-program/.

33. UNICEF, World Bank and World Health Organisation. *Nurturing Care for Early Childhood Development*. World Health Organisation, 2018. Available from: https://www.who.int/publications/i/item/9789241514064 (accessed 4 April 2025).

34. Segal L, Guy S, Furber G. What Is the Current Level of Mental Health Service Delivery and Expenditure on Infants, Children, Adolescents, and Young People in Australia? Aust N Z J Psychiatry. 2018;52:163–72. https://doi.org/10.1177/0004867417717796.

35. Luby J, Whalen D. Depression in Early Childhood. In CH Zeanah Jr. (ed.), *The Handbook of Infant Mental Health*. 4th ed. New York: The Guilford Press, 2019, 426–37.

36. Lyons S, Whyte K, Stephens R, Townsend H. *Developmental Trauma Close Up*. Beacon House Therapeutic Services and Trauma Team. 2020. Available from: https://beaconhouse.org.uk/wp-content/uploads/2020/02/Developmental-Trauma-Close-Up-Revised-Jan-2020.pdf.

37. Scottish Government. *Voice of the Infant Best Practice Guidelines and Infant Pledge*. Scottish Government, 2023. Available

38. McFadyen, A, Armstrong, VG, Masterson, K., Anderson, B. The Voice of the Infant. *Infant Observation.* 25 (2):104–22.
39. Parent Infant Partnership. *Rare Jewels.* Parent Infant Partnership, 2019. Available from: https://parentinfantfoundation.org.uk/our-work/campaigning/rare-jewels/ (accessed 4 April 2025).
40. PMHNS Care Pathways. *Scottish Perinatal Mental Health Care Pathways.* NHS Scotland, 2021. Available from: https://www.nn.nhs.scot/pmhn/wp-content/uploads/sites/11/2021/06/Care-Pathways-full.pdf.
41. Scottish Government. *Mental Health and Wellbeing Strategy.* Scottish Government, 2023. https://www.gov.scot/publications/mental-health-wellbeing-strategy/ (accessed 4 April 2025).
42. Brazelton TB, Koslowski B, Main M. The Origins of Reciprocity: The Early Mother-Infant Interaction. In M Lewis, LA Rosenblum (eds.), *The Effect of the Infant on Its Caregiver.* John Wiley, 1974, 49–76.
43. Beebe B. Mother-Infant Research Informs Mother-Infant Treatment. Psychoanal Stud Child. 2005;**60**:7–46.
44. Shulman G. Looking in the Right Way: The Use of Infant Observation as a Clinical Tool in Parent–Infant Psychotherapy with Parents with Severe Mental Health Difficulties. Infant Observation. 2016;**19**:97–119.
45. Rustin MJ. Observing Infants: Reflections on Methods. In L Miller, M Rustin, M Rustin, J Shuttleworth (eds.), *Closely Observed Infants.* Duckworth, 1989, 52–75.
46. Miller, L. Introduction. In L Miller, M Rustin, M Rustin, J Shuttleworth (eds.), *Closely Observed Infants.* Duckworth, 1989, 1–4.
47. Brazelton TB, Nugent JK. *Neonatal Behavioural Assessment Scale.* MacKeith Press, 1995.
48. Squires J, Bricker, D. *Ages & Stages Questionnaires®, Third Edition (ASQ®-3): A Parent-Completed Child Monitoring System.* Baltimore: Paul H. Brookes Publishing Co., 2009.
49. Larrieu J, Middleton M, Kelley A, Zeanah C. In CH Zeanah Jr. (ed.), *The Handbook of Infant Mental Health.* 4th ed. New York: The Guilford Press, 2019, 279–96.
50. Oates J, Gervai, J, Danis, I, Lakatos, K, Davies, J. Validation of the Mothers' Object Relations Scales Short-form (MORS-SF). JOPPPAH. 2018;**33**:38–50. Available from: https://www.morscales.org/publications/mors-sf-development/ (accessed 4 April 2025).
51. Achenbach T, Rescorla L. *Manual for the ASEBA Preschool Forms & Profiles.* Burlington: University of Vermont, Research Centre for Children, Youth, & Families, 2000.
52. NHS Lanarkshire. *Lanarkshire IMH Observational Indicator Set.* NHS Lanarkshire, 2021. Available from: https://www.nhslanarkshire.scot.nhs.uk/download/imh-observational-indicator-set.
53. Zeanah CH Jr, Zeanah PD. Infant Mental Health: The Clinical Science of Early Experience. In CH Zeanah Jr. (ed.), *The Handbook of Infant Mental Health.* 4th ed., IV Psychopathology. New York: The Guilford Press, 2019, 5–24.
54. Zero To Three. *DC:0–5 Crosswalk to DSM and ICD-10.* Zerotothree, 2016.
55. Nugent JK, Keefer CH, Minear S, Johnson L, Blanchard Y. *Understanding Newborn Behaviour and Early Relationships: The Newborn Behavioural Observations (NBO) System Handbook.* Brookes Publishing Co., 2007.
56. Hopkins J. Infant-Parent Psychotherapy. Journal of Child Psychotherapy. 1993;**19**:5–17.
57. Acquarone S. Life Is Like a Box of Chocolates: Interventions with Special-Needs Babies. In P Leach (ed.), *Transforming Infant Wellbeing: Research, Policy and Practice for the First 1001 Critical Days.* Routledge, 2018, 238–51.
58. Lieberman A, Ghosh Ippen C, Van Horn P. *Don't Hit my Mommy: A Manual for*

Child-Parent Psychotherapy with Young Children Exposed to Violence and Other Trauma. 2nd ed. Zerotothree, 2015.

59. Coyne J, Powell B, Hoffman K, Cooper G. The Circle of Security. In CH Zeanah Jr. (ed.), *The Handbook of Infant Mental Health*. 4th ed. New York: The Guilford Press, 2019, 500–13.

60. The Circle of Security International. *What Is the Circle of Security* [Internet]. Available from: https://www.circleofsecurityinternational.com/circle-of-security-model/what-is-the-circle-of-security/ (accessed 9 April 2025).

61. Kennedy H, Underdown A. Video Interaction Guidance: Promoting Secure Attachment and Optimal Development for Children, Parents and Professionals. In P Leach (ed.), *Transforming Infant Wellbeing: Research, Policy and Practice for the First 1001 Critical Days*. Routledge, 2018, 224–37.

62. National Institute of Health and Care Excellence. *Children's Attachment: Attachment in Children and Young People Who Are Adopted from Care, In Care or At High Risk of Going into Care. NG26*. National Institute of Health and Care Excellence, 2015. Available from: https://www.nice.org.uk/guidance/ng26/resources/childrens-attachment-attachment-in-children-and-young-people-who-are-adopted-from-care-in-care-or-at-high-risk-of-going-into-care-pdf-1837335256261 (accessed 4 April 2025).

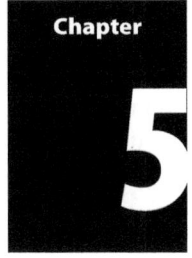

Chapter 5

Classification and Epidemiology

Josephine Holland, Kapil Sayal and Elena Garralda

Classification

Introduction

The classification of child and adolescent psychiatric disorders fulfils a need for communication between those involved with mental health services and is a requirement for services to function. The most widely used classification systems are the World Health Organisation's *International Classification of Diseases* (ICD 10th version (ICD-10), now being substituted by version 11) [1] and the American Psychiatric Association's *Diagnostic and Statistical Manual of Mental Disorders* (DSM-5) [2]. As outlined in their manuals, the descriptions of disorders aim to reflect current understanding and clinical consensus, assist in the communication and institution of evidence-based interventions and support mental health services practice [3].

As a result of a concerted effort to harmonise ICD and DSM classifications, recent versions are more similar – though not identical – conceptually and in diagnostic terms and descriptions. Their revisions over time have been guided by research evidence and wider considerations, such as suitability for administrative purpose, for example, billing for service use as well as the production of national statistics about mental disorders, so as to serve as an international common language for clinicians and researchers. Both classification systems aim to represent opinions of psychiatrists and other mental health personnel, and ICD-11 also aspires to assist with clinical and administrative practice in different settings and cultures.

In contrast with other branches of medicine, where diagnoses are supported by abnormal physical signs or laboratory findings, psychiatry focuses on the concept of disorder as represented by subjectively reported symptoms and observable sign clusters, involving patient distress and suffering as well as causing impairment and interference with activities. Both ICD and DSM define disorders categorically by the presence of a clinically recognisable set of symptoms or behaviours associated in most cases with impairment. They draw on abundant literature and clinical experience to inform assessment and treatment of disorders. Their overall philosophy has been one of refining the number of diagnosable disorders to leave the best validated and most clinically helpful; they also recognise multiple diagnoses/co-morbidity.

Categorical Versus Dimensional Classifications

A separation between early symptoms/signs and the presence of a disorder, while implicit in a categorical classification of disorders is not always clear-cut. Symptoms or changes that are precursors of disorders may be assessed and their severity graded in a dimensional way. This raises questions and debate about the advantages and disadvantages of dimensional versus dichotomous approaches to health problems and their management.

When is elevated blood pressure a disorder (e.g. hypertension) – calling for drug treatment? When are adolescent mood changes an expression of developmentally appropriate moodiness, an understandable situation-specific response to stressful relationships and when should they be regarded as an expression of a treatable depressive disorder? In response to these questions, rather than symptom counting, classificatory systems follow the taxonomical dichotomous tradition, aiming to describe the crucial symptoms that cluster together into clinically recognisable entities or disorders that open the way to potentially efficacious treatments.

Disorders are not necessarily mutually exclusive. They can overlap in terms of features, potential etiological factors and helpful treatments. As with the rest of medicine, psychiatric co-morbidities are not uncommon. Nevertheless, individual child psychiatric disorders as currently described – whether co-morbid or not – are distinct and valid enough in terms of aggregated clinical features and treatment implications; they are meaningful conceptually and have clinical utility [4].

In practice, the presentation and management of a child with the cluster of features characteristic of a depressive disorder can be easily differentiated by experienced clinicians from that of conduct disorder, autism or schizophrenia and accordingly official management guidelines such as those issued by NICE in the United Kingdom are usually disorder based.

Dimensional symptom rating scales can, however, be helpful as a screening tool for the possible presence of a clinically valid psychiatric disorder, in quantifying symptom severity, for measuring symptom change over time or in response to treatment and to help monitor clinical progress and outcomes. In the field of child psychiatry there are a wealth of rating scales to assess symptoms and features in a dimensional way. However, there are often important differences in the way rating scales are completed by parents, children and teachers and for clinical decision-making and to guide treatment they cannot substitute for clinical judgements on when these symptoms represent treatable categorical psychiatric disorders.

A challenge to current psychiatric classificatory systems came from the development of the quantitative, dimensional approach to diagnosis inherent in the Research Domain Criteria (RDoC), a paradigm launched over a decade ago as a potentially superior approach for the investigation of mental illness [5]. RDoC conceptualise normal human behaviour, emotions and cognition as dimensions, with mental illnesses representing dimensional extremes alongside prespecified neuropsychological dimensions. However, both the basis and clinical utility of the RDoC have been challenged, with claims that they have diverted attention away from the new neurobiology that is most relevant to psychiatric disease. RDoC may have value for understanding normal human psychology and for some conditions to be plausibly construed as extremes of normal variation, but for many serious mental illnesses, including dementia, autism, schizophrenia and bipolar disorder, they may be conceptually flawed. It is argued that rather than a deviation along dimensional axes of normal variation, psychiatric illnesses are most helpfully conceptualised as the result of complex but specific pathogenic processes that disrupt normal neurobiological function and normal patterns of cognition, emotion and behaviour [6].

The Role of Classification in CAMHS

Child psychiatric practice within Child and Adolescent Mental Health Services (CAMHS) attends to children and young people with the most severe and/or impairing difficulties and usually takes place in the context of multidisciplinary teams. This acknowledges the fact that disorders develop, manifest and are managed within the family and/or school environment, are closely linked to neurodevelopment, cognition and temperament and are influenced by physical health, psychosocial and socio-economic environment and that an understanding and management of these associated factors is essential for the assessment, management and prognosis of disorders.

In specialist CAMHS a combined categorical/dimensional approach is usually most effective in the joint framing and managing of problems. Because of their knowledge and training in medical and psychiatric disorders and in diagnostics, child and adolescent psychiatrists are ideally placed to provide categorical diagnoses that help make sense of distinct and impairing emotional and behavioural symptoms in children, to inform the choice of treatments and anticipate progress. Other multidisciplinary team members will have a central position in providing complementary psychological or social assessments, formulations and/or psychosocial interventions, some specific to the child's diagnosis but others more general and transdiagnostic. To address these various influences in clinical practice, diagnosis is helpfully complemented by a formulation of the difficulties, outlining the range of individual biological, psychosocial, familial and societal factors and influences for the development and maintenance of a particular disorder in an individual child.

A symptomatic approach to psychopathology can be helpful in non-specialist settings such as primary care or schools, to help identify children and young people with milder, subthreshold, or subsyndromal symptoms, who present with some but not all key diagnostic features but are at risk of developing disorders. For example, a substantial minority of adolescent general practice attenders, higher than expected from general population rates, are at risk from psychiatric disorders such as depression, and subsyndromal depressive symptoms are common [7]. Most consult for physical symptoms, reflecting the close links between physical and mental health. Identification of the presence and severity of depressive symptoms together with appropriate guidance offers an opportunity for non-specialist settings to both help reduce symptom levels and decrease the risk for the development of disorders.

Multiaxial Classification and Child and Adolescent Psychiatry

A multiaxial classification is one that involves several factors over and above the key psychiatric disorder. It aims to ensure that relevant psychological, biological, environmental and psychosocial factors are all considered when making a mental health diagnosis.

In child and adolescent psychiatry, the diagnostic classification system began as uniaxial, but the recognition of the impact of external factors for diagnoses gave impetus to the development of an ICD parallel multiaxial classification system, emphasising the broader biopsychosocial and ecological factors in children and adolescents presenting to mental health services [8]. In ICD-10 it consisted of Axis I: psychiatric syndromes; Axis II: specific disorders of development (such as speech and language, reading, motor development). Axis III: Intellectual level; Axis IV: associated medical conditions; Axis V: Associated abnormal psychosocial conditions including a range of psychosocial hazards (such as abnormal intrafamilial relationships, child abuse, family mental disorders, life events and other chronic stresses); Axis VI: Global level of social functioning.

ICD-11 does not support a multiaxial system. This is partly offset by ICD-11 allowing the use of psychiatric comorbidity: *'provided that the symptoms of co-morbid disorders are sufficiently extensive and impairing to justify more than one diagnosis and are not better explained by one single psychiatric disorder'*. ICD-11 has also introduced clinically relevant diagnostic *qualifiers* to help identify homogeneous subgroupings involving social, psychological and biological factors with management implications, the sort of information previously represented by the multiaxial system.

For example, the diagnosis of autism now involves the possibility of noting the presence of intellectual disability and language qualifiers. In ICD-10, multiaxial classification consisted of:

- Axis I: Psychiatric syndromes
- Axis II: Specific disorders of development (such as speech and language, reading and motor development)
- Axis III: Intellectual level
- Axis IV: Associated medical conditions
- Axis V: Associated abnormal psychosocial conditions, including a range of psychosocial hazards (such as abnormal intrafamilial relationships, child abuse, family mental disorders, life events and other chronic stresses)
- Axis VI: Global level of social functioning

Under ICD-11 the diagnosis would be autism with mild learning disability and language qualifiers, and co-morbid neurofibromatosis; relevant psychosocial factors would feature in the formulation of the problem.

Key Updates in ICD-11 and DSM-5

While ICD-11 and DSM-5 have not realised earlier hopes of a clinico-pathological aetiological approach to diagnosis, the changes introduced include detailed disorder descriptions (Clinical Descriptions and Diagnostic Guidelines in ICD-11) based as much as possible on existing practice and research findings; these can act as helpful memory aids and function in effect as mini-textbooks. There have also been several changes in terminology of disorder groups and individual disorders.

For child and adolescent psychiatry, a major change has been the introduction of a lifespan diagnostic approach and discontinuation of child-specific disorders; these are now redistributed with previously adult-only categories: Comments are added when a childhood onset carries clinical variations with it [9]. The lifespan strategy acknowledges that a considerable percentage of adult psychiatric disorders start to manifest in childhood or adolescence and that neuro-developmental or other childhood-onset problems often have recognisable adult manifestations.

Impairment of function has become a key feature across diagnoses. Lack of impairment does not imply absence of mental health difficulty, nor does it preclude the introduction of appropriate preventive strategies: it does however help set a useful threshold for specialist help-seeking, service provision and intervention. The introduction of *qualifiers* provides further useful information on case severity and complexity for prognosis and management. In fact, qualifiers involve severity ratings for a number of disorders. For example, a child with autism and intellectual disability/lack of language qualifiers may be expected to have more severe difficulties requiring more complex interventions than those without these qualifiers; the same may apply to low prosocial emotions qualifiers in children with CDs. Childhood irritability as a *qualifier* in a child with oppositional defiant disorder may alert to the need to consider anxiety or depressive disorders in differential diagnoses, and to the possibility of the oppositionality and irritability being a harbinger of a later mood disorder.

ICD-11 Changes from ICD-10

As part of the discontinuation of the 'Behavioural and Emotional Disorders with onset usually occurring in childhood and adolescence' ICD-11 has redistributed and made changes to disorders particularly relevant to this age group [10]. 'Separation Anxiety Disorder' and 'Selective Mutism' are now diagnosed within 'Anxiety and Fear-related disorders'. Feeding disorders of childhood have become part of a new 'Feeding and Eating Disorders' group, incorporating new 'Avoidant Restrictive Food Intake Disorder' (ARFID). Enuresis and Encopresis make up a new 'Elimination Disorders' group. ICD-10's 'Disorders of social functioning with onset specific to childhood and adolescence' (e.g. 'Reactive attachment' and 'Disinhibited attachment disorders of childhood') have been moved to 'Disorders specifically associated with stress' as 'Reactive attachment disorder' and 'Disinhibited social engagement disorder'.

The most distinct ICD 11 categories with a childhood onset are diagnosed within the Neurodevelopmental and Disruptive/Dissocial Groups.

– *Neurodevelopmental Disorders*

The neurodevelopmental disorders include ICD-10's 'Disorders of psychological development' but with a number of changes in terminology. For example, 'Pervasive Developmental disorders' (including Asperger's Syndrome and Atypical Autism categories) have been amalgamated and become 'Autistic Spectrum disorder' with *qualifiers* on intellectual development, language function and loss of previous acquired skills. Rett Syndrome and Disintegrative Disorder have been moved to the Diseases of the Nervous system causing regression. An important variation in the description of autistic spectrum disorders is the reduction of the previous three key features to two (social anomalies and restrictive interests), while merging these with the previous third key feature (language anomalies). Another modification has been the incorporation into the neurodevelopmental disorders group of Intellectual Disability and of the prior hyperkinetic disorder (now Attention Deficit Hyperactivity Disorder).

– *Disruptive/Dissocial Disorders*

Together with Oppositional Defiant Disorders, ICD-10's Conduct Disorders (now Conduct-Dissocial Disorders) are part of ICD-11's 'Disruptive and Dissocial Disorders'. They apply across the age range and have *qualifiers* variously including irritability, childhood versus adolescent onset and limited prosocial emotions. The 'Mixed disorder of conduct and emotions' category has been discontinued.

Comparison Between ICD-11 and DSM-5

Most disorders are now aligned across both systems, but there are some differences [11], over and above those in terminology such that ICD's *qualifiers* are termed *specifiers* in DSM-5.

Neurodevelopmental Disorders

Developmental Language Disorders: Alongside the reduced emphasis on language difficulties in autism, both classifications have highlighted a new developmental language anomaly, specifically affecting the pragmatic use of language ('the ability to understand and use language in social contexts, for example making inferences, understanding verbal humour and resolving ambiguous meaning') in individuals *without* autistic features. This has become the basis for a distinct Social (Pragmatic) Communication Disorder in DSM-5. However, ICD-11 considered there was not sufficient evidence for such a diagnosis. Given that most children with pragmatic language difficulties have other language deficits, ICD-11 has instead created a new pragmatic language *qualifier* within the Developmental Language Disorders.

Autism Spectrum Disorder (ASD): The diagnostic criteria in ICD-11 and DSM-5 are comparable, although DSM-5 is more descriptive of the deficits, and the examples given for 'restricted, repetitive and inflexible patterns of behaviour' are more characteristic of individuals with intellectual disability.

Attention Deficit Hyperactivity Disorder (ADHD): Diagnostic requirements are broadly comparable in both systems, but DSM-5 is more prescriptive in specifying a precise symptom count for diagnosis. Both require ADHD manifestations to be present by 12 years of age: ICD-11 calls for evidence of 'significant' prior inattention and/or hyperactivity–impulsivity symptoms, DSM-5 simply requires that 'several symptoms' be present in childhood.

Disruptive/Dissocial Disorders (ICD-11), Disruptive, Impulse Control and Conduct Disorders (DSM-5)

As well as Oppositional Defiant and Conduct Disorders, DSM-5 also includes in this group Impulse Control Disorders and Other Specific Disruptive Disorders or Personality Change due to another medical condition. ICD-11 instead has a separate Impulse Control Disorders group including Compulsive Sexual Behaviour Disorders and Secondary Impulse Control Syndrome.

Another difference between the systems concerns their *qualifiers/specifiers:* the new qualifier *with limited prosocial emotions* applies to both Oppositional Defiant and Conduct-Dissocial Disorder in ICD-11, but only to Conduct Disorder in DSM-5.

Oppositional Defiant Disorder (ODD): An important difference between the two systems concerns the *irritability qualifier* in ICD-11. Argumentative/defiant behaviour, vindictiveness and angry/irritable moods and behaviours (tantrums, often angry and resentful) are symptoms of ODD in both classification systems, but ICD-11 has also introduced a *chronic irritability/anger qualifier*. This is based on research evidence that it represents a separate construct, and on the unique associations of the irritability dimension of ODD in boys with a continuous pattern of mood and anxiety symptoms through adolescence and young adulthood.

To conceptualise this group of clinically impaired angry/irritable children, DSM-5 created a new disorder called 'Disruptive mood dysregulation disorder' (DMDD), which is part of the Depressive Disorders group. The ICD-11 working party considered there was insufficient evidence for a separate DMDD, because of limited reliability, lack of psychiatric consensus and high rates of overlap with other disorders, particularly ODD [12,13].

Concluding Comment

Psychiatric disorders are constructs, their utility, validity and reliability are relevant ongoing concerns [14,15,16] and these debates will continue to inform future diagnostic refinements. Diagnoses need to adapt and change in the light of new knowledge and expertise, including lived experience. Their ultimate goal remains one of integrating information, aiding communication between all those involved and affected and improving understanding and management of mental health problems.

Epidemiology

Introduction

There are challenges to understanding the true incidence and prevalence of psychiatric disorders among children and adolescents. As discussed earlier in this chapter, since psychiatric diagnosis is based upon a nuanced judgement incorporating symptoms, signs, distress and impact on a person's life and others, the measured prevalence of any disorder depends on where, when and how one looks for it. Over recent decades the UK has shown increased recognition of the importance of CAMHS and that a good understanding of the needs at a population level is essential. This has led to a number of large surveys within the UK looking at the mental health of children, adolescents and young adults.

Epidemiology Within the UK

When asked to self-rate how happy they were with their lives, the Department for Education's 'State of the Nation 2019: Children and Young People's Wellbeing' report [17] found that 84.9% of 10- to 15-year-olds and 82.9% of 16- to 24-year-olds were relatively happy with their lives; however, 5% and 3% in these age groups were relatively unhappy. Despite these high well-being scores, one-fifth of young people reported experiencing high levels of recent anxiety, suggesting that a small minority with recent anxiety still report feeling relatively happy with their lives. Overall ratings of wellbeing have decreased slightly since 2009, and these findings seem to be mainly driven by results from older children. Good Childhood report has been published annually for the past 10 years, this asks about specific reasons for unhappiness, their 2021 report finds increasing levels of unhappiness among 10- to 15-year-olds particularly around school and appearance, for example unhappiness with their school life has increased from 1:11 ten years ago to 1:8 today [18].

The Mental Health of Children and Young People (MHCYP) surveys have provided prevalence estimates of disorders, these were carried out in 1999 (19, covering the UK) with follow-up in 2002; 2004 (20, covering the UK) with follow-up in 2007 and 2017 (21, looking at England alone) with two further follow-up waves in 2020 [22] and 2021 [23]. The main surveys apply rigorous, detailed and consistent methods to assess for a range of mental or psychiatric disorders according to the ICD-10 diagnostic criteria [21] and DSM [24]. The recent follow-up waves are however based on a smaller cohort and assess *probable* mental disorder using an online Strengths and Difficulties Questionnaire [22,23].

The 2017 survey found that 1:8 (12.8%) 5- to 19-year-olds had a mental disorder; 1:20 (5.0%) 5- to 19-year-olds met the criteria for two or more mental disorders.

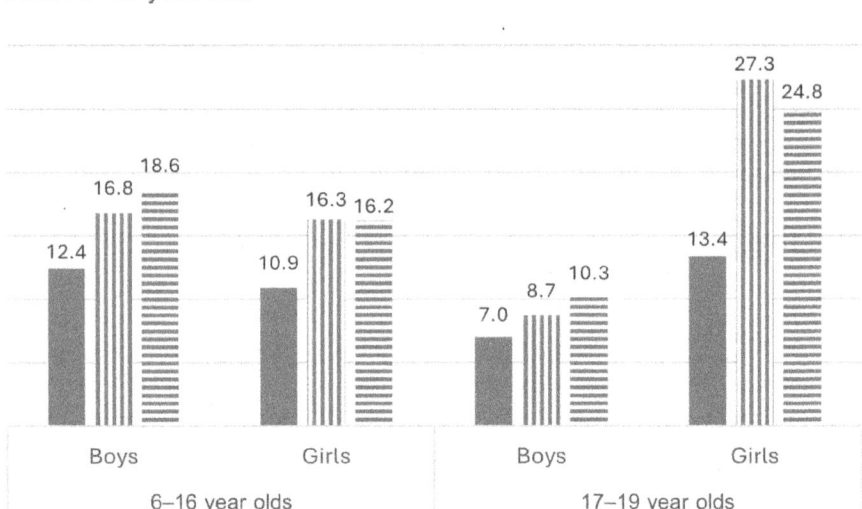

Figure 5.1 Percentage of children or young people with a probable mental disorder, by sex, 2017, 2020 and 2021. Mental health of children and young people in England, 2021: Wave 2 follow-up to the 2017 survey. Open Government Licence.

Since this survey series has been conducted at multiple timepoints using consistent methodology it allows exploration of longitudinal trends. There has been a slight increase in mental disorders in 5- to 15-year-olds over time (9.7% to 11.2%), in both girls and boys.

The follow-up waves have reported even higher rates, as shown in Figure 5.1, with 17.4% of 6- to 16-year-olds reporting probable mental disorder, with increases in both girls and boys. Among 17- to 19-year-olds rates have increased to 17.4% in 2021 from 10.9% in 2017, with a significant rise among young women.

Demographics and Correlates of Disorder

When broken down by age groups the overall prevalence of mental disorder increased with age, from 1:10 (9.5%) 5- to 10-year-olds, 1:7 (14.4%) 11- to 16-year-olds to 1:6 (16.9%) 17- to 19-year-olds. When this is further divided by sex, it shows that there is a clear relationship between increasing age and prevalence of mental disorder among girls (6.6% of 5- to 10-year-olds, 14.4% of 11- to 16-year-olds and 23.9% of 17- to 19-year-olds) but not among boys (12.2%, 14.3% and 10.3%, respectively).

The 2017 survey was the first time in these national surveys that the mental health of 2–4-year-olds was assessed and found 1:18 (5.5%) met criteria for a mental disorder, most commonly oppositional defiant disorder, autism spectrum disorder and sleep and feeding disorders.

In terms of correlates of disorder, the survey found that those who identified as lesbian, gay, bisexual, or with another sexual identity were more likely to have a mental disorder (34.9%) than those who identified as heterosexual (13.2%).

Rates of disorder in 5 -to 19-year-olds also differed between ethnic groups and tended to be higher in White British (14.9%) than Black/Black British (5.6%) or Asian/Asian British children (5.2%).

When assessed according to socio-economic status, overall disorder rates were higher in children whose parents were in receipt of low-income benefits. Emotional behavioural and autism spectrum disorder were more common in children living in lower income households; however, this pattern was not seen for hyperactivity or eating disorders. Higher rates of mental illness in young people were also associated with parental mental illness, adversity, low social support, poorer family functioning, poorer physical health and special educational needs.

Emotional Disorders

Emotional disorders are some of the most prevalent psychiatric disorders among children and adolescents [25]. They include anxiety disorders, mood disorders, obsessive compulsive disorder and post-traumatic stress disorder. Common symptoms such as worries, sadness and low self-esteem are experienced by a much larger percentage of children and young people; however, as noted earlier, to reach the diagnostic threshold for a disorder these symptoms need to be severe enough to cause distress to the young person or to cause an impairment in their functioning [1].

The 2017 MHCYP survey found that 1:12 (8.1%) 5- to 19-year-olds had an emotional disorder. Within this group, anxiety disorders were more common (7.2%) than depressive disorders (2.1%). It was this group of disorders that showed the most prominent change with age. When girls and boys were considered separately the overall rates within girls were higher (10.0%) than boys (6.2%); however, when the data are split by both sex and age group, it is clear that while boys show a rise in prevalence with age (4.6% in 5- to 10-year-olds, 7.1% in 11- to 16-year-olds and 7.9% in 17- to 19-year-olds), this increase with age is much more striking in girls (3.6%, 10.9% and 22.4%, respectively). These findings are in keeping with other studies. The Office of National Statistics found that 21% of 16- to 24-year-olds report symptoms of depression or anxiety, with rates higher in women than in men [29]. In 2014 the Adult Psychiatric Morbidity Survey found that anxiety disorders were more common in women aged 16 to 24 than other age and sex groups [26].

Comparing across timepoints showed that since 2004 there has been an increase in emotional disorders in both boys and girls aged 5 to 15 years. This is up from 4.3% in 1999 and 3.9% in 2004 to 5.8% by 2017.

In terms of correlates, the prevalence of emotional disorders was higher among those of white British ethnicity, lower socio-economic status and those with poorer parental mental health, of special educational needs and poorer physical health.

Hyperactivity Disorders

The behaviours that characterise hyperactivity disorders such as inattention, impulsivity and hyperactivity, are arguably common in many children and young people. However, for those with a diagnosable disorder these symptoms are present at a level that impairs functioning in more than one environment (e.g. home and school).

Since the MHCYP used ICD-10 criteria, the prevalence of hyperkinetic disorder is likely lower than the number of children diagnosed with ADHD (as defined in DSM-5, 3–5% [27]) due to more restrictive criteria.

The 2017 mental health survey found 1:60 (1.6%) 5- to 19-year-olds had a hyperactivity disorder, boys had higher rates (2.6%) than girls (0.6%). When split by age group, it was found that boys aged 11–16 showed the highest overall rates (3.2%).

When the groups were compared across ethnicities, white British children showed the highest prevalence (2.1%). The prevalence of hyperactivity disorder was also higher in groups with poorer physical health, poorer parental mental health, poorer family functioning and parents in receipt of disability or income benefits. Prevalence was not associated with household income or neighbourhood deprivation. The prevalence of hyperactivity disorders has remained roughly stable between 1999 and 2017.

Behavioural Disorders

Behavioural disorders, including ODD and conduct disorder are only diagnosed in childhood and characterised by persistent and repetitive patterns of disruptive and violent behaviour in which the rights of others and social norms are violated. A diagnosis of a behavioural disorder in childhood is associated with a higher likelihood of an adult diagnosis of antisocial personality disorder, substance-related disorders, drug use, mood and anxiety disorders and a higher rate of accidents [28].

In 2017, around 1:20 (4.6%) of those surveyed had a behavioural disorder, with higher rates in boys (5.8%) compared to girls (3.4%). ODD was the most common diagnosis, being found in 2.9% of children surveyed. As with hyperactivity disorders, behavioural disorders have shown a roughly stable prevalence over time between 1999 and 2017. When comparing between age groups, behavioural disorders showed a peak prevalence in 11- to 16-year-olds at 6.2%.

Behavioural disorders were more than seven times more prevalent in White British (5.7%) than Black/Black British (0.7%) and Asian/Asian British children (0.8%). Rates were also higher in young people with poorer physical health, parents with poorer mental health, poorer family functioning, lower household income and higher neighbourhood deprivation.

Other Disorders

In these national surveys, this group of disorders included ASD, eating disorders, tic disorders and a number of very low prevalence conditions. In 2017 about 1:50 (2.1%) 5- to 19-year-olds were identified with one of more of these types of disorder, 1.2% with ASD, 0.4% with an eating disorder and 0.8% with tics or another less common disorder. When the sexes were compared, ASD was more common among boys: 1.9% compared to 0.4% in girls. A higher percentage of girls (0.7%) had an eating disorder compared to boys (0.1%), and when comparison was made between age groups this showed increasing prevalence with increasing age (0.1% in 5- to 10-year-olds, 1.0% in 11- to 16-year-olds, 1.6% in 17- to 19-year-olds). The 2021 follow-up showed an increased prevalence of possible eating problems, when comparing the same measures between the two surveys (6.7% to 13.0% in 11- to 16-year-olds and from 44.6% to 58.2% in 17- to 19-year-olds).

For the disorders within this combined group, rates were higher among white British young people (2.7%) and lowest in Black/Black British (0.3%) young people, and also higher in those with poorer physical health, families with unhealthy functioning or where a parent had poor mental health. Children with ASD were more likely to live in lower income households and with a parent in receipt of benefits, but eating disorders showed no association with household income or parental receipt of benefits. Neither disorder was associated with neighbourhood deprivation.

Self-Harm and Suicide

Death by suicide is relatively uncommon among young people in the UK and figures have remained roughly stable, between 3.6 and 5.9 per 100,000 of the population, since 2000 [29]. Rates of death by suicide are around twice as frequent among males compared to females [30].

Self-harm (non-fatal self-injury or self-poisoning regardless of the intent of the act) is common in the UK and an increasing issue in young people [31]. It is the strongest risk factor for suicide [32]. The prevalence of self-harm in young people is described as an iceberg [30] with only a percentage presenting to services. Studies of hospital presentations with self-harm show higher rates among older adolescents (aged 12–14 years: males 98 and females 502 per 100,000 person-years; aged 15–17 years: males 371 and females 1287 per 100,000 person-years). The prevalence of self-harm (presenting to hospital and community-occurring) were higher in females compared to males, for example, aged 15–17 years: males 2598 per 100,000 person-years reporting a history of self-harm, females 8969 per 100,000 person-years [30].

Substance Misuse and Criminal Justice Contacts

The most recently published biannual NHS Digital survey of smoking, drinking and drug use among young people was completed in 2018 and surveyed 13 664 pupils in years 7–11 (mainly aged 11–15) [33]. This found that 2% of pupils were regular smokers, 3% occasional smokers, 3% used to smoke and 8% have tried smoking. This finding of 17% who have tried smoking was higher than the 11% found by the Health Survey for England 2019 (HSE) [34], an annual survey completed in people's homes. It is suggested that less young people are likely to admit to illicit behaviours when asked at home compared to surveys at school [33]. Although this was not significantly lower than the 2014 and 2016 surveys, there has been a general decline over time since 1996 when 22% were current smokers. The characteristics most strongly associated with current smoking were use of e-cigarettes, taking drugs and having friends who smoke.

When asked about alcohol, 6% reported drinking alcohol at least once a week and a further 11% between once a fortnight and once a month. However, the HSE 2019 reported that 15% of young people reported having ever tried alcohol [34]. These proportions were similar to those found in the 2016 survey. There was no significant difference between sexes, those with white ethnicity were most likely to have drunk alcohol in the last week (13% versus 3% of Black pupils and 1% of Asian pupils). The factors most strongly associated with recent alcohol consumption were having parents who do not discourage drinking, being in an older age group and recent drug use.

In 2018, 24% of pupils reported they had ever taken drugs, which was the same as 2016. There was no significant difference between sexes: Asian pupils were less likely to have taken drugs in the last year (13%) compared with mixed ethnicity (23%), white (17%) and black (18%) pupils. The factors most associated with drug use were smoking, drinking alcohol and having a family who do not discourage drug use. The most commonly used drug was cannabis (8% used within the past year compared to 13% in 2001). Type A drug use has been around 2–3% since 2010. The percentage of pupils perceiving that it was easy to get illegal drugs was 31%, this proportion has remained stable for the past 10 years. Pupils from more affluent families were more likely to have taken drugs in the last month (26% from the most affluent versus 20% in low affluence families).

The Youth Justice Statistics Report 2021 [35], covering England and Wales, showed just over 49,500 arrests of children (aged 10–17) for notifiable offences in that year. This was a decrease of 19% compared to the previous year and the lowest number of arrests of children since the time series began in 2011. Although it is likely that Covid-19 restrictions contributed to this decrease, the rates of child arrests have been falling. In 2021, there were also 20% fewer first-time entrants into the youth justice system, as well as fewer young people cautioned and sentenced. The number of young people sentenced and cautioned however, appears to have fallen among young people of white ethnicity, while the percentages of Asian (6% versus 4%), Black (12% versus 7%) and mixed ethnicity (10% versus 4%) young people receiving a sentence have increased since 2011. Over this decade, child first-time offences have fallen across all offence groups with the exception of possession of weapons offences.

Concluding Comment

Prior to the Covid-19 pandemic, large nationally representative surveys have shown increasing rates of emotional disorders, particularly among adolescent females, but rates of other disorders have remained stable. However, studies conducted since the beginning of the Covid-19 pandemic show this has had an impact on young people's mental health, but we are yet to fully understand its effects over the long term. In these national surveys, the differences in disorder rates by ethnicity are notable and might reflect methodological factors such as sampling or differences in reporting.

References

1. World Health Organisation. *International Statistical Classification of Diseases and Related Health Problems: ICD-11*. 11th ed. WHO, 2019.

2. American Psychiatric Association. *Diagnostic and Statistical Manual of Mental Disorders: DSM-5*. 5th ed. APA, 2013.

3. Garralda ME. ICD-11 – Comparison with DSM-5 and Implications for Child & Adolescent Psychiatric Disorders. In M Hodes, S Gau (eds.), *Positive Mental Health, Fighting Stigma and Promoting Resiliency for Children and Adolescents*. London: Academic Press/Elsevier, 2016, 15–35.

4. Rutter M, Pine D. Diagnosis, Diagnostic Formulations, and Classification. In A Thapar, D Pine, L Leckman, S Scott, M Snowling, E Taylor (eds.), *Rutter's Child and Adolescent Psychiatry* 6th ed. Wiley, 2015, 6–22.

5. Insel T, Cuthbert B, Garvey M, et al. Research Domain Criteria (RDoC): Toward A New Classification Framework for Research on Mental Disorders. Am J Psychiatry. 2010;**167**(7):748–51.

6. Ross CA, Margolis RL. Research Domain Criteria: Strengths, Weaknesses, and Potential Alternatives for Future Psychiatric Research. Mol Neuropsychiatry. 2019; **5**: 218–35.

7. Gledhill J, Garralda ME. Sub-syndromal Depression in Adolescents Attending Primary Care: Frequency, Clinical Features and Six Month Outcome. Soc Psychiatry Psychiatr Epidemiol. 2013;**48**:735–44.

8. Mayall M, McDermott B, Sadhu R, Husodo C. Multiaxial Classification in Child and Adolescent Mental Health – A Reaffirmation of Benefit and Practical Applications. Australas Psychiatry. 2021;**29**: 493–97.

9. Rutter M. Research Review: Child Psychiatric Diagnosis and Classification: Concepts, Findings, Challenges and Potential. J Child Psychol Psychiatry. 2011;**52**:647–60.
10. Reed GM, First MB, Kogan CS, et al. Innovations and Changes in the ICD-11 Classification of Mental, Behavioural and Neurodevelopmental Disorders. World Psychiatry. 2019; **18**(1):3–19.
11. First MB, Gaebel W, Maj M, et al. An Organization-and Category-Level Comparison of Diagnostic Requirements for Mental Disorders in ICD-11 and DSM-5. World Psychiatry. 2021; **20**(1):34–51.
12. Lochman JE, Evans SC, Burke JD, et al. An Empirically Based Alternative to DSM-5's Disruptive Mood Dysregulation Disorder for ICD-11. World Psychiatry. 2015;**14**:30–33.
13. Evans SC, Burke JD, Roberts MC, et al. Irritability in Child and Adolescent Psychopathology: An Integrative Review for ICD-11. Clin Psychol Rev. 2017;**53**:29–45.
14. Reed GM, Keeley JW, Rebello TJ, et al. Clinical Utility of ICD-11 Diagnostic Guidelines for High-Burden Mental Disorders: Results from Mental Health Settings in 13 Countries. World Psychiatry. 2018;**17**(3):306–15.
15. Evans SC, Roberts MC, Keeley JW, et al. Diagnostic Classification of Irritability and Oppositionality in Youth: A Global Field Study Comparing ICD-11 with ICD-10 and DSM-5. J Child Psychol Psychiatry. 2021;**62**(3):303–12.
16. Robles R, de la Peña FR, Medina-Mora ME, et al. ICD-11 Guidelines for Mental and Behavioral Disorders of Children and Adolescents: Reliability and Clinical Utility. Psychiatr Serv. 2022 Apr 1;**73**(4):396–402. https://doi.org/10.1176/appi.ps.202000830. Epub 2021 Aug 26. PMID: 34433288.
17. Department for Education. *State of the Nation 2019: Children and Young People's Wellbeing 2019.* Department for Education, 2019. Available from: https://assets.publishing.service.gov.uk/media/5f29457e8fa8f57acc8d8223/State_of_the_Nation_2019_young_people_children_wellbeing.pdf (accessed 3 February 2022).
18. The Children's Society. *The Good Childhood Report 2021.* The Children's Society, 2021. Available from: https://www.childrenssociety.org.uk/information/professionals/resources/good-childhood-report-2021 (accessed 3 February 2022).
19. Meltzer H, Gatward R, Goodman R, Ford T. Mental Health of Children and Adolescents in Great Britain. Int Rev Psychiatry. 2003;**15**(1–2):185–87.
20. Green H, McGinnity A, Meltzer H, Ford T, Goodman R. *Mental Health of Children and Young People in Great Britain.* London: Palgrave Macmillan, 2004.
21. NHS Digital. *Mental Health of Children and Young People in England, 2017 [PAS].* NHS England, 2018. Available from: https://digital.nhs.uk/data-and-information/publications/statistical/mental-health-of-children-and-young-people-in-england/2017/2017 (accessed 3 February 2022).
22. Vizard T, Sadler K, Ford T, et al. *Mental Health of Children and Young People in England, 2020: Wave 1 Follow Up to the 2017 Survey.* NHS, 2020 Oct 22. Available from: https://digital.nhs.uk/data-and-information/publications/statistical/mental-health-of-children-and-young-people-in-england/2020-wave-1-follow-up (accessed 4 April 2025).
23. Newlove-Delgado T, McManus S, Sadler K, et al. Child Mental Health in England Before and During the COVID-19 Lockdown. The Lancet. 2021;**8**(5):353–54.
24. Ford T, Goodman R, Meltzer H. The British Child and Adolescent Mental Health Survey 1999: The Prevalence of DSM-IV Disorders. JAACAP. 2003;**42**(10):1203–11.
25. Merikangas KR, Nakamura EF, Kessler RC. Epidemiology of Mental Disorders in Children and Adolescents. Dialogues Clin Neurosci. 2009;**11**(1):7–20.
26. Stansfeld, S, Clark C, Bebbington PE, King M, Jenkins R, Hinchliffe S. *Common Mental Disorders.* In S McManus, PE Bebbington, R Jenkins, T Brugha eds.,

Mental Health and Wellbeing in England: Adult Psychiatric Morbidity Survey. Leeds, UK: NHS Digital, 2014, 37–68.

27. Sayal K, Prasad V, Daley D, Ford T, Coghill D. ADHD in Children and Young People: Prevalence, Care Pathways, and Service Provision. The Lancet. 2018;5(2):175–86.

28. Theule J, Germain SM, Cheung K, Hurl KE, Markel C. Conduct Disorder/Oppositional Defiant Disorder and Attachment: A Meta-analysis. J Dev Life Course Criminol. 2016;2(2):232–55.

29. Office of National Statistics. *Young People's Wellbeing.* Office for National Statistics, 2017. Available from: https://www.ons.gov.uk/releases/youngpeopleswellbeing2017 (accessed 4 April 2024).

30. Geulayov G, Casey D, McDonald KC, et al. Incidence of Suicide, Hospital-Presenting Non-fatal Self-Harm, and Community-Occurring Non-fatal Self-Harm in Adolescents in England (the Iceberg Model of Self-Harm): A Retrospective Study. The Lancet. 2018;5(2):167–74.

31. Morgan C, Webb RT, Carr MJ, et al. Incidence, Clinical Management, and Mortality Risk Following Self-Harm Among Children and Adolescents: Cohort Study in Primary Care. BMJ. 2017 Oct 18;**359**:j4351.

32. Hawton K, Bale L, Brand F, et al. Mortality in Children and Adolescents Following Presentation to Hospital After Non-fatal Self-Harm in the Multicentre Study of Self-Harm: A Prospective Observational Cohort Study. Lancet Child Adolesc Health. 2020;4(2):111–20.

33. NHS Digital. *Smoking, Drinking and Drug Use Among Young People, England 2016.* Leeds: NHS Digital, 2017a. Available from: https://files.digital.nhs.uk/07/49FE46/sdd-2016-rep-cor.pdf (accessed 3 February 2022).

34. NHS Digital. *Health Survey for England 2016.* Leeds: NHS Digital, 2017b. https://digital.nhs.uk/data-and-information/publications/statistical/health-survey-for-england/health-survey-for-england-2016 (accessed 4 April 2025).

35. Youth Justice Board/Ministry of Justice Statistics Bulletin. *Youth Justice Statistics, 2015/16: England and Wales.* Ministry of Justice, 2017. Available from: https://digital.nhs.uk/data-and-information/publications/statistical/health-survey-for-england/health-survey-for-england-2016 (accessed 4 April 2025).

Chapter 6

Law in Relation to Children and Young People

Tina Irani, John O'Brien and Shermin Imran

Introduction

Clinicians navigating the legislation when working with young people and their families in the UK may need to use several relevant frameworks of legislation at the same time. This may appear complex in practice, for example, when legislation affecting CYP may have different age cut-offs in relation to restrictions and freedoms, along with a relative lack of case law for some specific issues.

Clinicians need to consider how a young person's development across multiple domains, for example, cognitive, emotional, moral, social and so on, can have an impact upon their decision-making. Clinicians who work with children and young people often also work with parents or their local authority statutory equivalents, as well as other statutory and non-statutory agencies, to help find the best outcomes for children and young people (CYP). This requires good knowledge of legal frameworks, competence in working within complex multi-agency systems and being able to understand and work with different perspectives around an issue.

This chapter specifically discusses aspects of the law in relation to children and adolescents (all those under 18 years) including the Human Rights Framework, Mental Capacity Act 2005, Children Act 1989 (amended 2004), Mental Health Act (amended 2007) and Criminal Justice Act (2003) within England and Wales. We have not addressed the differences in legislation in Northern Ireland or Scotland but have commented on distinct issues where relevant.

Human Rights Act 1998

Human rights, described by the United Nations Universal Declaration, are rights inherent to all human beings, regardless of race, sex, nationality, ethnicity, language, religion, or any other status. Human rights include the right to life and liberty, freedom from slavery and torture, freedom of opinion and expression, the right to work and education, and many more.

The UK Human Rights Act 1998[1] defines the obligations for governments to act in certain ways or to refrain from certain acts, to promote and protect human rights and fundamental freedoms of individuals or groups. This sets out a legal duty for public authorities in the UK including National Health Service (NHS), courts, schools, police and so on, to respect and protect human rights.

When working with CYP in mental health settings, human rights also referred to as 'Articles' in the Human Rights Act 1998 in the UK are sometimes questioned or challenged. It is important to note the human rights can be 'Absolute' rights that cannot be interfered with nor restricted, or 'non-absolute' rights that may be restricted but only after careful consideration to ensure that this is done in a lawful, legitimate and proportionate way, for example, the issue of 'blanket' bans or restrictions where adherence to principles of least restrictive practice in caring for CYP needs to be ensured. Other examples include absolute rights like right to life (Article 2), for instance, in managing a suicidal person, right not to be tortured or treated in an inhuman or degrading way (Article 3), right to a fair trial (Article 6) right to respect for private and family life, home and correspondence (Article 8) as well as other non-absolute ones like right to liberty and security (Article 5), right to peaceful enjoyment of possessions (Article 1), for example, relevant in managing access to smartphones in inpatient units.

Principles of good practice in working with CYP and families when making decisions around their human rights include; involving them in decision making as much as possible, establishing the facts and impact of any care decisions, identifying which rights are being affected and whether these are absolute or not, ensuring decisions impacting on their non absolute rights are lawful, legitimate and proportionate, recording any decisions or changes that need to be made and reviewing these at regular intervals.

The Mental Capacity Act 2005

The Mental Capacity Act 2005 (MCA) [2] is applicable for young people aged 16 and 17 years in England and Wales. The principles of the MCA remain the same for this age group as in adults, that is, assuming they have capacity; ensuring all practicable steps taken to support CYP making their own decisions; not treating a person as lacking the capacity to make a decision just because they make an unwise decision; decisions made for someone who lacks capacity are made in their best interests; any interventions must be least restrictive in terms of their rights and freedoms.

Likewise, when assessing capacity in young people (16–17 years) the standard '2 stage test' is followed – (i) do they have an impairment of their mind or brain?, (ii) does the impairment mean that the person is unable to make a specific decision when they need to? The second stage must include assessing the young person to decide if they can understand the information relevant to the specific decision, including advantages, risks and longer-term impact; retain that information; use or weigh up that information to make the decision; and communicate their decision. If a person cannot meet one or more of these, they are deemed to lack capacity. As is the case with adults, capacity in young people can fluctuate over time, hence needs regular reviews.

When supporting young people to make decisions it is important to explain and present information in a way appropriate to their age and developmental level, to consider asking parents and other experts like speech and language therapists to help with communication in complex issues and to carefully consider issues like particular time and location where a young person might feel more at ease.

In English and Welsh law, there was previously no system prescribed by law to authorise the detention of individuals who could not give informed consent to an informal admission into a hospital or care home, known as the 'Bournewood gap' from R v Bournewood Community and Mental Health NHS Trust [3]. This contravened Article 5 of the Human Rights Act, Right to liberty and security, and resulted in an amendment in legislation to include Deprivation of Liberty Safeguards (DoLS). Although considered a helpful piece of legislation, in practice it was sometimes poorly implemented and left vulnerable people lacking appropriate legal safeguards. In addition, it was also not inclusive for CYP as it only applied to 18-year-olds or older.

The Mental Capacity Amendment Act 2019 plans to replace the DoLS with Liberty Protection Safeguards (LPS) in England and Wales, applicable also to 16- and 17-year-olds. Where the DoLS or the LPS (once in practice) do not apply due to age, any decisions that are required to go through Court judgement should be captured through High Court/Court of Protection Inherent Jurisdiction.

Consent and Competency

Psychiatrists are often asked to assess CYP capacity to make decisions about their own treatment. Furthermore, treatment of mental health conditions may also occur under the Mental Health Act 1983 (amended 2007) [5] and a degree of overlap may be seen across legislation in cases, some of these practical issues are considered in this section.

Anyone above the age of 16 is considered to have the capacity to consent or refuse their treatment unless otherwise indicated, whereas if young people under the age of 16 wish to receive treatment without their parent or carers' consent or even knowledge, they need to be assessed if they are Gillick competent. Gillick Competence and Fraser Guidelines refer to the guidelines set out by Lord Fraser in his judgement of the Gillick v West Norfolk and Wisbech Area Health Authority in the House of Lords [4] that related specifically to contraceptive advice.

While capacity is assumed to be present, competence needs to be proven via an assessment of a young person regarding their understanding and retention of information, weighing up and communicating their decision. Like capacity, competence is very much specific to the decision being made and the assessor needs to ensure consent is not given under duress. The young person should be encouraged to discuss it with their parents and if there is a difference in opinion between the two, a second opinion could be sought. If the young person is not Gillick competent, in most cases consent from parents or carers is sought before proceeding with the care.

The principal of Gillick competence also applies to refusing medical treatment unless refusing treatment endangers their life or may result in permanent harm, in which case this can potentially be overruled. If during the assessment concerns arise regarding safety of the young person, advice from a local authority should be sought.

Principles of confidentiality in sharing information for medical practitioners from the General Medical Council (GMC) apply to assessment of Gillick competence when delivering treatment and care. Where there are safeguarding concerns or a risk of harm to self or others, information may need to be shared by psychiatrists even without the consent of the young person and/or their parent [7].

Scope of Parental Responsibility

The MHA code of practice [8] covers the role of the person with parental responsibility (PR) with regard to decision-making around the confinement of a child under 16 who lacks Gillick competence to hospital and consenting to treatment on their behalf. While no Court authorisation is needed, sufficient consideration must be given to ensure that the person with PR is exercising their rights appropriately. If there are concerns about their own capacity and/or intent, then legal advice should be sought, and the Mental Health Act may need to be used ensuring appropriate safeguards for the young person.

The clinician also needs to determine whether this is a decision that a person with PR should reasonably be expected to make, that the decision is being made in the best interest of the child and whether there any factors that might undermine the validity of parental consent. When it is established that a particular decision can be authorised by a parent, this is described to fall within the 'scope of parental responsibility'.

The UK Supreme Court, however, has confirmed in the case of Child D [6] that the deprivation of liberty of a young person aged 16 or 17, who lacks capacity, is so far different from the experience of their capacitous peers that the deprivation of their liberty must be recognised, the court ruled that parents cannot authorise their deprivation of liberty. Since LPS cannot be used for those under 16 years of age in England and Wales, the young person's rights must currently be protected by application to the Court of Protection for an order authorising their deprivation of liberty. This case explores the interfaces between the MCA, the Children Act 1989 and Gillick competence, and is recommended for further study by anyone facing complex decisions about a young person lacking capacity.

Treatment Under the Mental Health Act 1983 (Amended 2007) (MHA)

Section 63 of MHA [5] states that an approved clinician under the act can provide medical treatment irrespective of whether or not a detained patient has capacity to refuse such treatment, to be able to provide necessary medical treatment for the mental disorder from which they are suffering. This section can also potentially be used to treat people with physical health conditions where their decision-making has been affected by their mental health. Case law has established that a range of acts ancillary to the core mental disorder treatment are allowed under S63.

To help with the decision-making in a young person (aged 16+), if they are assessed to have capacity then the MCA does not apply. If they are detained under the MHA and are refusing treatment for their physical health condition due to, or secondary to, a symptom of their mental disorder (does not have to be the mental disorder that they have been detained for), then S63 can potentially be used.

Children Act 1989

The Children Act 1989 [9] is the legal framework in the UK that sets out the duties of the local authorities in looking after the welfare and safeguarding of the child (anybody under the age of 18 is considered a child). This includes questions regarding the upbringing and/or the administration of the child's property and so on.

Some of the relevant sections for child and adolescent mental health psychiatrists, including for example, S17 - Child in Need, place a general duty on all local authorities to assess the needs of a child and ensure appropriate support for the family to safeguard and promote the welfare of the child in need.

S20 of the Children Act enables voluntary accommodation of the child and places the responsibility on the local authority to provide accommodation in the event of the child not having a person who has PR for them or the person with PR is unable to care for them and has given permission for such accommodation.

S25 of the Children Act applies to Secure Accommodation Order for a child who is being 'looked after' by a local authority and, if not placed in secure accommodation, are at risk of absconding and if they were to abscond are likely to suffer from significant harm. Furthermore, if they were to be kept in at unrestricted accommodation, they are likely to injure themselves or others. This is a particularly relevant section to consider for young people with high-risk behaviours in the community. However, the threshold is extremely high and there are very limited secure accommodation placements available across the UK. Therefore there is a need to ensure all possible efforts have been made to support them in the community before considering secure accommodation.

S31 of the Children Act relates to Care and Supervision under a full care order, the application for which is made to the court by the designated local authority when there is concern with regard to a risk of harm. The court would only make the order if satisfied that the child concerned is suffering or likely to suffer from significant harm and that the harm or likelihood of harm is attributed to the care given to the child or that the child is beyond parental control. Of note, no order can be made with respect to a child who has reached the age of 17, or 16 in the case of child who is married.

S44 is an Emergency Protection Order (EPO) allowing for a child to be removed to provide immediate short-term protection. The local authority (or any person) can apply to the family court for an EPO where the court is satisfied that there is reasonable cause to believe that the child is likely to suffer 'significant harm' if not removed to accommodation provided by the applicant; or does not remain in the place in which the child is being accommodated; or S47 Enquiries (necessary to decide whether to take any action to safeguard a child at risk of serious harm) are being frustrated by unreasonable refusal of access to the child; and the local authority has reasonable cause to believe that access is needed as a matter of urgency.

The local authority is granted PR for the child, which enables the child to be removed to other accommodation or to remain in a place where they are being accommodated (e.g. a hospital or foster placement). An application for an EPO is a serious step taken only after the court must be satisfied that this is both necessary and proportionate at the time. The role of a psychiatrist might be to provide an opinion with regard to harm that the child might have suffered or is likely to suffer and to occasionally advise on therapeutic interventions to support the young person.

Mental Health Act 1983 (Amended 2007)

The Mental Health Act for England and Wales (MHA) [5] does not have a lower age limit and is applicable to CYP. This includes both Part II, 'Compulsory Admission to Hospital and Guardianship', often referred to as 'civil sections', and Part III, 'Patients Concerned in Criminal Proceedings or Under Sentence', sometimes referred to as the 'forensic sections', key sections summarised in Table 6.1 (see also Figure 6.1 for application of Part III).

MHA Assessments for young people require medical recommendation by two doctors (one of whom is S12 approved), as well as an Approved Mental Health Practitioner who ultimately makes the application for detention under the Act. Ideally, when assessing young people, one of the doctors should be a child and adolescent psychiatrist.

Furthermore, children and young people have to meet the same 'statutory criteria' for detention under the MHA as adults that they have a mental disorder of nature or degree that requires hospital admission AND it is necessary for the health or safety of the patient or for the protection of other persons that they should receive such treatment, and it cannot be

Table 6.1 Key sections in Part III of the MHA

MHA section	Notes	Duration
2	Admission for assessment	Up to 28 days
3	Admission for treatment	Up to 6 months
	Can be renewed, initially for 6 months, then for a further 12-month period at a time	
35	**Remand (transfer) to hospital for report on accused's mental condition**	28 days
	Can be renewed for further 28 days, for a total of no more than 12 weeks	
	Treatment is not covered by this Section	
36	**Remand (transfer) of accused person to hospital for treatment**	28 days
	Can be renewed for further 28 days, for a total of no more than 12 weeks	
37 (+/- S41)	**Hospital Order (with or without S41 restrictions)**	Up to 6 months
	Given after conviction by Crown or Magistrates court. Can be renewed, initially for 6 months, then for a further 12-month period at a time	
	A S37 is largely similar to S3	
38	**Interim Hospital Order**	Initial period of up to 12 weeks
	Given after conviction	
	Typically used where there is evidence that it may be appropriate for a subsequent hospital order S37 to be made	
	Can be extended by 28 days at a time to a maximum of 12 months	
47/49 48/49	**S47: Transfer of a sentenced prisoner to hospital for treatment**	
	S48: Transfer of a remand prisoner to hospital for treatment	
	These sections come with a S49 restriction direction. The S47/49 and S48/49 transfer 'warrants' require authorisation and oversight from the Secretary of State via the Ministry of Justice. In practice this means that the AC cannot authorise S17 leave or discharge. For those on S47/49, when the release date for their original custodial sentence is reached, the S47/49 automatically changes to a 'Notional S37'. This means that the patient can be managed similar to a S37 hospital order, and the AC can authorise leave and discharge	
41 & 49	Restriction Directions	

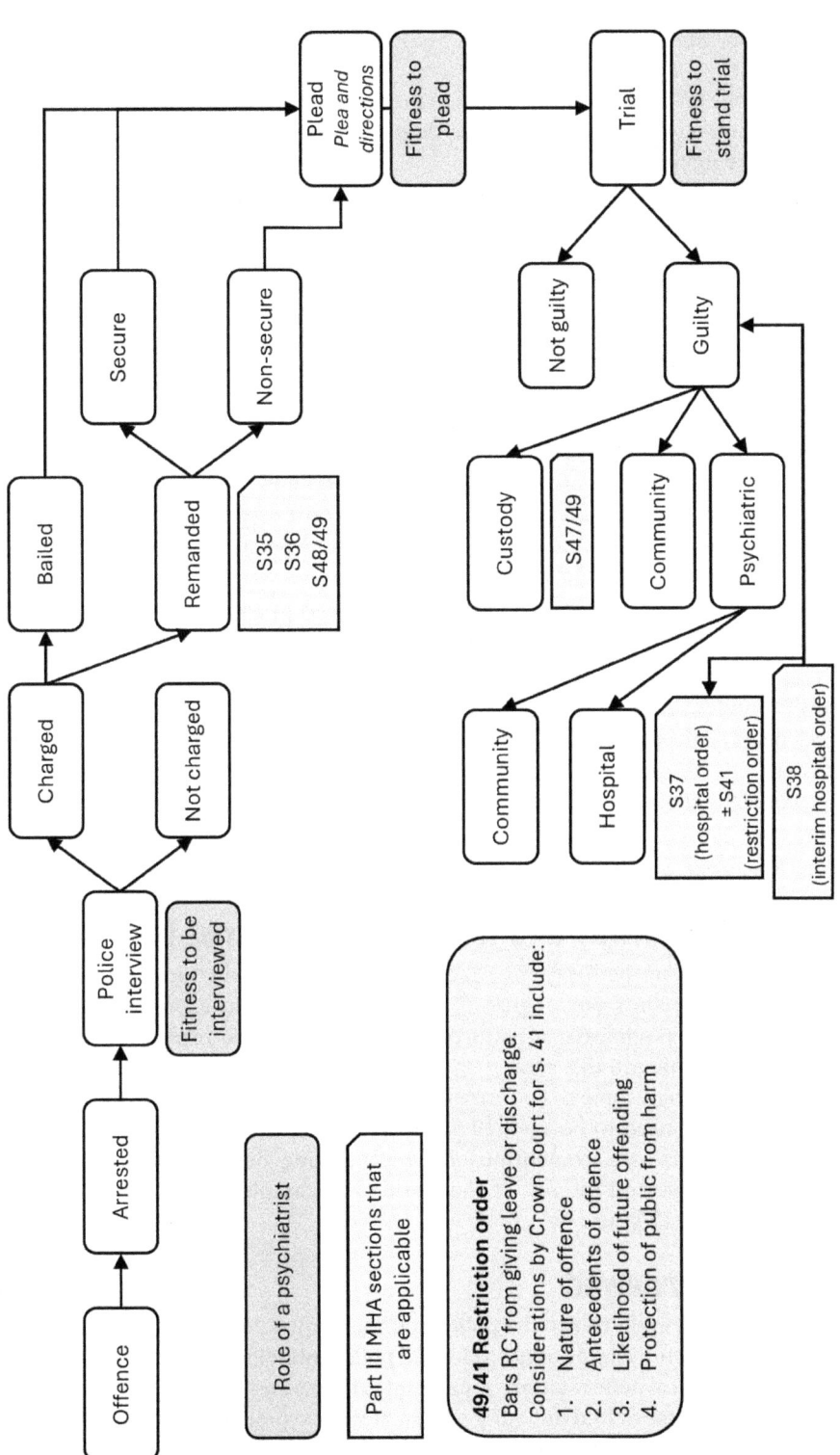

Figure 6.1 Criminal justice system pathway

provided unless they are detained under this section AND that appropriate treatment is available.

With regard to the term 'nature', this refers to the specific mental disorder, its prognosis, chronicity and response to treatment. Whereas 'degree' refers to the current presentation or manifestation of the mental disorder.

When children and young people are detained in hospital under the MHA, similar to adults they will all have an allocated Approved Clinician. Their role is to ensure that necessary assessment and treatment is made available to the patient. They are also responsible for providing evidence (written reports and oral) for hospital managers hearings and tribunals, authorising leave and discharge, and renewing a Section. A new mental health bill to make provisions to amend the MHA is currently passing through UK parliament. Amendment aims to enhance patient advocacy and least restrictive care environment.

S37 - Guardianship Order

In cases where a young person has attained the age of 16 years and the risk requires a level of supervision but not necessarily treatment in hospital, the court may place the young person under the Guardianship of a local social service authority or a person approved by the local authority, if they meet the following criteria:

1. On the written or oral evidence of two registered medical practitioners, the offender is suffering from a mental disorder;
2. The mental disorder is of a nature or degree that warrants his reception into guardianship under this Act; and
3. Having regard to all the circumstances including the nature of the offence and the character and antecedents of the offender, and to the other available methods of dealing with them, the most suitable method of disposing of the case is by means of an order under this section.

The court must be satisfied that the young person will be received by the local authority before making the order.

Criminal Justice Pathway and Role of a Psychiatrist for CYP

The criminal justice system pathway may require the expertise of child and adolescent psychiatrists at various points (see Figure 6.1). Although a forensic psychiatrist is not necessarily required, the psychiatrist is required to work within their expertise and should have experience and training in this area.

For children and young people to be formally involved in the criminal justice system in England and Wales they need to be aged 10 years or over, known as the 'age of criminal responsibility'. This remains a contentious issue generating debate as this age varies significantly across Europe and the rest of the world, for example, in Scotland the age of criminal responsibility is 12 years.

Fitness to Be Interviewed

After arrest by the police, and prior to the police and the Crown Prosecution Service (CPS) making a decision whether to charge or not, a formal police interview should take place [10]. This will usually be at a local police station. A psychiatrist can be asked to give an opinion on 'fitness to be interviewed' for a child or young person, it is good practice for this to be carried out between a child and adolescent psychiatrist. This is important to prevent miscarriages of justice and to make sure that the police and CPS can obtain admissible evidence that can potentially later be used in a trial, as well as prevent any harm to the young person or deterioration in their mental state caused by the interview process.

When assessing a person in custody regarding their fitness for a police interview, the psychiatrist should explore issues such as:
- whether the person understands the police caution
- whether the person's mental state affects their capacity to be accurate and tell the truth
- how the person's physical or mental state might affect their ability to understand the nature and purpose of the interview, to comprehend what is being asked and to appreciate the significance of any answers given and make rational decisions about whether they want to say anything
- the extent to which the person's replies may be affected by their physical or mental condition in representing a rational and accurate explanation of their involvement in the offence
- how the nature of the interview, which could include particularly probing questions, might affect the person

If a young person (or anyone who is deemed to be 'mentally vulnerable') is fit for police interview, they need to have an appropriate adult with them in addition to their solicitor. The appropriate adult is often a social worker, but could be a relative, guardian or a carer though not anyone employed by the police. They should have some experience in dealing with people with mental health difficulties and their role includes:
- to advise the person being interviewed
- to observe whether the interview is being conducted properly and fairly
- to facilitate communication with the person being interviewed

Diversion

If a young person in police custody is deemed unwell and needs to be admitted ('diverted') to hospital directly from the police station, a MHA assessment might be requested to assess whether they meet the statutory criteria for detention in hospital for assessment/treatment (see also MHA section).

When assessing for diversion to hospital, mental health provision available in custodial settings (secure children's homes, Secure Schools, Secure training centres and YOIs) should also be considered if this may be able to meet the needs of the young person.

If at the time of diversion to hospital the young person has not yet been interviewed by the police, plans should be put in place to enable a police interview taking place at a later date in hospital or a local police station, to ensure that criminal justice system processes continue in parallel to the hospital admission.

Transfer of a Young Person from Custodial Settings

If charged following police interview, a young person may be placed on remand (for more serious offences or if the risk of harmful re-offending is high). While on remand, if they require transfer to hospital to assess and treat their mental illness, a transfer might be made to a medium secure inpatient unit under the MHA, S48/49. S48/49 requires two medical recommendations from S12-approved practitioners under the MHA and a warrant from the Ministry of Justice (MoJ). S49 (often referred to as 'restrictions') means that the AC cannot grant leave or discharge without approval from the MoJ. When in hospital, a young person can appeal against their detention in hospital to a mental health tribunal. If they are deemed not to be detainable in hospital, they could be returned to a custodial setting.

If a young person is served a custodial sentence and then becomes unwell in the custodial estate, requiring transfer to hospital for assessment and/or treatment, S47/49, is used with conditions like S48/49 described in the previous section. Furthermore, if detained in hospital under S47/49 requiring ongoing treatment and the sentence release date is reached, the MHA status changes from S47/49 to S37N ('a notional 37', or a 'notional hospital order'). At this point, the 'restrictions' (S49) are no longer in place and the responsibility for leave (S17) and discharge remain with the AC.

Assisting a Young Person Through the Court Process

A psychiatrist may be asked via the court (CPS or young person's defence legal team) to give their independent opinion on issues such as whether they are fit to plead, stand trial, or on suitable 'disposal options' if a young person was found guilty having either 'done the act or made the omission' when not fit to plead. This should be formally requested and the psychiatrist's 'instructions' should be clear and agreed in advance.

Fitness to plead is assessed using the Pritchard criteria, as for adults, however young people at different stages of development or those suffering with a mental health problem, either/both affecting their fitness to plead is important to consider. The Pritchard criteria are as follows:

- Understand the nature of the charge.
- Understand the difference between pleading guilty and not guilty.
- Follow the course of proceedings on the trial.
- Challenge any jurors to whom they may object.
- Understand the evidence presented in the court.
- Instruct their legal representatives properly.

If considered fit to plead, the young person is supported by their legal team to enter a plea in court, for example, a 'normal' trial if they plead not guilty or a 'Trial of Facts' if the young person is found unfit to plead, which may result in the person either acquitted, or found to have 'done the act or made the omission', that is, the term 'guilty' is not used in these circumstances. When this is the case, the disposal options are limited to a hospital order or a guardianship order (only for those above the age of 16) in the care of the local authority.

Clinicians need to also consider how to help a young person in their 'effective participation' [11] in court. This may include advice to best communicate with the young person in clear, concise and simple language, taking more time to explain difficult issues and checking that they understand, more frequent breaks and other recommendations to make the court environment more tolerable for the young person. Appointing an intermediary could be considered who can assist the young person in court in explaining court procedure, supporting them to give evidence.

Psychiatrists (and other specialists) can also be asked for their opinion on a person's fitness to stand trial and in addition to the issues described in this subsection, they should also consider whether the person is mentally (or physically) well enough to be able to attend and participate in court proceedings.

Disposals

Once a person has been found guilty there are several options of disposal [11] available that may be recommended by psychiatrists. These include (please also see Figure 6.1), S37 - Hospital order or S37/41 - Hospital order with Restriction requiring oversight from the Secretary of State/Home Office for the AC to approve leave and discharge from this hospital, which is most likely a 'conditional discharge', usually from a mental health tribunal. The conditions are likely to address treatment needs in the community. If these conditions are not met, or the person's mental state deteriorates then they could be recalled to hospital.

S38 – Interim hospital order may be used when the need for hospital treatment (e.g. S37) may need to be tested, hence S38 provides a period of time in hospital (initially not exceeding 12 weeks, but extendable for up to 28 days at a time for up to 12 months) to evaluate the person's response to hospital treatment. At the end of the S38 period the young person will return to Court for final sentencing and recommendations from the psychiatrists as to whether hospital is needed in the long term (e.g. S37) or not could also be considered (see Figure 6.1).

Other Provisions of Part III MHA

S35 and S36 can be used by the court for people who are awaiting trial. This allows the person to be admitted to hospital for a report (S35) or treatment (S36). This is for up to 12 weeks. At the end of 12 weeks the person returns to court, typically with further recommendations from the psychiatrists involved.

If a person is given a custodial sentence, and later they are deemed to require treatment in hospital, they can be transferred to hospital under S47/49. Of note, if a person requires transfer to hospital while on remand (unsentenced), S48/49 would be used.

Dangerousness

It is not uncommon for psychiatrists to be asked to comment on 'dangerousness'. However, it is important to remember that the assessment of dangerousness is a 'judgement of the court'. This is important for courts as there are specific sentences available to them when the criteria for determining dangerousness is met. Specified offences that are considered include violent and sexual offences that carry a lengthy maximum sentence. For young people, a sentence for dangerousness can apply if they are defined as being a 'significant risk to members of the public of serious harm occasioned by the commission of further specified offences', serious harm being described as 'death, serious personal injury, whether physical or psychological'. To do this, the court must consider all information available about the nature and circumstances of the offence, information about patterns of behaviour related to the offence and other relevant information about the young person.

For the court to determine dangerousness, there are principles that should be followed for young people including:
- The risk must be significant, also described as noteworthy of 'considerable amount or importance'.

- Consideration of characteristics of current and previous behaviour patterns, responses to previous disposals, social factors and the young person's developmental level and presentation (e.g. maturity, mental state, attitudes, etc.).
- A pre-sentence report should be completed by the Youth Offending team and a medical report also be completed if concerns arise regarding their mental health.
- That dangerousness should not be assumed, even when behaviour has been deemed to be dangerous before.

Psychiatric Defences

In the UK, in order to be convicted of an offence, there needs to be evidence beyond reasonable doubt that the accused person carried out the criminal act (actus reus – 'guilty act') and that there was 'criminal' intention or risk of a harmful outcome (mens rea – 'guilty mind'). Specific psychiatric defences can be available to reduce or remove responsibility in the UK. These include:

- Insanity at the time of the offence: Mc Naughton Rules from case R v Mc Naughton [12] govern the law of insanity in England and Wales, which relates to the accused's understanding of the wrongfulness of the alleged act and their knowledge as to whether the alleged act is contrary to the law. If at the time of committing the act, the accused was determined to suffer from a defect of reason from a disease of the mind so that they did not know that what they were doing was wrong, this could be used successfully as a defence.
- Diminished Responsibility: Applies to murder charges to reduce this to manslaughter/culpable homicide. This is important as a murder conviction automatically results in a life sentence. Diminished Responsibility is described as an abnormality of mental functioning that must have substantially impaired the defendant's ability to do one or more of the following: understand the nature of the defendant's conduct; form a rational judgement; exercise self-control.
- Automatism: A person commits an offence when the body was not deemed to have been in control of the mind so that the person was in a state where they were capable of the action but not conscious of what they were doing. In these circumstances the person would not have 'mens rea'. There are mainly two types:

    Insane automatism: If behaviour is likely to recur (e.g. associated with sleep walking, brain tumour or epilepsy, etc.), which may lead to verdict of not guilty by reason of insanity, and

    Sane Automatism where cause was extrinsic (e.g. a reflex reaction or due to concussion or confusional state, etc.), which may lead to full acquittal.

- Infanticide: When a woman by any wilful act or omission causes the death of her child (under 12 months of age) but at the time of the act or omission the balance of her mind was disturbed by her not having fully recovered from the effect of giving birth to the child, or the effect of lactation after the birth of the child. This might be used when the mother has been suffering with mental illness such as postnatal depression. If used this reduces the charge of murder to manslaughter.

Court System and Custodial Estate for Children and Young People

Youth Courts

There was a recognition that adult courts were intimidating and difficult arenas for young people. In 1847, the Juvenile Offenders Act was the first legislation to distinguish between adults and children in the justice system. Children under 14 years were to be tried summarily in a magistrate's court for lesser offences.

The current youth courts are a special type of magistrates' courts for children and young people between the ages of 10 and 17 years. They either have three magistrates (who are laypeople) or a district judge.

It is a less formal court where no wigs are worn, no members of the general public are allowed, and the young person is addressed by their first name. An appropriate adult needs to be present and can be the parent or a guardian.

It is expected that summary cases and more serious indictable offences start in the youth court but will be then transferred to Crown court. Sentencing through youth courts includes community sentence and Detention and training orders. If a hospital order is recommended, the case will often be transferred to Crown court.

Crown Courts

Young people under the age of 18 years are only tried in the Crown court for an indictable offence and where the likely sentence is detention for more than 2 years. These include the following 8 exceptions:

1. If jointly charged with an Adult.
2. Charged with the offence of Homicide.
3. A young person over the age of 16 charged with a firearms offence subject to a mandatory minimum sentence of 3 years.
4. Charged with Grave crimes with a possible sentence of more than 2 years' detention.
5. Charged with Terrorism offences.
6. Charged with a serious or complex fraud.
7. Notice given in a child case where the witness is a child (this is rarer and exceptional).
8. Where a child or young person is charged with a specified offence, and the court considers that the child or young person would meet the criteria for a sentence under the 'dangerous offender' provisions.

Family Courts

All matters relating to family cases are dealt with in the family courts or the family division of the High court. The judges normally do not wear judicial robes, and the proceedings are more informal.

Custodial Estate for Young People

As of April 2022, the secure custodial estate comprised three types of institution:

Table 6.2 Secure Estate for young people statistics

Secure Estate	Age range	Legislative framework	Capacity	Gender
Secure children's homes	10 to 17	Children Act and criminal justice	14	all
Secure training centres	12 to 17	Criminal justice	3 (2 closed)	all
Youth offender institutions	15 to 17 18 to 21	Criminal justice	5	Mainly male
Secure colleges	12 to 18	Criminal justice	1	all

1. Secure children's homes (SCHs) that accommodate vulnerable children, typically aged 10 to 17, in small establishments with a higher staff-to-child ratio.
2. Young offender institutions (YOIs), which are bigger establishments, typically accommodating children aged 15 to 17, are more similar in design to adult prisons.
3. Secure training centres (STCs) that are designed to be bigger than SCHs but smaller than YOIs. STCs typically accommodate children aged 12 to 17 who are too vulnerable for a YOI.

A new secure school/college setting is under development in the UK. The Youth Justice Board details regular statistics and trends for all children in custody in England and Wales. The Secure Estate for young people is described in Table 6.2.

Some Variations in the Devolved Nations

The age of criminal responsibility in Scotland is 12 years (Age of Criminal Responsibility (Scotland) Act 2019). Most offences committed by children between the ages of 12 and 16 years will be dealt with by early intervention or the children's hearings system (Criminal Procedure (Scotland) Act 1995). If it is a more serious crime like murder or rape, this can be taken through the courts.

The age of criminal responsibility in Northern Ireland is 10 years of age (Criminal Justice (Northern Ireland) Order 1998). Children are treated differently than adults and like the English system are dealt by youth court and for the most serious offences they may have to appear in Crown court.

References

1. HM Government, *Human Rights Act*. HM Government, 1998. Available from: https://www.legislation.gov.uk/ukpga/1998/42/contents (accessed 30 August 2024).
2. HM Government, *Mental Capacity Act*. HM Government, 2005. Available from: https://www.legislation.gov.uk/ukpga/2005/9/contents (accessed 30 August 2024).
3. R (L) v Bournewood Community and Mental Health NHS Trust [1998] UKHL 24; [1999] AC 458; [1998] 3 All ER 289; [1998] 3 WLR 107; [1998] 2 FLR 550; [1998] 2 FCR 501; [1998] Fam Law. 1998 June 25;592. Available from: http://www.bailii.org/uk/cases/UKHL/1998/24.html.

4. Gillick v West Norfolk and Wisbech AHA [1985] UKHL 7. http://www.bailii.org/uk/cases/UKHL/1985/7.html.
5. HM Government, *Mental Health Act*. HM Government, 1983 (amended 2007). Available from: https://www.legislation.gov.uk/ukpga/1983/20/contents (accessed 30 August 2024).
6. D (A Child) (Rev2) [2019] UKSC 42. http://www.bailii.org/uk/cases/UKSC/2019/42.html.
7. General Medical Council. *Confidentiality and Sharing information, Good Medical Practice*. General Medical Council, 2024. Available from: https://www.gmc-uk.org/professional-standards/professional-standards-for-doctors/protecting-children-and-young-people/confidentiality-and-sharing-information (accessed 10 September 2024).
8. Department of Health. *The Mental Health Code of Practice: 1983*. Department of Health, 2015 (updated 2017). Available from: https://assets.publishing.service.gov.uk/media/5a80a774e5274a2e87dbb0f0/MHA_Code_of_Practice.PDF (accessed 30 August 2024).
9. HM Government, *Children Act*. HM Government, 1989. Available from: https://www.legislation.gov.uk/ukpga/1989/41/contents (accessed 30 August 2024).
10. Ventress MA, Rix KJB, Kent JH. Keeping PACE: Fitness to Be Interviewed by the Police. Adv. Psychiatr. Treat. 2008;**14**(5):369–81. https://doi.org/10.1192/apt.bp.107.004093.
11. Branston G, Norton H. *Youth Defendants in the Crown Court*. October 2023. Judicial College, 2023.
12. Mc Naughton's case [1843] UKHL J16. http://www.bailii.org/uk/cases/UKHL/1843/J16.html.

Chapter 7

What Does a Good Assessment in Children and Adolescents Look Like?

Kishan Sharma[†] and Rachel Elvins

Introduction

The success or failure of a patient's journey in mental health services often hinges on the difficulties being accurately identified and formulated. Hence assessments in child and adolescent psychiatric practice are one of the more complex clinical tasks that one needs to master. It requires many attributes and skills from the clinician; a sense of curiosity about the family and their journey, like Columbo, a doggedness to get to the bottom of the 'problem' and like Sherlock Holmes a power of observation and inferencing, and a keen intellect directed towards putting all the information together to explain the present. All this to be done with a compassion for the suffering of the family and the child and skills to engage the family in what can be sometimes a difficult and convoluted process. For a trainee or a practitioner this may seem a bit daunting, as after all no one person can have all the attributes mentioned above. But learning is a lifelong process, skills can be acquired and with practice comes ability. Empathy develops with experience and a desire to do the best for the people who come to us for help. Viewed in this sense, the psychiatric assessment can be both intellectually stimulating and fulfilling to the practitioner and hopefully will instil trust and a sense of being understood for the patients. It is also worth remembering that sometimes assessments are not a single process but can happen sequentially across development with evidence gathered over a period. This is particularly true of neurodevelopmental and behavioural difficulties [1].

Purpose of the Assessment

What Is It For

The format of an assessment in Child and Adolescent Psychiatry can vary depending on the stage of the patient journey or the referral reason; for example an assessment when the patient/family first present to Child and Adolescent Mental Health Services (CAMHS) might look different to an assessment for a particular condition. The overall goals of the assessment however should be as follows:

To establish a rapport and working relationship with the patient: 'the therapeutic alliance'.

To obtain the relevant information in a manner that fosters openness and honesty.

To arrive at an understanding of the presenting difficulties in collaboration with the patient/family.

To jointly formulate a management plan in accordance, as far as is possible, with the goals and wishes of the patient.

Although the main goal of an assessment is not treatment, assessments can in themselves be therapeutic. The child and family should experience a feeling of being heard and listened to, of being understood, their difficulties empathised with and a feeling of hope for recovery. These also help in the development of a therapeutic relationship, which is key in psychiatric practice [2].

Who Is It For

Psychiatry trainees and practitioners will recognise the inherent dilemmas in an assessment process where the family and clinician may have differing goals, for example, the family may present with concerns about how to manage oppositional and dysregulated behaviours in a child, but the clinician may be trying to find out if there is an underlying problem such as ADHD. Sometimes the child may see no problem in the concerns expressed by the parents for example in eating disorders where the young person (YP) may deny any such symptoms. Lastly, there may be differing purposes between professionals. The social worker referring the family may want an assessment of the child's mental health whereas the psychiatrist may formulate that the social circumstances are giving rise to difficulties. It is always worth bearing in mind who has the concerns and what the assessment is driven by. Ultimately the assessment is about finding an adequate explanation for the difficulties experienced by children and young people (CYP) and family. In this regard it is always useful to facilitate a shared understanding of the problems that need to be addressed including that of the assessor, so that everybody is clear about the further process of management. This may take some time but is worth investing in.

In the vignette in Box 7.1 the priorities of each of the parties involved may be different. Please make a note of what you think each member may expect from the assessment including the assessor.

What Does It Involve

Broadly, an assessment involves a direct conversation or interaction with the patient, information obtained from other sources and observations in the clinic. It is essential to have a structure or systematic process to collect this information. The overall psychiatric history-taking follows the structure with which psychiatric trainees are already familiar (Box 7.2). Within this an effort should be made to gather information from different sources including parents and carers, school and other professionals involved, if appropriate. (As long as any consent/confidentiality issues have been addressed.) Direct interaction includes

---

Box 7.1 – Case Vignette

A 14-year-old boy was referred by the social worker to CAMHS requesting a psychiatric assessment. The concerns were ongoing difficulties with the young person's aggression at home and school, risky behaviours such as going missing from home and attempts to harm himself. The boy lived with his parents who had mental health difficulties themselves with another young child to care for. School was worried that the YP was not achieving and seemed very 'moody' with poor interaction in school and thought he might have autism spectrum condition. During the assessment it transpired that the YP did not really like school as he was targeted by older peers, and the YP's parents were struggling to manage the aggression at home.

> **Box 7.2 – Structure of Routine Psychiatric History Taking**
>
> Introductions
> Presenting complaints
> History of presenting complaints
> Past psychiatric history/involvement with mental health services
> Developmental history
> Medical history
> Family history
> Education history
> Social/personal history
> Forensic history
> Substance misuse
> Mental state examination
> Formulation and risk assessment

aspects of history and mental state/physical examination. Ability to carry out daily living activities, school performance, peer interactions and home circumstances are some of the examples of information that can be obtained from parents and other professionals such as teachers or social workers. Validated and standardised questionnaires may be used to elicit symptom profiles. In addition, an assessment may involve semi-structured activities in the clinic as well as observation of the child's behaviour and interaction both with assessor and the person accompanying the CYP to the clinic.

Multidisciplinary approach to assessments: On some occasions such as specialist clinics and assessment of specific conditions such as autism, assessments can involve a multidisciplinary team. The key here is good planning and joined-up working to reduce delays between one assessment to the next and ensuring not to duplicate or omit key information.

Setting the Scene

It is important to remember that this may be the first time a child, young person or a family has come to see a mental health professional. It is vital that they feel comfortable to talk about topics that are personal and sensitive in nature.

Preparation

Being prepared with the details of the patient (name, age, preferred pronouns, etc.) and familiarising yourself with the information already known helps to gain the family's confidence and shows that the practitioner is interested. Being ready with any questionnaires you might want to use and having knowledge of the clinic space will help.

The environment should be conducive to an assessment. The room should be free of clutter and seats arranged in a way to ensure comfortable conversation. Attention should be paid to the smells, sounds and lighting in the room. Opening the blinds to let the light come in or having a lamp for example can make a difference to the ambience and to the mood of the patient. Consideration should be given to developmentally appropriate spaces, both for teenagers and younger children. Appropriate toys/drawing materials/books may be helpful.

Any need for interpretation services should be identified before seeing the family. It is not generally appropriate to allow or expect children to interpret for other family members, and professionals should always be used where possible. Cultural considerations should also be considered before seeing the family and accommodated where possible and appropriate.

The practitioner should make sure they are comfortable as well. It is difficult to carry out a proper assessment on a rumbling stomach!

Introductions

The assessment generally starts by a round of introductions. Even though this might appear to be a formality, it plays an important role in helping the patient understand the professional and the role of an assessor at the time. For example the practitioner might introduce herself as 'I am X and I am here to talk to you about your worries' or that 'I am here to see how we can help you with your difficulties'. Introductions from the family will also help to know who has accompanied the child as this might not always be obvious, such as step-parents or carers. This will also help to clarify if the accompanying adult has parental responsibility.

Confidentiality

It is important to have a statement of confidentiality explaining what it involves to both the young person and to the parents. In accordance with the principles enshrined in the General Medical Council's Good Practice document [3] confidentiality can only be broken if there is an imminent risk of serious harm to the patient or others or if there are safeguarding concerns. In clinical practice this usually results in having an agreement with the young person and the parents about information that would be considered confidential and that can be disclosed based on the guidance. This will help the YP feel at ease to talk freely. It also reduces parents' anxiety and to trust that the practitioner will disclose information that relate to risk or safety so that they are well informed. When copying or sending letters to other professionals, be mindful of what is necessary for them to be aware of and what should be omitted, for example, it is not necessary or usually helpful to include family histories in letters to schools, but for the GP this could be useful information. Sending draft letters to young people/families and asking them to check for accuracy or making an agreement about what should be shared can be helpful in these circumstances.

Older children and teenagers should always be offered an opportunity to speak to you without their parent/carer being present. Some older teenagers may choose to attend the clinic by themselves. In this instance it is important to establish early on how to contact parents or carers in the event of a serious risk or safeguarding issue and what information may need to be shared or kept confidential.

Principles in Assessments of Children and Adolescents

History-Taking

All assessments begin with gathering information about the person/family in the clinic and the nature of their difficulties. Though history-taking in child and adolescent psychiatry follows a familiar structure (Box 7.2), the emphasis that one places on various aspects of history-taking may be different than when talking to adult patients. Triadic consultations (child or young person with parent/carer) need particular care and structure so that essential information is gathered, and each party feels listened and attended to. Some families may attend with other professionals, for example social workers or teachers. These interactions need structuring, and more time may be required. Thought should be given to which information can be obtained in this setting, and how it will help in formulation or differential diagnosis.

It is helpful to show an interest in the young person or child and to get to know them better before launching into questions about their problem. A social history first, asking them about their hobbies/interests, extracurricular activities and friendships or relationships can be an icebreaker. Doing this will also obtain important information that can be used later, such as exploring anhedonia in depression or anxiety related to social situations. By the end of this one should also have some understanding of the child and family's current environment both at home and school.

The presenting problems can then be explored in detail in a way familiar to all psychiatric trainees. The focus will be on the onset and progression of the difficulties, its pervasiveness and its impact on functioning. The principle of open-ended questions and encouragement to describe the experiences should be maintained but bearing in mind that some primary school-age children might not have the language or developmental understanding to describe their thoughts or experiences comprehensively. For example, in obsessive compulsive disorders the compulsions may be accurately described but not clear-cut obsessive thoughts apart from a vague feeling of discomfort [4].

As with history of the presenting problems in adults, comorbidities should be explored as well as daily functioning. Hence if someone presents with social anxiety, other aspects of anxiety [5] as well as mood and other psychiatric symptoms should be explored as well as effects on sleep, appetite and general functioning. Similarly, one should screen for developmental disorders (e.g. tics, ADHD, autism, etc.).

More time may be devoted to the developmental history. This is especially important in developmental disorders but all other emotional and behavioural problems as well. Mental disorders may present in different ways in children versus adults. Some show homotypic continuity through childhood, for example, anxiety, or heterotypic, that is, as precursors of other disorders. For example, poor self-control can be associated with later diagnosis of behavioural disorder. Knowledge of expected cognitive, emotional and social milestones as well as physical development is important, as well as an understanding of the presentations of common disorders in both sexes at various ages.

The goal should be to obtain a clear idea of developmental trajectory of the child/YP from childhood to the present. Typically, this can be done in sections of pregnancy and early years (up to age of 18 months–2 years, toddler years from 2 to 4 years), early primary school years 5–8 years and later childhood (8–11 years and adolescent years). Children go through transitions at these times and particular aspects of their development become relevant through these stages. Early temperament and attachment behaviours are typically explored between the ages of 18 months and 4 years, social development and friendships from 4 to 5 years through to primary school and so on. One of the other purposes of taking a good developmental history is to chart the current problem through development. Anxiety may be present itself as inhibited temperament and separation anxiety in school, peer related or social anxiety in primary school years or Generalised Anxiety Disorder later [5].

An educational history is valuable as children spend a large part of their day in schools and school environment plays a big part in the child's social and emotional development. A history of school performance, the support that is offered, relationship with peers and academic attainments are important as well as school moves and the reasons behind it, for example a child with undiagnosed ADHD may have moved different schools due to disruptive behaviour. Difficulties may not be reported accurately if the school is naturally already making some accommodations but have not gone through a formal process to do this, for example, carrying out an educational psychology review.

It is important to remember when requesting information from education or social care professionals that you are asking for an accurate *description* (not an opinion) of a child's behaviour in both structured and unstructured times in school. Questionnaires and outcome measures can help with this task. Teachers, support staff, educational psychologists and social care staff can all be sources of useful information. Educational processes can seem complicated, and it is important that psychiatric trainees familiarise themselves with school structures, how schools support special educational and health needs and the requirements from health care professionals to support statutory assessment (e.g. assessment for an Education, Health and Care Plan). It is equally important for doctors to familiarise themselves with local social care and safeguarding structures and processes.

Intellectual disabilities (both specific and general) may not be identified by schools or may be identified later in a child's development. Again, consideration of expected milestones and expected progress at school can help the clinician screen for such difficulties and seek more information/refer appropriately if this is suspected.

Mental State Examination

The mental state examination deserves special mention as it is not only vitally important in the assessment of children and young people but is also something that may be overlooked or not fully attempted when compared to adult patients. As before, the structure of the mental state examination is like that of adults (Box 7.3). **The key practice is to notice and accurately record the observations without making specific assumptions as to the cause of these behaviours.** We start by observing the appearance and behaviour of the CYP in the clinic and paying attention to their language/conversation, mood and their thought processes. We may also attempt a brief cognitive examination and determine their insight into their difficulties. How this might be approached and assessed is largely dependent on the developmental level of the child. In this context it will also be important to mention that 'play based assessments' are often employed in the mental state and behavioural assessments of very young children. Conversation or play with the child or the YP must be attempted, and even a negative response will give important clues to behaviours related to attachment or separation anxiety. Mental state examination happens independently but also in the context of the presenting problems and the history given. Some examples are given below, but this list is not exhaustive.

Appearance and Behaviour

Any concern about the general conditions of the CYP should immediately capture attention. A dishevelled or an unkempt child, injury marks, an older teenager with smell of alcohol or cannabis, scars or cuts and so on should be followed up appropriately. For a short while, the child or the YP in the clinic becomes the most interesting object in the room and

> **Box 7.3 – Mental State Examination**
>
> Appearance (distinctive features, grooming, clothing, hygiene).
>
> Behaviour (eye contact, posture, body language/gestures, rapport/social engagement, attitude to assessment, arousal level, unusual features, hypo/hyperactivity, anxious/aggressive).
>
> Mood and affect (low mood, anhedonia, hopelessness, etc.).
>
> Speech (tone, quantity, volume, speech rate, ease of conversation).
>
> Cognition (level of consciousness, memory, attention/concentration, orientation in time, place and person).
>
> Thoughts (content – e.g. delusions, preoccupations, ED ideas, depressive thoughts, self-harm/suicidal/harm to others/obsessions/anxiety.
>
> Process (coherence of ideas).
>
> Perception (dissociation, illusions, hallucinations).
>
> Insight (total, partial, none, evidence of ambivalence towards treatment and getting better).

every effort should be made to capture the image in detail. A good way to do this is to imagine that you will need to describe the child to another person. Like Sherlock Holmes, if you don't know what you are looking for you are unlikely to find it, hence a good knowledge of childhood psychopathology will supplement the observational skills.

Speech and Language

A careful and detailed attention to the child's language and speech helps to understand underlying mental states and possible neurodevelopmental conditions. Examples include abnormalities in tone or stereotyped speech in autism. Excessive talking may be a sign of anxiety or ADHD or paucity or retardation of speech in depression.

Mood

One should comment on both a subjective description of mood states and what is objectively observed. Enquiring into mood states can also be an opportunity to explore other emotional states (particularly in young children) such as feeling happy, sad or worried. The assessment of affect apart from giving important clues to emotional disorders is also important in developmental disorders such as autism where impairment in communication of affect is a typical feature.

Thoughts

The observation and assessment of thoughts also proceed along the same lines as adults such as paying attention to the form of thought patterns and the content themselves. Trainees in adult psychiatry are familiar with delusional ideas and thought disorder in psychotic illnesses. Other examples include chaotic thought processes in ADHD/anxiety, slowed-down thoughts or lack of understanding in intellectual disability or an excessive focus on a particular interest in autism.

The contents of the thoughts form a vital part of mental state examination in child psychiatry. The trainee needs to explore the child's mental representations of their life,

> **Box 7.4 – Activity**
>
> Go back to the Case Vignette described in Box 7.1, and make a note of things you want to observe and elicit when seeing the boy in the clinic.

important relationships and of the self in an engaging and sensitive manner, in conversation and or in play. One needs to be aware that in young children or low functioning autistic children, it may not always be that easy to elicit cognitions related to mood states such as what makes them anxious or worried or obsessions associated with compulsive behaviours.

A brief examination of cognitive function can be done in the clinic but the practicality of this is variable. One generally gets a sense of the child's cognitive ability through other means than direct testing in the clinic. Of course, when one suspects organic pathology as in assessing suspected intoxicated adolescents in A&E or in an acute psychotic episode an examination of cognitive status is important.

Insight

Insight is typically assessed as an understanding of the condition and its formulation by the patient but also the need for treatment and outcomes. Within this framework insight may not be easy to assess and determine in young children but attempts should be made.

Assessment of Risk

Though a detailed description of risk assessment is beyond the scope of this chapter, a good psychiatric assessment always encompasses an assessment of risk. When assessing risk it is good to remember that risk is more than just self-harm/suicidal risk. It is important to assess risk in several other areas in which the child and young person functions. These may include risks related to vulnerability – such as exploitation, victims of aggression, drug or alcohol misuse, risk related to dropping out/excluded from education and risk to property and other related forensic risks. In this context, a concurrent assessment of the psychosocial risk factors is essential to come to a holistic understanding of the presenting problems. They can be protective as well as offer a chance to intervene. They may be related to personal experiences such as abuse, bullying, poor care giving or environmental risk factors such as socio-economic circumstances and the family lifestyle, the neighbourhood, opportunities to pursue leisure activities, parental ill health or drug misuse. The importance of these risk factors is in their interaction with the genetic makeup and individual characteristics to give rise to psychopathology through development [6]. As such it is helpful to understand the effects these adversities have had on the YP and the family unit and how they have managed to cope with them.

Risk assessment tools for self-harm/suicide have been found to have limited clinical utility[7] and their use is not recommended by the National Institute of Health and Care Excellence [8].

Principles in Assessment of Parents/Carers and Families

One of the important areas that child psychiatric practice differs to adult practice is the fact that parents play a larger part in the reporting of difficulties and in the implementation of any treatment plan. The mental health difficulties of CYP influences and is influenced by the social and emotional environment of the family, its functioning and relationship and interactions among family members. The family can contribute to resilience and be a protective factor or equally could play a part in the maintenance of the problem [9]. For a more in-depth discussion on the impact of parental mental and physical health see Stein and Harold [10]. Parental responsibility (PR) and who has it is important to establish early on, as the person with PR may not be in the assessment but may need to be contacted to gather consent to treatment for example.

The Genogram

An accurate three-generation genogram is a vital component of a comprehensive first assessment. Psychiatry trainees should be familiar with and be able to draw a basic genogram. Relevant information can be gained from taking a thorough history of family composition/whoever is involved in care and support, and the chronology of changes to the family structure. It also helps to identify genetic loading of certain traits and disorders relevant to the assessment.

History of Parental Health and Education

Detailed information regarding both the medical and mental health problems in family members, both present and historical will be important. For example a history of parental depression/stress **may** point to an impaired dynamics/suboptimal emotional environment at home [11]. It helps to know whether parents went to mainstream schools, whether they received any support in school or struggled with their behaviours. This might give clues as to possible genetic susceptibility in the case of learning disability or developmental disorders or an estimate of parental learning and functioning that might have implications on current management.

Parental Beliefs About the Reasons for Child's Difficulties

Parental beliefs about the child's difficulties are important indicators for family functioning/parental interactions, outcomes of the assessment and the child's functioning. A parent who might blame oneself for the cause of the child's difficulties may feel guilty. Equally a parent who centres all the difficulties in the child may be less amenable to exploring environmental or systemic factors. This can also be apparent in parental histories where the information given can be coloured based on one's beliefs. This may also drive some parental help seeking behaviour.

Similarly, obtaining information about parental experiences of illness, its impact on the family and treatment history will be helpful as they may be factors in acceptance or otherwise of formulation/diagnosis and adherence to treatment.

Observation of Parent–Child Interaction in the Clinic – Parental Responses

One of the most important observation skills that a practitioner of child mental health needs to develop is that of parent and child interaction, even though the clinic is an artificial environment. Particular attention should be paid to emotional relatedness such as how does the child share delight/sadness, sharing of interests and so on, with the parent and how the parent responds. Does the parent set appropriate boundaries in the clinic and how does the child respond? Is the parent appropriately concerned or overly anxious? If there is more than one parent accompanying the child, it is important to observe how the two relate to each other.

Physical Examination

An understanding of normal physical development and morphology is equally important as is that of typical behaviour. The physical examination can be considered in two parts. One is the simultaneous observation of the child's physical appearance and movements and abilities, and the other is a formal physical examination. Observations include stature and proportions, any unusual facial features, movement and gait, pigmentation or marks/signs of injury and bruising and so on. These give important clues for investigating the underlying problem such as a genetic syndrome/neurological condition or to signs of abuse or general malnutrition as in anorexia nervosa. Observations of movement/writing skills may point to hypermobility or poor coordination, often associated with neurodevelopmental disorders. Instances where a formal physical examination can be undertaken are assessing nutritional states in eating disorders or monitoring children on antipsychotics or ADHD medication.

All psychiatric trainees should be able to conduct a routine physical examination including a basic neurological examination and to do this regularly to keep up their skills. The basic physical examination should include a general physical examination along with measurement of head circumference (plotted on a centile chart) where indicated. Measurement of height, weight and BP/pulse as well as listening to heart sounds should be done where indicated and referred to specialist care as appropriate. If one suspects dysmorphology or a genetic syndrome, one might refer to paediatrics or to the local genetics department for a more detailed examination.

Other Means of Assessments

It is true that bulk of the assessment happens in a clinical setting when interviewing children and families in face-to-face appointments. In the way current CAMHS services are structured where multiple practitioners in different settings with differing levels of experience and seniority may be involved in the assessments of the child, the use of standardised measures either in the form of structured/semi-structured interviews or questionnaires is commonly employed to make the assessments more structured and information gathered in a consistent way.

Tools to Interview Parent/Carers

These can be respondent based or interviewer based. The respondent-based tool such as the Diagnostic Interview for Children (DISC) [12] are more rigid and does not give flexibility to ask around the questions already in the tool. These do not require a high level of training. Interviewer-based semi-structured interviews are more helpful as they allow the clinicians to explore around each topic based on their clinical judgement. This does require some training on the examiners' part. Examples of these assessments include the Child and Adolescent psychiatric assessment [13], the Autism Diagnostic Interview – Revised (ADI-R) [14] or the ADHD clinical evaluation [15]. Each approach has its strengths, and a combination of the two approaches that includes an 'expert judgement' is the Development and Well-Being Assessment [16].

Services commonly employ questionnaires to screen for disorders prior to diagnosis or for ongoing treatment monitoring. **A common mistake is to assume that scores on the screening questionnaire contributes to diagnosis, but outcomes on the screening tools rely on their sensitivity and specificity and population prevalence of the disorder. Hence it is important for psychiatric trainees to be aware of the usefulness and limitations of screening instruments** (Table 7.1). The evidence for the utility of digital technology is still developing though young people are reported to engage well in this format [17].

Table 7.1 Commonly used screening instruments in child psychiatry (various sources)

Disorder/problem	Questionnaire	Age group (yrs)	Version	Usage
ADHD + related disorders (ODD/CD/aggression, etc.)	SNAP-IV	6–18	Parent and teacher Short and long versions	Cut-off scores for caseness/severity (mild, moderate and severe) Use for initial screening and symptom monitoring
	Conners 3	6–18	Parent, teacher and self Short and long versions	T Scores/clinical cut-offs/severity Use for initial screening and short version for symptom monitoring
	ADHD rating scale	5–18 + adults	Parent and teacher ratings	For screening and monitoring response to treatment
Autism	Social Communication Questionnaire (SCQ)	4 +	Lifetime and current version Lifetime version parent/carer rated	Cut-off for possible ASD/autism Useful as screening tool
	Social Responsiveness Scale (SRS)	4–18	Parent and teacher ratings	T Scores indicating overall severity of autism-related symptoms + individual dimensions
Anxiety and depression	Revised Child Anxiety and Depression Scale (RCADS)	8–18	Parent and self-rated	Gives clinical thresholds for anxiety disorders and depression Use for screening and symptom monitoring
	Moods and Feelings Questionnaire (MFQ)	8–18	Long and short Parent and self-rating	Symptoms of depression in the last 2 weeks. Total score. No cut-offs. Best used to monitor change

Table 7.1 (cont.)

Disorder/ problem	Questionnaire	Age group (yrs)	Version	Usage
	Spence Children's Anxiety scale	8–15	Parent and self-report versions	Subscales for specific anxiety disorders. Has an online self-scoring version
Eating disorders	Eating Disorders Examination – Questionnaire (EDE-Q)	14 +	Self-reported	Adapted from EDE. Gives four subscales (restraint, eating, shape and weight concerns). Use for assessment and monitoring
General psychopathology	Strengths and Difficulties Questionnaire (SDQ)	3–16	Parent/teacher and self-Report versions	Widely used. Best for screening for broad psychopathology Useful impact supplement

Observational Assessments

Most observations in the assessment are carried out in the context of a mental state examination. However, sometimes it is helpful to accurately and systematically record observations including observation of the behaviour in response to tasks. A commonly employed observational paradigm is a playground or a classroom observation of a child's behaviour. Though this can be done by a competent practitioner who knows what to look for, the Manchester Inventory for Playground Observation [18] is an example of a tool to systematically record playground behaviour.

Another popular semi-structured clinical observational assessment done with children is the Autism Diagnostic Observation Schedule (ADOS) [19] which requires training and is used concurrently with the ADI-R. Similarly the Manchester Child Attachment Story Task is a structured play-based assessment to determine the nature of attachment in children up to 8 years of age [20].

Specialist Assessments

Some assessments are not done by psychiatrists but nonetheless psychiatrists will direct the need for these additional specialist assessments to be undertaken by the wider team. Hence, it is good to be aware of the indications for these assessments and how you can use them to inform psychiatric assessments and outcomes.

Assessments of Cognitive Functioning

Most assessments of cognitive functioning in children are undertaken by educational psychologists for purposes of assessments of learning and support required in school. These take the form of 'ability' assessments such as a the Wechsler Intelligence Scale for children-Fifth Edition (WISC-V) or tests of 'attainment' such as the Wechsler Individual Attainment Test. It is important for psychiatry trainees to understand in what circumstances and for what purposes schools might request these assessments (see above paragraph) and how to obtain copies of reports if they will assist in the psychiatric formulation. Nonetheless, it is often clinically useful to have an estimate of the child's abilities and developmental level as some of the behaviours assessed by child psychiatrists, such as inattention or social skills, are assessed against the child's general intellectual development. In addition, children with ASC or ADHD, for example, may have a discrepant cognitive profile. It is important when we are assessing a child with intellectual disability to understand their profile of strengths and weaknesses in order to plan interventions (e.g. children with poor auditory processing may need visual prompts.

Speech and Language Assessments (SAL)

The SAL assessment in psychiatric practice is usually a part of an holistic assessment of a CYP's developmental difficulties. It is important to distinguish what could be a specific language impairment compared to a deficit in social communication or a purely communication deficit as opposed to autism. Where speech and language therapists may be involved independently in the community, obtaining copies of the assessment or having a conversation with them can greatly enhance our understanding of the CYP difficulties.

Occupational Therapy Assessment (OT)

OT assessments are increasingly being recognised for their value in helping us understand not only a CYP's daily functional skills but a breadth of developmental difficulties such as motor control deficits and sensory symptoms. They often provide an avenue for meaningful interventions such as sensory diet, motor planning resources and adaptations to daily living, which are especially valuable in CYP with intellectual disabilities.

Formulation and Diagnosis

The time now comes to put together all the assessments that have been done into a coherent narrative that not only explains the concerns and observed difficulties but points to potential avenues for intervention. Traditionally a formulation or a diagnosis are the two ways to go about this, but a combined one is the best. A formulation attempts to pull together all the relevant factors in the patient's presentation and weave them into a coherent narrative-based explanation of the difficulties in that particular patient. The formulation is ideally done with the patient and family but practically a formulation may be arrived at which is then shared and fine tuned in collaboration with the family. The formulation is also a way of strengthening the rapport with the family, helping them to buy in and engage with the treatment process [21]. A diagnosis set outs to identify the core features in the presentation that helps to 'categorise' the problem into known psychiatric disorders. It is a way to convey this message in broad impersonal terms, in a way that makes sense for other professionals and treatment planning. If one has more proclivity towards a diagnostic system, the multiaxial system of diagnosis, either ICD orDSM, is an attempt to bring together additional relevant factors akin to a formulation. A formulation or a diagnosis may be preferred depending on the scenario where they may be helpful, parent preference and the presenting problem. Psychiatric trainees should make an effort to do both, that is, have a differential diagnosis and a preferred one as well as attempt a formulation.

One of the first hurdles that come the way of child psychiatry trainees is the variability and sometimes the contradictory information that appears when gathering info from different sources. For example the school questionnaire may show very few features of ADHD whereas parent questionnaires may show high levels of difficulties. In these scenarios, it is helpful to have a system to make sense of this information and how much importance should be given to which source. Psychiatric trainees and practitioners should persist in their efforts to establish the pervasiveness of difficulties as this is essential for a psychiatric diagnosis. Hence, in the presence of contradictory information, more avenues to obtain samples of reported difficulties should be sought such as observing a child in school or requesting specialist assessments. It is helpful to be aware that children in different settings may genuinely show slightly different behaviours and different people involved with the child see different things. For example a teacher may observe a slightly different set of difficulties or differing intensity of similar difficulties, compared to a clinician in the clinic or a parent at home [22]. However, one still needs to explain the apparent contradictions within the overall formulation much like a pieces of a jigsaw puzzle.

One of the core competencies of psychiatry training is to recognise one's limitations and take action accordingly and trainees and practitioners should always seek supervision/not hesitate to request a second opinion if it is not possible to reach a conclusion in spite of all the above efforts.

Formulations can be done in various ways depending on the background and the preferences of the practitioner. The following are examples of commonly used methods to arrive at a formulation.

4 Ps – Predisposing, Precipitating, Perpetuating and Protective

The condition of the patient can be explained by identifying the components of aforementioned areas and then weaving them together to come to an explanation. This approach has the advantage of not just underlying factors but also identifying areas of resilience that can be used to build on in treatment.

Bio Psycho Social

First introduced by Engel [23], the bio psycho social approach to formulations is a popular one where an effort is made to identify the strengths and weaknesses in all aspects of a patient's life and history. Biological factors include medical/genetics factors, psychological factors include current state of mind and thought patterns and social factors include the state of home/school environment, parenting, socio-economic status and so on. The advantage of this approach is to help the practitioner think holistically about the patient's difficulties and also has the added advantage of mapping intervention onto similar biopsychosocial domains.

> **Box 7.5 – Formulation Activity**
>
> Try and apply the above models of formulation to explain the presentation of the young person we came across earlier. For example in the 4 Ps model, the predisposing factors are parental mental health difficulties and possibly change in family composition whereas the same can be explained as biological vulnerability in terms of the biopsychosocial model.

Developmental

This approach preferred by developmentalists has the advantage of answering the 'why' question at a proximate level. It weaves together vulnerability and early adversity and how they interact with development and further life events leading to psychopathology. It brings together evidence-based pathways of development while at the same time identifying the unique life trajectory of the individual.

Managing expectations: Though this is not directly related to assessment skills, it is an important aspect of child psychiatric practice and one that really sets the tone of future relationship with services. Understandably, in matters relating to CYP there may be high levels of worry and anxiety on the part of parents and professionals, but the desire to make a lasting and significant difference is also great. This is of course the aspiration of every clinician but realistically one must understand the limitations on one's practice. It is best to be open and honest about the impact of individual treatments and the evidence base. For example, medications for conditions such as ADHD and psychotic disorders have strong evidence behind them; less so medicines for eating disorders and the core symptoms of ASC. That said, the strength of psychiatric practice is to be able to empathise with the patient, take a holistic view of patients' difficulties through a multidisciplinary approach to assessments and most importantly as a consequence, offer treatment in more than one domain.

Feedback on Assessments

Where doing an assessment accurately and comprehensively is more of a science using evidence-based tools, applying logic and observational skills and having knowledge of the subject, feeding back the outcome to families and conveying the right message is an art, honed through practice. Feeding back the outcome is not just about letting families know what the end product of the assessment is but is a communication that takes into account parental expectations and views, the context in which the assessment was conducted and the implications of the outcome both for the child/young person and the family. Sometimes it may take more than one session and might involve involving other members of the team. The outcome can be a negative or a positive depending on the parental expectations. A lack of diagnosis at the end of the assessment might mean that the family feels that their difficulties are not being recognised, and they will not get any help. Equally, for some families, a diagnosis might mean stigma and a notion of disability. Formulations can be equally divisive, if the formulation involves significant systemic influences, parents might feel blamed and sometimes formulation on its own might not mean much for a patient who is looking for a name or a 'label' for the difficulties they experience.

Feedback of the assessments is best done face-to-face with the family and to involve the young person where possible. It is good to take the family through their journey within the service highlighting the reasons for various assessments done at that point in time and explaining the outcomes. The final impressions should be conveyed in a sensitive manner with the clinician being aware of the personal journey of the family and the implications of the diagnosis. For example many families may be relieved at the diagnosis of autism as they have been given an explanation for their child's difficulties, but some families may be worried about the impact of such a diagnosis on life and further education and social functioning.

Families come to services with a particular set of difficulties, and potential solutions should be part of the feedback process. Where possible families should be signposted to relevant support groups. Information given regarding websites may help, and support that is available both with in the service and outside should be discussed. Where there is clear indication for intervention such as an antidepressant medication, this should be part of the feedback. Time should be given to families to process the information and opportunity given to ask questions or clarify. The importance of getting the buy-in from the child or young person regarding the diagnosis or formulation cannot be stressed enough, as this leads to greater insight and better engagement with treatment which predicts outcome [24].

Summary

To summarise, the psychiatric assessment is probably the most important starting point for the patient in their engagement with services. An accurate and comprehensive assessment minimises further surprises down the road and reduces the chances of premature discharge and revolving door scenarios. As discussed, it requires skills of observation, interaction and knowledge of child development and subject matter on the part of the examiner. It requires the practitioner to be open minded and work with different professionals and incorporate conflicting information. Above all, crucial to a good assessment is an interest in the person in front of us and a curiosity about their journey to this point. Ultimately, a good assessment that reasonably summarises the available evidence, which is greeted with nods of approval and statements like 'that makes sense' from the family, gives the family and young person a hope for change. To be willing partners in the next step of the journey is a satisfying experience.

References

1. Rutter M, Kim-Cohen J, Maughan B. Continuities and Discontinuities in Psychopathology Between Childhood and Adult Life. J Child Psychol Psychiatry. 2006;47:276–95.
2. Green J. Annotation: The Therapeutic Alliance – A Significant but Neglected Variable in Child Mental Health Treatment Studies. J Child Psychol Psychiatry. 2006;47:425–35.
3. General Medical Council. *Confidentiality: Good Practice in Handling Patient Information.* 2017. Available from: https://www.gmc-uk.org/professional-standards/the-professional-standards/confidentiality (accessed 24 March 2025).
4. Grados, A Labuda, MC, Riddle MA, Walkup JT. Obsessive-Compulsive Disorder in Children and Adolescents. Int Rev Psychiatry. 1997;9:83–98.
5. Beesdo K, Knappe S, Pine DS. Anxiety and Anxiety Disorders in Children and Adolescents: Developmental Issues and Implications for DSM-V. Psychiatr Clin North Am. 2009;32:483–524.
6. Assary E, Vincent JP, Keers R, Pluess M. Gene-Environment Interaction and Psychiatric Disorders: Review and Future Directions. Semin Cell Dev Biol. 2018;77:133–43.
7. Quinlivan L, Cooper J, Meehan D, et al. Predictive Accuracy of Risk Scales Following Self-Harm: Multicentre,

8. National Institute for Health and Care Excellence. *Self-Harm: Assessment, Management and Preventing Recurrence, NICE guideline NG225*. National Institute for Health and Care Excellence, 2022. Available from: https://www.nice.org.uk/guidance/ng225 (accessed 4 April 2025).

9. Harold GT, Sellers R. Annual Research Review: Interparental Conflict and Youth Psychopathology: An Evidence Review and Practice Focused Update. J Child Psychol Psychiatry. 2018;59:374–402.

10. Stein A, Harold G. Impact of Parental Psychiatric Disorder and Physical Illness. In A Thapar, DS Pine, JF Leckman, S Scott, MJ Snowling, EA Taylor (eds.), *Rutter's Child and Adolescent Psychiatry*. 6th ed. John Wiley & Sons Ltd., 2018, 352–63.

11. Smith M. Parental Mental Health: Disruptions to Parenting and Outcomes for Children. Child Htmlent Glyphamp Asciiamp Fam Soc Work. 2004;9:3–11.

12. Shaffer D, Fisher P, Lucas CP, Dulcan MK, Schwab-Stone ME. NIMH Diagnostic Interview Schedule for Children Version IV (NIMH DISC-IV): Description, Differences from Previous Versions, and Reliability of Some Common Diagnoses. J Am Acad Child Adolesc Psychiatry. 2000;39:28–38.

13. Angold A, Costello EJ. The Child and Adolescent Psychiatric Assessment (CAPA). J Am Acad Child Adolesc Psychiatry. 2000;39:39–48.

14. Lord C, Rutter M, Le Couteur A. Autism Diagnostic Interview-Revised: A Revised Version of a Diagnostic Interview for Caregivers of Individuals with Possible Pervasive Developmental Disorders. J Autism Dev Disord. 1994;24:659–85.

15. Young S. *ADHD Child Evaluation: A Diagnostic Interview of ADHD in Children*. Psychology Services Limited, 2015. Available from: https://www.adhdfoundation.org.uk/wp-content/uploads/2024/02/Dr-Susan-Young-ACE-ADHD-RATING-SCALES-INFORMATION-AND-LIN KS-ADHDF-website-text-Feb-2024.pdf (accessed 4 April 2025).

16. Goodman R, Ford T, Richards H, Gatward R, Meltzer H. The Development and Well-Being Assessment: Description and Initial Validation of an Integrated Assessment of Child and Adolescent Psychopathology. J Child Psychol Psychiatry. 2000;41:645–55.

17. Punukollu M, Marques M. Use of Mobile Apps and Technologies in Child and Adolescent Mental Health: A Systematic Review. Evid Based Ment Health. 2019;22:161–66.

18. Gibson J, Hussain J, Holsgrove S, Adams C, Green J. Quantifying Peer Interactions for Research and Clinical Use: The Manchester Inventory for Playground Observation. Res Dev Disabil. 2011;32:2458–66.

19. Lord C, Risi S, Lambrecht L, et al. [No title found]. J Autism Dev Disord. 2000;30:205–23.

20. Green J, Stanley C, Smith V, Goldwyn R. A New Method of Evaluating Attachment Representations in Young School-Age Children: The Manchester Child Attachment Story Task. Attach Hum Dev. 2000;2:48–70.

21. Baird J, Hyslop A, Macfie M, Stocks R, Van der Kleij T. Clinical Formulation: Where It Came From, What It Is and Why It Matters. BJPsych Adv. 2017;23:95–103.

22. Garcia-Rosales A, Vitoratou S, Faraone SV, et al. Differential Utility of Teacher and Parent–Teacher Combined Information in the Assessment of Attention Deficit/Hyperactivity Disorder Symptoms. Eur Child Adolesc Psychiatry. 2021;30:143–53.

23. Engel GL. The Biopsychosocial Model and the Education of Health Professionals? Ann N Y Acad Sci. 1978;310:169–81.

24. Segarra R, Ojeda N, Peña J, et al. Longitudinal Changes of Insight in First Episode Psychosis and Its Relation to Clinical Symptoms, Treatment Adherence and Global Functioning: One-Year Follow-Up from the Eiffel Study. Eur Psychiatry. 2012;27:43–49.

Neurodevelopmental Disorders in Children and Young People

Catherine J. Gregory, Hannah Slevin and Shruti Garg

Introduction

'Neurodevelopmental disorders' (NDDs) are an umbrella term for a heterogeneous group of conditions that begin early in the developmental period and likely persist throughout one's lifetime. They may affect both cognitive and social communication development, and display sex differences with males more likely to be affected [1]. Many of these conditions co-occur, suggesting a shared underlying neurobiological aetiology. These conditions may be distinguished from other childhood disorders such as anxiety or mood disorders, in that they are developmental in origin and lack the episodic course. NDDs are thought to affect up to 10% of children in the UK [2]. Children with NDDs frequently present to Children and Adolescent Mental Health Services (CAMHS), where the developmental disability may either be the primary presenting problem or co-occur with other emotional or behavioural difficulties.

The classification of NDDs has been problematic and subject to much debate. There have been important changes in this diagnostic category in ICD-11 as compared to ICD-10, summarised in Table 8.1. Despite these changes, it can be argued that this diagnostic category is no longer clinically useful, given the widely heterogeneous conditions included, with varying presenting symptomatology. Furthermore, the language used to describe these diagnostic categories is radically at odds with the social model of disability advocated by those with lived experiences, such that these conditions are not 'disorders' but rather brain differences that are part of a continuum rather than a deficit. 'Neurodiversity' is the preferred term used to describe the experience of neurological variance outside the cognitive norm. The language used matters to parents and patients as it helps define whether individuals experience inclusion and opportunities, and redefines the power imbalances between clinicians and service users. While we use the ICD-11 language to describe the conditions in this chapter, our own clinical practice is consistent with the neurodiversity-affirming language.

Case Examples

We illustrate the approach taken for the assessment of NDDs using the two following case examples.

Case 1

Muhammad, an 8-year-old boy, was brought to clinic by his parents. His mother had a history of epilepsy and was on Valproate during pregnancy. Muhammad was born at term, with no delivery complications. He had trigonocephaly, epicanthic folds, a flat nasal

Table 8.1 Differences between ICD-10 and ICD-11 classification of neurodevelopmental disorders

ICD-10 Disorders of psychological development	ICD-11 Neurodevelopmental disorders
	6A00 Disorders of intellectual development
F80 Specific developmental disorders of speech and language	**6A01 Developmental speech or language disorders**
F80.0 Specific speech articulation disorder	6A01.0 Developmental speech sound disorder
F80.1 Expressive language disorder	6A01.1 Developmental speech fluency disorder
F80.2 Receptive language disorder	6A01.2 Developmental language disorder
F80.3 Acquired aphasia with epilepsy (Landau-Kleffner syndrome)	6A01.20 Developmental language disorder with impairment of receptive and expressive language
F80.8 Other developmental disorders of speech and language	6A01.21 Developmental language disorder with impairment of mainly expressive language
F80.9 Developmental disorder of speech and language, unspecified	6A01.22 Developmental language disorder with impairment of mainly pragmatic language
	6A01.23 Developmental language disorder with other specified language impairment
	6A01.Y Other specified developmental speech or language disorders
	6A01.Z Developmental speech or language disorders, unspecified
F84 Pervasive developmental disorders	**6A02 Autism Spectrum Disorder**
F84.0 Childhood autism	6A02.0 Autism spectrum disorder without disorder of intellectual impairment and with mild or no impairment of functional language
F84.1 Atypical autism	6A02.1 Autism spectrum disorder with disorder of intellectual development and with mild or no impairment of functional language
F84.2 Rett Syndrome	6A02.2 Autism spectrum disorder without disorder of intellectual development and with impaired functional language
F84.3 Other childhood disintegrative disorder	6A02.3 Autism spectrum disorder with disorder of intellectual development and with impaired functional language
F84.4 Overactive disorder associated with mental retardation and stereotyped movements	6A02.5 Autism spectrum disorder with disorder of intellectual development and with absence of functional language
F84.5 Asperger's syndrome	6A02.Y Other specified autism spectrum disorder
F84.8 Other pervasive developmental disorders	6A02.Z Autism spectrum disorder, unspecified
F84.9 Pervasive developmental disorder, unspecified	

F81 Specific developmental disorders of scholastic skills
F81.0 Specific reading disorder
F81.1 Specific spelling disorder
F81.2 Specific disorder of arithmetic skills
F81.3 Mixed disorder of scholastic skills
F81.8 Other developmental disorders of scholastic skills
F81.9 Developmental disorder of scholastic skills, unspecified

F82 Specific developmental disorder of motor function

F83 Mixed specific developmental disorders

Behavioural and emotional disorders with onset usually occurring in childhood and adolescence

F90 Hyperkinetic disorders
F90.0 Disturbance of activity and attention
F90.1 Hyperkinetic conduct disorder
F90.8 Other hyperkinetic disorders
F90.9 Hyperkinetic disorder, unspecified

Behavioural and emotional disorders with onset usually occurring in childhood and adolescence

F95 Tic disorders
F95.0 Transient tic disorder

6A03 Developmental learning disorder
6A03.0 Developmental learning disorder with impairment in reading
6A03.1 Developmental learning disorder with impairment in written expression
6A03.2 Developmental learning disorder with impairment in mathematics
6A03.3 Developmental learning disorder with other specified impairment of learning
6A03.Z Developmental learning disorder, unspecified

6A04 Developmental motor coordination disorder

6A05 Attention deficit hyperactivity disorder
6A05.0 Attention deficit hyperactivity disorder, predominantly inattentive presentation
6A05.1 Attention deficit hyperactivity disorder, predominantly hyperactive-impulsive presentation
6A05.2 Attention deficit hyperactivity disorder, combined presentation
6A05.Y Attention deficit hyperactivity disorder, other specified presentation
6A05.Z Attention deficit hyperactivity disorder, presentation unspecified

6A06 Stereotyped movement disorder

8A05.0 Primary tics or tic disorders (primary classification elsewhere)
8A05.00 Tourette syndrome
8A05.1 Chronic motor tic disorder
8A05.2 Chronic phonic tic disorder
8A05.3 Transient motor tics

Table 8.1 (cont.)

ICD-10 Disorders of psychological development	ICD-11 Neurodevelopmental disorders
F95.1 Chronic motor or vocal tic disorder	8A05.0Y Other specified primary tics or tic disorders
F95.2 Combined vocal and multiple motor tic disorder (de la Tourette)	8A05.Z Primary tic or tic disorders, unspecified
F95.8 Other tic disorders	
F95.9 Tic disorder, unspecified	
	6E60 Secondary neurodevelopmental syndrome
F88 Other disorders of psychological development	6A0Y Other specified neurodevelopmental disorders
F89 Unspecified disorder of psychological development	6A0Z Neurodevelopmental disorders, unspecified

bridge and a shallow philtrum. Following discharge, he struggled to feed and gain weight. As he progressed to solid food, he was a picky eater, preferring only 'beige' food. His motor and language milestones were delayed, and he walked at 24 months. He developed single words by 36 months and phrase speech by 4 years. He started nursery at 30 months but struggled to separate from his mum. In Reception, he was quiet and compliant. However, he struggled with phonics and writing, and the school put extra support in place for him. In primary school, he was on the periphery of friendship groups. He circled the playground at lunch time, only joining in when encouraged to do so. His mum reported that he rarely played, preferring to watch YouTube videos about dinosaurs. He was clumsy and often fell over, preferred to use his fingers while eating, and struggled to clean himself after using the toilet. He needed prompting to get ready for school and often his mum found him daydreaming if she did not hurry him up.

Case 2

Olivia is a 15-year-old girl who presented to the clinic with her mother. She was a bright young person, academically able and a competitive dancer. Olivia described that she struggled to fit in and had often wondered what was 'wrong' with her. Her mother described Olivia's highly structured routine during the week, dancing up to 2 hours every evening and travelling to dance competitions at the weekends. Her mother described that Olivia was keen to have close friends, but struggled to fit in with her peers. She was often blunt and condescending of her peers, disapproving of their choice of clothes and make-up. She lacked an understanding of how some of her comments might hurt others. A careful neurodevelopmental history revealed that although she met her developmental milestones, her childhood language mostly mimicked that of characters in favourite TV shows, and she was extremely sensitive to environmental noise. As she grew older, she struggled to understand sarcasm, idioms or the meaning behind others' comments. She had received a course of Cognitive Behavioural Therapy in the past for anxiety, which was impacting on her school attendance. In recent months, she had begun to develop repetitive blinking, twitching of her neck and shoulders and regular grunting, all of which she tried to suppress at school. Her main concern was that this was beginning to impact her dancing performance.

Neurodevelopmental Assessment

Crucial stages of a neurodevelopmental assessment include obtaining a detailed developmental history, careful observation of the child and obtaining collateral information, particularly from the child's educational setting. A multidisciplinary assessment approach is key. The clinician should be alerted to the likelihood of co-occurring conditions, as NDDs rarely occur in isolation and often overlap. Indeed, research suggests that as many as 50% of children meeting criteria for one neurodevelopmental disorder also meet criteria for at least one other [3].

Multidisciplinary Approach for Assessment of NDDs

A neurodevelopmental assessment is best carried out using a multidisciplinary approach. An assessment by the Community Paediatrics Service is crucial if concerns arise about the child's physical health and to rule out underlying genetic conditions that may increase the likelihood of NDDs. Certain genetics conditions have a high prevalence of NDDs, such as Fragile X, Tuberous Sclerosis and Neurofibromatosis Type 1 [4], but these will present relatively infrequently to clinicians in mental health settings.

A Speech and Language Therapy assessment can provide an understanding of the child's core language and social communication abilities. Hearing and visual impairments should be screened to check for any concerns about speech development or inattention. If underlying learning difficulties are suspected, a psychometric assessment is indicated to assess for core learning abilities to highlight specific aspects of learning that require additional support. An Occupational Therapist is well placed to assess co-ordination or sensory processing difficulties. Collateral information, including reports from teachers, can provide crucial insights into the child's academic attainment, peer interactions, attention, concentration and behaviour.

Developmental History

A careful developmental history should be obtained by the clinician, to identify when concerns first began to emerge and how these have changed or progressed over time [4]. This should include assessment of exposure to alcohol or drugs in utero, prematurity and perinatal infections. [5]. As in Case 1, exposure to Valproate and other antiepileptics are known to cause Foetal Valproate Syndrome with an increased likelihood of co-occurring autism, ADHD and learning disability [6]. Other important areas to consider include the progression of the pregnancy and the birth of the child (including gestational age, method of delivery, delivery complications and condition of the child at birth, including whether any neonatal resuscitation or time in intensive care was required). Attainment of motor, language and social developmental milestones in the first years of life, and any evidence of delay, should be explored. The temperament of the child, difficulties with feeding or toilet training and physical health issues are also important areas to elicit.

The clinician should seek to develop an understanding of how the child began to interact with other children as they grew older, and whether there were any associated difficulties such as struggling to form and maintain friendships, overly intrusive interaction, lack of imaginative play or repetitive rituals. The child's use of language, including reciprocal conversation, understanding of sarcasm or idiom and overly literal interpretation of language should be explored. Parents/carers may recall feedback from nursery or school settings about their child's development, learning, attention and peer interactions. Asking to see previous school reports if available can be useful if the parent cannot recall early educational feedback.

Psychosocial Assessment and Family History

The clinician should explore the psychological development and current mental state of the child, considering differential or co-occurring diagnoses such as conduct disorders, anxiety, depression, obsessive compulsive disorder and attachment disorders [4]. Specifically enquiring about tics is important, both in terms of diagnosis, co-morbidity and treatment planning.

The domains of sleep and appetite are important to explore. Sleep disturbance is highly prevalent in children with NDDs, presenting as either insomnia or hypersomnia [7]. Children with ASD may exhibit particular rigidity in relation to food preferences, while understanding the appetite of children with ADHD is important given that stimulant medications may impair appetite and thereby cause weight loss.

A sensitive exploration of the psychosocial environment of the child can reveal difficulties such as parental mental illness or substance misuse, traumatic experiences such as abuse and neglect, bereavements, housing difficulties and parental involvement with the Criminal Justice System. Understanding these factors means that multi-agency support can be offered to the child and their family. Moreover, research suggests that ACEs and neurodevelopmental conditions often co-exist and have an additive effect on harmful child health outcomes [8].

Obtaining a family history, including family members with NDDs, other mental health illnesses and genetic conditions is important as NDDs are highly heritable [9]. Screening for consanguinity between parents or grandparents is relevant, as this may increase the risk of autosomal recessive genetic conditions.

Observation of the Child

Clinicians should engage with and observe the child, either in-clinic or an educational setting. A mental state assessment should be carried out to assess for underlying anxiety and mood. Impulsive or compulsive behaviours, sensory sensitivities and rituals may be apparent. The child's play and topics of interest can be elicited through providing toys, drawing materials and engaging in joint play. Observing the child both in structured settings (such as the classroom) and unstructured settings (such as the playground) can be extremely helpful in understanding communication and social interaction skills, behaviour including impulsivity and the ability to maintain attention and gross and fine motor abilities. Finally, a referral to clinical genetics may be considered if there are signs of dysmorphology.

Evidence suggests that autistic characteristics in female children may present in ways that differ from traditional diagnostic criteria, leading to under-recognition of ASD [10]. As in Case example 2, autistic females may have similar levels of social motivation as non-autistic females, but find it more difficult to maintain longer-term friendships than autistic males [11]. Moreover, autistic female children are more likely than males to experience internalising difficulties such as anxiety and depression [10].

Rating Scales and Assessments

Various validated self-report questionnaires are available to assist with the diagnosis of NDDs, all of which have varying sensitivities and specificities. For ADHD, the SNAP-IV, Conners Rating Scales or ADHD Rating Scale are commonly used in clinical practice [12,13,14]. These can be completed by parents/carers or teachers. For ASD, the SCQ (Social Communication Questionnaire) and SRS (Social Responsiveness Scale) can also be completed by parents/carers and teachers[15,16].

In terms of clinician-led assessments, the Quantified Behavioural test is a computer-based assessment that examines core ADHD symptoms of hyperactivity, impulsivity and inattention. It is used as an adjunct as part of a clinical assessment, and also in evaluating the impact of treatment for ADHD [17]. For ASD, the ADI-R (Autism Diagnostic Interview Revised) is a semi-structured interview for parents [18]. The ADOS-2 (Autism Diagnostic Observation Schedule) is a semi-structured assessment of social communication, social interaction and imaginative play. Different modules are used depending on the expressive communication level of the child [19].

It should be remembered that rating scales and clinician-led assessments are not diagnostic in themselves, but used to add further evidence to a clinical diagnosis of ASD or ADHD.

Neurodevelopmental Disorders

Autism Spectrum Disorder

ASD is characterised in ICD-11 by pervasive difficulties with social communication and interaction as well as excessive restricted and repetitive behaviours [20]. These are clearly outside the limits of normal variation expected for age and intellectual development, and cause significant impairment in functioning. These difficulties will arise during the early developmental period but in some individuals the diagnosis may only be recognised later in life, as social demands increase in complexity. ASD is characterised as a 'spectrum disorder' because these difficulties can manifest and impact differentially between individuals and across the lifespan. Examples of social communication and interaction difficulties might include difficulties understanding and modulating behaviour in social situations, difficulties in holding reciprocal conversation, or in forming and sustaining relationships. Restrictive and repetitive behaviours may include sensory sensitivities, excessive adherence to routine or intense interests. The prevalence of ASD is around 1% [21], with 4-fold higher rates in males compared to females [22]. ASD is commonly co-morbid with other NDDs, psychiatric disorders such as depression and anxiety, and disorders of intellectual development [23].

The heritability of ASD is estimated to be between 50% and 90%, with a 10-fold higher likelihood with an affected sibling [24], suggesting that genetic factors play a substantial role in its aetiology. A large number of genetic variants, each conferring a small increased risk [25] including genes involved in neurotransmitter signalling, epigenetics and synaptogenesis [26] have been implicated in ASD. Genetic conditions such as Fragile X, Tuberous Sclerosis and Neurofibromatosis 1 are associated with higher rates of ASD [27]. Perinatal environmental factors that increase the likelihood of ASD include preterm birth, obstetric complications such as hypoxic injury, increasing maternal and paternal age, maternal exposure to alcohol and medications such as valproic acid, infections during pregnancy such as rubella and maternal conditions such as diabetes [28,29]. For a comprehensive review of ASD genetics, please see Manoli and State [30].

Pathological Demand Avoidance

Pathological Demand Avoidance (PDA) is a term used to describe a set of behaviours including resistance to routine daily demands with socially manipulative strategies of avoidance, along with social difficulties, lability of mood and obsessive behaviour [31]. Clinicians are likely to encounter this term used by parents and families to refer to the difficulties faced by their children, although it does not appear as a diagnostic entity in the ICD-11 or DSM-V, and its existence as a separate diagnostic entity is controversial. Overlap with ASD is well recognised, but it has been argued that there are features distinct from ASD including an equal prevalence between girls and boys, the prominence of socially manipulative behaviour, a comfort with role playing and fantasy and a positive response to unpredictability [32]. Proponents argue that PDA responds to an approach distinct from that of ASD, emphasising flexibility, spontaneity and sensitivity to the child's needs [32].

Other authors have argued that there is insufficient evidence for the validity of PDA as an independent diagnosis. Rather, it has been argued that it can best be seen as part of the spectrum of difficulties seen in ASD, and that assessment of these difficulties should take place within a wider neurodevelopmental assessment, including a thorough exploration of challenging behaviours [31]. For a review of this condition, we refer the reader to Green et al [31].

Attention Deficit Hyperactivity Disorder

ADHD is characterised in ICD-11 by pervasive difficulties with inattention and/or impulsivity and hyperactivity, beyond that expected for age and level of intellectual ability, and which cause significant impairment in functioning [20]. The diagnosis is subdivided according to whether difficulties are predominantly inattentive, hyperactive-impulsive or both. Onset of symptoms must have occurred before the age of 12, although the diagnosis may only be made later in life. Inattention may manifest as difficulties including distractibility, inability to sustain concentration on a given task, forgetfulness or disorganisation. Impulsivity can manifest as interrupting, difficulty in waiting their turn, it can manifest in younger children as concerns over road safety or, in the case of adolescents, risk-taking behaviour. Hyperactivity may present as excessive activity, difficulty remaining seated or excessive fidgeting. ADHD is associated with adverse outcomes including impairment of social relationships, poor school attainment, criminality and substance misuse. It often co-occurs with other neurodevelopmental and psychiatric disorders [33]. In the UK, the prevalence of ADHD is estimated to be 3–4%, with a male to female ratio of 3:1 [34]. Twin studies have shown high heritability of ADHD ranging from 74% to 88% [35], with reports of a 9-fold increased risk with an affected sibling [36]. ADHD is a polygenic disorder, with overlap between the genetic risk of ADHD and other NDDs and psychiatric disorders [35,37,38]. Several genes have been reported to be involved in the aetiology; for a comprehensive review see Faraone and Larsson [39]. Environmental factors that increase the likelihood of ADHD include preterm birth, maternal use of medications such as valproic acid in pregnancy, maternal conditions such as pre-eclampsia and obesity, exposure to environmental toxins such as phthalates and lower socio-economic status [33].

Specific Disorders of Development and Language

These disorders arise in the developmental period and describe specific difficulties that significantly impair functioning and are below the expected level for age and general intellectual ability.

Developmental Speech or Language Disorders

Developmental speech or language disorders are characterised by ICD-11 as difficulties in the understanding, production or use of language [20]. These disorders are further subcategorised as follows:

- *Developmental speech sound disorder* refers to difficulties with the production of speech and errors in pronunciation.
- *Developmental speech fluency disorder* refers to disruption of the flow or rate of speech.
- *Developmental language disorder* is characterised by difficulties with the understanding, production or use of language and is further subdivided according to whether the

difficulties are predominantly expressive or also affect receptive (understanding of) language. A further subdivision, a new addition in ICD-11, refers to 'impairment of mainly pragmatic language' which is characterised by difficulties in the understanding and use of language in a social context. This should not be used if the child's difficulties are better explained by ASD.

Developmental Learning Disorder

Developmental learning disorders are characterised in ICD-11 as 'significant and persistent difficulties in learning academic skills', markedly below the level expected for age and intellectual functioning, and causing a significant impact on functioning [20]. They are subdivided according to whether the main difficulty lies with reading, writing or mathematics.

Developmental Motor Coordination Disorder

Developmental motor coordination disorder, also known as dyspraxia, is characterised in ICD-11 by impairment in the acquisition and execution of gross and fine motor skills, significantly below the expected level for age and intellectual functioning [20]. There is increasing evidence that impaired executive functioning is also a feature of dysphraxia, including difficulties with working memory, inhibition and attention, although this does not form part of the diagnostic criteria [40]. Prevalence is estimated to be around 5% [41]. The cause of these disorders is unclear and is likely to be multifactorial. There is evidence for heritability of these conditions, and a number of genetic variations have been implicated [42], although genome-wide association studies have generally failed to find variants of significance [43]. Environmental factors such as low birth weight or preterm birth are predictors of dyspraxia [40]. Dyspraxia often co-occurs with other NDDs such as ADHD (50% co-occurrence), which poses diagnostic challenges given some of the symptom overlap such as attention difficulties [41].

Primary Tics or Tic Disorders

These disorders are primarily categorised in ICD-11 under 8A05 'tic disorders' under the umbrella of movement disorders in diseases of the nervous system. However, they also appear under NDDs. Tics are characterised in ICD-11 as 'sudden, rapid, non-rhythmic, and recurrent movements or vocalisations' [20]. In order to diagnose chronic tics, they must be present for at least 1 year, although they may present with a waxing and waning course. *Tourette syndrome* is characterised by the presence of both chronic motor and vocal tics, with onset during the developmental period. *Chronic motor tic disorder* and *chronic phonic tic disorder* are characterised by the presence of solely motor or vocal (phonic) tics, respectively. Motor tics present for less than 1 year are characterised as *transient motor tics*.

The prevalence of tics has been reported as 19–24% in children, with the prevalence of Tourette syndrome of 0.4–3%. Like other NDDs, they are 3-fold more common in males [44]. Tourette syndrome is commonly comorbid with other neurodevelopmental and psychiatric conditions, in particular ADHD and obsessive-compulsive disorder (OCD), with evidence for a shared underlying genetic risk factors [44,45].

Dysfunction of neurotransmission, particularly dopamine, has been implicated in the pathophysiology of tics [46,47,48]. Perinatal environmental factors such as maternal alcohol and smoking and low birth weight have been associated with tic disorders, but evidence is conflicting [44]. There is limited evidence for a condition known as paediatric autoimmune neuropsychiatric disorders, associated with acute onset of tics or OCD following streptococcal infection, although the existence of this as a diagnostic entity remains controversial [44,49].

Summary of the Key Differences Between ICD-10 and ICD-11

The progression from ICD-10 to ICD-11 has brought with it a number of changes to the classification of NDDs, mirroring those seen in DSM-V [50]. The term 'Autism Spectrum Disorder' in ICD-11 replaces a range of diagnoses present in ICD-10 (childhood autism, atypical autism and Asperger syndrome). ICD-11 recognises subtypes of ASD based on co-occurring intellectual or functional language impairment. ICD-11 also removes the requirement for onset before the age of 3 years, recognising that symptoms may not be manifest until later, when social demands exceed inherent capacity. The term 'attention deficit hyperactivity disorder' replaces the diagnosis of hyperkinetic disorders used in ICD-10 and removes the requirement for onset of symptomatology before the age of 5 years. Importantly, consistent with empirical evidence and clinical practice, a diagnosis of ASD and ADHD can be made concurrently, which was precluded in ICD-10.

Treatment Approaches

General Principles

Psychoeducation for both the parent/carer and the young person is crucial in the management of NDDs, to enable an understanding of the difficulties the young person may encounter and how best to support them [51,52]. Environmental modifications should be considered as the first line and will depend on the difficulties the young person experiences. These may include a lower stimulus environment, such as access to a quiet room at school, support during unstructured play times and the use of ear defenders if sensitivity to noise is present. Aids such as visual timetables and simple steps to support understanding, such as breaking instructions down into steps with visual prompts, can be helpful [51].

Management of NDDs should be multidisciplinary in approach. Liaison with education providers is important and consideration should be given to whether they would benefit from specialist assessment of their educational needs. Input from Speech and Language Therapy may be beneficial to make recommendations to support the young person's pragmatic understanding and use of language, and this is often accessed via education. Young people presenting with significant sensory sensitivities or impairment of motor skills may benefit from assessment by Occupational Therapy, which can make recommendations to support them in these areas.

Children with NDDs, particularly ASD, can sometimes present with challenging behaviours. A thorough functional assessment of such behaviours should be carried out to identify the antecedent interpersonal and environmental triggers for these behaviours [51]. Environmental modifications and psychosocial interventions are recommended as first line. The use of medication to manage challenging behaviour should be limited to situations where such interventions have failed and where the behaviour presents significant distress or risk. Antipsychotic medication such as risperidone or aripiprazole can be used in such situations and should be short term and reviewed frequently [25,51].

Co-morbid psychiatric disorders should be actively considered and treated as appropriate. Interventions such as cognitive behaviour therapy (CBT) may need to be modified [51]. The first line of management of sleep disturbance should be a thorough assessment of the sleep difficulties by means of a sleep diary, sleep hygiene advice and consideration of any modifiable factors that may be affecting sleep [51]. If sleep disturbance persists, melatonin can be considered, which may be helpful in reducing sleep-onset latency[51,53].

Interventions for Specific Disorders

Autism Spectrum Disorder

A number of psychosocial interventions have been developed, aimed at modifying the interactions between the caregiver and child, with the hope that this may translate to improved social interaction more generally. The field has been hampered by significant heterogeneity between studies and poor methodological quality, but there is some evidence that such interventions can improve caregiver communicative responsiveness, sensitivity and synchrony [54]. It is less clear whether this translates into improved social communication on the part of the child and still less whether this is generalisable across other contexts.

A range of compounds targeting neurobiological pathways implicated in the pathogenesis of ASD have been studied, including glutamatergic antagonists such as memantine, Gama-Aminobutyric Acid agonists such as arbaclofen, agents enhancing dopamine activity such as methylphenidate, selective serotonin reuptake inhibitors and oxytocin. Evidence for the efficacy of such drugs is limited and does not currently support the use of medication to treat the core symptoms of ASD in clinical practice [25,54].

The best evidence for psychosocial intervention is Preschool Autism Communication Treatment. This targets social communication and interaction difficulties by improving parental sensitivity to their child's communication through the use of video feedback, and by teaching positive communication strategies [27]. A complete review of current psychosocial interventions is included in the reviews by Green et al and Gosling et al [27,55].

Attention Deficit Hyperactivity Disorder

There is good evidence to support the efficacy of medications for ADHD, particularly for the efficacy and tolerability of methylphenidate in children and adolescents, supporting its use as first-line medication as per NICE (National Institute for Health and Care Excellence UK) guidance [52,56,57]. Methylphenidate (and alternatives such as dexamfetamine or its prodrug lisdexamfetamine) is a stimulant medication, acting primarily as a dopamine and noradrenaline reuptake inhibitor to boost activity in the prefrontal cortex and improve executive functioning [58]. Side effects include nausea, headaches, reduced appetite and weight loss, sleep disturbance, emotional lability and potential stimulant effects on the heart, such as raised pulse and blood pressure [58]. Baseline assessment, including cardiovascular assessment and regular monitoring of height, weight, blood pressure and pulse, must be carried out [52,57]. Non-stimulant medications are advised by NICE as second line therapies [52]. Atomoxetine is a noradrenaline reuptake inhibitor, with additional effects on dopamine reuptake in the prefrontal cortex. Guanfacine is an alpha-2 adrenergic agonist which enhances noradrenergic transmission in the prefrontal cortex [58]. NICE guidance recommends ADHD-focused parent-training and environmental modifications as first line for children under the age of 5, but states that medication can be considered as second line following specialist opinion [52]. For children aged 5 and over, it recommends medication be considered if significant impairment remains after environmental modification (although it acknowledges that the use of medication in children aged 5, or under, constitutes 'off-label' use).

A number of non-pharmacological interventions have been studied in relation to ADHD, but the quality of the evidence base is generally poor [59]. Behavioural training for parents is reported to reduce oppositional behaviours and promote positive parenting strategies, but evidence for an improvement in the core symptoms of ADHD is poor [60]. Studies of neurofeedback techniques and cognitive training have shown conflicting results [59]. The evidence base around dietary interventions is insufficient, although a small benefit of supplementation with free fatty acids has been reported [61].

Specific Disorders of Development and Language

The evidence base around interventions for specific disorders of development and language is limited, with significant heterogeneity of inclusion criteria and interventions trialled. Young people with developmental speech or language disorders should receive input from Speech and Language Therapy. A meta-analysis of speech and language interventions for children with primary speech and language disorder noted these limitations but reported efficacy for expressive difficulties and limited evidence for receptive difficulties [62]. Young people with developmental learning disorders can be assessed within school, and may benefit from specialist assessment by an Educational Psychologist. Young people with developmental motor coordination disorder should receive input from Occupational Therapy.

Tic Disorders

The first-line treatment for tic disorders is recommended to be psychoeducation and behavioural interventions, with evidence for the efficacy of Habit Reversal Training (which aims to increase awareness of tics and encourage the expression of a physically incompatible response to prevent its occurrence) and Exposure and Response Prevention (suppressing the tics in a graded fashion) [63]. Medication can be considered if the tics cause distress or impair functioning, but the evidence base is generally poor, with some evidence for efficacy of aripiprazole, risperidone, clonidine and guanfacine, the latter two particularly where tics are comorbid with ADHD [64,65]. This is an 'off-label' use of such medication. Early evidence for median nerve stimulation as a possible treatment for tics is emerging [66].

Conclusion

In summary, NDDs are a heterogeneous group of conditions that are commonly encountered within CAMHS and often co-occur within an individual child. Advances have been made in recent years in our understanding of these conditions, although the interplay of underlying genetic, neurobiological and environmental factors in the aetiology remains to be fully elucidated. The evidence base for some treatments is well established; however, non-pharmacological interventions in particular require further research focus. Assessment and treatment approaches require a multidisciplinary approach, placing the needs and concerns of the child and family at the centre.

References

1. Bolte S, Neufeld J, Marschik PB, Williams ZJ, Gallagher L, Lai MC. Sex and Gender in Neurodevelopmental Conditions. Nat Rev Neurol. 2023;**19**(3):136–59.

2. Alexander RT, Langdon PE, O'Hara J, et al. Psychiatry and Neurodevelopmental Disorders: Experts by Experience, Clinical Care and Research. Br J Psychiatry. 2021;**218**(1):1–3.

3. Kaplan BJ, Dewey DM, Crawford SG, Wilson BN. The Term Comorbidity Is of Questionable Value in Reference to Developmental Disorders: Data and Theory. J Learn Disabil. 2001;**34**(6):555–65.

4. National Institute for Health and Care Excellence. *Autism Spectrum Disorder in Under 19s: Recognition, Referral and Diagnosis*. National Institute for Health and Care Excellence, 2011. Available from: https://www.nice.org.uk/guidance/cg128.

5. Mithyantha R, Kneen R, McCann E, Gladstone M. Current Evidence-Based Recommendations on Investigating Children with Global Developmental Delay. Arch Dis Child. 2017;**102**(11):1071–76.

6. Clayton-Smith J, Bromley R, Dean J, et al. Diagnosis and Management of Individuals with Fetal Valproate Spectrum Disorder: A Consensus Statement from the European Reference Network for Congenital Malformations and Intellectual Disability. Orphanet J Rare Dis. 2019;**14**(1):180.

7. Robinson-Shelton A, Malow BA. Sleep Disturbances in Neurodevelopmental Disorders. Curr Psychiatry Rep. 2016;**18**(1):6.

8. Gajwani R, Minnis H. Double Jeopardy: Implications of Neurodevelopmental Conditions and Adverse Childhood Experiences for Child Health. Eur Child Adolesc Psychiatry. 2023;**32**(1):1–4.

9. Gidziela A, Ahmadzadeh YI, Michelini G, et al. A Meta-analysis of Genetic Effects Associated with Neurodevelopmental Disorders and Co-occurring Conditions. Nat Hum Behav. 2023;**7**(4):642–56.

10. Hull L, Petrides KV, Mandy W. The Female Autism Phenotype and Camouflaging: A Narrative Review. Rev J Autism Dev Disord. 2020;**7**(4):306–17.

11. Hiller RM, Young RL, Weber N. Sex Differences in Autism Spectrum Disorder Based on DSM-5 Criteria: Evidence from Clinician and Teacher Reporting. J Abnorm Child Psychol. 2014;**42**(8):1381–93.

12. Bussing R, Fernandez M, Harwood M, et al. Parent and Teacher SNAP-IV Ratings of Attention Deficit Hyperactivity Disorder Symptoms: Psychometric Properties and Normative Ratings from a School District Sample. Assessment. 2008;**15**(3):317–28.

13. Conners CK, Pitkanen J, Rzepa, SR. Conners 3rd Edition (Conners 3; Conners 2008). In JS Kreutzer, J DeLuca, B Caplan (eds.), *Encyclopedia of Clinical Neuropsychology*. 3rd ed. New York: Springer, 2011, 675–78.

14. DuPaul GJ, Reid R, Anastopoulos AD, Lambert MC, Watkins MW, Power TJ. Parent and Teacher Ratings of Attention-Deficit/Hyperactivity Disorder Symptoms: Factor Structure and Normative Data. Psychol Assess. 2016;**28**(2):214–25.

15. Constantino JN, Abbacchi AM, Lavesser PD, et al. Developmental Course of Autistic Social Impairment in Males. Dev Psychopathol. 2009;**21**(1):127–38.

16. Rutter M, Bailey, A, Lord C. *The Social Communication Questionnaire*. Western Psychological Services, 2003.

17. National Institute for Health and Care Excellence. *QbTest for the Assessment of Attention Deficit Hyperactivity Disorder (ADHD)*. National Institute for Health and Care Excellence, 2023. Available from: https://www.nice.org.uk/advice/mib318.

18. Lord C, Rutter M, Le Couteur A. Autism Diagnostic Interview-Revised: A Revised Version of a Diagnostic Interview for Caregivers of Individuals with Possible Pervasive Developmental Disorders. J Autism Dev Disord. 1994;**24**(5):659–85.

19. Lord C, Risi S, Lambrecht L, et al. The Autism Diagnostic Observation

Schedule-Generic: A Standard Measure of Social and Communication Deficits Associated with the Spectrum of Autism. J Autism Dev Disord. 2000;30(3):205–23.
20. World Health Organisation. *ICD-11 for Mortality and Morbidity Statistics*. World Health Organisation, 2022. Available from: https://icd.who.int/browse11/l-m/en.
21. Baird G, Simonoff E, Pickles A, et al. Prevalence of Disorders of the Autism Spectrum in a Population Cohort of Children in South Thames: The Special Needs and Autism Project (SNAP). Lancet. 2006;368(9531):210–15.
22. Maenner MJ, Shaw KA, Baio J, et al. Prevalence of Autism Spectrum Disorder Among Children Aged 8 Years – Autism and Developmental Disabilities Monitoring Network, 11 Sites, United States, 2016. MMWR Surveill Summ. 2020;69(4):1–12.
23. Bougeard C, Picarel-Blanchot F, Schmid R, Campbell R, Buitelaar J. Prevalence of Autism Spectrum Disorder and Co-morbidities in Children and Adolescents: A Systematic Literature Review. Front Psychiatry. 2021;12:744709.
24. Sandin S, Lichtenstein P, Kuja-Halkola R, Larsson H, Hultman CM, Reichenberg A. The Familial Risk of Autism. JAMA. 2014;311(17):1770–77.
25. Howes OD, Rogdaki M, Findon JL, et al. Autism Spectrum Disorder: Consensus Guidelines on Assessment, Treatment and Research from the British Association for Psychopharmacology. J Psychopharmacol. 2018;32(1):3–29.
26. Rodriguez-Gomez DA, Garcia-Guaqueta DP, Charry-Sánchez JD A, et al. A Systematic Review of Common Genetic Variation and Biological Pathways in Autism Spectrum Disorder. BMC Neurosci. 2021;22(1):60.
27. Green J, Garg S. Annual Research Review: The State of Autism Intervention Science: Progress, Target Psychological and Biological Mechanisms and Future Prospects. J Child Psychol Psychiatry. 2018;59(4):424–43.
28. Ornoy A, Weinstein-Fudim L, Ergaz Z. Prenatal Factors Associated with Autism Spectrum Disorder (ASD). Reproductive Toxicology. 2015;56:155–69.
29. Muhle RA, Reed HE, Stratigos KA, Veenstra-VanderWeele J. The Emerging Clinical Neuroscience of Autism Spectrum Disorder: A Review. JAMA Psychiatry. 2018;75(5):514–23.
30. Manoli, DS, State, MW. Autism Spectrum Disorder Genetics and the Search for Pathological Mechanisms. Am J Psychiatry. 2021;178(1):30–38.
31. Green J, Absoud M, Grahame V, et al. Pathological Demand Avoidance: Symptoms but Not a Syndrome. Lancet Child Adolesc Health. 2018;2(6):455–64.
32. O'Nions E, Viding E, Greven CU, Ronald A, Happé F. Pathological Demand Avoidance: Exploring the Behavioural Profile. Autism. 2014;18(5):538–44.
33. Faraone SV, Banaschewski T, Coghill D, et al. The World Federation of ADHD International Consensus Statement: 208 Evidence-Based Conclusions about the Disorder. Neurosci Biobehav Rev. 2021;128:789–818.
34. National Institute for Health and Care Excellence. *Attention Deficit Hyperactivity Disorder: Clinical Knowledge Summary*. National Institute for Health and Care Excellence, 2023. Available from: https://cks.nice.org.uk/topics/attention-deficit-hyperactivity-disorder/ (accessed 4 April 2025).
35. Faraone SV, Larsson H. Genetics of Attention Deficit Hyperactivity Disorder. Mol Psychiatry. 2019;24(4):562–75.
36. Chen W, Zhou K, Sham P, et al. DSM-IV Combined Type ADHD Shows Familial Association with Sibling Trait Scores: A Sampling Strategy for QTL Linkage. Am J Med Genet B Neuropsychiatr Genet. 2008;147B(8):1450–60.
37. Demontis D, Walters RK, Martin J, et al. Discovery of the First Genome-Wide Significant Risk Loci for Attention Deficit/Hyperactivity Disorder. Nat Genet. 2019;51(1):63–75.

38. Brainstorm C, Anttila V, Bulik-Sullivan B, et al. Analysis of Shared Heritability in Common Disorders of the Brain. Science. 2018; 360(6395):eaap8757.

39. Faraone SV, Larsson H. Genetics of Attention Deficit Hyperactivity Disorder. Mol Psychiatry. 2019;24(4):562–75.

40. Meachon EJ, Zemp M, Alpers GW. Developmental Coordination Disorder (DCD): Relevance for Clinical Psychologists in Europe. Clin Psychol Eur. 2022;4(2):e4165.

41. Blank R, Barnett AL, Cairney J, et al. International Clinical Practice Recommendations on the Definition, Diagnosis, Assessment, Intervention, and Psychosocial Aspects of Developmental Coordination Disorder. Dev Med Child Neurol. 2019;61(3):242–85.

42. Kang C, Drayna D. Genetics of Speech and Language Disorders. Annu Rev Genomics Hum Genet. 2011;12(1):145–64.

43. Graham SA, Fisher SE. Understanding Language from a Genomic Perspective. Annu Rev Genet. 2015;49(1):131–60.

44. Ueda K, Black KJ. A Comprehensive Review of Tic Disorders in Children. J Clin Med. 2021;10(11):2479.

45. Yang Z, Wu H, Lee PH, et al. Investigating Shared Genetic Basis Across Tourette Syndrome and Comorbid Neurodevelopmental Disorders Along the Impulsivity-Compulsivity Spectrum. Biol Psychiatry. 2021;90(5):317–27.

46. Greydanus DE, Tullio J. Tourette's Disorder in Children and Adolescents. Transl Pediatr. 2020;9(Suppl 1):S94–S103.

47. Levy AM, Paschou P, Tümer Z. Candidate Genes and Pathways Associated with Gilles de la Tourette Syndrome-Where Are We? Genes (Basel). 2021;12(9):1321.

48. Buse J, Schoenefeld K, Münchau A, Roessner V. Neuromodulation in Tourette Syndrome: Dopamine and Beyond. Neurosci Biobehav Rev. 2013;37(6):1069–84.

49. Set KK, Warner JN. Tourette Syndrome in Children: An Update. Curr Probl Pediatr Adolesc Health Care. 2021;51(7):101032.

50. Stein DJ, Szatmari P, Gaebel W, et al. Mental, Behavioral and Neurodevelopmental Disorders in the ICD-11: An International Perspective on Key Changes and Controversies. BMC Med. 2020;18(1):21–.

51. National Institute for Health and Care Excellence. *Clinical Guideline CG170: Autism Spectrum Disorder in Under 19s: Support and Management*. National Institute for Health and Care Excellence, 2013. Available from: https://www.nice.org.uk/guidance/cg170.

52. National Institute for Health and Care Excellence. *NICE Guideline NG87: Attention Deficit Hyperactivity Disorder: Diagnosis and Management*. National Institute for Health and Care Excellence, 2018. Available from: https://www.nice.org.uk/guidance/ng87.

53. Wilson S, Anderson K, Baldwin D, et al. British Association for Psychopharmacology Consensus Statement on Evidence-Based Treatment of Insomnia, Parasomnias and Circadian rhythm Disorders: An Update. J Psychopharmacol. 2019;33(8):923–47.

54. Green J, Garg S. Annual Research Review: The State of Autism Intervention Science: Progress, Target Psychological and Biological Mechanisms and Future Prospects. J Child Psychol Psychiatry. 2018;59(4):424–43.

55. Gosling CJ, Cartigny A, Mellier BC, Solanes A, Radua J, Delorme R. Efficacy of Psychosocial Interventions for Autism Spectrum Disorder: An Umbrella Review. Mol Psychiatry. 2022;27(9):3647–56.

56. Cortese S, Adamo N, Del Giovane C, et al. Comparative Efficacy and Tolerability of Medications for Attention-Deficit Hyperactivity Disorder in Children, Adolescents, and Adults: A Systematic Review and Network Meta-analysis. Lancet Psychiatry. 2018;5(9):727–38.

57. Bolea-Alamañac B, Nutt DJ, Adamou M, et al. Evidence-Based Guidelines for the Pharmacological Management of Attention Deficit Hyperactivity Disorder: Update on Recommendations from the British Association for

Psychopharmacology. J Psychopharmacol. 2014;28(3):179–203.

58. Mechler K, Banaschewski T, Hohmann S, Häge A. Evidence-Based Pharmacological Treatment Options for ADHD in Children and Adolescents. Pharmacol Ther. 2022;230:107940.

59. Coghill D, Banaschewski T, Cortese S, et al. The Management of ADHD in Children and Adolescents: Bringing Evidence to the Clinic: Perspective from the European ADHD Guidelines Group (EAGG). Eur Child Adolesc Psychiatry. 2023;32(8):1337–61.

60. Daley D, van der Oord S, Ferrin M, et al. Behavioral Interventions in Attention-Deficit/Hyperactivity Disorder: A Meta-Analysis of Randomized Controlled Trials Across Multiple Outcome Domains. J Am Acad Child Adolesc Psychiatry. 2014;53(8):835–47, 847.e1–5.

61. Stevenson J, Buitelaar J, Cortese S, et al. Research Review: The Role of Diet in the Treatment of Attention-Deficit/Hyperactivity Disorder – An Appraisal of the Evidence on Efficacy and Recommendations on the Design of Future Studies. J Child Psychol Psychiatry. 2014;55(5):416–27.

62. Law J, Garrett Z, Nye C. Speech and Language Therapy Interventions for Children with Primary Speech and Language Delay or Disorder. Cochrane Database Syst Rev. 2003;2003(3):CD004110.

63. Andrén P, Jakubovski E, Murphy TL, et al. European Clinical Guidelines for Tourette Syndrome and Other Tic Disorders-Version 2.0. Part II: Psychological Interventions. Eur Child Adolesc Psychiatry. 2022;31(3):403–23.

64. Roessner V, Eichele H, Stern JS, et al. European Clinical Guidelines for Tourette Syndrome and Other Tic Disorders-Version 2.0. Part III: Pharmacological Treatment. Eur Child Adolesc Psychiatry. 2022;31(3):425–41.

65. Besag FM, Vasey MJ, Lao KS, Chowdhury U, Stern JS. Pharmacological Treatment for Tourette Syndrome in Children and Adults: What Is the Quality of the Evidence? A Systematic Review. J Psychopharmacol. 2021;35(9):1037–61.

66. Iverson AM, Arbuckle AL, Ueda K, et al. Median Nerve Stimulation for Treatment of Tics: Randomized, Controlled, Crossover Trial. J Clin Med. 2023;12(7):2545.

Intellectual Disabilities in Children and Young People

Mark Lovell and Ashley Liew

Introduction

Intellectual Disabilities are common, and children or young people with ID may present to Children and Adolescent Mental Health Services (CAMHS) for assessment or for the treatment of co-occurring conditions. Intellectual Disabilities have been known by many names over the years. Unfortunately, they have often ended up as pejoratives, so terminology has needed to progress. With each iteration, the words used have become more descriptive and less insulting. There are still differences in preference regarding which terms to use, though internationally in both research and clinically, the term of choice is currently Intellectual Disability [1]. Descriptors are person first rather than condition first, so it is a person with an intellectual disability.

What Is an Intellectual Disability?

An Intellectual Disability (ID) is defined by 2 main parameters: (1) an Intelligence Quotient (IQ) more than 2 standard deviations below the mean and (2) adaptive functioning, also 2 standard deviations below the mean (see Figure 9.1) These have to have been evident in the developmental period, that is, childhood [2].

Definition of IQ

IQ is defined as Mental age / Chronological age x 100. This equation generally only works within the developmental period. When in adulthood, the mental age (developmental age) may not progress further, and while chronological age increases, IQ doesn't decrease as you get older, so adjustments are made to the IQ equation to maintain stability as people age. Historically it was considered to be a stable construct over time; however, IQ results may vary depending on the test used, the circumstances in which it was conducted and may be affected by variations in developmental trajectories with not all children developing in the same ways. IQ is made up of a variety of cognitive skills and these vary depending upon the test used, For example, verbal reasoning, non-verbal reasoning, working memory and processing speed. The separate domains are combined to give an overall IQ.

Definition of Adaptive Behaviours

Adaptive behaviours relate to the behaviours and skills required to function in daily life and normally vary based upon chronological age and developmental expectations. They include communication (e.g. written, receptive and expressive skills), daily living skills (e.g. personal,

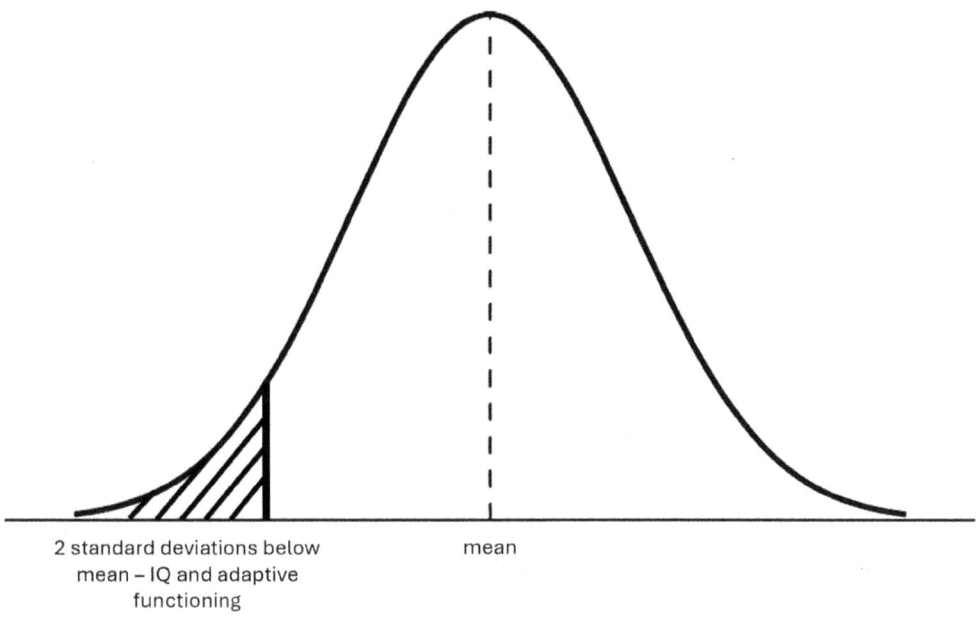

Figure 9.1 Normal distribution indicating ID at 2 standard deviations below mean

at home and in the community) and socialisation skills (e.g. play, occupation, coping, interpersonal skills and relationships).

Previously, diagnosing an ID often focused on specific IQ cut-offs with differences between the 2 major classification systems with ICD-10 [3] having a cut-off of 69 and below and DSM-IV [4] a cut-off of 70 and below. The newer systems of ICD-11 [5] and DSM-5 [2] use standard deviations and centiles as their cut-offs, though in practice they equate to the same equivalent levels of developmental delay.

4 Levels of ID

There are 4 levels of ID with a provisional level that can apply whenever firm diagnosis of either of the 4 levels cannot be made.

Mild

Intellectual functioning and adaptive behaviour are approximately 2 to 3 standard deviations below the mean (approximately 0.1 – 2.3 percentile), based on appropriately normed, individually administered standardised tests. Difficulties will be exhibited in the acquisition and comprehension of complex language concepts and academic skills. Most master basic self-care, domestic and practical activities. Appropriate support may be required in adulthood to live independently or sustain employment.

Moderate

Intellectual functioning and adaptive behaviour are approximately 3 to 4 standard deviations below the mean (approximately 0.003 – 0.1 percentile), based on appropriately normed, individually administered standardised tests. Language and capacity for acquisition of academic skills vary but are generally limited to basic skills. Some may manage basic self-care, domestic and practical activities. Considerable consistent support may be required to achieve independent living and employment as adults.

Severe
Intellectual functioning and adaptive behaviour are approximately 4 or more standard deviations below the mean (less than approximately the 0.003rd percentile), based on appropriately normed, individually administered standardised tests. Very limited language and capacity for acquisition of academic skills are demonstrated. There may also be motor impairments and daily support is required in a supervised environment for adequate care, basic self-care skills may be acquired with intensive training.

Profound
Intellectual functioning and adaptive behaviour are found to be approximately 4 or more standard deviations below the mean (approximately less than the 0.003rd percentile), based on individually administered appropriately normed and standardised tests. Very limited communication abilities are demonstrated and the capacity for acquisition of academic skills is restricted to basic concrete skills. Co-occurring motor and sensory impairments or common and daily support in a supervised environment is often required for adequate care.

Note that standardised tests of intelligence cannot reliably or validly distinguish among individuals with intellectual functioning below the 0.003rd percentile, thus Severe and Profound Disorders of Intellectual Development are differentiated exclusively on the basis of adaptive behaviour differences.

Provisional
A Provisional Disorder of Intellectual Development is when there is evidence of a Disorder of Intellectual Development, but the individual is an infant or child under the age of 4, making it difficult to ascertain whether the observed impairments represent a transient delay. This is sometimes referred to as Global Developmental Delay. The diagnosis can also be given in individuals 4 years of age or older when evidence is suggestive of a Disorder of Intellectual Development but it is not possible to conduct a valid assessment of intellectual functioning and adaptive behaviour owing to motor or communication impairments, sensory or physical impairments (e.g. blindness, pre-lingual deafness), severe behavioural problems or the presence of another Mental, Behavioural or Neurodevelopmental Disorder that interferes with assessment [5].

Causes of Intellectual Disabilities
The specific cause for most children's ID is usually unknown, but may include a range of factors that interfere with brain development and/or functioning. These factors include:

Genetics
Studies demonstrate that below average intelligence is heritable [6], and certain genetic conditions are associated with a higher prevalence of ID. Examples include:
- Down Syndrome (Trisomy 21)
- Fragile X Syndrome (due to a mutation of the FMR1 gene)

- Smith-Magenis Syndrome (due to a microdeletion of chromosome 17p12)
- Phenylketonuria (resulting in an inborn error of metabolism)
- Tuberous Sclerosis

Interesting examples of genetic conditions include Prader-Willi Syndrome (due to a paternal derived deletion at 15q11-13 or uniparental disomy) that results in mainly Mild-Moderate ID and Angelman Syndrome (due to a maternal derived deletion at 15q11-13 or a mutation of the UBE3A gene) that results in mainly Severe-Profound ID.

Environmental

These include difficulties at birth like being deprived of oxygen, being born pre-term or at a low birth weight. Maternal infections when pregnant such as rubella and toxoplasmosis can also increase ID in the infant. Maternal consumption of alcohol can result in Fetal Alcohol Spectrum Disorder that may also present with ID although this is often mild in degree [7]. Other factors after birth, such as experiencing the complications of an infection, for example, meningitis or measles, sustaining a serious head injury or being exposed to toxic substances like lead, can also cause ID.

Assessment of Intellectual Disabilities

IQ Measurement

IQ is measured using standardised psychometric tests. These are tests that have been researched to measure with a high level of specificity and sensitivity. They have specific tests and subtests that measure different components of cognition, for example, verbal comprehension, fluid reasoning, visuo-spatial, processing speed and working memory. The results are standardised to different populations and there are different language versions available. Results are presented with 95% confidence intervals and care should be taken to ensure that the results are interpretable. It is possible to underscore, but far less likely for there to be an overscore (but not impossible on some of the subtests, where guessing can inflate a score). Examples of tests are the Wechsler Intelligence Scale for Children (WISC)©, Wechsler Preschool and Primary Scale of Intelligence, Wechsler Adult Intelligence Scale, Wechsler Nonverbal Scale of Ability and British Ability Scales. Typically, psychologists administer these tests, although there are some abridged tests that can be carried out by other professionals, for example, the Quick Test [8] or Kaufman Brief Intelligence Test. Unfortunately, these are not validated for children and adolescents.

Adaptive Behaviours Measurement

Adaptive Behaviours can be measured using standardised tools such as the Vineland Adaptive Behaviour Scales [9] or Adaptive Behaviour Assessment System [10]. Sometimes formal testing may not be possible, for example if psychometric tests or psychometric testing expertise is not available or a child either declines to do a test or is unable. On these occasions, all forms of developmental information may be used to conclude a likelihood of an ID, even though an actual level will not be possible to diagnose.

The IDIDA2H© framework [11] can act as a guide to collecting information and making decisions or plans and is set out as follows:

A- **Academic Information.** Are they operating at less than 70% of their chronological age? Has there been enough engagement and opportunity with learning to have progressed.
B- **Adaptive Behaviours.** What is the developmental equivalence of their daily living skills. Is it at less than 70% of expected?
C- **Formal Cognitive Testing.** Is it globally delayed, or specific delays more than 2 standard deviations below the mean? Is there evidence from formal testing? Is it consistent over time. Did the child engage with the tests? Are the results interpretable?
D- **Developmental Information.** Most are significantly delayed from birth, unless there are reasons for a significant deterioration in development after a normal developmental period, for example, a head injury.
E- **Environmental Factors.** Are there reasons external to the child for delays in development, for example, neglect, non-attendance at school.
F- **Other Factors.** Are there any other reasons for delays, for example, genetic conditions related to brain development, severe epilepsy or exposure to neurotoxins.
G- **Global Impression.** Is it likely the child has, or hasn't got an ID? Or, is more information needed to make a decision. For younger children, a provisional diagnosis of ID may be required (previously called global developmental delay).

Investigations like blood tests and genetic testing may also be considered if there are features on history and examination that may indicate a possible cause or identification of a genetic syndrome [12].

Differential Diagnoses and Co-occurring Disorders

The main differential diagnoses for an ID are other neurodevelopmental disorders. This is because any condition that affects the development of the brain will lead to delays or differences in the way an individual thinks or acts. This results in overlaps in the developmental presentations of the different neurodevelopmental disorders, despite each having separate diagnostic criteria. In addition to this, they also commonly co-occur.

Figure 9.2 below shows the prevalence of Mental Disorders as categorised by the ICD-10.

Autism Spectrum Disorder (ASD)

Autism was covered in more detail in Chapter 8 – Neurodevelopmental Disorders in Children and Young People. Many of the symptoms and signs of autism are normal at a younger developmental stage from the communication differences to the repetitive behaviours, interests, imagination, play and sensory preferences. Autism co-occurs with ID in about 50% of autistic children [13] and can resemble ID even if IQ is above ID range owing to the communication delay and difficulties in adaptive behaviours. Refusal to engage with non-preferred tasks or to generalise learnt skills may also lead to an overlap in presentation with ID through difficulties in learning new skills and non-engagement with education and subsequent lowered academic progress [14].

Attention Deficit Hyperactivity Disorder (ADHD)

ADHD was covered in more detail in Chapter 8. ADHD is more common in ID, but all three major symptom clusters of ADHD (poor attention, hyperactivity and impulsivity) are normal at a younger developmental stage so developmental age/stage needs to be kept in

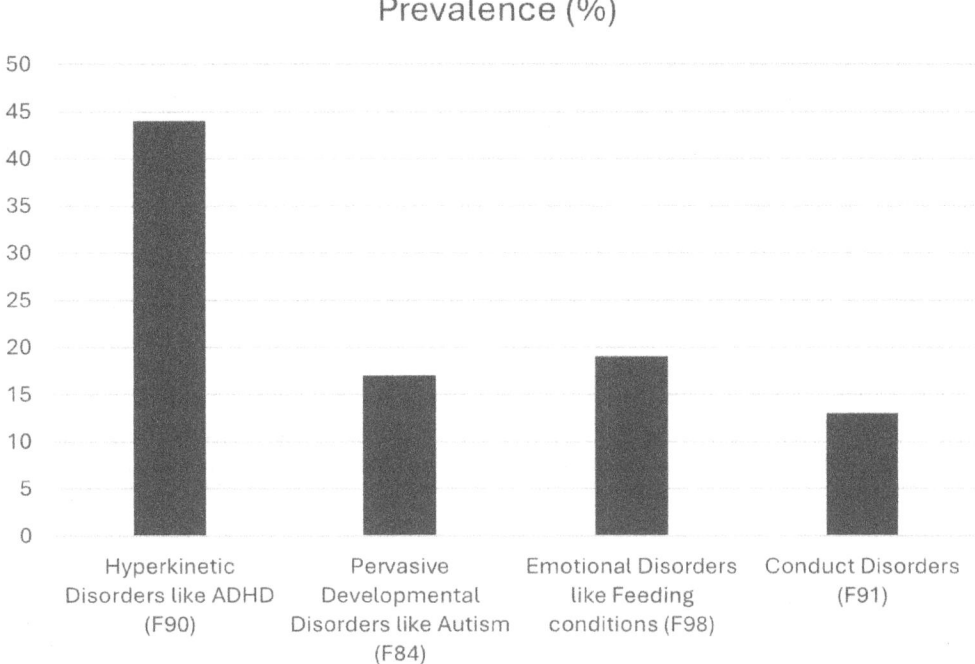

Figure 9.2 Prevalence of mental disorders by ICD-10 category – adapted from data in P Strømme, TH Diseth, Prevalence of Psychiatric Diagnoses in Children with Mental Retardation: Data from a Population-Based Study. *Dev. Med. Child Neurol.* 2007;42:266–70.

mind [15]. This results in ADHD being both a differential diagnosis for ID and also a co-occurring disorder. ADHD has evidence-based treatments so it is important that its presence is correctly identified to meet needs.

Developmental Speech and Language Disorders
Severe language disorders may be part of the developmental delays as part of ID, but may also present similarly to ID with language affecting so many components of intellect [16]. Generally other delays wouldn't be present if the disorder is solely language based.

Developmental Coordination Disorder (DCD)
DCD is a specific coordination disorder affecting fine and gross motor skills. This is more common alongside other neurodevelopmental disorders, as well as having a potential to be mistaken for the developmental delays in motor development that may occur in those who are globally delayed [17]. If the delays are solely motor based, then other significant delays would not be expected. However, deficits in motor coordination may affect coordination of play and the ability to make friendships based upon exercise-based play. The fine motor issues may affect academic performance and show as more significant scholastic delays if not appropriately supported.

Developmental Learning Disorders

Developmental learning difficulties, otherwise known as specific learning difficulties, may resemble ID owing to their effects on academic performance. By definition, they do not lead to global developmental delays, but rather specific delays that may also occur within the context of an ID. However, they can resemble ID owing to the effects on academic performance and potentially on the components of psychometric tests that use the skills that are directly affected by the specific learning difficulty. Developmental Learning Disorders may have wide-ranging academic effects including reading, writing and arithmetic. They can co-occur with ID and should also be considered as a differential diagnosis for ID.

Borderline Intellectual Functioning

Borderline intellectual functioning (intellectual functioning between 1 and 2 standard deviations below the mean) is not a 'diagnosable disorder' but will lead to generalised developmental delays including IQ and adaptive functioning, but not at the level of an ID. Of course, with measurements having 95% confidence intervals, there will be an overlap in the confidence intervals between the top end of an ID and the bottom end of 'normal' function.

Mental Health Disorders

These disorders are more common in children and adolescents with ID [18] and the key issue is that they may present atypically compared to a neurotypical child. Often cognitive and language-based symptoms are 'simplified' owing to the developmental delays. The young person may find it difficult to express their experiences and may lack the vocabulary and emotional awareness to describe their symptomatology. The biological symptoms and signs of disorders or behavioural change may also be the dominant presentation, which may lead to diagnostic uncertainty.

Anxiety is by far the most common clinical presentation [19]. This may be specific, for example, phobias, PTSD, OCD or more generalised. It is often linked to levels of understanding, need for routine and communication difficulties. Presentations can vary from a child clearly reporting that they are anxious or afraid and this being linked to clear triggers, through to somatic presentations of stomach aches, diarrhoea, urinary frequency or headaches, particularly in those with more severe ID.

Mood Disorders may also develop, particularly during adolescence. Many young people with ID suffer from additional losses, with bereavements and associated symptomatology through to *Depression*. These additional losses may appear trivial to outside observers but may have significant impacts particularly when understanding that the needs for routine and communication are factored in. Changes of significant carers may occur frequently with little warning and peers may also have life-limiting conditions, so bereavements may occur more commonly than for most children. The more able children with ID may be able to express their mood state more clearly, but like anxiety often it is changes in behaviour such as being less motivated, isolating or somatic symptoms that present, for example, changes in appetite, sleep, energy or weight. Often the child may be crying more or appearing sad without clear triggers [20].

Bipolar Affective Disorder is a rare disorder in children with ID, like the neurotypical population. It is more likely to start in adolescence and may be difficult to distinguish from trigger-related emotional responses, immaturity of emotions and other co-occurring neurodevelopmental disorders, for example, ADHD or autism from the core symptomatology or sequelae of those disorders in addition to the ID, for example, attention, activity levels, impulsivity. Access to depressive or manic thought processes may be difficult owing to levels of language (receptive and expressive) limiting the descriptions of symptomatology or understanding of the questions during a psychiatric history and mental state examination [21].

Psychosis/Schizophrenia may also occur within the context of ID. Like the other mental health disorders symptomatology may be simplified, for example, noises/simple phrases heard as auditory hallucinations or lower-level paranoia rather than florid psychotic phenomenology that often requires a greater degree of imagination skills and language ability. Negative symptomatology may resemble depression, grief reactions or if co-occurring autism, the presentation of the autism [22]. The key here is to establish whether there has been a change and if any clear triggers are present. There are conditions like velo-cardio-facial syndrome (22q11 deletions syndrome, DiGeorge syndrome) that increase the likelihood of psychosis and ID.

Personality Disorders are less common in children with ID owing to the delays in personality development often being more about temperament and behavioural presentations. In those with milder levels of ID, they may present more like the non-ID population.

Addictions are no different to the rest of the population and may include alcohol, drugs, gambling or other addictions, for example, pornography, internet or gaming. They are not so common in children with ID owing to often limited exposure to them, supervision and support being in place. Iatrogenic causes for addictions may occur with the prescribing of addictive medications, for example, benzodiazepines.

Behavioural Disorders

These include oppositional behaviours (less severe or lesser impact on society, mostly breaking rules) through to conduct disorder (more severe, greater impact on society, moving into breaking laws). Though technically a child with ID may present with these types of behaviours, often they are not given a specific diagnosis since it generally requires a higher degree of understanding of rules and laws to consciously break them.

Behaviours that Challenge others is the description of a set of behaviours and not a diagnosis. These are common, particularly in the more severe levels of ID. They are defined as 'Behaviour of such an intensity, frequency or duration as to threaten the quality of life and/or the physical safety of the individual or others and is likely to lead to responses that are restrictive, aversive or result in exclusion' [23]. They may pose risks to the child or others or limit access to community activities. They usually represent a response to distress, but may also be linked to self-stimulation and lack of meaningful activity.

Self-harm/self-injurious behaviour is again not a diagnosis per se, and more often are presenting symptoms and signs of distress in children with ID that may be linked to a mental or physical health disorder or in response to an environmental or communication factor. Self-harm with suicidal intent or to relieve distress may be more commonly seen in the more able, whereas self-injurious behaviour (a subset of behaviours that challenge others) is generally more common in those with more severe levels of ID [24].

Physical Health Aspects

Children and adolescents with ID may present more frequently with physical disorders. These include sensory impairments of hearing and sight (including cerebral visual impairments) [25]. The risk of physical disabilities is also heightened [26]. Certain genetic syndromes like Smith-Magenis Syndrome commonly present with other physical disorders in addition to ID like cardiovascular disorders (e.g. ventricular septal defects and arrhythmias), ocular defects (e.g. iris and corneal abnormalities) and genitourinary malformations [27]. Common ailments like discomfort (from a fever or constipation) or pain (from reflux or headache) may present as behaviours that challenge, due to limitations in communicating these symptoms verbally.

Neurological disorders are by far the largest group of conditions that may present in conjunction with having ID, particularly if the child has severe-profound ID [28]. Epilepsy is a prominent example and in addition to some focal seizures presenting as mood or behavioural difficulties, seizures that are poorly controlled or the adverse effects of anti-seizure medication, may also be causes for or exacerbate behaviours that present in the child with ID [29]. Epilepsy may also present more frequently as part of the genetic syndrome associated with ID, for example Angelman Syndrome and Tuberous Sclerosis [30]. Sleep disorders also present frequently in children with ID [31], and are often associated with higher levels of challenging behaviours [32]. Children with ID who experience pain also display snoring and other sleep-disordered breathing difficulties [33].

Unfortunately, children with ID face greater challenges in accessing health services [34]. An important consideration is the concept of 'diagnostic overshadowing' where the behaviours exhibited by a child with ID to communicate symptoms of a physical disorder, are ignored and attributed to the ID itself [35]. 'Diagnostic overshadowing' or not making reasonable adjustments (e.g. giving more time to complete a physical examination) are significant reasons for the difficulties in accessing health services. Even once a child with ID is admitted to hospital to treat a physical condition, they experience inequalities in their clinical quality and safety outcomes [36].

Assessment of Co-occurring Conditions

Adaptations to ICD-10 criteria for adults with ID from mental health and behavioural disorders were described in DC-LD. Unfortunately, this did not cover children and adolescents, but the principles of the ICD-10 criteria are similar albeit within a developing child. For ICD-11 there is an intention to create a new version including children and adolescents with ID, to map onto the ICD-11 mental health and behavioural disorder descriptions.

The main reasonable adjustments required for the assessment of mental health and behavioural disorders for children and adolescents with ID are:
- Simplify any questions asked.
- Check understanding.
- Account for the developmental stage of the child – cognitive, language, emotional and adaptive behavioural expectations.
- Often third-party information is required rather than direct from the child (parent, carer, teacher).
- Observe the child in different settings in addition to psychiatric history.

- Allow extra time.
- Adjust diagnostic thinking to place more emphasis on biological rather than psychological symptoms/signs.
- Assessment outcomes may lead to a formulation in addition to a diagnosis.

Clinical formulations should consider attendant biological, psychological and social factors cross referenced with presenting, predisposing, precipitating, perpetuating and protective factors, as well as a consideration of the risks to self and others.

Treatment of Co-occurring Conditions

There is no treatment for ID specifically, rather interventions are about understanding, supporting and making reasonable adjustments to assist the person in any aspect of their life where they have difficulties, to enable them to have the most productive, positive life experience possible with as much independence as feasible. In addition, any support should build upon skills, knowledge and abilities to develop these as best as possible within the limits of the disability [21].

Most treatments therefore are for co-occurring conditions, disorders or diseases. Interventions may be biological, psychological or social. In ID, they are often more likely to be provided in the reverse order, that is social, psychological then biological. Often reasonable adjustments and modifications are required to these treatments and interventions. In the same way as adjustments are made to their assessment, similar approaches are required for treatments.

Social Interventions

- Interventions may be environmental rather than psychological or biological, for example, establishing routine, increasing predictability, removal or management of external triggers.
- Interventions, for example, respite or home support may be to allow parent/carer recouperation to increase resilience or sleep.
- Interventions may be provided via a parent or carer, for example, parent-led CBT, sleep or behavioural management.

Psychological Interventions

- Simplify any talking that therapy had offered.
- Check any understanding as therapy progresses.
- Account for the developmental stage of the child – cognitive, language, emotional and adaptive behavioural expectations to direct the style of therapeutic intervention, for example, the use of art or music.
- Often therapeutic intervention or advice may be provided to a third party rather than direct to the child (parent, carer, teacher).
- Changes and improvements may be behavioural or biological in their presentation rather than psychological.
- Allow extra time for processing in a therapeutic session.
- Repetition of talking therapies may be required.
- Longer duration of interventions may be required.

Biological Interventions
- Physical health interventions may be required, for example, for pain, discomfort or painful conditions such as constipation, resulting in behavioural changes or mental health disorders such as anxiety or mood.
- Medications for mental health disorders are the same as for those children without ID; however, lower doses may often be required, along with a slower pace of increasing dose and additional monitoring for side effects.
- Medication, used often in other neurodevelopmental conditions like Melatonin to treat sleep disorders, is safe and effective when used in children with ID [37].
- Physical health monitoring is important; however, exposure work may be required to achieve this in children that refuse to have measurements taken. At times if it is not possible, a balance of risks may be considered to decide if it is more risky to not monitor physical parameters versus not treating a disorder.
- Consideration of not overprescribing medications and ensuring the appropriateness of them is paramount.

Legislation
- Competency or Capacity may be considered to establish if a young person can consent to an assessment or intervention. If not, then available legislation may be needed to protect rights and act in someone's best interests to assent on their behalf rather than the child directly consenting, for example, the use of the Children Act [38], the Mental Capacity Act [39] or the Mental Health Act [40] in England and Wales.

Research and Future Directions
Most of the risk factors and causes for ID are shared with other physical and mental disorders presenting in childhood – as such, public heath approaches and supporting research (e.g. to reduce the incidence or impact of prematurity) will have the greatest influence in reducing ID and associated difficulties [41]. Genetic research has advanced by an incredible leap over the last decade and next-generation sequencing methods including whole genome sequencing, combined with other clinical information on bioinformatics platforms, are allowing even greater precision in the identification and understanding of relevant genetic factors. This will also allow the subsequent use of gene-editing techniques and the design of more effective disease models for research [42].

Contemporary research using large sets of digital data and machine learning approaches have already helped identify more detailed health profiles in people with Fragile X Syndrome [43], and have incredible potential to assist more accurate diagnosis, investigate underlying mechanisms and interrogate clinical outcomes from more pragmatic clinical populations at scale [44]. There is an urgent need for more clinical trials of all forms of treatments (e.g. medication, psychological, behavioural and communication interventions) especially for children with severe ID, as there is practically no good quality research evidence [45].

Conclusions
It is important to identify an intellectual disability to ensure that the rights and needs of the child or young person are met. Mental health and other neurodevelopmental disorders are

more common and are often masked or missed. Making diagnoses and offering appropriate treatments may require reasonable adjustments (modifications). More research is required in this area to ensure that appropriate evidence-based approaches are used and extrapolation from non-ID child and adolescent research or adult ID research does not continue.

References

1. Schalock RL, Luckasson R, Tassé MJ. The Contemporary View of Intellectual and Developmental Disabilities: Implications for Psychologists. *Psicothema.* 2019;31(3):223–28.

2. American Psychiatric Association. *Diagnostic and Statistical Manual of Mental Disorders.* 5th ed., text rev. American Psychiatric Association, 2022. Available from: https://www.appi.org/dsm (accessed 5 April 2025).

3. World Health Organisation. *ICD-10: International Statistical Classification of Diseases and Related Health Problems.* 2nd ed., 10th rev. World Health Organisation, 2004. Available from: https://iris.who.int/handle/10665/42980 (accessed 5 April 2025)

4. American Psychiatric Association. *Diagnostic and Statistical Manual of Mental Disorders.* 4th ed. American Psychiatric Association, 1994. Available from: https://archive.org/details/diagnosticstatis00amer_0 (accessed 5 April 2025). (Please note only available via archive as updated to DSM-5.)

5. World Health Organisation. *International Statistical Classification of Diseases and Related Health Problems.* 11th ed. World Health Organisation, 2019. Available from: https://www.who.int/standards/classifications/classification-of-diseases (accessed 5 April 2025).

6. Plomin R, Spinath FM. Intelligence: Genetics, Genes, and Genomics. J. Pers. Soc. Psychol. 2004;**86**:112–29.

7. Wozniak JR, Riley EP, Charness ME. Clinical Presentation, Diagnosis, and Management of Fetal Alcohol Spectrum Disorder. Lancet Neurol. 2019;**18**:760–70.

8. Ammons RB, Ammons CH. The Quick Test (QT): Provisional Manual. Psychol Rep. 1962;**11**:111–61.

9. Sparrow SS, Cicchetti DV. The Vineland Adaptive Behavior Scales. In CS Newmark (ed.), *Major Psychological Assessment Instruments.* Vol. **2**. Allyn & Bacon, 1989, 199–231.

10. Harrison PL, Oakland T. Adaptive Behavior Assessment System: Third Edition. In JS Kreutzer, J DeLuca, B Caplan (eds.), *Encyclopedia of Clinical Neuropsychology.* Springer International Publishing, 2018, 57–60.

11. ACAMH. IDIDA2H. 2018. Available from: https://www.acamh.org/app/uploads/2018/10/IDIDA2H-Long-Version.pdf.

12. Amor DJ. Investigating the Child with Intellectual Disability: Investigating Intellectual Disability. J. Paediatr. Child Health. 2018;**54**:1154–58.

13. Postorino V, Fatta LM, Sanges V, et al. Intellectual Disability in Autism Spectrum Disorder: Investigation of Prevalence in an Italian Sample of Children and Adolescents. Res. Dev. Disabil. 2016;**48**:193–201.

14. Thurm A, Farmer C, Salzman E, Lord C, Bishop S. State of the Field: Differentiating Intellectual Disability from Autism Spectrum Disorder. Front. Psychiatry. 2019;**10**:526.

15. Clark B, Bélanger SA. ADHD in Children and Youth: Part 3 – Assessment and Treatment with Comorbid ASD, ID, or Prematurity. Paediatr. Child Health. 2018;**23**:485–90.

16. Marrus N, Hall L. Intellectual Disability and Language Disorder. Child Adolesc. Psychiatr. Clin. N. Am. 2017;**26**:539–54.

17. Straub L, Bateman BT, Hernandez-Diaz S, et al. Neurodevelopmental Disorders Among Publicly or Privately Insured Children in the United States. JAMA Psychiatry. 2022;**79**:232–42.

18. Strømme P, Diseth TH. Prevalence of Psychiatric Diagnoses in Children with Mental Retardation: Data from a Population-Based Study. Dev. Med. Child Neurol. 2007;42:266–70.

19. Maïano C, Coutu S, Tracey D, et al. Prevalence of Anxiety and Depressive Disorders Among Youth with Intellectual Disabilities: A Systematic Review and Meta-analysis. J. Affect. Disord. 2018;236:230–42.

20. Eaton C, Tarver J, Shirazi A, et al. A Systematic Review of the Behaviours Associated with Depression in People with Severe–Profound Intellectual Disability. J. Intellect. Disabil. Res. 2021;65:211–29.

21. Siegel M, McGuire K, Veenstra-VanderWeele J, et al. Practice Parameter for the Assessment and Treatment of Psychiatric Disorders in Children and Adolescents with Intellectual Disability (Intellectual Developmental Disorder). J. Am. Acad. Child Adolesc. Psychiatry. 2020;59:468–96.

22. Foss-Feig JH, Velthorst E, Smith L, et al. Clinical Profiles and Conversion Rates Among Young Individuals with Autism Spectrum Disorder Who Present to Clinical High Risk for Psychosis Services. J. Am. Acad. Child Adolesc. Psychiatry. 2019;58:582–28.

23. Royal College of Psychiatrists. *Challenging Behaviour: A Unified Approach*. Royal College of Psychiatrists, 2007. Available from: https://www.rcpsych.ac.uk/docs/default-source/improving-care/better-mh-policy/college-reports/college-report-cr144.pdf?sfvrsn=73e437e8_2 (Accessed 5 April 2025)

24. Symons FJ, Devine DP, Oliver C. Self-Injurious Behaviour in People with Intellectual Disability: Editorial. J. Intellect. Disabil. Res. 2012;56:421–26.

25. Bradley E, Bolton P. Episodic Psychiatric Disorders in Teenagers with Learning Disabilities with and Without Autism. Br J Psychiatry. 2006;189:361–66.

26. Dunn K, Rydzewska E, Fleming M, Cooper S-A. Prevalence of Mental Health Conditions, Sensory Impairments and Physical Disability in People with Co-occurring Intellectual Disabilities and Autism Compared with Other People: A Cross-Sectional Total Population Study in Scotland. BMJ Open. 2020;10:e035280.

27. Rinaldi B, Villa R, Sironi A, Garavelli L, Finelli P, Bedeschi MF. Smith-Magenis Syndrome – Clinical Review, Biological Background and Related Disorders. Genes. 2022;13:335.

28. Amiet C, Gourfinkel-An I, Bouzamondo A, et al. Epilepsy in Autism is Associated with Intellectual Disability and Gender: Evidence from a Meta-Analysis. Biol. Psychiatry. 2008;64:577–82.

29. Lewis J, Tonge B, Mowat D, Einfeld S, Siddons H, Rees V. Epilepsy and Associated Psychopathology in Young People with Intellectual Disability. J. Paediatr. Child Health. 2000;36:172–75.

30. Leung HTT, Ring H. Epilepsy in Four Genetically Determined Syndromes of Intellectual Disability. J. Intellect. Disabil. Res. 2013;57:3–20.

31. Tietze A-L, Blankenburg M, Hechler T, et al. Sleep Disturbances in Children with Multiple Disabilities. Sleep Med. Rev. 2012;16:117–27.

32. Scheithauer MC, Zarcone J. Evaluating the Relationship Between Sleep and Problem Behavior in Children with Disabilities. Behav Analysis Practice. 2015;8:27–36.

33. Breau LM, Camfield CS. Pain Disrupts Sleep in Children and Youth with Intellectual and Developmental Disabilities. Res. Dev. Disabil. 2011;32:2829–40.

34. Nageswaran S, Parish SL, Rose RA, Grady MD. Do Children with Developmental Disabilities and Mental Health Conditions Have Greater Difficulty Using Health Services than Children with Physical Disorders? Matern Child Health J. 2011;15:634–41.

35. Underwood JFG, DelPozo-Banos M, Frizzati A, Rai D, John A, Hall J. Neurological and Psychiatric Disorders Among Autistic Adults: A Population

Healthcare Record Study. *Psychol Med.* 2023;**53**(12):5663-73.

36. Mimmo L, Harrison R, Travaglia J, Hu N, Woolfenden S. Inequities in Quality and Safety Outcomes for Hospitalized Children with Intellectual Disability. Develop Med Child Neuro. 2022;**64**:314-22.

37. Abdelgadir IS, Gordon MA, Akobeng AK. Melatonin for the Management of Sleep Problems in Children with Neurodevelopmental Disorders: A Systematic Review and Meta-analysis. Arch. Dis. Child. 2018;**103**:1155-62.

38. HM Government. *Children Act.* HM Government, 1989. Available from: https://www.legislation.gov.uk/ukpga/1989/41/contents (accessed 5 April 2025)

39. HM Government. *Mental Capacity Act.* HM Government, 2005. Available from: https://www.legislation.gov.uk/ukpga/2005/9/contents#:~:text=Mental%20Capacity%20Act%202005%20is%20up%20to%20date,Inability%20to%20make%20decisions%204.%20Best%20interests%204A (accessed 5 April 2025).

40. HM Government. *Mental Health Act.* HM Government, 1983. Available from: https://www.legislation.gov.uk/ukpga/1983/20/contents (accessed 5 April 2025).

41. Totsika V, Liew A, Absoud M, Adnams C, Emerson E. Mental Health Problems in Children with Intellectual Disability. Lancet Child Adolesc. Health. 2022;**6**:432-44.

42. Ilyas M, Mir A, Efthymiou S, Houlden H. The Genetics of Intellectual Disability: Advancing Technology and Gene Editing. F1000Res. 2020;**9**:22.

43. Movaghar A, Page D, Scholze D, et al. Artificial Intelligence-Assisted Phenotype Discovery of Fragile X Syndrome in a Population-Based Sample. Genet. Med. 2021;**23**:1273-80.

44. Gupta C, Chandrashekar P, Jin T, et al. Bringing Machine Learning to Research on Intellectual and Developmental Disabilities: Taking Inspiration from Neurological Diseases. J Neurodevelop Disord. 2022;**14**:28.

45. Vereenooghe L, Flynn S, Hastings RP, et al. Interventions for Mental Health Problems in Children and Adults with Severe Intellectual Disabilities: A Systematic Review. BMJ Open. 2018;**8**:e021911.

Chapter 10

Antisocial Behaviours in Young People

Paul A. Tiffin and Oliver O'Mara

Antisocial behaviour, as the terms suggests, is that which violates society's morals, ethics and laws. Thus, to some extent, its definition is socially and culturally constructed. Nevertheless, there are behaviours that are universally condemned by societies, such as property theft or damage, threatened or actual violence (not justified by self-defence) and dishonesty. The usefulness of diagnostic labelling of young people with behaviours that challenge has been questioned. This is partly due to concerns that such categorisation locates the problem solely in the child. Indeed, oppositionality and aggression can be an understandable response to trauma and adverse social environments. Moreover, professionals working in child and adolescent mental health services (CAMHS) vary in their views of antisocial behaviour as an issue meriting input from such teams. Some see the role of child psychiatry as restricted to identifying and managing comorbid conditions, such as ADHD, that may be perceived as more 'treatable'. Putting such controversies aside, the impact of conduct issues on a young person, their family and society at large is profound. A diagnosis of conduct disorder is strongly associated with poor educational and occupational achievement, social isolation, substance misuse, contact with criminal justice and worsened mental health both in adolescence and into adulthood [1]. Economically, one Finnish study estimated the average lifetime costs to society for severe conduct problems to be €44,348 per individual [2]. Given these considerations this chapter summarises the definition and categorisation of childhood conduct issues, highlighting key points about what is currently known about the epidemiology and aetiology of such syndromes. The main approaches to assessment and management are also outlined.

Definition and Categorisation

Oppositional Defiant Disorder

Where persistent antisocial behaviour, or other behaviours that challenge carers are present in younger children these may be categorised as 'Oppositional Defiant Disorder' (ODD). The diagnosis of 'oppositional disorder' was first introduced in the DSM-III [3]. The ICD-11 [4], in keeping with DSM-V, defines ODD as a persistent pattern, lasting more than 6 months, of markedly defiant, disobedient, provocative or spiteful behaviour. A fuller summary of the ICD-11 diagnostic categories and definitions for ODD are detailed in Table 10.1. Neither ICD-11 nor DSM-V have an upper age cut-off for the definition of ODD, though the label tends to be applied to younger children (i.e. under 10 years) with less severe antisocial behaviours. Diagnostically, ODD is mainly differentiated from conduct disorder by the latter involving impingement of others' rights and violation of age-appropriate social norms.

Table 10.1 ICD-11 categories and (abbreviated) definitions related to the diagnosis of 'Oppositional defiant disorder' (ODD). Note 'unspecified' diagnostic subcategories are not included here

ICD–11 Code	Diagnostic (sub)category with summarised definition
6C90	**Oppositional defiant disorder – general diagnostic requirements** Persistent pattern (e.g. ≥6 months) of markedly defiant, disobedient, provocative or spiteful behaviour, out of keeping with the individual's developmental level, not restricted to interaction with siblings. May manifest in persistent angry or irritable mood and severe temper outbursts. Results in significant impairment in personal, family, social, educational, occupational or other areas of functioning.
6C90.0	**Oppositional defiant disorder with chronic irritability-anger** Characterised by prevailing, persistent angry or irritable mood, without provocation, often with severe temper outbursts, present nearly every day are across multiple settings and are not restricted to the parental/carer relationship.
6C90.01	**Oppositional defiant disorder with chronic irritability-anger with limited prosocial emotions** As for 6C90.00 but with 'callous and unemotional' characteristics (lack of empathy, remorse, guilt, sensitivity and concern for others' distress; relative indifference to the probability of punishment and poor school/work performance in school or work; limited expression of authentic positive emotions).
6C90.1	**Oppositional defiant disorder without chronic irritability-anger** Features argumentative, and defiant behaviour, without chronic irritability-anger.
6C90.10	**Oppositional defiant disorder without chronic irritability-anger with limited prosocial emotions** As for 6C90.1 with 'callous and unemotional' characteristics.
6C90.11	**Oppositional defiant disorder without chronic irritability-anger with typical prosocial emotions** Fulfils the requirements for 6C90.1 without 'callous and unemotional' characteristics.

Conduct Disorder

The diagnostic categorisation of 'conduct disorder' only appeared relatively recently in DSM-IV. However, in 1902 George Still had published a description of children he postulated as having a 'Defect of moral control as a morbid manifestation, without general impairment of intellect and without physical disease' [5]. Sill noted many features of conduct disorder, as currently defined, including persistent aggression, dishonesty and failure to learn from punishment.

Conduct disorder is now labelled 'conduct-dissocial disorder' within ICD-11, under the 'disruptive behaviour or dissocial disorders' section. As in ICD-10, conduct-dissocial disorder is broadly defined as ' ... *repetitive and persistent pattern of behaviour in which the basic rights of others ... age-appropriate societal norms, rules, or laws are violated* ... '. Table 10.2 summarises fuller descriptions and diagnostic subcategories of conduct-dissocial disorder. Both childhood (prior to 10 years) and adolescent-onset can be specified, with the

Table 10.2 A summary of the ICD-11 diagnostic criteria for the main conduct-dissocial disorder [4]. Note 'unspecified' diagnostic subcategories are not included here

ICD–11 Code	Diagnostic (sub)category with summarised definition
6C91	**Conduct-dissocial disorder – general definition** Repetitive, persistent patterns of behaviour where the basic rights of others or societal norms, rules, or laws are violated (e.g. aggression towards people, animals or property, deceitfulness, theft, etc.). The severity results in significant impairment in personal, family, social, educational, occupational or other areas of functioning. Behaviours must have been present for 12 months or more.
6C91.0	**Conduct-dissocial disorder, childhood onset** Features must be present during childhood prior to adolescence (e.g. before 10 years) and have endured 12 months or more.
6C91.00	**Conduct-dissocial disorder, childhood onset with limited prosocial emotions** As for 6C91.0 with 'callous and unemotional' characteristics (see Table 1; 6C90.01).
6C91.01	**Conduct-dissocial disorder, childhood onset with typical prosocial emotions** As for 6C91.0 without 'callous and unemotional' characteristics.
6C91.1	**Conduct-dissocial disorder, adolescent onset** No features evident before 10 years of age.
6C91.10	**Conduct-dissocial disorder, adolescent onset with limited prosocial emotions** As for 6C91.1 with 'callous and unemotional' characteristics.
6C91.11	**Conduct-dissocial disorder, adolescent onset with typical prosocial emotions** As for 6C91.1 without 'callous and unemotional' characteristics.

earlier subcategories relating to the context (i.e. family, socialised, etc.) discarded. Importantly, the specifier 'with limited (or "typical") prosocial emotions' (LPE) has now been added. DSM-V also includes this LPE specifier for conduct disorder, which is intended to reduce the heterogeneity within diagnostic subcategories and improve prognostic accuracy [6,7,8]. The LPE specifier is closely related to the concept of 'callous-unemotionality' and emerging psychopathy (see Table 10.2 for descriptors).

Impulse Control Disorders

ICD-11 contains a section relating to 'impulse control disorders', providing some harmonisation with DSM-V, which describes and defines a similar set of conditions. These are characterised by repeated failures to resist an impulse to perform an act that is experienced as immediately rewarding to the individual but results in longer-term harm. These behaviours result in distress and/or impairment of functioning to the individual or others. They are thus conceptualised as 'behavioural addictions' and include *pyromania*, *kleptomania*, *compulsive sexual behaviour* disorders and *intermittent explosive disorder* (IED) [9]. They are generally differentiated from other offending behaviours by the lack of apparent external motivating factors. For example, an urge to set a fire in pyromania is driven by the reward of experiencing the fire or its effects itself, rather than say, revenge.

IED may be especially relevant in terms of the prevalence and nature of aggressive behaviour in under-18s. In IED there are repeated brief episodes of verbal or physical aggression, grossly out of proportion to any actual or perceived provocation. IED differs from other impulse control disorders in several ways; there is usually no appetitive urge before, or hedonic reward after the behavioural outburst. These episodes do not occur in the context of chronic irritability, as can occur in ODD, which is itself an exclusion criteria for IED, according to ICD-11. Nevertheless, IED can, where appropriate, be diagnosed in the presence of other conditions, including conduct-dissocial disorder, unless the latter better explains the aggressive outbursts [4].

Personality Disorder

Changes to ICD-11 and DSM-V have been made to the categorisation of 'personality disorder' with no lower age limits for the diagnosis. A dimensional approach, with differing gradings of severity, ranging from personality 'difficulty' to 'severe personality disorder'. The trait domain of 'dissociality' is that most relevant to conduct disorder. Others such as 'disinhibition' and 'negative affectivity' may also be relevant. ICD-11 still allows the specification of a 'borderline pattern qualifier'. Indeed, females exhibiting marked antisocial behaviour commonly also display emerging 'borderline personality traits', including suicidality [10]. A diagnosis of personality disorder should not be considered permanent. However, the application of this categorisation by CAMHS, who rarely make this controversial diagnosis, will require a cultural shift.

Epidemiology of Conduct Problems in Young People

In the UK approximately 1 in 20 (4.6%) 5–19-year-olds are likely to meet the criteria for a behavioural disorder, with rates higher in boys (5.8%) than girls (3.4%) [11]. These rates are internationally fairly consistent. The pooled global rate for disruptive disorders is estimated as 5.7% [12]. There are some lifetime continuities between disruptive behaviour issues. However, findings from the Great Smoky Mountain study suggested that transition from ODD to conduct disorder is relatively uncommon; around 20% of 9-year-olds with conduct disorder had a history of ODD, though this was only true of around 2% of 13-year-olds [13]. In contrast, roughly half of those with conduct disorder may later reach the criteria for antisocial personality disorder [14], though some research reports lower rates of continuity [15]. Moreover, a diagnosis of conduct disorder is associated with a range of undesirable outcomes, such as failure to complete high school (odds ratio (OR) = 2.7), substance use disorders (OR = 2.1) and violent criminality (OR = 3.5) compared to young people without the diagnosis [16]. In addition, the US-based National Comorbidity Survey observed that around 7.8% of adolescents met the DSM-IV criteria for lifetime IED, with the aggressive behaviours tending to persist across time [17]. Moreover, there is some evidence that around 20% of young people with a diagnosis of ADHD or conduct disorder may also reach the criteria for IED [18].

Comorbid developmental and mental health issues are prevalent in disruptive behaviour disorders. Rates of coexisting ADHD are especially high with younger onset conduct problems. Of those with a diagnosis of conduct disorder around a third, or more, of young people may have clinically significant post-traumatic stress, depression [19] and anxiety symptoms [20]. Around 12% of individuals with an autism spectrum condition (ASC) may also have a disruptive, impulse-control, or conduct disorder [21]. It is less clear what the prevalence of ASC is in conduct disordered young people, though many have social and communication issues. For example around 25–40% of young people with offending behaviours may have a speech and language disorder, with 'pragmatic language' issues (relating to the social use of language) prominent [22]. Literacy issues are also common in this population with one study of detained young people reporting that half met the criteria for 'dyslexia' [23].

Aetiology

Interacting biological, psychological and social factors all play a role in the development of antisocial behaviours.

Biological Factors

The hereditability of conduct problems is estimated to be around 50% [24]. There seem to be a number of genes that influence different aspects of antisocial behaviour (e.g. oppositionality versus aggression) with differential effects across the early life-course [25]. A number of candidate genes have been identified with much interest in 'warrior genes', associated with callous-unemotional traits. The original, and most researched of these, is the gene associated with expression of the activity of monoamine oxidase A (MAO-A), which breaks down catecholamines in the synaptic cleft. The allele associated with low MAO-A activity is associated with an increased risk of criminality [26].

A number of prenatal risk factors have also been identified for conduct disorder including maternal smoking, alcohol and drug use [27], as well as stress and anxiety during pregnancy [28]. Birth complications are associated with conduct problems, though this link may be mediated by impaired intellectual ability [29].

Brain structure and functioning, neurophysiological and psychophysiological differences have also been demonstrated between conduct and non-conduct disordered youth. Children with ODD or conduct disorder tend to have a reduced cortisol response to stress, and a flattened daily secretion profile [30]. Conduct disordered young people tend to have reduced physiological arousal in response to stress, such as reduced heart rate [31]. Brain imaging studies show that youths with conduct issues have relatively reduced grey matter volumes in certain cortical and subcortical regions [32]. Functional imaging studies have shown fairly consistent anomalies in activation levels in brain regions associated with emotional processing in children with ODD and conduct disorder [33]. However, this may differ between young people with conduct problems with and without prominent callous-unemotional traits. Specifically, those without such traits may show increased responses to threat-related stimuli (e.g. an image of an aggressive male), explaining a tendency to reactive aggression. In contrast, those with prominent callous-unemotional traits may show decreased activation in brain regions associated with empathy, the presence of which can inhibit antisocial behaviour.

Psychosocial Factors

Neurocognitive deficits have been noted in young people with conduct problems, including the recognition of emotional expressions and empathy [34], especially in those with prominent callous-unemotional traits [35]. Young people with conduct issues tend to be more reckless, and influenced by potential rewards, rather than punishments, when making decisions [36].

Risk factors relating to adverse social environments may include dysfunctional parenting, characterised by harsh, coercive but inconsistent disciplining [37], as well as more extreme neglect, abuse and exposure to trauma such as domestic abuse [38]. Community-level risk factors include associations with antisocial peers and adults, relative poverty and local crime [39].

Interaction Between Genetic and Environmental Factors

The biopsychosocial factors outlined above frequently seem to interact, often synergistically. For example, the genetic vulnerabilities, and notably the presence of the low-activity MAO-A allele, manifest mainly in the presence of childhood adversity [24]. Moreover, parental genes associated with antisocial behaviour will provide children with an inherited vulnerability and the adverse early environment associated with conduct problems. Parenting quality may also be an important 'buffering' factor for children with prominent callous-unemotional traits [40].

The use of newer statistical approaches has been helpful in untangling the predominant direction of causality for putative factors associated with antisocial behaviour, though the effects of some may be smaller than initially estimated [41].

Assessment

The principles of effective assessment in CAMHS are outlined in Chapter 8. NICE also provides some specific guidance to inform initial and comprehensive assessment [42]. Information should be sought from a variety of sources, including education, carers and other involved agencies. These often include social care, and agencies linked to the criminal justice system (youth justice services, police, etc.). Table 10.3 depicts some of the domains that should be covered when assessing a young person with behaviours that challenge, providing examples of structured instruments that can support assessment. A trauma-informed perspective is often valuable [43]. Specifically, it is important to consider how exposure to acute and chronic traumas, as well as poor, neglectful or abusive care will have affected the neurobiological as well as social, emotional and psychological development of the young person. As indicated in Table 10.3, this perspective can be useful in deriving a general, and risk, formulation. It is also important to identify if antisocial behaviours are driven by a disorder of impulse control (see earlier). In such cases the focus will need to be largely placed on intrinsic motivations and drivers for the behaviours. Management plans should then emerge from initial formulations.

Structured instruments are available that support the screening for clinically significant behaviours that challenge. In general recognition of conduct problems is best achieved via a comprehensive clinical assessment. However, screening may still have a role in recognising younger children who may benefit from targeted prevention work, at school and home. For example, the Strengths and Difficulties Questionnaire (SDQ) has both a scale related to *conduct problems* [44] and can be thought of as generally measuring two dimensions relating to externalising (behavioural) and internalising (emotional) issues [45]. However, for routine care, structured instruments are mainly useful for eliciting and quantifying issues in specific areas. This can include the identification of comorbid developmental or mental health issues such as ADHD or autism spectrum

Table 10.3 A summary of the areas that should be covered when assessing conduct issues in children and young people, including examples of structured tools that may be helpful

Domain	Examples of specific areas of enquiry	Examples of potentially helpful structured tools
Presenting problem/s	- Who referred and what triggered referral? - Are concerns equally shared by family, school and social care, etc.? - Is there an immediate risk of harm to the young person or others? (i.e. urgency).	Teacher form of the Strengths and Difficulties Questionnaire (SDQ) [44]
Previous mental health history and interventions	- Have previous diagnoses been made? - Previous contact with mental health services? - What interventions have been tried? - How (in)effective have these been, and why? - How has previous support been viewed by all involved?	Not applicable
Family background and history	- Family history of mental health or developmental issues? - Quality of early care environment? - Exposure to trauma, neglect or abuse? - Prenatal exposure to drugs or alcohol? - Previous social services involvement? - Previous parental substance misuse or criminality? - Any positive experiences reported?	The Trauma Symptom Checklist in Childhood [72] The Adverse Childhood Experiences (ACE) Scale [73] The Benevolent Childhood Experiences (BCEs) Scale [74]
Current social circumstances	- Who lives at home? - Current parenting quality - Quality of household relationships (e.g. parental conflict) - Risks posed to other young people, or vulnerable adults, in the home - What outside agencies have been involved? (e.g. those relating to domestic abuse, anti-terrorism and child exploitation) - Nature of peer group - Hobbies, interests and skills - Parental substance (mis)use - Family social and economic situation - Nature of internet/social media usage - Missing from home episodes, and response	The Family Perceptions Scale (FPS) [75]
Substance use	- Early onset substance misuse? - Substances tried/used regularly - Pattern of alcohol/substance use - Motivators for substance use?	Young People's Drug Use Screening Tool [76]

Table 10.3 (cont.)

Domain	Examples of specific areas of enquiry	Examples of potentially helpful structured tools
	- Parental attitudes towards substances - 'Vaping' (e-cigarettes) and energy drink use - Funding for substance use/'drug debts'	
Educational history and functioning	- Previous educational settings, plans, support and engagement - Educational assessment results and cognitive profile - Specific or generalised learning problems suspected or identified - Any antisocial behaviours observed - Educational management of behaviours that challenged - School safety plan present? - Peer and staff relationships in education	The Wechsler Intelligence Scale for Children-Fifth Edition (WISC-V) [77]
Developmental and attachment profiles	- Developmental milestones (e.g. walking unaided) achieved within normal range? - Delays or anomalies in social and communication skills - Any specific delays in motor or cognitive functioning? - Selective attention and concentration (e.g. ADHD) - Maternal post-natal mental health or bonding issues - Number of caregivers and their emotional availability	The Autism Diagnostic Interview- Revised (ADI-R) [78] The Autism Diagnostic Observation Schedule (ADOS) [79] The Conners ADHD Questionnaire [80]
Personality Development	- How would the young person themselves, and others, describe their emerging personality? - To what extent is the young person perceived as being likeable to adults and other young people? - Is there any evidence for the presence of emerging callous-unemotional traits? - To what extent is the young person sensation-seeking, risk-taking and easily bored?	The Inventory of Callous-Unemotional Traits (ICU) [81] The Antisocial Process Screening Device [82] The Psychopathy Checklist-Youth Version (PCL-YV) [83]
Physical problems and relevant medical history	- History of head injury or cerebral insults - Nutrition and body weight - Medication adherence and side effects - Risk-taking behaviour with health implications (unsafe sex, substance use, etc.)	Not applicable

Table 10.3 (cont.)

Domain	Examples of specific areas of enquiry	Examples of potentially helpful structured tools
Forensic history	- Previous cautions, convictions, warnings or police involvement - Trajectory of offending - Likely internal and external drivers of offending - Response to previous sanctions or conditions imposed - Current youth justice service input - Likely detection of offending behaviours - Person's view of any offending and its consequences	Not applicable
Risk evaluation	- Current risks to their own safety (i.e. self-harming behaviours or suicidal ideation) - Risks that others may pose to the young person (e.g. criminal exploitation, neglect, abuse, peer victimisation) - Risks to safety of others and property (e.g. nature, severity and frequency of aggression) - Likely targets for aggression/antisocial behaviour? - Fire setting behaviours - Potentially harmful sexualised behaviours - Current safety plan and likely effectiveness	The Structured Assessment of Violence Risk in Youth (SAVRY) [84] Short-Term Assessment of Risk and Treatability: Adolescent Version (START:AV) [85] Functional Analysis in Care Environments-Child and Adolescent Risk-Assessment Suite [84] The Juvenile Sex Offender Assessment Protocol-II [86]
Formulation	- Risk formulation: summary of nature and magnitude of risks, likely targets and approximate timescale for risk forecast - General formulation: how primary presenting problem is understood in context of any biological, psychological and social factors identified - Can antisocial behaviours be understood as valid responses to adverse environments, and seen as useful by the young person? - Consider potential predisposing, precipitating, perpetuating and protective factors	

conditions, or emerging callous-unemotional personality traits. Some of these instruments, such as the Psychopathy Checklist-Youth Version (PCL-YV), require training, while others, such as the Inventory of Callous-Unemotional Traits (ICU), do not. Example tools are listed in Table 10.3.

Management

Psychopharmacology

Although commonly prescribed for reactive and impulsive aggression, the evidence for the sustained effectiveness of psychotropics in this regard is weak. There are some studies that demonstrate the short-term (up to 6 to 12 weeks) anti-aggressive effects of risperidone, especially in young people with relatively low cognitive ability [46]. There are also some suggestions that augmentation of stimulants and parent training with risperidone may reduce aggression for up to 12 weeks in children with ADHD [47]. Thus, risperidone should be regarded only as a short-term measure, with weight gain and hyperprolactinaemia being common and frequently problematic adverse effects [42]. There is insufficient evidence to support the use of other second-generation antipsychotics [48]. A number of low-quality studies exist, evaluating the potential of mood stabilisers, such as carbamazepine and valproate, to reduce aggression in young people, with mixed results [49]. Likewise there is inadequate evidence to recommend the alpha-2-adrenergic agonist clonidine as an anti-aggressive/anti-impulsive agent [50].

However, pharmacotherapy may still be indicated for comorbid conditions, for example, the use of stimulants for coexisting ADHD. In this respect, a number of studies report a reduction in aggression in young people meeting the criteria for both ADHD and conduct disorder [51]. There is currently no firm evidence base to guide pharmacological treatment of disorders of impulse control in adolescents. However, findings from some clinical trials in adults suggested that oxcarbazepine and fluoxetine may be effective in IED, and naltrexone for kleptomania [52]. Lastly, depression and anxiety are also relatively common in young people with behaviours that challenge [53]. These may evade identification due to the 'diagnostic overshadowing' of the externalising problems. Thus, selective serotonin reuptake inhibitors, such as fluoxetine, may be considered where psychological approaches have been ineffective, in accordance with the National Institute for Health and Care Excellence (NICE) Guidelines [54].

Psychosocial Approaches

Psychosocial approaches to antisocial behaviour are the mainstay of management.
The common, core components across interventions for antisocial behaviour are:
- psychoeducation for parents and young people
- increasing parenting skills and warmth
- positive reinforcement of desirable behaviours
- providing negative, but non-aggressive consequences to behaviours that challenge
- improving family functioning and the quality of communication
- increasing associations with prosocial peers
- improving social, emotional and problem-solving skills
- increasing community support

All interventions are typically taught via in-session modelling, role-play and 'homework'. Other elements observed to be associated with positive intervention outcomes were: *therapist adherence to the intervention model, therapeutic alliance, creating a family focus* and *delivery in the home*. Additionally, caregiver key ingredients included: *putting the problem into words, recognising and adjusting expectations, responding with sensitivity* and *youth seeing the family commitment*. The main challenge in implementing these approaches is engaging young people and families, who may have had negative experiences with services and be mistrustful or sceptical about professional input [55]. This is highlighted by frequently low recruitment and retention rates in studies [56].

Naturally, the provision of psychosocial interventions does not preclude practical actions, such as providing additional social support to a family, including respite care for a child. In some cases, where child safeguarding or other marked risks are identified, a change in care arrangements may have to be considered.

For younger children (3–11 years), NICE recommends parent/carer training [42]. This emphasises the first four components outlined above, and to some extent, the fifth. There is evidence from meta-analysis that parent management training is clinical [57] and cost-effective [58] in reducing childhood behaviours that challenge. Findings from a separate network meta-analysis suggested that, at least for younger children, more focused programmes were generally more effective. Specifically, those with only behaviour management components showed, on average, the largest effect sizes. For prevention work, those with only behaviour management and parental self-management seemed to be the most effective approach [59]. NICE also recommends targeting young people who may be at risk of conduct disorder for work around emotional regulation and problem solving [42].

For those aged over 12, young person-focused approaches, such as social and cognitive problem-solving programmes are frequently helpful. Here the emphasis is on a detailed ('functional') analysis of antisocial behaviours, exploring its antecedents and consequences from behaviouralist and cognitive perspectives. Thinking patterns that may increase aggression are also collaboratively challenged, for example, the idea that aggressive responses are always 'helpful in getting what you want'. Such programmes usually include training to improve emotional regulation, problem-solving and effective communication [60]. A meta-analytic study report that, on average, CBT-based interventions have large effect sizes for externalising problems in young people with diagnoses of ODD or conduct disorder. Indeed, around half the participants in the included study were 'in remission' following treatment [61]. Although evidence is generally lacking, CBT has also been used to treat impulse control disorders [62].

Antisocial behaviours are problematic for families and society, and systemic approaches are typically required. In this regard multimodal interventions should be offered to 11- and 17-year-olds who fulfil the criteria for conduct disorder and generally show moderate effect sizes [63]. Multimodal interventions are manualised approaches with a family focus, based on a social learning model, and involving various systems around the individual (education, youth justice, community, etc.). It is intensively delivered (three or more sessions per week) by trained case managers over three or more months [42].

Multisystemic therapy (MST) is a multimodal approach based on family therapy. While earlier, US-based, studies reported long-term clinical and cost-effectiveness of MST compared to management as usual [64], later studies have not always observed such positive impacts [65,66]. Thus, to summarise, there is insufficient quality of evidence to recommend one particular approach over another in adolescents with antisocial behaviours [67].

Consequently, psychosocial interventions, with components of known overall efficacy, should be tailored according to individual needs and the available resources. Nevertheless, there is evidence that some attempted approaches, such as military-style 'boot camps', are both ineffective and potentially actually increase offending [68]. Other specific therapies may be indicated for comorbidity, including depression and the sequelae of trauma. Other psychotherapies may be available in the future. These may focus on improving emotional processing [69] or mentalisation ability [70]. There is also the possibility of increased digital therapy delivery [56].

Summary

Conduct issues are common in young people, impact substantially on individuals, families and society and are often associated with developmental and mental health disorders. Interacting biological, psychological and social factors all play roles in the aetiology of antisocial behaviour. In terms of treatment, medication should be generally reserved for comorbid conditions, where indicated, and effective psychosocial approaches share some common active 'ingredients', though a specific therapy cannot be recommended. However, interventions that are highly focused, frequent and of longer duration, that target younger children are likely to be the most effective [71].

References

1. Colman I, Murray J, Abbott RA, et al. Outcomes of Conduct Problems in Adolescence: 40 Year Follow-Up of National Cohort. BMJ. 2009;**338**:a2981.

2. Rissanen E, Kuvaja-Köllner V, Elonheimo H, Sillanmäki L, Sourander A, Kankaanpää E. The Long-Term Cost of Childhood Conduct Problems: Finnish Nationwide 1981 Birth Cohort Study. J Child Psychol Psychiatry. 2022 Jun;**63**(6):683–92.

3. Ghosh A, Ray A, Basu A. Oppositional Defiant Disorder: Current Insight. Psychol Res Behav Manag. 2017;**10**:353–67.

4. World Health Organisation. *ICD-11 for Mortality and Morbidity Statistics*. 11th ed. World Health Organisation, 2018.

5. Still GF. The Goulstonian Lectures. Some Abnormal Psychical Conditions in Children. The Lancet. 1902;**159**(4104):1163–68.

6. Regier DA, Kuhl EA, Kupfer DJ. The DSM-5: Classification and Criteria Changes. World Psychiatr. 2013;**12**(2):92–98.

7. Jambroes T, Jansen LMC, Vermeiren RRJM, et al. The Clinical Usefulness of the New LPE Specifier for Subtyping Adolescents with Conduct Disorder in the DSM 5. Eur Child Adolesc Psychiatry. 2016;**25**(8):891–902.

8. Vanwoerden S, Reuter T, Sharp C. Exploring the Clinical Utility of the DSM-5 Conduct Disorder Specifier of 'with Limited Prosocial Emotions' in an Adolescent Inpatient Sample. Compr Psychiatry. 2016;**69**:116–31.

9. Grant JE, Atmaca M, Fineberg NA, et al. Impulse Control Disorders and 'Behavioural Addictions' in the ICD-11. World Psychiatr. 2014;**13**(2):125–27.

10. Szewczuk-Bogusławska M, Kaczmarek-Fojtar M, Adamska A, Frydecka D, Misiak B. Assessment of the Association Between Non-suicidal Self-Injury Disorder and Suicidal Behaviour Disorder in Females with Conduct Disorder. BMC Psychiatry. 2021;**21**(1):172.

11. NHS Digital. *Mental Health of Children and Young People in England 2017*. Leeds: NHS Digital, 2017. Available from: https://digital.nhs.uk/data-and-information/publications/statistical/mental-health-of-children-and-young-people-in-england/2017/2017 (accessed 5 April 2025).

12. Polanczyk GV, Salum GA, Sugaya LS, Caye A, Rohde LA. Annual Research Review: A Meta-analysis of the Worldwide Prevalence of Mental Disorders in Children and Adolescents. J Child Psychol Psychiatry. 2015;56(3):345–65.
13. Rowe R, Costello EJ, Angold A, Copeland WE, Maughan B. Developmental Pathways in Oppositional Defiant Disorder and Conduct Disorder. J Abnorm Psychol. 2010;119(4):726–38.
14. Simonoff E, Elander J, Holmshaw J, Pickles A, Murray R, Rutter M. Predictors of Antisocial Personality. Continuities from Childhood to Adult Life. Br J Psychiatry. 2004;184:118–27.
15. Copeland WE, Shanahan L, Costello EJ, Angold A. Childhood and Adolescent Psychiatric Disorders as Predictors of Young Adult Disorders. Arch Gen Psychiatry. 2009;66(7):764–72.
16. Erskine HE, Norman RE, Ferrari AJ, et al. Long-Term Outcomes of Attention-Deficit/Hyperactivity Disorder and Conduct Disorder: A Systematic Review and Meta-Analysis. J Am Acad Child Adolesc Psychiatry. 2016;55(10):841–50.
17. McLaughlin KA, Green JG, Hwang I, Sampson NA, Zaslavsky AM, Kessler RC. Intermittent Explosive Disorder in the National Comorbidity Survey Replication Adolescent Supplement. Arch Gen Psychiatry. 2012;69(11):1131–39.
18. Emil FC. Intermittent Explosive Disorder as a Disorder of Impulsive Aggression for DSM-5. Am J Psychiatry. 2012;169(6):577–88.
19. Ingoldsby E, Kohl G, McMahon R, Lengua L, Conduct Problems Prevention Research Group. Conduct Problems, Depressive Symptomatology and their Co-occurring Presentation in Childhood as Predictors of Adjustment in Early Adolescence. J Abnorm Child Psychol. 2006;34(5):603–21.
20. Connor DF, Ford JD, Albert DB, Doerfler LA. Conduct Disorder Subtype and Comorbidity. Ann Clin Psychiatry. 2007;19(3):161–68.
21. Hossain MM, Khan N, Sultana A, Ma P, McKyer ELisako J, Ahmed HU, et al. Prevalence of Comorbid Psychiatric Disorders Among People with Autism Spectrum Disorder: An Umbrella Review of Systematic Reviews and Meta-analyses. Psychiatry Res. 2020;287:112922.
22. Anderson SA, Hawes DJ, Snow PC. Language Impairments Among Youth Offenders: A Systematic Review. Child Youth Serv Rev. 2016;65(C):195–203.
23. Kirk J, Reid G. An Examination of the Relationship Between Dyslexia and Offending in Young People and the Implications for the Training System. Dyslexia. 2001;7:77–84.
24. Jaffee SR, Caspi A, Moffitt TE, Dodge KA, Rutter M, Taylor A, et al. Nature × Nurture: Genetic Vulnerabilities Interact with Physical Maltreatment to Promote Conduct Problems. Dev Psychopathol. 2005;17(1):67–84.
25. Wesseldijk LW, Bartels M, Vink JM, van Beijsterveldt CEM, Ligthart L, Boomsma DI, et al. Genetic and Environmental Influences on Conduct and Antisocial Personality Problems in Childhood, Adolescence, and Adulthood. Eur Child Adolesc Psychiatry. 2018;27(9):1123–32.
26. Brunner HG, Nelen M, Breakefield X, Ropers H, Van Oost BA. Abnormal Behavior Associated with a Point Mutation in the Structural Gene for Monoamine Oxidase A. Science. 1993;262(5133):578–80.
27. Ruisch IH, Dietrich A, Glennon JC, Buitelaar JK, Hoekstra P. Maternal Substance Use During Pregnancy and Offspring Conduct Problems: A Meta-analysis. Neurosci Biobehav Rev. 2018;84:325–36.
28. MacKinnon N, Kingsbury M, Mahedy L, Evans J, Colman I. The Association Between Prenatal Stress and Externalizing Symptoms in Childhood: Evidence from the Avon Longitudinal Study of Parents and Children. Biol Psychiatry. 2018;83(2):100–108.

29. Liu J, Raine A, Wuerker A, Venables PH, Mednick S. The Association of Birth Complications and Externalizing Behavior in Early Adolescents: Direct and Mediating Effects. J Res Adolesc. 2009;19(1):93–111.

30. Fairchild G, van Goozen SHM, Stollery SJ, et al. Cortisol Diurnal Rhythm and Stress Reactivity in Male Adolescents with Early-Onset or Adolescence-Onset Conduct Disorder. Biol Psychiatry. 2008;64(7):599–606.

31. Herpertz SC, Mueller B, Qunaibi M, Lichterfeld C, Konrad K, Herpertz-Dahlmann B. Response to Emotional Stimuli in Boys with Conduct Disorder. Am J Psychiatry. 2005;162(6):1100–107.

32. Noordermeer SDS, Luman M, Oosterlaan J. A Systematic Review and Meta-analysis of Neuroimaging in Oppositional Defiant Disorder (ODD) and Conduct Disorder (CD) Taking Attention-Deficit Hyperactivity Disorder (ADHD) Into Account. Neuropsychol Rev. 2016;26(1):44–72.

33. Alegria, AA, Radua, J, Rubia, K. Meta-Analysis of fMRI Studies of Disruptive Behavior Disorders. Am J Psychiatry. 2016;173(11):1119–30.

34. Stevens D, Charman T, Blair R. Recognition of Emotion in Facial Expressions and Vocal Tones in Children with Psychopathic Tendencies. J Genet Psychol. 2001;162(2):201–11.

35. Martin-Key N, Brown T, Fairchild G. Empathic Accuracy in Male Adolescents with Conduct Disorder and Higher Versus Lower Levels of Callous-Unemotional Traits. J Abnorm Child Psychol. 2017;45(7):1385–97.

36. Sonuga-Barke EJS, Cortese S, Fairchild G, Stringaris A. Annual Research Review: Transdiagnostic Neuroscience of Child and Adolescent Mental Disorders–Differentiating Decision Making in Attention-Deficit/Hyperactivity Disorder, Conduct Disorder, Depression, and Anxiety. J Child Psychol Psychiatry. 2016;57(3):321–49.

37. Moore AA, Silberg JL, Roberson-Nay R, Mezuk B. Life Course Persistent and Adolescence Limited Conduct Disorder in a Nationally Representative US Sample: Prevalence, Predictors, and Outcomes. Soc Psychiatry Psychiatr Epidemiol. 2017;52(4):435–43.

38. Greenwald R. The Role of Trauma in Conduct Disorder. J Aggress Maltreat Trauma. 2002;6(1):5–23.

39. Boden JM, Fergusson DM, Horwood LJ. Risk Factors for Conduct Disorder and Oppositional/Defiant Disorder: Evidence from a New Zealand Birth Cohort. J Am Acad Child Adolesc Psychiatry. 2010;49(11):1125–33.

40. Waller R, Hyde LW. Callous–Unemotional Behaviors in Early Childhood: Measurement, Meaning, and the Influence of Parenting. Child Dev Perspect. 2017;11(2):120–26.

41. Jaffee SR, Strait LB, Odgers CL. From Correlates to Causes: Can Quasi-experimental Studies and Statistical Innovations Bring Us Closer to Identifying the Causes of Antisocial Behavior? Psychol Bull. 2012;138(2):272–95.

42. National Institute for Health and Care Excellence. *Antisocial Behaviour and Conduct Disorders in Children and Young People: Recognition and Management-Clinical Guideline [CG158]*. London, NICE: 2013.

43. Raja S, Hasnain M, Hoersch M, Gove-Yin S, Rajagopalan C. Trauma Informed Care in Medicine: Current Knowledge and Future Research Directions. Fam Community Health. 2015;38(3):216–26.

44. Goodman R, Ford T, Simmons H, Gatward R, Meltzer H. Using the Strengths and Difficulties Questionnaire (SDQ) to Screen for Child Psychiatric Disorders in a Community Sample. Br J Psychiatry. 2000;177(6):534–39.

45. Goodman A, Lamping DL, Ploubidis GB. When to Use Broader Internalising and Externalising Subscales Instead of the Hypothesised Five Subscales on the Strengths and Difficulties Questionnaire (SDQ): Data from British Parents, Teachers and Children. J Abnorm Child Psychol. 2010;38(8):1179–91.

46. Ipser J, Stein DJ. Systematic Review of Pharmacotherapy of Disruptive Behavior Disorders in Children and Adolescents. Psychopharmacology. 2007;**191**(1):127–40.

47. Findling RL, Townsend L, Brown NV, Arnold LE, Gadow KD, Kolko DJ, et al. The Treatment of Severe Childhood Aggression Study: 12 Weeks of Extended, Blinded Treatment in Clinical Responders. J Child Adolesc Psychopharmacol. 2017;**27**(1):52–65.

48. Loy JH, Merry SN, Hetrick SE, Stasiak K. Atypical Antipsychotics for Disruptive Behaviour Disorders in Children and Youths. Cochrane Database Syst Rev. 2017;**8**(8):CD008559.

49. Pringsheim T, Hirsch L, Gardner D, Gorman DA. The Pharmacological Management of Oppositional Behaviour, Conduct Problems, and Aggression in Children and Adolescents with Attention-Deficit Hyperactivity Disorder, Oppositional Defiant Disorder, and Conduct Disorder: A Systematic Review and Meta-analysis. Part 2: Antipsychotics and Traditional Mood Stabilizers. Can J Psychiatry. 2015;**60**(2):52–61.

50. Pisano S, Masi G. Recommendations for the Pharmacological Management of Irritability and Aggression in Conduct Disorder Patients. Expert Opin Pharmacother. 2020;**21**(1):5–7.

51. Patel BD, Barzman DH. Pharmacology and Pharmacogenetics of Pediatric ADHD with Associated Aggression: A Review. Psychiatr Q. 2013;**84**(4):407–15.

52. Tahir T, Wong MM, Maaz M, Naufal R, Tahir R, Naidoo Y. Pharmacotherapy of Impulse Control Disorders: A Systematic Review. Psychiatry Res. 2022;**311**:114499.

53. Polier GG, Vloet TD, Herpertz-Dahlmann B, Laurens KR, Hodgins S. Comorbidity of Conduct Disorder Symptoms and Internalising Problems in Children: Investigating a Community and a Clinical Sample. Eur Child Adolesc Psychiatry. 2012;**21**(1):31–38.

54. National Institute for Health and Care Excellence. *Depression in Children and Young People: Identification and Management- NICE Guideline [NG134]*. London: NICE, 2019.

55. McDonald RJ, Signal T, Canoy D. Family Therapy for Conduct Disorder: Parent/Caregiver Perspectives on Active Ingredients. Aust N Z J Family Ther. 2021;**42**(2):160–73.

56. Dadds MR, Sicouri G, Piotrowska PJ, Collins DAJ, Hawes DJ, Moul C, et al. Keeping Parents Involved: Predicting Attrition in a Self-Directed, Online Program for Childhood Conduct Problems. J Clin Child Adolesc Psychol. 2019;**48**(6):881–93.

57. Michelson D, Davenport C, Dretzke J, Barlow J, Day C. Do Evidence-Based Interventions Work When Tested in the 'Real World?' A Systematic Review and Meta-analysis of Parent Management Training for the Treatment of Child Disruptive Behavior. Clin Child Fam Psychol Rev. 2013;**16**(1):18–34.

58. Sampaio F, Barendregt JJ, Feldman I, Lee YY, Sawyer MG, Dadds MR, et al. Population Cost-Effectiveness of the Triple P Parenting Programme for the Treatment of Conduct Disorder: An Economic Modelling Study. Eur Child Adolesc Psychiatry. 2018;**27**(7):933–44.

59. Leijten P, Melendez-Torres G, Gardner F. Research Review: The Most Effective Parenting Program Content for Disruptive Child Behavior—A Network Meta-analysis. J Child Psychol Psychiatry. 2022 Feb;**63**(2):132–42.

60. Hogue A, Bobek M, MacLean A. Core Elements of CBT for Adolescent Conduct and Substance Use Problems: Comorbidity, Clinical Techniques, and Case Examples. Cogn Behav Pract. 2020;**27**(4):426–41.

61. Riise EN, Wergeland GJH, Njardvik U, Öst L-G. Cognitive Behavior Therapy for Externalizing Disorders in Children and Adolescents in Routine Clinical Care: A Systematic Review and Meta-analysis. Clin Psychol Rev. 2021;**83**:101954.

62. Grant JE, Odlaug BL. Impulse control disorders. In D McKay, JS Abramowitz, S Taylor (eds.), Cognitive-Behavioral

63. Gatti U, Grattagliano I, Rocca G. Evidence-Based Psychosocial Treatments of Conduct Problems in Children and Adolescents: An Overview. Psychiatry Psychol Law. 2019;26(2):171–93.
64. Curtis NM, Ronan KR, Borduin CM. Multisystemic Treatment: A Meta-analysis of Outcome Studies. J Fam Psychol. 2004;18(3):411–19.
65. Fonagy P, Butler S, Cottrell D, Scott S, Pilling S, Eisler I, et al. Multisystemic Therapy Versus Management As Usual in the Treatment of Adolescent Antisocial Behaviour (START): 5-year Follow-Up of a Pragmatic, Randomised, Controlled, Superiority Trial. Lancet Psychiatry. 2020;7(5):420–30.
66. Littell JH, Pigott TD, Nilsen KH, Green SJ, Montgomery OLK. Multisystemic Therapy® for Social, Emotional, and Behavioural Problems in Youth Age 10 to 17: An Updated Systematic Review and Meta-analysis. Campbell Syst Rev. 2021;17(4):e1158.
67. Bakker M, Greven C, Buitelaar J, Glennon J. Practitioner Review: Psychological Treatments for Children and Adolescents with Conduct Disorder Problems–A Systematic Review and Meta-analysis. J Child PsycholPsychiatry. 2017;58(1):4–18.
68. Petrosino A, Turpin-Petrosino C, Hollis-Peel ME, Lavenberg JG. 'Scared Straight' and Other Juvenile Awareness Programs for Preventing Juvenile Delinquency. Cochrane Database of Syst Rev. 2013(4): CD002796.
69. Javdani S, Sadeh N, Donenberg GR, Emerson EM, Houck C, Brown LK. Affect Recognition Among Adolescents in Therapeutic Schools: Relationships with Posttraumatic Stress Disorder and Conduct Disorder Symptoms. Child Adolesc Ment Health. 2017;22(1):42–48.
70. Taubner S, Hauschild S, Kasper L, Kaess M, Sobanski E, Gablonski T-C, et al. Mentalization-Based Treatment for Adolescents with Conduct Disorder (MBT-CD): Protocol of a Feasibility and Pilot Study. Pilot Feasibility Stud. 2021;7(1):1–10.
71. Tiffin PA, Kaplan C. Dangerous Children: Assessment and Management of Risk. Child Adolesc Ment Health. 2004;9(2):56–64.
72. Briere J. *Trauma Symptom Checklist for Children: Professional Manual*. Odessa, FL: Psychological Assessment Resources Inc., 1996.
73. Finkelhor D, Shattuck A, Turner H, Hamby S. Improving the Adverse Childhood Experiences Study Scale. JAMA Pediatr. 2013;167(1):70–75.
74. Narayan AJ, Rivera LM, Bernstein RE, Harris WW, Lieberman AF. Positive Childhood Experiences Predict Less Psychopathology and Stress in Pregnant Women with Childhood Adversity: A Pilot Study of the Benevolent Childhood Experiences (BCEs) Scale. Child Abuse Negl. 2018;78:19–30.
75. Tiffin PA, Kaplan C, Place M. Brief Report: Development of the Family Perceptions Scale: A Novel Instrument for Evaluating Subjective Functioning in the Families of Adolescents. J Adolesc. 2011;34(3):593–97.
76. Turning Point, Suffolk County Council. *Young People's Drug Use Screening Tool (DUST)*. Turning Point & Suffolk County Council, 2015. Available from: https://www.turning-point.co.uk/services/suffolk-drug-and-alcohol-service (accessed 5 April 2025).
77. Wechsler D. Wechsler Intelligence Scale for Children-Fifth Edition. Administration and scoring manual (5th). London: Pearson, 2014.
78. Rutter M, Le Couteur A, Lord C. *ADI-R: Autism Diagnostic Interview-Revised (ADI-R)*. Los Angeles, CA: Western Psychological Services, 2003.
79. Lord C, Risi S, Lambrecht L, et al. The Autism Diagnostic Observation Schedule – Generic: A Standard Measure of Social and Communication Deficits Associated with

the Spectrum of Autism. J Autism Dev Disord. 2000;**30**(3):205–23.

80. Conners CK. The Conners. 3rd ed. North Tonawanda, NY: Multi-Health Systems, 2009.

81. Kimonis ER, Frick PJ, Skeem JL, et al. Assessing Callous–Unemotional Traits in Adolescent Offenders: Validation of the Inventory of Callous–Unemotional Traits. Int J Law Psychiatry. 2008;**31**(3):241–52.

82. Vitacco MJ, Rogers R, Neumann CS. The Antisocial Process Screening Device: An Examination of Its Construct and Criterion-Related Validity. Assessment. 2003;**10**(2):143–50.

83. Kosson DS, Cyterski TD, Steuerwald BL, Neumann CS, Walker-Matthews SJ. The Reliability and Validity of the Psychopathy Checklist: Youth Version (PCL: YV) in Nonincarcerated Adolescent Males. Psychol Assess. 2002;**14**(1):97–109.

84. Vincent GM, Chapman J, Cook NE. Risk-Needs Assessment in Juvenile Justice: Predictive Validity of the SAVRY, Racial Differences, and the Contribution of Needs Factors. Crim Justice and Behav. 2011;**38**(1):42–62.

85. Sher MA, Warner L, McLean A, Rowe K, Gralton E. A Prospective Validation Study of the START: AV. J Forensic Pract. 2017;**19**(2):115–29.

86. Prentky RA, Righthand S. The Juvenile Sex Offender Assessment Protocol-II (J-SOAP-II). In KS Douglas, RK Otto (eds.), *Handbook of Violence Risk Assessment*. 2nd ed. International Perspectives on Forensic Mental Health. New York: Routledge/Taylor & Francis Group, 2021, 294–321.

Chapter 11

Attachment, Anxiety Disorders and Experience of Trauma in Children and Adolescents

Emma Williams and Bridie Gallagher

Attachment

The theory of how attachment evolves, and the four attachment styles, have been described in detail in Chapter 2 – 'Normal Childhood Development: Theories and Influence'. An overview of the four attachment styles is summarised in Table 11.1.

Attachment Disorders: Reactive Attachment Disorder (6B44) and Disinhibited Social Engagement Disorder (6B45)

In the ICD-11, [1] disorders of attachment are categorised under 'Disorders specifically associated with stress'. In a shift from the ICD-10, the current diagnostic description of Reactive Attachment Disorder (RAD) does not list specific symptoms. Instead, it summarises that it is a disorder *'characterized by grossly abnormal attachment behaviours in early childhood, occurring in the context of a history of grossly inadequate childcare (e.g. severe neglect, maltreatment, institutional deprivation)'*. A newly added category of Disinhibited Social Engagement Disorder (DSED) features a parallel diagnostic description, but refers to *'grossly abnormal* social *behaviour'*, as opposed to *attachment* behaviour, originating from the same inadequate childcare experiences.

The two disorders are differentiated by the behaviours that occur because of an individual's early attachment experiences. RAD is concerned primarily with the absence of certain attachment behaviours; such as not seeking comfort in times of distress, or not responding to comfort when it is offered. These absences lead to a pervasive pattern of withdrawn and inhibited behaviour from the child. In comparison DSED describes social behaviours that are deemed to be outside of the norm. In this instance a child displays behaviour with unknown adults that is overly familiar and lacks the attachment strategy associated with a safe haven, where a child 'checks back' with a familiar caregiver in an unfamiliar or stressful setting.

The ICD-11 instructs that RAD and DSED should only be diagnosed in childhood, after the age of 9 months, and only if features were observed prior to the age of 5 years. This can make diagnostic attempts difficult in older children, particularly where accurate histories or historians are not available. Neither should be diagnosed if a child also has a diagnosis of an Autism Spectrum Disorder and both are seen as a potential precursor to the diagnosis of Complex PTSD. This is unsurprising, as a history of childhood maltreatment (which would constitute grossly inadequate childcare) is a common experience for young people who meet the criteria for the newly established C-PTSD diagnosis.

Table 11.1 Overview of attachment styles

Attachment style	Parent/carer behaviour	Internal working model	Childhood	Adolescence
Secure	Consistent and predictable Sensitive, responsive, available, nurturing and comforting	I am lovable I am effective Others are available, dependable, caring and loving 'I am ok and you are ok'	Develops an understanding of own and others' emotions Can learn via play and develops social skills	Develops skills in managing stress Able to share feelings with others Sense of self-esteem and confidence
Insecure – Avoidant	Consistently unresponsive Rejecting, dismissive, controlling, intrusive Expressions of closeness are punished, ignored or shut down	I am unlovable I am better off looking after myself Others do not respond to my distress Others are rejecting or intrusive 'I am ok, you are not ok'	Undemanding of carers Supresses emotions Avoids closeness Self-sufficient (outside of developmental norm)	Self-reliant and orientated by achievement May appear 'regulated' but manages emotions by dismissing them Avoidant of interdependent relationships
Insecure – Anxious/Ambivalent	Inconsistent (sometimes responsive and sometimes unavailable) Inconsistency reinforces persistence	I am unlovable I have to draw attention to get my needs met Others cannot be trusted Others are unreliable 'You are ok, I am not ok'	Intensifies attachment strategies to ensure they are noticed, to gain closeness Struggle to utilise comfort effectively when provided Anger when needs not met	Pre-occupied with others' availability in relationships May crave attention or approval from others May express high levels of anxiety or fear
Disorganised	Frightening	I am scared I am out of control Others are scary Others are overwhelming 'I am not ok, you are not ok'	Confused behaviour Fearful and helpless Cannot trust others Appears shut down May appear angry or manipulative (as desperate to find a sense of control)	Controlling Avoids closeness Distressed in relationships Dissociative coping Cannot share internal world with others

The Wider Relevance of Attachment in Child and Adolescent Psychiatry

The diagnostic rate for attachment disorders is low, and Children and Adolescent Mental Health Services (CAMHS) clinicians are more likely to encounter children and young people described as having *attachment difficulties* rather than disorders. There is a vast amount of research linking attachment insecurity with mental health difficulties in childhood, adolescence and adulthood.

Insecure attachments should be viewed as a 'general vulnerability' to, rather than a cause of, mental health problems where attachment security interacts with other biopsychosocial factors, including temperament, life experiences and intelligence [2]. It is thought that individuals with insecure attachments rely on secondary attachment strategies to manage emotions. These strategies are described as either hyperactivating or deactivating depending on the style of insecure attachment [3]. Individuals with anxious attachments are more likely to engage in hyperactivating strategies to achieve a sense of closeness with caregivers. In comparison those with avoidant attachments would be more likely to employ deactivating methods to avoid closeness with others and deny attachment needs.

Several meta-analyses have explored the relationship between attachment and mental health difficulties in young people. Findings showed that an insecure attachment style is moderately linked to anxiety, with ambivalent attachment most significantly associated and the relationship at its strongest during adolescence [4]. Insecure attachment was also significantly associated with depression [5] in both children and adolescence, leading to a recommendation that attachment should be considered and addressed as part of treatment for depression in this population. Secure attachments are shown to protect young people from developing PTSD symptoms following experiences of sexual trauma [6], with insecurely attached individuals more at risk of developing difficulties associated with dissociation, anxiety, depression and anger as a consequence of childhood sexual abuse [7]. For further exploration of the role of attachment in child and adolescent mental health please see Chapter 3 – Risk Factors for Psychopathology in Children and Young People.

Trauma

Post-traumatic Stress Disorder

PTSD is characterised by an anxiety response, following a traumatic event. Initial diagnostic criteria specified that the traumatic event, acting as a catalyst for PTSD, could encompass both civilian and military experiences, but made no reference to intrafamilial traumas, such as childhood abuse or domestic violence. The symptomatic response leads to feelings of threat, experiences of hyperarousal and concerns about ongoing safety. Children with PTSD are likely to present with dreams about the trauma, reliving via play, loss of interest in enjoyable activities, problems concentrating, behavioural difficulties, physical health complaints and expressing fears about their safety [8]. Adolescents with PTSD are more likely to experience substance misuse, physical health problems and academic difficulties and are more at risk of emotional and behavioural dysregulation and suicide [9].

Prevalence and Causes of PTSD

A comprehensive epidemiological study found that almost a third (31%) of children and adolescents across England and Wales had been exposed to a traumatic event prior to the age of 18 [10]. The most commonly reported traumas were Network Traumas; the exposure to trauma impacting on a significant other within their network, for example, death or imprisonment (28%), interpersonal assaults or threats of assaults (22%) and accident or injury (19%). Of the third exposed to traumatic events, one-quarter went on to experience symptoms of PTSD, giving an overall prevalence estimation of 7.8%.

Despite traumatic events in childhood being common, the comparable prevalence of PTSD symptoms is lower, suggesting that most childhood traumas do not result in PTSD [10, 11]. Young people are more likely to develop PTSD following interpersonal traumas such as peer bullying or adult maltreatment [10] with the highest levels occurring after physical violence or sexual trauma, following repeated traumas, within the context of family adversity and pre-existing anxiety [11] and for girls [12].

Complex Trauma

Herman [13] originally proposed the concept of *Complex Trauma* as a response to prolonged exposure to multiple or repeated traumatic events in early childhood, outlining that PTSD as a diagnosis did not capture additional observed difficulties such as somatisation, dissociation, changes to affect, identity and relationships and increased risk of further harm (from self or others). Original definitions of complex trauma focused primarily on the traumas that may occur within family relationships, including childhood sexual, physical and emotional abuse, neglect and exposure to domestic violence. The concept was then expanded to encapsulate other types of prolonged trauma; including exposure to war and conflict, being held as a prisoner of war and being the victim of trafficking or resettlement as a refugee. Complex Trauma is now also used to capture the reaction some individuals have in response to single '*calamitous*' traumas, such as prolonged torture, gang rape or witnessing another's death [14].

ICD-11: Post-traumatic Stress Disorder (6B40) and Complex Post-traumatic Stress Disorder (6B41)

The 11th edition of the ICD [1] includes two distinct but related conditions: PTSD and the newly formulated Complex Post Traumatic Stress Disorder (C-PTSD) categorised under 'Disorders specifically associated with stress'.

The new figuration of PTSD is made up of three symptom clusters. Firstly, the individual must re-experience the trauma as if it is happening again in the present moment, usually through flashbacks and nightmares. Secondly, the individual should be employing avoidance as a tactic to evade reminders of the trauma. This avoidance could be *environmental*, not going to a certain place, *relational*, not spending time with certain people, or *psychological*, not thinking about or allowing feelings about the event. Finally, the person must still feel persistently under threat; describing feelings of jumpiness and hypervigilance to what is happening, either externally in their environment, or internally in their body.

The newly added diagnosis of C-PTSD is characterised by the three elements of PTSD *plus* additional difficulties in self-organisation. The individual must experience persistent and significant difficulties in emotion regulation (affective disorganisation). This may include the inability to experience positive emotions, intense reactions in response to mild stress (either violent outbursts, heightened emotional states, dissociation or emotional numbing) and self-destructive behaviour as a method of coping. They must also hold a view

Table 11.2 Diagnostic criteria for PTSD and C-PTSD

	PTSD	C-PTSD
Exposure to a threatening or horrifying event	✓	✓
Re-experiencing of the trauma in the present	✓	✓
Avoidance of factors likely to remind an individual of the trauma	✓	✓
Persistent sense of remaining under threat and being hypervigilant to harm	✓	✓
Pervasive difficulties in regulating affect	✗	✓
Persistently negative beliefs about oneself	✗	✓
Significant and persistent difficulties in maintaining close relationships	✗	✓
These disturbances must have a significant impact on an individual's functioning	✓	✓

of oneself that is negative, which may stem from feelings of worthlessness, guilt, shame or a negative perception of how they managed themselves in response to or during the trauma. Finally, they must have difficulties maintaining relationships, with a tendency to avoid social interactions, and difficulties trusting others.

The diagnostic criteria of PTSD and C-PTSD is shown in Table 11.2.

Assessing Trauma in Children and Adolescents: Special Considerations

Asking Difficult Questions

Clinicians are encouraged to explore an individual's trauma history during assessment, with the acknowledgement that a significant proportion of people who seek help from mental health services do so because of the indirect or direct consequences of trauma [15]. This is further emphasised in the principles of trauma-informed care, which promotes a shift from 'what is wrong with you' to 'what has happened to you' [16]. Clinicians frequently report anxiety about asking questions about childhood trauma, even within adult populations, with many finding such questions even more difficult with children and adolescence. All young people accessing mental health services should be asked about their history of adverse childhood experiences. Questions should be posed in a developmentally appropriate way, and metaphors and euphemisms should be avoided. It is also important to give the child the opportunity to answer this question alone wherever possible, particularly in situations where the clinician suspects a history of trauma or safeguarding concerns related to the child that may not be disclosed by the caregiver.

Assessing Very Young Children

A meta-analysis of PTSD prevalence in under-6s found that following a traumatic event, the prevalence of PTSD was similar to rates in older children and adults, as long as developmentally appropriate criteria were applied [17]. Assessment in very young children can be impeded by immature cognitive or language capabilities, which makes it difficult to rely solely on the child's self-report for the three core criteria across both diagnoses (re-experiencing, avoidance and hypervigilance). Clinicians need to incorporate caregiver reports and observations and pay particular attention to trauma manifestations through repetitive play, drawings, re-enactments and stories. Further indicators of trauma in the very young *may include* the presence of inhibited and disinhibited behaviours, such as regression of skills, excessive crying, age-inappropriate fears and behavioural outbursts [1].

Differential Diagnoses

A common question following reports of the introduction of the C-PTSD diagnosis related to how this condition would be differentiated from existing diagnoses of personality disorder. A close examination of the ICD-11 criteria [1] and studies examining both the overlap and discrepancies helps to answer this question. In summary:

- A diagnosis of C-PTSD specifically requires both a history of trauma, and the typical PTSD symptoms of avoidance, intrusions and experiences of reliving [18] whereas a diagnosis of personality disorder does not.
- Individuals with C-PTSD are likely to hold a persistently negative view of themselves whereas people with a diagnosis of personality disorder may hold a view of self that oscillates between overly negative and overly positive or grandiose [18].
- In C-PTSD individuals are avoidant of relationships due to mistrust and a fear of getting hurt [19] as opposed to individuals with a diagnosis of personality disorder who may show fluctuations in their relationships with idealised and rejecting patterns of interaction.
- When the diagnostic criteria for both C-PTSD and personality disorder are met, only the diagnosis of C-PTSD should be given, unless there is a strong rationale for the additional diagnosis adding to the clinical picture in a way that C-PTSD does not already capture [18].
- Individuals with a personality disorder diagnosis are more likely than those with C-PTSD to engage in repetitive self-injurious or suicidal behaviours to regulate emotions [15].

All the studies examining the differences between the diagnostic profiles of C-PTSD and personality disorder are with adults. It is therefore critical to take note of the developmental considerations within the ICD-11 [1]:

- Adolescents are particularly likely to engage in risky and impulsive behaviours because of the emotional dysregulation and interpersonal difficulties at the core of C-PTSD. This includes behaviours associated with risk to self (substance misuse, unsafe sex and self-injury) and risk to others. This suggests that self-injurious and other risk behaviours should not be taken as evidence of a personality disorder over C-PTSD in a process of differential diagnosis *in adolescents*.
- A similar caution should be held when differentiating between PTSD and personality disorder, as again young people are more likely than adults to use self-harm or substance misuse as a coping strategy for the core features of PTSD (e.g. to manage the constant feelings of arousal associated with threat, flashbacks or nightmares).

In summary, if a young person has experienced a trauma, displays the PTSD indicators of re-experiencing, avoidance and hypervigilance and has difficulties in managing emotions, sustaining relationships and a persistently negative sense of self, many professionals working in CAMHS would conceptualise these difficulties under the lens of C-PTSD.

Anxiety Disorders

Causes

A developmental psychopathology approach to understanding the aetiology of anxiety disorders describes several complex transactions between protective and risk factors, both within the child and their environment. Vasey and Dadds [20] highlighted the key concepts of multideterminism, mulitifinality and equifinality. Multideterminism suggests that there will be multiple causal influences in the development of anxiety; and few will be either necessary or sufficient on their own. Multifinality suggests that a single factor can have multiple outcomes and equifinality suggests there can be numerous routes to any given outcome. For example, a traumatic experience involving an animal (a direct conditioning experience) may cause specific phobia in one child and no disorder in another. Another child may receive fear information regarding the same animal and develop specific phobia without the direct conditioning experience. The outcome will depend upon the complex interaction between multiple internal and external factors, including but not limited to attachment style, temperament and parental support. The developmental psychopathology framework suggests it is erroneous to look for a single cause or maintaining factor in childhood anxiety.

'Normal' Childhood Fears

The anxiety disorder classifications are aligned with normal fears that develop through childhood and adolescence that naturally reduce or disappear as the child develops increased reasoning and emotion regulation skills. For example, it is typical for young children to be scared of the dark, thunderstorms, or a number of specific fears akin to a specific phobia, for example, spiders. Separation anxiety is also normal as young children begin to spend more time outside the home and need to develop relationships and accept soothing and regulation from caring adults other than their immediate family. During adolescence a focus on the opinions of peers is crucial to the core task of this developmental period; finding their role within the community and their friendship group and developing intimate relationships with peers. The focus on the evaluation from others during this stage means that anxiety in this period is most likely to be social in nature. Muris et al [21] used the DSM criteria to look at the severity of 'normal' childhood fears in 290 8–13-year-olds and found that 23% met criteria for a disorder, with clinical levels of impairment.

Disorder Categories

There has been debate regarding the usefulness of applying the different diagnostic categories to children and adolescents. Rutter [22] argued convincingly for the clinical utility of collapsing the different categories into 'Anxiety Disorder', as the majority of children met criteria for 3 or more disorders and treatment does not differ across the categories. However, when studying the onset, course and sequelae of anxiety in childhood there are persistent disorder-specific patterns that emerge, which are argued to be both clinically and conceptually useful – for example Separation Anxiety is a better predictor of adult psychopathology than other disorder categories [23]. While most anxiety disorders share core

Table 11.3 Overview of anxiety disorders

Anxiety disorders	Core differentiating criteria
Generalised anxiety disorder (6B00)	Persistent and uncontrollable worry about a variety of everyday events and situations. Worry may be accompanied by a general sense of foreboding, physical manifestations of anxiety, tiredness and difficulties concentrating.
Separation anxiety disorder (6B05)	Excessive fear and accompanying distress about being separated from or losing an attachment figure. The fears are in excess of what is developmentally expected and have an impact on the child's functioning or independence.
Social anxiety disorder (6B04)	Excessive and preoccupying fears of behaving or appearing in a way that leads to being negatively judged by, or humiliated, in front of others. Fears may lead to a focus on excessive self-evaluation, self-monitoring and avoidance behaviours.
Specific phobia (6B03)	Overwhelming and persistent fear of a situation, object, animal or place that is disproportionate and debilitating. Fear may be accompanied by avoidant behaviours.
Panic disorder (6B01)	Unexpected and unpredictable anxiety attacks in the absence of a clear trigger. Panic attacks are often accompanied by a fear of further attacks and a misinterpretation of the physical symptoms of anxiety such as 'I am having a heart attack' or 'I am going to die'.
Obsessive compulsive disorder (6B20)	Intrusive obsessional thoughts that are unwanted, distressing and often ego-dystonic. Thoughts are a trigger to compulsive behaviours or rituals that are carried out in order to reduce the distress caused by the obsessions.
Body dysmorphic disorder (6B21)	Persistent worries about body image where an individual is distressed and preoccupied about certain, often imperceptible or imagined, negative aspects of their appearance.

features of physical symptoms of fight, flight, freeze response, negative foreboding cognitions and hypervigilance, there are differentiating factors, summarised in Table 11.3.

Prevalence

A meta-analysis of the prevalence of anxiety through early childhood to late adolescence [23] reviewed over 50 epidemiological studies of 2–18-year-olds, using statistical methods to combine large quantities of prevalence data from studies of varying design (see Table 11.4). The findings demonstrate that anxiety disorders are highly prevalent throughout childhood and adolescence and that these estimates are stable and reliable in adolescence despite differing populations and methods employed. It is notable that the percentage of young people reporting that they suffer from anxiety disorders is not markedly different to some of the large studies of anxiety prevalence rates in adulthood [24].

Longitudinal data from the Avon Longitudinal Study demonstrates much lower rates of any anxiety disorder with only approximately 2–3 of every 100 children at any one time in middle childhood to early adolescence, with prevalence being highest at the age of 10 [25].

Table 11.4 Prevalence of anxiety disorders [26]

	Age 6–12 years				Age 13–18 years			
Anxiety disorders	Mean (%)	SE (%)	2.5%	97.5%	Mean (%)	SE (%)	2.5%	97.5%
Any	12.3	5.4	7.1	28.2	11.0	0.5	10.3	12.2
GAD	1.7	1.2	0.9	5.0	1.9	0.5	1.3	3.3
Separation anxiety	3.9	1.5	2.6	8.5	2.3	0.9	1.4	4.8
Social anxiety	2.2	2.2	1.0	8.8	5.0	1.3	3.5	8.4
Specific phobia	6.7	3.6	4.0	18.0	6.7	1.6	4.7	10.9
Panic disorder	1.5	3.2	0.2	8.9	1.1	0.3	0.7	1.8

Age at Onset

The high prevalence of anxiety in children and adolescents leads to the assumption that many anxiety disorders have their first onset in this period. Costello et al [23] attempted to include age at onset in their review; however, only the authors' study [26] had assessed and reported age at onset for anxiety disorders in the diagnostic interview. This study reported the median age of onset for any anxiety disorder as 8 years old, significantly below reports from adult studies, for example, 11 years [27]. When examining the median and interquartile ranges for each disorder, the findings demonstrate that most disorders have their onset before the age of 10, with only panic and agoraphobia onsetting later (12 and 18 years respectively).

Course and Outcomes

There are contradictory findings regarding whether anxiety disorders in children are merely transitory or have a chronic course and relationship with adult psychopathology. It has previously been believed that anxiety disorders remit quickly, with several clinical population studies supporting this hypothesis [28, 29]. An examination of risk factors in preschool children pinpointed anxious *symptoms* (along with child temperament) in pre-schoolers, as the best predictor of anxiety symptoms at 6 and 8 years old [36] suggesting that early symptoms are important predictors of later psychopathology. In longer term follow-up (10 to 11 years old) parent-reported internalising and externalising symptoms at preschool uniquely predict their diagnostic counterpart (DSM-IV disorder). Mesman and Koot [31] similarly reported that children with parent-reported internalising symptoms in kindergarten have a 3-fold odds of meeting diagnostic criteria for an anxiety or depressive disorder in pre-adolescence.

Continuity of Disorders

The testing of ecological models of anxiety by Mian et al. [30] suggest that child factors (symptoms) are far better predictors of later anxiety than external factors, so the hypothesis that the association between early symptoms and later psychopathology is the product of a third social or family factor (e.g. social disadvantage or insecure attachment) seems less likely.

The contention that anxiety is not persistent and is usually transitory has been supported by a number of short-term follow-up studies of clinical samples that have shown the vast majority of children to be free of their primary anxiety diagnosis within a short period of time, leading to the conclusion that the course of childhood anxiety disorders is remitting and less malignant than the course of adult disorders [28,29,32,33]. The issue with these studies is that they use a single diagnostic follow-up over a relatively short period (18 months to 5 years) to ascertain whether the participant is 'well' or remains ill, they also often focus upon only one disorder; for example Cantwell and Baker [32] examined Obsessive Compulsive Disorder (OCD) and Foley et al. [33] looked at separation anxiety. Alternatively the other studies do not distinguish between outcomes of the different anxiety disorders and examine 'any anxiety disorders' making comparisons difficult.

A naturalistic study carried out by Carballo and colleagues [34] in paediatric psychiatric clinics in Spain, followed nearly 2000 children over 14 years. They report the persistence of most anxiety disorders (particularly social anxiety and specific phobias) to be very high. Over 80% received the same diagnosis at 75% of consultations (minimum number of consultations was 3). In adolescents the persistence was lower (between 60% and 70%). This is still very high in comparison to the other clinical studies cited and may reflect the large sample size offering greater accuracy, or alternatively may be a result of the naturalistic design and human reasoning, with clinicians being increasingly likely to reassign a diagnosis once they have previously recorded it, and those who remit not attending clinic, which could lead to an artificial inflation of the persistence of the disorders.

Beesdo-Baum et al. [35] propose that early anxiety does not have a linear course, instead anxiety disorders remit and change their symptom profile through the course of development, but leave the young person at an increased risk of later psychopathology. They present data from 4 waves of assessment in the Dresden study reporting data from a 10-year follow-up of the sample of 14–24-year-olds. Analysis of the data provided further evidence to support the contention that anxiety has an unstable course in adolescence, with many disorders having only moderate stability across the follow-up periods. However, it also clearly demonstrates that although anxiety may remit in the short term, heterotypic continuity is high; anxiety in adolescence is a significant risk factor for anxious and depressive psychopathology in adulthood. Ten-year follow-up at 23–34 years demonstrated that a sizeable proportion (35–41%) of adolescents met criteria for the same anxiety disorder (strict homotypic continuity) and only 10–14% were without psychopathology, with 70% suffering from an emotional disorder (depression or anxiety). Of those who were diagnosed with social anxiety at baseline only 13% were free of psychopathology at 10 years; 35% met criteria for social anxiety (strict homotypic continuity) and 64% were diagnosed with an anxiety or depressive disorder (heterotypic continuity). When examining generalised anxiety disorder and PTSD, no one diagnosed at baseline was free from psychopathology at 10 years. It is notable that both generalised anxiety and PTSD sample sizes were small, as these are rare disorders in this age group; however, this is still a clinically important finding.

Interventions

Anxiety Disorders

NICE, the National Institute for Health and Care Excellence, recommends that psychological interventions are effective, and the least intrusive treatment for anxiety disorders in children and young people, and they should be first-line treatments as opposed to pharmacological intervention. Evidence-based psychological approaches include both low-intensity approaches (guided self-help) and more intensive psychological therapies delivered by trained and accredited therapists (e.g. CBT).

Specific guidelines for social anxiety [36] propose 8–12 45-minute sessions of group or individual CBT (social skills training, psychoeducation and graded exposure to feared social situations) with the involvement of families to be considered and prioritised for all, but with the parents of children under 7-years-old being targeted for intervention rather than the child. Similarly, parents should be offered a group intervention that supports them to encourage exposure to feared situations and promote their child's social skills. Pharmacological treatment is expressly written as treatments that should not be offered for under-18s who present with social anxiety.

OCD and Body Dysmorphic Disorder guidelines [37] similarly promote the primary use of CBT; either in low-intensity guided self-help, for mild impairment, or individual CBT where there is moderate or severe impairment. The involvement of parents and carers is thought to be beneficial to treatment outcomes; however, the method of this involvement is not so clearly specified.

PTSD

NICE guidelines advise not to offer drug treatments to young people aged under 18 years for prevention or treatment of PTSD; however, drug treatment may be used for a comorbid mental health condition informed by the relevant evidence base. NICE guidelines also suggest we should not provide psychologically informed debriefing as this can increase the incidence of disordered responses to trauma [8]. Active monitoring should be considered for those within 1 month of experiencing trauma or those who have subclinical symptoms (not causing impaired functioning). The guidelines identify benefits of group interventions for those experiencing large-scale shared trauma but specify that this must be based on a manualised CBT treatment delivered by trained practitioners. All children and young people presenting with symptoms 1 month after the traumatic event should be considered for individual Trauma Focused CBT (TFCBT), carried out over a course of 8–12 sessions. The therapeutic intervention should focus on supporting the young person to process and make meaning from the trauma and encourage their exposure to feared situations/stimuli, as well as providing psychoeducation about trauma reactions. EMDR is also recommended for children who cannot or will not engage in TFCBT. The International Society of Traumatic Stress Studies guidelines for the prevention and management of PTSD [38] report an increase in strong evidence for TFCBT, for children, and for caregivers alongside children, as well as EMDR for children and adolescents. There is also an increasing evidence base for the use of Narrative Therapy in refugee children (KIDNET), with a randomised controlled trial (RCT) demonstrating its effectiveness in reducing and sustaining reduction in chronic PTSD symptoms following only 8 sessions of intervention [39].

The NICE guidelines do not cover children under 8 years; however, evidence from an early stage RCT [40] highlighted that an adapted form of cognitive focused trauma-based therapy can be effective in the treatment of PTSD in 3- to 8-year-olds who have experienced a single incident trauma. The therapy limited the amount of exposure intervention, focusing primarily on cognitive aspects of intervention, such as restructuring the trauma narrative and remedying unhelpful coping responses. The authors called for a larger trial of its effectiveness, emphasising the importance of these early positive responses in an age group where there is often a lack of therapeutic intervention available.

C-PTSD

General consensus regarding the treatment options for C-PTSD appears to favour a staged approach, with a primary focus on stabilisation of mood and installation of safe coping strategies prior to moving forward with any memory or reprocessing work, akin to what would usually be offered for PTSD. However, some have concerns regarding the delay in moving to the processing stage of therapeutic intervention [41], arguing that affect can be stabilised through the reprocessing elements of trauma, and does not therefore need to be a primary target for intervention. There is a limited number of studies investigating the efficacy of treatments for C-PTSD in young people; however, it is hoped that this will change with the inclusion of the diagnosis within the ICD-11. Retrospective analysis of existing trial data has shown some efficacy for the use of TFCBT in young people who were deemed to have met the criteria for C-PTSD, with both PTSD and C-PTSD responding equally well [42]. However, it is notable that despite significant improvement, the young people with C-PTSD retained significantly more symptomatic than the PTSD group, suggesting a higher symptomatic impairment at the start and end of treatment. This highlights the importance of further research into effective treatments for C-PTSD in young people, particularly for those who experience dissociation, self-harm, express suicidal ideation or present as a risk to others, as these individuals are often absent from research data. The International Society for Traumatic Stress Studies Guidelines for the Prevention and Treatment of Post-Traumatic Stress Disorder guidelines [38] highlight that despite an increasing evidence base for certain interventions, there should be no one-size-fits-all approach to trauma treatment. The importance of a comprehensive assessment, followed by a discussion regarding the intervention options, with both the individual and parent/caregiver, was reiterated.

New Developments: Online CBT

Computerised CBT is a well-established treatment option for mild to moderate mental health problems in adults; primarily targeted at those receiving primary care interventions for stress, anxiety and depression. With the increased focus on young people's mental health and the disparity between the numbers reporting difficulties and those accessing treatment, computerised interventions for young people are felt to be promising as a means of increasing access to therapy. There are additional benefits of reduced clinician time that allows re-allocation of therapist resources to the most complex cases and proposed cost-effectiveness.

A recent meta-analysis explored the effectiveness of online CBT for young people under the age of 18 who met the criteria for an anxiety disorder, based upon a diagnostic interview [43]. The review identified that online CBT had a moderate effect on the remission of anxiety disorders compared to control groups, when measured by clinicians, a small effect regarding parent report and no effect in relation to self-report. The review highlighted the importance of involving young people in the development of online therapeutic interventions and cautioned against the narrative that young people prefer to seek help online. The review directed further studies to compare online CBT against both purely face-to-face CBT and a mixed approach combining both online and face-to-face sessions. Previous research into CBT for social anxiety showed promising results when guided online CBT was supplemented by online sessions for parents and in-person group exposure sessions [44].

In the treatment of trauma, the NICE guidelines [8] recommend offering computerised TFCBT *for adults*, where it is the patient preference. However, this is only indicated where there is no evidence of dissociation or known risk to self or others. There is no current NICE guidance regarding the use of computerised TFCBT for children or adolescents; however, there is a current trial underway hosted by the Institute of Psychiatry, exploring the effectiveness of online TFCBT for young people who have experienced single incident trauma.

Concluding Remarks

A significant proportion of young people today identify problems relating to anxiety and trauma. It is hoped that the development of C-PTSD assists clinicians in the accurate assessment and formulation of children and adolescents that have experienced complex trauma and/or repeated adverse childhood experiences. Interventions for young people experiencing anxiety disorders, disrupted attachments or PTSD/C-PTSD should all have some focus on developing a young person's skills in managing distress, improve their confidence in problem-solving and increase exposure to positive emotions. Insecure attachments play a key role in child and adolescent psychopathology, and interventions designed to treat difficulties in this client group should also focus on improving the quality and security of a young person's attachments. Clinicians must also be sensitive to the potential cognitive difficulties faced by young people who have experienced trauma and adversity and be willing to adapt services appropriately. This includes having the time to orientate a young person to the environment and the relationship, a willingness to go at the child's pace and an ability to flex the service offer in response to delays in assessment and treatment.

References

1. World Health Organisation. *The ICD-11 Classification of Mental and Behavioural Disorders: Clinical Descriptions and Diagnostic Guidelines*. World Health Organisation, 2022.
2. Mikulincer M, Shaver PR. An Attachment Perspective on Psychopathology. World Psychiatry. 2012;**11**(1):11–15.
3. Cassidy J, Kobak RR. Avoidance and Its Rrelation to Other Defensive Processes. In J Belsky & T Nezworski, *Clinical implications of attachment*. Lawrence Erlbaum Associates, 1988.
4. Colonnesi C, Draijer EM, Stams GJ, Van der Bruggen CO, Bogels SM, Noon MJ. The Relationships Between Insecure Attachment and Child Anxiety. J Clin Child Adolesc Psychol. 2011;**40**(4):630–45.
5. Spruit A, Goos L, Weenink N, et al. Attachment and Depression in Children and Adolescents: A Multi-level Meta-analysis. Clin Child Fam Psychol Rev. 2020;**23**(1):54–69.
6. Jardin C, Venta A, Newlin E, Ibarra S, Sharp C. Secure Attachment Moderates the Relation of Sexual Trauma with Trauma Symptoms Among Adolescents from an Inpatient Psychiatric Facility. J Interpers Violence. 2017;**32**:1565–85.
7. Ensink K, Fonagy P, Normandin L, Rozenberg A, Marquez C, Godbout N. Post-traumatic Stress Disorder in Sexually Abused Children: Secure Attachment as a Protective Factor. Front Psychol. 2021;**12**:1–10.
8. NICE. *Post-Traumatic Stress Disorder*. NICE, 2018. Available from: https://www.nice.org.uk/guidance/NG116 (accessed 6 April 2025).

9. Nooner KB, Linares O, Batinjane J, Kramer RA, Silva R, Cloitre M. Factors Related to Posttraumatic Stress Disorder in Adolescence. TVA. 2012;13(3):153–66.

10. Lewis SJ, Arseneault L, Caspi A, et al. The Epidemiology of Trauma and Post-traumatic Stress Disorder in a Representative Cohort of Young People in England and Wales. Lancet Psychiatry. 2019;6:247–56.

11. Copeland WE, Keeler G, Angold A, Costello J. Traumatic Events and Posttraumatic Stress in Childhood. Arch Gen Psychiatry. 2007;64:577–84.

12. Alisic E, Zalta AK, van Welsel F, et al. Rates of Post-traumatic Stress Disorder in Trauma-Exposed Children and Adolescents: Meta-analysis. Br J Psychiatry. 2018;204(5):335–40.

13. Herman, J. Complex PTSD: A Syndrome in Survivors of Prolonged and Repeated Trauma. J Trauma Stress. 1992;5(3):377–91.

14. Courtois CA. Complex Trauma, Complex Reactions: Assessment and Treatment. Psychol Psychotherapy. 2004;41(4):412–25.

15. Cloitre M, Galvert DW, Weiss B, Carlson EB, Bryant RA. Distinguishing PTSD, Complex PTSD and Borderline Personality Disorder: A Latent Class Analysis. Eur J Psychotraumatol. 2014;5:1–10.

16. Sweeney A, Filson B, Kennedy A, Collinson L, Gillard S. A Paradigm Shift: Relationships in Trauma-Informed Mental Health Services. BJPsych Advances. 2018;24(5):319–33.

17. Woolgar F, Garfield H, Dalgleish T, Meiser-Stedman R. Systematic Review and Meta Analysis: Prevalence of Posttraumatic Stress Disorder in Trauma-Exposed Preschool-Aged Children. J Am Acad Child Adolesc Psychiatry. 2022;61(3):366–77.

18. Felding SU, Mikkelsen LB, Bach B. Complex PTSD and Personality Disorder in ICD-11: When to Assign One or Two Diagnoses? Australas Psychiatry. 2021;29(6):590–94.

19. Brewin CR, Cloitre M, Hyland P, et al. A Review of Current Evidence Regarding the ICD-11 Proposals for Diagnosing PTSD and Complex PTSD. Clin Psychol Rev. 2017;58:1–15.

20. Vasey MW, Dadds M. *The Developmental Psychopathology of Anxiety*. Oxford University Press, 2001.

21. Muris P, Meesters C, Merckelbach H, Hulsenbeck P. Worry in Children Is Related to Perceived Parental Rearing and Attachment. Behav Res Ther. 2000;38:487–97.

22. Rutter M. Research Review: Child Psychiatric Diagnosis and Classification: Concepts, Findings, Challenges and Potential. J Child Psychol Psychiatry. 2011;52(6):647–60.

23. Costello EJ, Egger HL, Copeland WE, Erkanli A, Angold A. The Developmental Epidemiology of Anxiety Disorders: Phenomenology, Prevalence, and Comorbidity. In WK Silverman & AP Field (eds.), *Anxiety Disorders in Children and Adolescents*. 2nd ed. Cambridge University Press: 2011, 56–75.

24. Alonso J, Angermeyer MC, Bernert S, et al. Prevalence of Mental Disorders in Europe: Results from the European Study of the Epidemiology of Mental Disorders (ESEMeD) Project. Acta Psychiatr Scand Suppl. 2004;109:21–27.

25. Gallagher SB. *Epidemiology of Childhood Anxiety: Longitudinal Perspectives*. DClinPsy thesis. School of Psychology, University of Leeds, 2011.

26. Costello EJ, Mustillo S, Erkanli A, Keeler G, Angold A. Prevalence and Development of Psychiatric Disorders in Childhood and Adolescence. Arch. Gen. Psychiatry. 2003;60:837–44.

27. Kessler RC, Berglund P, Demler O, Jin R, Merikangas KR, Walters EE. Lifetime Prevalence and Age-of-Onset Distributions of DSM-IV Disorders in the National Comorbidity Survey Replication. Arch Gen Psychiatry. 2005;62(6):593–602.

28. Aschenbrand SG, Kendall PC, Webb A, Safford SM, Flannery-Schroeder E. Is Childhood Separation Anxiety Disorder

a Predictor of Adult Panic Disorder and Agoraphobia? A Seven-Year Longitudinal Study. J Am Acad. Child Adolesc Psychiatry. 2003;42(12):1478–85.
29. Last CG, Perrin S, Hersen M, Kazdin AE. A Prospective Study of Childhood Anxiety Disorders. J Am Acad Child Adolesc Psychiatry. 1996;35:1502–10.
30. Mian ND, Wainwright L, Briggs-Gowan MJ, Carter AS. An Ecological Risk Model for Early Childhood Anxiety: The Importance of Early Child Symptoms and Temperament. J Abnorm Child Psychol. 2011;39(4):501–12.
31. Mesman J, Bongers IL, Koot HM. Preschool Developmental Pathways to Preadolescent Internalizing and Externalizing Problems. J Child Psychol Psychiatry. 2001;42(5):679–89.
32. Cantwell DP, Baker L. Stability and Natural History of DSM-III Childhood Diagnoses. J Am Acad Child Adolesc Psychiatry. 1989;28(5):691–700.
33. Foley DL, Pickles A, Maes HM, Silberg JL, Eaves LJ. Course and Short-Term Outcomes of Separation Anxiety Disorder in a Community Sample of Twins. J Am Acad Child Adolesc Psychiatry. 2004;43(9):1107–14.
34. Carballo JJ, Baca-Garcia E, Blanco C, et al. Stability of Childhood Anxiety Disorders Diagnoses: A Follow Up Naturalistic Study in Psychiatric Care. Eur Child Adolesc Psychiatry. 2010;19:395–403.
35. Beesdo-Baum K, Hoffler, M, Gloster, AT, et al. The Structure of Common Mental Disorders: A Replication Study in a Community Sample of Adolescents and Young Adults. Int J Methods Psychiatr Res. 2009;18(4):204–20.
36. NICE. *Social Anxiety Disorder: Recognition, Assessment and Treatment*. NICE, 2013. Available from: https://www.nice.org.uk/guidance/cg159 (accessed 6 April 2025).
37. NICE. *Obsessive-Compulsive Disorder and Body Dysmorphic Disorder: Treatment*. NICE, 2005. Available from: https://www.nice.org.uk/Guidance/CG31 (accessed 6 April 2025).
38. Bisson JI, Berliner L, Cloitre M, et al. The International Society for Traumatic Stress Studies New Guidelines for the Prevention and Treatment of Post-Traumatic Stress Disorder: Methodology and Development Process. J Trauma Stress. 2019;32:475–83.
39. Ruf M, Schauer M, Neuner F, Catani C, Schauer E, Elbert, TE. Narrative Exposure Therapy for 7-to-16-Year-Olds: A Randomized Controlled Trial with Traumatized Refugee Children. J Trauma Stress. 2010;23(4):437–45.
40. Hitchcock C, Goodall B, Wright I, Boyle A, Johnston D, Dunning D. The Early Course and Treatment of Post-traumatic Stress Disorder in Very Young Children: Diagnostic Prevalence and Predictors in Hospital Attending Children and a Randomized Proof of Concept Trial of Trauma Focused Cognitive Therapy, for 3- to 8-Year-Olds. J Child Psychol Psychiatry. 2022;63(1):58–67.
41. de Jongh A, Resick PA, Zoellner LA, et al. Critical Analysis of the Current Treatment Guidelines for Complex PTSD in Adults. Depress Anxiety. 2016;33:359–69.
42. Sachser C, Keller F, Goldbeck L. Complex PTSD as Proposed for ICD-11: Validation of a New Disorder in Children and Adolescents and Their Response to Trauma-Focused Cognitive Behavioural Therapy. J Child Psychol Psychiatry. 2017;58(2):160–68.
43. Cervin M, Lundgren T. Technology-Delivered Cognitive-Behavioral-Therapy for Pediatric Anxiety Disorders: A Meta-analysis of Remission, Posttreatment Anxiety, and Functioning. J Child Psychol Psychiatry. 2022;63(1):7–18.
44. Nordh M, Vigerland S, Ost LG, et al. Therapist-Guided Internet-Delivered Cognitive-Behavioural Therapy Supplemented with Group Exposure Sessions for Adolescents with Social Anxiety: A Feasibility Trial. BMJ Open. 2017:7(12):1–11.

Chapter 12

Self-Harm and Suicide in Young People

Mindy Reeves, Eleni Frisira and David Kingsley

Introduction

Self-harm and suicidal behaviours in children and young people pose a significant public health concern. These behaviours, although heterogeneous, are increasingly common in this age group [1]. Self-harm is a transdiagnostic symptom and can be a manifestation of a number of emotional or mental health difficulties. Self-harm is associated with adverse future outcomes, including poor educational and employment outcomes, and early death by suicide or non-suicide related causes (e.g. accidents or assaults) [2,3]. This chapter outlines key concepts and terminology related to self-harm and suicide, reviewing the aetiology, epidemiology, risk assessment and management.

Terminology and Meaning

A number of terms and definitions are used in clinical practice and relevant literature. Self-harm or self-injurious behaviour can occur in the context of suicidal ideation but may also be unrelated to it. Non-suicidal self-injury or self-harm is the act of purposefully inflicting a physical injury to one's own body without suicidal intent [4,5]. Suicidal ideation describes the thought process of envisioning one's own death and suicide. Sometimes the term includes planning for a suicidal act, while at other times it is limited to individuals considering the idea of suicide before the planning stage [6]. Suicidality is an umbrella term that includes thoughts of attempting or completing suicide, and suicidal behaviours. It is thought that self-harm represents a spectrum of risk within a continuum of such behaviours [7,8]. At one end of the spectrum, young people may engage in self-harm as a coping mechanism for developmental stressors whereas at the other end, self-harm may be indicative of a real intent to end conscious life [8]. Self-harm and suicide are often the result of a complex interplay of multiple individual and contextual factors that cannot be easily generalised [9].

Aetiology and Association with Mental Health Conditions

Young people are more likely to self-harm if they have a mental health condition. These include mood disorders, anxiety disorders, OCD, BDD, psychotic illnesses and ADHD. As such, self-harm may be interpreted as a risk indicator for the development of one of these conditions [10]. Self-harm is common in autism, and studies have indicated that the problem may affect as many as 24% [11]. Autistic people may find it difficult to recognise, manage and express their emotions – alexithymia. These individuals may feel frustrated, anxious and depressed. Low mood and impulsivity have been noted as risk factors for self-harm in at least one autistic sample [11]. Importantly, however, not all young people who self-harm will have an established diagnosis. In a UK study, only one-third of young people had a recorded mental health condition. In the same study, depression increased the odds of both self-harm and suicide more than other diagnostic categories (self-harm: OR (odds ratio) 7.9; 95% CI (confidence interval) 7.8–8.2; suicide: OR 7.4; 95% CI 5.5–9.9) [12]. This is consistent with previous literature showing a strong independent association with depression and with anxiety [13,14]. Self-harm is also linked to alcohol and substance misuse, possibly due to both being used as maladaptive coping strategies by young people [15,16].

Self-harm is often associated with patients who meet criteria for a diagnosis of borderline personality disorder (BPD), many of whom may have experienced significant psychological trauma due to sexual abuse or other maltreatment. Individuals with BPD report engaging in self-harm behaviours as a coping mechanism to manage intense emotional distress. Early signs of BPD often include self-harm and suicidality, which are significant indicators of current and future risk [17]. However, in child and adolescent psychiatry, the link between self-harm, suicidality and BPD is often obscured, given clinicians' reluctance to diagnose BPD in young people. Predictive validity for diagnosis in young people is similar to adults [18] and a diagnosis facilitates the patient and their family receiving appropriate evidence-based treatment and helpful information about their condition as well as accessing support groups. Hesitancy to diagnose, often due to concern about the stigma attached to the 'personality disorder' label, can lead to erroneous diagnoses being made, such as of depression, and ineffective treatment being given for the wrong disorder [19]. This reluctance makes it difficult to accurately estimate the prevalence of BPD in this age group. Underreporting and misdiagnosis may lead to a lack of provision of targeted interventions for high-risk behaviours as lack of diagnostic clarity and consensus obscures resource allocation needs [19].

Some clinicians tend to opt for an alternative diagnosis of Complex Post-Traumatic Stress Disorder (C-PTSD), which requires criteria for PTSD to be met in addition to symptoms in domains of emotion regulation, self-identity and relational capacities. For many years researchers have debated whether C-PTSD is actually PTSD with comorbid BPD [20]. However, it has been shown that individuals with C-PTSD are distinguishable from those with BPD and there are some notable clinical differences with treatment implications. Individuals with C-PTSD experience a severe but stable negative self-concept whereas those with BPD report shifts in their self-image, vacillating between highly positive and highly negative self-perceptions. In C-PTSD relational difficulties are characterised by a tendency to avoid and have difficulty maintaining relationships, particularly during periods of conflict or high emotion, whereas BPD is associated with rapid engagement followed by ups and downs, or idealisation and denigration of relationships. Although emotion regulation difficulties are central to both C-PTSD and BPD, their expression can be different, with suicidal behaviours and self-harm a core feature of BPD in contrast to C-PTSD. C-PTSD does not require the presence of either problem for diagnosis for which preliminary data indicate rates of these issues are substantially lower. It is also important to note that a significant minority of patients with BPD have not disclosed psychological trauma, so they would not, by definition, be eligible for a diagnosis of C-PTSD.

There is an overlap between potential determinants related to self-harm and suicide. A large population-based study has recently been completed in the UK that has identified several risk factors to completed suicide [21] but these can also be associated with self-harm. These include mental health disorders, educational stressors, physical health illnesses, bullying and substance misuse. Comorbidity of different mental disorders further increases the risk [22]. The rise in self-harm and suicide rates has occurred alongside an increase in both the number of young people seeking mental health services and the prevalence of mental health disorders in this population. Clinical samples, taken from inpatient or outpatient samples, have higher rates of self-harm and suicide compared to community populations, which could be related to selection bias of people with more co-morbid mental health difficulties or a higher prevalence of females in clinical samples [23]. Previous self-harm has often been present in individuals who have attempted or completed suicide [24]. Some young people have described using self-harm as a way to manage negative emotions or the burden of an external environment that can seem hard to control [25].

Family adversity includes an array of difficulties that may negatively affect mental health such as poverty, separation or divorce, and childhood abuse or neglect. There has been a decrease in the household income for 20% of young people in the past 5 years [26]. Children and young people who have parents with mental illness have a higher chance of developing their own mental health difficulties [12]. Lower levels of parental educational achievement have also been found to be associated [24].

The digital world and social media have introduced additional stressors to some young people including pressures to achieve lifestyles and body images that are displayed online by social influencers. The internet has created an imaginary world that has likely increased the feeling of rejection in many young people along with negatively contributing to poor body image and comparisons of personal value, which can lead to depressive symptoms [27]. The internet is often used to research methods of suicide and can encourage young people to engage in suicidal acts. Exposure to self-harm online has been found to negatively influence self-harming behaviours [28]. The internet can be positive, and some young people can find online support such as group forums helpful when they are struggling, particularly as it provides an 'anonymous' place for young people to seek support when they may be embarrassed to speak about self-harm with their family or friends.

There are some studies that demonstrate differences in the presentation of self-harm and suicide between the male and female gender, although limited research is currently available for the child and adolescent population. Girls often reported relationship problems as a main reason of self-harm while boys typically had difficulties in educational or work settings [20]. The majority of studies suggest that while suicide attempts occur more frequently with females, that males are more likely to complete suicide [29].

Epidemiology

The prevalence of self-harm among young people has been rising [9], and suicide is one of the leading causes of death for individuals aged 10–19 in England and Wales [30]. Internationally, the lifetime prevalence rates of self-harm in the general adolescent population range between 14% and 23% [1,5,31]. In England, around 10% of the non-clinical population of children and young people aged 8 to 16 years have attempted to self-harm [1]. In the same year, almost a third of the young people in this age group with a probable mental health condition had tried to harm themselves, highlighting that self-harm is more prevalent in those affected by co-morbid mental health conditions than the general population [32]. In response to the public health concern about rising suicide rates, the NHS five year forward plan [33] set a target of reducing suicide rates in England by 10% by 2020. However, there has been no statistically significant reduction in suicide rates since this time. In response, in 2023 the UK government published a 5-year cross-sector strategy for suicide prevention in England [34], which includes specific actions in relation to children and young people, such as expanding mental health support in schools, funding mental health leads in schools, tackling bullying, including suicide and self-harm prevention in the school curriculum and promoting the health and well-being of looked-after children, including care leavers up to age 25.

Self-harm is a risk factor for future suicidality. Young people who have self-harmed once are more likely to repeatedly injure themselves and subsequently die by suicide [31]. With increasing frequency of suicidal ideation, the likelihood of suicide attempts also increases [35]. In the UK, the rate of suicide for individuals between the ages of 15 and 19 is 5.1 per 100,000 [36].

Multiple risk factors have been identified in relation to self-harm and suicide in youth (Table 12.1). With the transition from childhood to adolescence comes an increase in rates of self-harm, although some of the self-harm behaviours present in adolescence will regress spontaneously [14]. Adolescence is considered a period in one's lifetime when the risk of self-harm and suicide increases the most, marking a particularly vulnerable period [37]. Studies looking at the longitudinal course of non-suicidal self-harm have shown that prevalence peaks in adolescent years followed by a decline in young adulthood [38], meaning that health care services dealing with young people under 18 are likely to encounter higher rates of self-harm.

Table 12.1 Risk factors for self-harm and suicide

		Risk factors for self-harm	Risk factors for suicide
1.1	Demographic	Female gender	Male gender
2.1	Psychological	Mood disorders	Mood disorders
2.2		Anxiety disorders	Other severe mental health conditions like psychosis
2.3		Borderline personality traits	History of self-harm
2.4		History of trauma or abuse	History of trauma or abuse
2.5		Previous incidents of self-harm	Previous suicide attempts
3.0	Social	Bullying	Bullying
3.1		Substance abuse	Substance abuse
3.2		Poor family dynamics	Family history of suicide or mental illness
3.3		Lack of social support	Lack of social support
3.4		Living in a single-parent home	Stressful life events including academic pressures or bereavement
3.5		Siblings	Suicide related internet use
3.6			Availability of means

Adolescents who self-harm are 30 times more likely to die by suicide than those who do not [39]. Self-harm was reported in 52% of people aged under 20 that died by suicide [39]. Females are more at risk of self-harm than males, although studies have shown modest differences in the strength of gender association with self-harm. However, males appear to be more likely to die by suicide, with a male to female ratio of about 2.5:1. Across all types of self-harm, adolescent females are about 1.5 times more likely than adolescent males to engage in self-harm behaviours [31], but the effect of gender on self-harm likelihood varies depending on method of self-harm used [40]. The gender pattern appears to be somewhat different in younger children compared to that of older adolescents, with a preponderance of males up to the age of 10 years and similar numbers of males and females at age 11 years before a marked switch to considerably more females than males at the age of 12 years, a phenomenon that may be associated with the onset of puberty [41]. Young people who are LGBT are also at increased risk of self-harm, suicidal thoughts and attempts [42]. According to NCISH data, 5% of suicide deaths involved individuals who identified as LGB, and 1% as trans (including transgender, transsexual and non-binary). Self-harm seems to be present across all ethnic groups and may in fact be more prevalent in all minority groups, implying that it may be the social experience of being part of a minority group rather than being of a particular ethnicity that is the key factor [43].

Methods

Young people use different methods to inflict self-harm. Most people who repeatedly self-harm tend to use more than one method over time [44]. The list reviewed in this chapter is non-exhaustive. Methods can include poisoning, scratching, cutting, tattooing, headbanging, foreign object swallowing or inserting in body orifices/under skin, bloodletting, gassing, self-hitting, suspended or non-suspended ligatures, drowning, jumping, burning or wound aggravation [45].

The methods of self-harm vary by a number of factors. In both clinical and non-clinical populations, most studies report cutting as the most common method used by young females (usually using razors, knives or broken pieces of glass) [45,46]. Across people who have engaged in self-harm behaviours, approximately 70–90% of them have used cutting [47]. Following cutting, other common types are burning, headbanging and hitting oneself. Hitting is more common among young males [48]. Interfering with wound healing has also been reported as a prevalent type of non-suicidal self-harm [49]. Another study showed poisoning by overdose to be one of the most common types of self-harm behaviour among young females [50]. Young people with a learning disability typically engage in slightly different patterns of self-harm, such as repeated rhythmic headbanging [51].

For completed suicide, the most common method is hanging [21]. The second most common methods for females are poisoning by overdose or ingestion of toxic liquid such as pesticides; for males it is poisoning closely followed by use of firearms [52,53]. Other common types of suicide include jumping in front of a moving object, use of a sharp object or drowning [52]. Over the last two decades, there has been an increase in all types of suicide, with hanging and suffocation showing the largest rise [54].

There is a growing body of evidence describing how disordered eating can be used as a form of self-harm behaviour [55,56]. Disordered eating can include restricting dietary intake, bingeing, purging or excessive exercising [57]. Although these behaviours are part of the core features of eating disorders such as anorexia or bulimia nervosa, they can occur outside these diagnostic categories. Some young people describe that restrictive eating serves as a means to inflict harm to their bodies, therefore being used as a method to self-harm, a means of communicating distress, an avoidance of puberty due to past sexual trauma or a way of dissociating due to the cognitive blunting caused by starvation. Self-harm and dietary restriction may therefore share common functions and possibly be used interchangeably by some young people [58]. There is likely to be a bidirectional relationship between non-suicidal self-harm and restrictive eating, as the presence of either increases the risk of the other [56]. In a population admitted to a mental health hospital or an intensive community treatment team, almost 30% exhibited disordered eating symptoms as a means of self-harm [57]. As such, screening for and treating disordered eating symptoms in young people with a history of self-harm is increasingly important.

Formulation of Self-Harm

Self-harm and suicide are multidimensional and complex behaviours and there are different reasons why young people choose to engage in them [9]. These are not always well understood, but it is important that the underlying reasons are explored, beyond superficial acknowledgement of the behaviour or the resulting injury. Formulation overlaps with diagnosis but has a broader focus. It is the process of systematically gathering and integrating information in a way that leads to a full understanding of the patient's difficulties and strengths. A formulation should encompass biological, social and psychological perspectives. It should draw on information from a wide range of sources including the patient, family members, observations by staff, medical records, community-based professionals from health, education or social care and sometimes the results of medical tests or psychometric measures. This information should then be integrated into a coherent narrative that explains the origins of the patient's difficulties and what may be perpetuating them. This understanding then forms the basis for treatment planning. Crucially, a formulation should always be developed, discussed and, ideally, agreed with the patient.

In developing a formulation for a young person who has been engaging in self-harming or suicidal behaviour, it is important to consider predisposing factors, such as psychological trauma, psychosocial or family issues or substance misuse. Precipitating factors may relate to recent traumatic or distressing events or the recent onset of a mental disorder that needs treatment. Perpetuating factors may be continuing issues in the child or young person's life that are causing ongoing distress, and which may need to be addressed if the distress – and hence the associated self-harm risk – are to be reduced. Protective factors, which can be worked with to reduce risk and prevent future harm, may include positive parental or peer relationships.

Often children and young people who harm themselves use this as a strategy for emotional regulation [59]. Self-harm can commonly be a manifestation of heightened distress, self-punishment or a 'cry for help' [60]. A qualitative study with female patients outlined intrapersonal reasons for self-harm such as 'to communicate distress', 'to suppress distressing thoughts' or to 'relieve tension' [61]. Recognising self-harm as a transdiagnostic issue is crucial for clinicians, as it emphasises the importance of evaluating this behaviour within the context of multiple mental health difficulties or diagnoses. This approach ensures that treatment plans are not merely symptom-focused but are designed to address the deeper psychological drivers behind self-harm, potentially improving therapeutic outcomes.

Previous adverse experiences often play a role in the development of self-harming behaviours. Children and young people who have experienced trauma may be using self-harm as a way to regulate trauma-related memories [62]. As trauma can often lead to a poor sense of self and self-worth, trauma survivors often internalise strong feelings of shame and blame leading them to believe they are deserving of being hurt [63]. Self-harm may therefore be reinforced by allowing the person to escape aversive feelings of shame and guilt [59].

There is evidence suggesting an addictive component to self-harm, related to an increase in the levels of dopamine during self-injury [64]. This rise in dopamine in response to pain is linked to a physiological sense of relief, reinforcing the behaviour. Both functional and structural neuroimaging differences have been observed in young people who repeatedly self-harm, especially in areas involved in emotional regulation and salience, mainly the fronto-limbic pathways [65]. Such changes include localised reduction in grey matter, reduced microstructure of white matter or generalised hypoactivity of these areas that is disrupted by the dopamine surges during a self-harming episode [65,66,67].

Risk Assessment

The multiplicity of risk factors and the difficulties in quantifying risks in regard to self-harm and suicide has made it difficult if not impossible to create a reliable single risk assessment classification tool [68]. NHS England guidelines do not support the use of standardised risk assessments as predictors of self-harm or suicide attempts [69]. The National Institute for Health and Care Excellence UK (NICE) updated the guidelines on self-harm in 2022 [70]. NICE advises against the use of standardised risk assessment tools to make future predictions about self-harm or to inform care planning [70]. Risks should no longer be categorised as high, medium or low as these are too reductive and have been shown to be inaccurate. The sensitivity of using risk stratification is limited and studies have demonstrated that a significant number of individuals classified as 'low or medium' risk of suicide were reported to die by suicide later [71]. Risk assessment tools can make it harder for individuals to build a therapeutic relationship with their mental health team [24]. The use of tools that rely on a tick box approach contributes to a lack of individualisation in the formulation, understanding and consequent care of the young person.

A more personalised approach to risk assessment that develops a detailed risk formulation and safety plan can lead to a more holistic understanding of the individual's strengths, difficulties and risk factors, taking into account any early warning signs and triggers for self-harm or suicidal behaviour [70]. Interviews that contribute to risk formulation should include discussion of the detail of the suicidal act, including a description of suicide ideation, lethality, intent/motivation at the time and current intent. Previous suicidal behaviours and triggers should be explored. There should be an exploration of any history parental mental illness or suicidal behaviour, difficult family relationships or losses in the family. A history of physical, emotional and sexual abuse is also important: although it may be present it may not have been disclosed. Poor school attendance, disaffection from school, bullying and feeling isolated from or different to their peers should be explored. Sometimes a persistent feeling of being 'different' may relate to undiagnosed autism. Finally, it is important to get a sense of the young person's intentions and ability to keep themselves safe and the support that they may be able to access from family or peers can help them to do so. The appraisal of both the risk factors and potential triggers for future self-harm as well as the motivation of the young person to keep themselves safe should be assessed as well as the availability of support from family, peers or others within the young person's network.

Collaborative and therapeutic approaches towards the formulation of risks will help practitioners and young people work together to identify patterns of behaviours related to self-harm and suicidal thoughts so that interventions can be developed to support the young person to use alternative methods of managing negative emotions [37].

Interventions

Overall, there is a limited body of evidence available to support the efficacy of interventions for self-harm and suicidality in children and young people. In mild cases, it is important to avoid over-medicalising the situation – self-harm that may be a 'cry for help' from a young person struggling with issues in school, family or with peers, may only need a 'listening ear' from a supportive teacher, parent/carer or peer. Support groups may exist locally or online that can help young people to feel that they are not alone and that there are others who can support them from their own lived experience. Primary support may include online information, crisis services that offer contact via telephone or texting and school-based interventions. Offering a high standard of clinical care can of itself decrease self-harming behaviour and suicidal ideation, but this will look different across services.

Children and young people who engage in self-harming behaviours often find it challenging to engage in treatment [72]. Clinic-based Children and Adolescent Mental Health Services (CAMHS) services, operating only during office hours, are not well suited to meeting the needs of young people who self-harm or who may find it difficult to trust professionals, particularly if they have a history of trauma. They are more likely to reach a crisis out of hours when services are less available. As such, they require services that are responsive and flexible and, where possible, provided by consistent professionals who can build a relationship with the young person. Service models should be influenced by the principles of Trauma Informed Care [73].

Crisis teams and intensive home-based services are becoming more available in CAMHS, which is welcome, and they are reducing the incidence of inappropriate and unhelpful hospital admissions. As relational difficulties are a key component of these disorders, support should, where possible, be provided by professionals known to the young person and who are aware of their histories. This will increase the likelihood of effective engagement and de-escalation of risks. The 24/7 telephone support included in DBT-A, which ensures that a known professional is available to the young person at all times, is a good example of flexible and relational support for this client group. Remote contact interventions such as sending letters and texts or making phone calls can offer benefits that include reducing social isolation [72].

NICE suggests that everyone should receive a psychosocial assessment by a trained professional as soon as possible following an incident of self-harm or suicidal attempt [70]. Ongoing care needs should be identified, and a safety plan should be co-developed with the young person. Co-existing conditions should be taken into account when identifying appropriate interventions [70]. Developing individualised and clear diagnosis and formulation, including an understanding of the psychosocial needs for each young person, will help to tailor interventions to their needs.

Interventions for self-harm and suicidality include psychological treatment, pharmacological treatment or a combination of both. Psychological interventions can help consider a variety of issues that include addressing risk factors, increasing coping skills and improving self-esteem. The availability of specific psychological therapies will vary dependent on geography.

Dialectical Behaviour Therapy (DBT) was developed for the management of BPD but can also be helpful in the management of self-harm. This therapy involves individual and group work including learning skills and having access to individual support on a 24/7 basis. An adaptation has been developed for adolescents, and multiple Randomised Controlled Trialshave demonstrated that DBT-A offers the best efficacy for reducing self-harm and suicidal thoughts [74]. DBT-A led to a reduction in the repetition of self-harm during treatment compared to receiving conventional treatment [72]. DBT-A has been successfully used in inpatient settings and studies have shown decreased frequency of self-harm in adolescent units as a result [75].

Mentalisation-based treatment adapted for adolescents [76] has also been shown to be more effective than treatment as usual in reducing self-harm in patients presenting to community services (85% female). This improvement was explained by increased mentalisation and reduced attachment avoidance and reflected a reduction in emergent BPD symptoms and traits.

CBT has been shown to reduce self-harm in adult populations, but the available research has not shown a similar benefit in adolescents [72]. Making adaptations to CBT for this population could lead to more positive outcomes.

There is some evidence that family-based therapies can address family stressors and behaviours of the child and their parents or carers, which should lead to a reduction in self-harm and suicidal thoughts, although there is not enough research available to support this theory [72]. A family approach will not be appropriate for everyone including some cases of abuse and neglect.

Pharmacological treatments should be selected based on underlying mental health disorders or co-morbid conditions and include antidepressants, antipsychotics and mood stabilisers. Anxiolytics should be used with caution and only for short periods if indicated. Safety plans that include safe storage and utilisation of medication should be put in place, including consideration of the use of preparations that pose lower risk of overdose. Antidepressants should be used with caution, particularly where the pattern of mood is more of fluctuant 'emotional dysregulation' more consistent with BPD rather than the persistent low mood typical of depression, as there is a risk of antidepressants increasing impulsivity that may lead to an increased risk of self-harm and suicidal acts [27].

Hospital admissions should be avoided in most instances, as they can be counterproductive leading to escalated and more chronic patterns of risky behaviour. However, where a young person is deemed to be at imminent significant risk of suicide or life-changing self-harm that cannot be safely managed in the community, a brief crisis admission to a General Adolescent Unit or CAMHS PICU may be life-saving. Patients can become more dependent during inpatient stays, particularly when more restrictive measures are adopted such as enhanced observations, which can increase risks and reduce the motivation for a young person to manage their risks independently. The use of restraints and intramuscular injections of medication can be experienced by young people with histories of psychological trauma as re-traumatising events. Making changes to the ward environment that includes limiting access to certain areas and offering therapeutic activities during both the day and the evening for patients has been shown to reduce incidents of self-harm [75]. Staff members should be offered training to encourage problem-solving for specific incidents that might occur, along with time for allocating time to staff for reflective practice to consider challenging situations that occur on an inpatient ward. Taking the time to educate staff has also been shown to decrease self-harm in the inpatient unit [75].

A small minority of patients with extreme levels of suicidality or self-harm cannot be safely managed outside of specialist settings. Low Secure CAMHS units offer longer-term therapeutic interventions that can assist young people to engage in therapeutic work, which often will involve processing trauma – trauma can be the 'fuel' that perpetuates self-harming behaviour and self-denigrating feelings. Such settings also offer rehabilitation work to assist young people who may have been in hospital for long periods to rebuild the skills and confidence to manage themselves safely and effectively in the community. Similarly, some young people with chronic high risks to self who require ongoing intensive support may benefit from residential care settings supported by specialist mental health to avoid delayed discharges from hospital and to assist them in their recovery journeys into the community.

References

1. Farkas BF, Takacs ZK, Kollárovics N, Balázs J. The Prevalence of Self-Injury in Adolescence: A Systematic Review and Meta-analysis. Eur Child Adolesc Psychiatry. 2024 Oct;33(10):3439–58.
2. Singhal A, Ross J, Seminog O, Hawton K, Goldacre MJ. Risk of Self-Harm and Suicide in People with Specific Psychiatric and Physical Disorders: Comparisons Between Disorders Using English National Record Linkage. J R Soc Med. 2014;107(5):194–204. https://doi.org/10.1177/0141076814522033. PMID: 24526464; PMCID: PMC4023515.
3. Mars B, Heron J, Crane C, et al. Clinical and Social Outcomes of Adolescent Self Harm: Population Based Birth Cohort Study. BMJ. 2014;349:g5954. https://doi.org/10.1136/bmj.g5954. PMID: 25335825; PMCID: PMC4205277.
4. American Psychiatric Association. *Diagnostic and Statistical Manual of Mental Disorders (DSM-5)*. 5th ed. Arlington: American Psychiatric Association, 2013.
5. Xiao, Q, Song, X, Huang, L, Hou, D, Huang, X. Global Prevalence and Characteristics of Non-suicidal Self-Injury Between 2010 and 2021 Among a Non-clinical Sample of Adolescents: A Meta-analysis. Front Psychiatry. 2022;13:912441. https://doi.org/10.3389/fpsyt.2022.912441.
6. Harmer B, Lee S, Duong TVH, Saadabadi A. *Suicidal Ideation* [Internet]. Treasure Island, FL: StatPearls Publishing, 2024 Jan–. PMID: 33351435.
7. Fox F, Stallard P, Cooney, G. GPs Role Identifying Young People Who Self-Harm: A Mixed Methods Study. Fam Pract. 2015;32(4):415–19. https://doi.org/10.1093/fampra/cmv031.
8. Bailey D, Wright N, Kemp L. Self-Harm in Young People: A Challenge for General Practice. Br J Gen Pract. 2017;67(665):542–43. https://doi.org/10.3399/bjgp17X693545. PMID: 29192098; PMCID: PMC5697528.
9. Townsend E. Time to Take Self-Harm in Young People Seriously. Lancet Psychiatry. 2019;6(4):279–80. https://doi.org/10.1016/S2215-0366(19)30101-4.
10. Reichl C, Kaess M. Self-Harm in the Context of Borderline Personality Disorder. Curr Opin Psychol. 2021;37:139–44. https://doi.org/10.1016/j.copsyc.2020.12.007.
11. Licence L, Oliver C, Moss J, Richards C. Prevalence and Risk-Markers of Self-Harm in Autistic Children and Adults. J Autism Dev Disord. 2020 Oct;50(10):3561–74. https://doi.org/10.1007/s10803-019-04260-1. PMID: 31655964; PMCID: PMC7502049.
12. Cybulski L, Ashcroft DM, Carr MJ, et al. Risk Factors for Nonfatal Self-Harm and Suicide Among Adolescents: Two Nested Case-Control Studies Conducted in the UK Clinical Practice Research Datalink. J Child Psychol Psychiatry. 2022 Sep;63(9):1078–88. https://doi.org/10.1111/jcpp.13552. Epub 2021 Dec 4; PMID: 34862981.

13. Gulbas LE, Hausmann-Stabile C, De Luca SM, Tyler TR, Zayas LH. An Exploratory Study of Nonsuicidal Self-Injury and Suicidal Behaviors in Adolescent Latinas. Am J Orthopsychiatry. 2015;85:302–14.

14. Moran P, Coffey C, Romaniuk H, et al. The Natural History of Self-Harm from Adolescence to Young Adulthood: A Population-Based Cohort Study. Lancet. 2012;379(9812):236–43. https://doi.org/10.1016/S0140-6736(11)61141-0. PMID: 22100201.

15. Moran P, Coffey C, Romaniuk H, Degenhardt L, Borschmann R, Patton GC. Substance Use in Adulthood Following Adolescent Self-Harm: A Population-Based Cohort Study. Acta Psychiatrica Scandinavica. 2015;131(1):61–68 https://doi.org/10.1111/acps.12306.

16. Steeg S, Mok P. Substance Misuse Disorder Linked to High Risk of Self-Harm. Lancet. 2022;7(2):110–11. https://doi.org/10.1016/S2215-0366(19)30532-2.

17. Brickman LJ, Ammerman BA, Look AE, et al. The Relationship Between Non-suicidal Self-Injury and Borderline Personality Disorder Symptoms in a College Sample. Bord Personal Disord Emot Dysregul. 2014;1:14. https://doi.org/10.1186/2051-6673-1-14.

18. Bornovalova MA, Hicks BM, Iacono WG, McGue M. Stability, Change, and Heritability of Borderline Personality Disorder Traits from Adolescence to Adulthood: A Longitudinal Twin Study. Dev Psychopathol. 2009;21(4):1335–53. https://doi.org/10.1017/S0954579409990186. PMID: 19825271; PMCID: PMC2789483.

19. Kingsley D. Debate: Child and Adolescent Mental Health Professionals Have a Responsibility to Diagnose Personality Disorder. Child Adolesc Ment Health. 2022;27:196–98. https://doi.org/10.1111/camh.12557.

20. Cloitre M. ICD-11 Complex Post-traumatic Stress Disorder: Simplifying Diagnosis in Trauma Populations. Br J Psychiatry. 2020 Mar;216(3):129–31. https://doi.org/10.1192/bjp.2020.43. PMID: 32345416.

21. Rodway C, Tham SG, Ibrahim S, Turnbull P, Kapur N, Appleby L. Children and Young People Who Die by Suicide: Childhood-Related Antecedents, Gender Differences and Service Contact. BJPsych Open. 2020;6(3):e49.

22. Sadath A, Troya MI, Nicholson S, et al. Physical and Mental Illness Comorbidity Among Individuals with Frequent Self-Harm Episodes: A Mixed-Methods Study. Front. Psychiatry. 2023;14:1121313. https://doi.org/10.3389/fpsyt.2023.1121313.

23. Nixon MK, Cloutier, P, Jansson SM. Nonsuicidal Self-Harm in Youth: A Population-Based Survey. CMAJ. 2008;178(3):306–12.

24. Knipe D, Padmanathan P, Newton-Howes, G, Chan L, Kapur N. Suicide and Self-Harm. Lancet. 2022;399(10338):1903–16. https://doi.org/10.1016/S0140-6736(22)00173-8.

25. Uh S, Dalmaijer E, Sigzdaite R, Ford T, Astle DJ. Two Pathways to Self-Harm in Adolescence. Am Acad Child Adolesc Psychiatry. 2021;60(12):1491–500.

26. Newlove-Delgado T, Marcheselli F, Williams T, et al. *Mental Health of Children and Young People in England, 2022 – Wave 3 Follow Up to the 2017 Survey*. NHS Digital, 2022.

27. Dubicka B, Martin J, Firth J. Editorial: Screen Time, Social Media and Developing Brains: A Cause for Good or Corrupting Young Minds. Child and Adol Mental Health. 2019;24(3):203–204. http://doi.org/10.1111/camh.12346.

28. Hetrick SE, Subasinghe A, Anglin K, et al. Understanding the Needs of Young People Who Engage in Self-Harm: A Qualitative Investigation. Front Psychol. 2020;10:2916. https://doi.org/10.3389/fpsyg.2019.02916.

29. Miranda-Mendizabal A, Castellví P, Parés-Badell O, et al. Gender Differences in Suicidal Behavior in Adolescents and Young Adults: Systematic Review and Meta-analysis of Longitudinal Studies. Int J Public Health. 2019 Mar;64(2):265–83. https://doi.org/10.1007/s00038-018-1196-1. Epub 2019 Jan 12. PMID: 30635683; PMCID: PMC6439147.

30. Royal College of Paediatrics and Child Health. *State of Child Health.* London: RCPCH, 2020. Available from: stateofchildhealth.rcpch.ac.uk (accessed 6 April 2025).

31. Lucena NL, Rossi TA, Galvão Azevedo LM, Pereira M. Self-Injury Prevalence in Adolescents: A Global Systematic Review and Meta-analysis. Children Youth Serv Rev. 2022;**142**:1–11. https://doi.org/10.1016/j.childyouth.2022.106634.

32. NHS England. *Mental Health of Children and Young People in England, 2023 – Wave 4 Follow Up to the 2017 Survey.* Official statistics, Survey. London: NHS England, 2023.

33. NHS England. *NHS Five Year Forward View* [Internet]. NHS England, 2014. Available from: http://www.england.nhs.uk/wp-content/uploads/2014/10/5yfv-web.pdf.

34. Department of Health and Social Care. *Suicide Prevention in England: 5-Year Cross-Sector Strategy* [Internet]. Department of Health and Social Care, 2023. Available from: https://www.gov.uk/government/publications/suicide-prevention-strategy-for-england-2023-to-2028/suicide-prevention-in-england-5-year-cross-sector-strategy.

35. Miranda R, Ortin A, Scott M, Shaffer D. Characteristics of Suicidal Ideation that Predict the Transition to Future Suicide Attempts in Adolescents. J Child Psychol Psychiatry. 2014 Nov;**55**(11):1288–96. https://doi.org/10.1111/jcpp.12245. Epub 2014 May 15. PMID: 24827817; PMCID: PMC4821401.

36. Office for National Statistics. *Suicide Rate in England and Wales in 2022, by Age Group* [Internet]. Office for National Statistics, 2023. Available from: https://www.ons.gov.uk/peoplepopulationandcommunity/birthsdeathsandmarriages/deaths/bulletins/suicidesintheunitedkingdom/2022registrations (accessed 6 April 2025).

37. Hawton K, Bale L, Brand F, et al. Mortality in Children and Adolescents Following Presentation to Hospital After Non-fatal Self-Harm in the Multicentre Study of Self-Harm: A Prospective Observational Cohort Study. Lancet Child Adolesc Health. 2020;**4**(2):111–20.

38. Plener PL, Schumacher TS, Munz LM, et al. The Longitudinal Course of Non-suicidal Self-Injury and Deliberate Self-Harm: A Systematic Review of the Literature. Bord Personal Disord Emot Dysregul. 2015;**2**(2). https://doi.org/10.1186/s40479-014-0024-3.

39. University of Manchester. *National Confidential Inquiry into Suicide and Homicide by People with Mental Illness (NCISH). Suicide by Children and Young People.* Manchester: University of Manchester, 2017. https://sites.manchester.ac.uk/ncish/ (accessed 6 April 2025).

40. Bresin K, Schoenleber M. Gender Differences in the Prevalence of Nonsuicidal Self-Injury: A Meta-analysis. Clin Psychol Rev. 2015;**38**:55–64. https://doi.org/10.1016/j.cpr.2015.02.009.

41. Geulayov G, Casey D, Bale L, et al. Self-Harm in Children 12 Years and Younger: Characteristics and Outcomes Based on the Multicentre Study of Self-Harm in England. Soc Psychiatry Psychiatr Epidemiol. 2022;**57**(1):139–48. https://doi.org/10.1007/s00127-021-02133-6. Epub 2021 Jul 19. PMID: 34282487; PMCID: PMC8761160.

42. Espelage DL. Suicidal Thoughts and Behaviors Among LGBTQ Youth: Meta-Analyses and a Systematic Review. Arch Suicide Res. 2019;**25**(1):1–37 https://doi.org/10.1080/13811118.2019.1663329.

43. Roberts RE, Chen YR, Roberts CR. Ethnocultural Differences in Prevalence of Adolescent Suicidal Behaviours. Suicide Life Threat Behav. 1997;**27**:208–17.

44. Lurigio AJ, Nesi D, Meyers SM. Nonsuicidal Self Injury Among Young Adults and Adolescents: Historical, Cultural and Clinical Understandings. Soc Work Ment Health. 2024;**22**(1):122–48.

45. Beckman K, Mittendorfer-Rutz E, Waern M, Larsson H, Runeson B, Dahlin M. Method of Self-Harm in Adolescents and Young Adults and Risk of Subsequent Suicide. J Child Psychol Psychiatry. 2018;**59**(9):948–56. https://doi.org/10.1111/jcpp.12883.

46. Brown RC, Plener PL. Non-suicidal Self-Injury in Adolescence. Curr Psychiatry Rep. 2017;**19**(3):20. https://doi.org/10.1007/s11920-017-0767-9.

47. Nock MK, Favazza AR. Nonsuicidal Self-Injury: Definition and Classification. In MK Nock (ed.), Understanding Nonsuicidal Self-Injury: Origins, Assessment, and Treatment. Washington, DC: American Psychological Association, 2009, 9–18.

48. Barrocas AL, Hankin BL, Young JF, Abela JR. Rates of Nonsuicidal Self-Injury in Youth: Age, Sex, and Behavioral Methods in a Community Sample. Pediatrics. 2012;**130**(1):39–45. https://doi.org/10.1542/peds.2011-2094.

49. Poudel A, Lamichhane A, Magar KR, et al. Non Suicidal Self Injury and Suicidal Behavior Among Adolescents: Co-occurrence and Associated Risk Factors. BMC Psychiatry. 2022;**22**:96.

50. Patra BN, Sen MS, Sagar R, Bhargava R. Deliberate Self-Harm in Adolescents: A Review of Literature. Ind Psychiatry J. 2023 Jan-Jun;**32**(1):9–14.

51. Favazza AR. *Bodies Under Siege: Self-Mutilation, Nonsuicidal Self-Injury, and Body Modification in Culture and Psychiatry*. Baltimore, MD: The Johns Hopkins University Press, 2011.

52. Manders B, Windsor-Shellard B. *Suicides in England and Wales: 2019 Registrations*. Census return for England and Wales [Internet]. Office for National Statistics, 2019. Available from: https://www.ons.gov.uk/peoplepopulationandcommunity/birthsdeathsandmarriages/deaths/bulletins/suicidesintheunitedkingdom/2019registrations#suicide-methods.

53. Kõlves K, de Leo D. Suicide Methods in Children and Adolescents. Eur Child Adolesc Psychiatry. 2017;**26**(2):155–64. https://doi.org/10.1007/s00787-016-0865-y. Epub 2016 May 18. PMID: 27194156.

54. Ormiston CK, Lawrence WR, Sulley S, et al. Trends in Adolescent Suicide by Method in the US, 1999-2020. JAMA Netw Open. 2024;**7**(3). https://doi.org/10.1001/jamanetworkopen.2024.4427.

55. Wang SB, Fox KR, Boccagno C, et al. Functional Assessment of Restrictive Eating: A Three-Study Clinically Heterogeneous and Transdiagnostic Investigation. J Abnorm Psychol. 2021 Oct;**130**(7):761–74. https://doi.org/10.1037/abn0000700. PMID: 34780230; PMCID: PMC8597895.

56. Kiekens G, Claes L. Non-Suicidal Self-Injury and Eating Disordered Behaviors: An Update on What We Do and Do Not Know. Curr Psychiatry Rep. 2020;**22**(12):68. https://doi.org/10.1007/s11920-020-01191-y.

57. Washburn JJ, Soto D, Osorio CA, Slesinger NC. Eating Disorder Behaviors as a Form of Non-suicidal Self-Injury. Psychiatry Res. 2023;**319**. https://doi.org/10.1016/j.psychres.2022.115002.

58. Muehlenkamp JJ, Suzuki T, Brausch AM, Peyerl N. Behavioral Functions Underlying NSSI and Eating Disorder Behaviors. J. Clin. Psychol. 2019;**75**:1219–32. https://doi.org/10.1002/jclp.22745.

59. Sheehy K, Noureen A, Khaliq A, et al. An Examination of the Relationship Between Shame, Guilt and Self-Harm: A Systematic Review and Meta-analysis. Clin Psychol Rev. 2019;**73**:101779.

60. Scoliers G, Portzky G, Madge N, et al. Reasons for Adolescent Deliberate Self-Harm: A Cry of Pain and/or a Cry for Help? Findings from the Child and Adolescent Self-Harm in Europe (CASE) Study. Soc Psychiatry Psychiatr Epidemiol. 2009;**44**:601–607.

61. Hawton K, Saunders KE, O'Connor RC. Self-Harm and Suicide in Adolescents. Lancet. 2012;**379**:2373–82. https://doi.org/10.1016/S0140-6736(12)60322-5.

62. Nester MS, Boi C, Brand BL, Schielke HJ. The Reasons Dissociative Disorder Patients Self-Injure. Eur J Psychotraumatol. 2022;**13**(1):2026738.

63. Yakeley J, Burbridge-James W. Psychodynamic Approaches to Suicide and Self-Harm. BJPsych Advances. 2018;**24**(1):37–45. https://doi.org/10.1192/bja.2017.6.

64. Worley J. Self-Injury as an Addictive Disorder. J Psychosoc Nurs Ment Health

Serv. 2020;**58**(6):13–16. https://doi.org/10.3928/02793695-20200513-03.

65. Kaess M, Hooley JM, Klimes-Dougan B, et al. Advancing a Temporal Framework for Understanding the Biology of Nonsuicidal Self-Injury: An Expert Review. Neurosci Biobehav Rev. 2021;**130**:228–39.

66. Ando A, Reichl C, Scheu F, et al. Regional Grey Matter Volume Reduction in Adolescents Engaging in Non-suicidal Self-Injury. Psychiatry Res Neuroimaging. 2018;**280**:48–55. https://doi.org/10.1016/j.pscychresns.2018.08.005.

67. Wilde M. *Understanding and Working Through Self-Harm*. Unpublished manuscript, PSYCH 307: Writing Within Psychology. Department of Psychology, Brigham Young University, 2022.

68. Laye-Gindhu A, Schonert-Reichl KA. Nonsuicidal Self-Harm Among Community Adolescents: Understanding the 'Whats' and 'Whys' of Self-Harm. J Youth Adolesc. 2005;**34**(5):447–57. https://doi.org/10.1007/s10964-005-7262-z.

69. Graney J, Hunt IM, Quinlivan L, et al. Suicide Risk Assessment in UK Mental Health Services: A National Mixed-Methods Study. Lancet Psychiatry. 2020 Dec;7(12):1046–53. https://doi.org/10.1016/S2215-0366(20)30381-3. Epub 2020 Nov 12. PMID: 33189221.

70. National Institute for Health and Care Excellence (NICE). *Self-Harm: Assessment, Management and Preventing Recurrence* [Internet]. NICE NG225. NICE, 2022. https://nice.org.uk/guidance/ng225 (accessed 6 April 2025).

71. Hawton K, Lascelles K, Pitman A, Gilbert S, Silverman M. Assessment of Suicide Risk in Mental Health Practice: Shifting from Prediction to Therapeutic Assessment, Formulation, and Risk Management. Lancet Psychiatry. 2022;**9**(11):922–28. https://doi.org/10.1016/S2215-0366(22)00232-2.

72. Witt KG, Hetrick SE, Rajaram G, et al. Interventions for Self-Harm in Children and Adolescents. Cochrane Database Syst Rev. 2021;7 3(3). https://doi.org/10.1002/14651858.CD013667.pub2.

73. Emsley E, Smith J, Martin D, Lewis NV. Trauma-Informed Care in the UK: Where Are We? A Qualitative Study of Health Policies and Professional Perspectives. BMC Health Serv Res. 2022;**22**(1):1164. https://doi.org/10.1186/s12913-022-0846 1-w. PMID: 36104750; PMCID: PMC9473455.

74. Kothgassner OD, Robinson K, Goreis A, Ougrin D, Plener PL. Does Treatment Method Matter? A Meta-analysis of the Past 20 Years of Research on Therapeutic Interventions for Self-Harm and Suicidal Ideation in Adolescents. Bord Personal Disord Emot Dysregul. 2020;7:9. https://doi.org/10.1186/s40479-020-00123-9.

75. Nawaz RF, Reen G, Bloodworth N, Maughan D, Vincent C. Interventions to Reduce Self-Harm on In-patient Wards: Systematic Review. BJPsych Open. 2021;7(3). https://doi.org/10.1192/bjo.2021.41.

76. Rossouw TI, Fonagy P. Mentalization-Based Treatment for Self-Harm in Adolescents: A Randomized Controlled Trial. J Am Acad Child Adolesc Psychiatry. 2012;**51**(12):1304–13. https://doi.org/10.1016/j.jaac.2012.09.018.

Chapter 13

Mood Disorders in Young People

Amy McCulloch, Stephen Connery Adams, Aditya Sharma and Bernadka Dubicka

Depression

Introduction
Depression is among the leading causes of illness and disability in children and adolescents [1], and can be associated with significant impairment [2], increased loneliness [1,3], increased risk of suicide [1,2], poor educational attainment [4], lower odds of being employed in adulthood [3] and higher risk of mental illness as an adult [3]. Prior to the Covid-19 pandemic, the WHO reported that worldwide, around 20% of all children and adolescents had a mental health disorder and around half of all adult mental health disorders begin before the age of 14 [5]. In the UK, the rate of probable mental health disorders in children and young people increased from 1:9 in 2017 to 1:6 in 2020, and this increase was largely accounted for by the increase in emotional disorders [6].

Epidemiology
The lifetime prevalence of Major Depressive Disorder (MDD) and severe MDD in adolescence have been estimated as 11.0% and 3.0%, respectively [2]. Rates of depression increase significantly in older adolescents [2], with a greater increase in girls than boys [2,7]. There is a lack of current UK data on adolescent depressive disorder; however, the Mental Health of Children and Young People in England Survey (2017) found that 8.1% of 5–19-year-olds, and 22.4% of 17–19-year-old girls had an emotional disorder (anxiety disorders, depressive disorders and mania/bipolar affective disorder) [7]. This study also reported that rates of emotional disorders have increased since 2004 [7].

Although clinical observations and retrospective patient accounts of depressive symptoms beginning in infancy are well described, there are insufficient empirical data available to validate a clinical syndrome in children younger than the age of 3 [8]. Depressive syndromes in preschool age children arise at a similar prevalence to that identified in pre-adolescent children [9].

Diagnosis and Clinical Features
About half of adolescents with a mood disorder will experience an onset of symptoms before the age of 13 [10]. Impairment in functioning is necessary for a diagnosis of depression to be made. Adolescents are more likely than children to present with significant hopelessness, anergia, hypersomnia, weight loss and serious suicidal acts [11]. Children are more likely than adolescents to present with symptoms that started following a specific event or preoccupation [11].

Table 13.1 Depression symptoms in ICD-11 and DSM-5

ICD-11 criteria [12]	DSM-5-TR criteria [13]
Depressed mood or diminished interest in activities occurring most of the day, nearly every day for at least 2 weeks accompanied by symptoms such as - difficulty concentrating - feelings of worthlessness - excessive or inappropriate guilt - hopelessness - recurrent thoughts of death or suicide - changes in appetite or sleep - psychomotor agitation or retardation - reduced energy or fatigue	At least one core symptom most of the day, nearly every day for 2 weeks: - depressed mood or irritability - loss of interest or pleasure Plus associated symptoms (minimum of 5 symptoms in total, including core symptoms): - weight loss or gain or failure to make expected weight gain - insomnia or hyposomnia - fatigue - psychomotor agitation or retardation - worthlessness or excessive/inappropriate guilt - decreased concentration - thoughts of death/suicide
No history of manic, mixed or hypomanic episode (bipolar disorder)	No history of manic or hypomanic episode
ICD-11 includes codes for single episodes of depression and recurrent depressive disorders, coded as mild, moderate or severe, depending on severity of symptoms and impact on functioning. Moderate and severe episodes are further divided by the presence or absence of psychotic symptoms	DSM-5 includes diagnoses of subthreshold, mild, moderate and severe depression plus dysthymia (subthreshold depression for 2 years) and seasonal affective disorder. DSM-5-TR includes the option to diagnose a mood disorder alongside a psychotic disorder if the mood symptoms are not explained by the psychotic disorder

As core depressive symptomatology shows continuity across the lifespan, neither ICD-11 nor DSM-5 specifies a lower age limit within its diagnostic criteria for MDD [8] (Table 13.1).

Comorbidity in adolescent depression is very common. In a trial of psychotherapy in UK Children and Adolescent Mental Health Services (CAMHS; IMPACT trial), 48% of adolescents with depression had at least one other psychiatric disorder and 13% had two other disorders [14]. The most common comorbid disorders were Generalised Anxiety Disorder (21.3%), social phobia (13.1%) and Oppositional Defiant Disorder (9.5%) [14].

Rating Scales

The National Institute for Health and Care Excellence UK (NICE) recommend the use of youth-specific rating scales for symptoms of depression [15]. There are many different measures available, some are youth-specific with a good evidence base, others lack evidence of validity [16,17]. The Beck Depression Inventory [18] has good evidence as a screening tool [19], the Kiddie Schedule for Affective Disorders and Schizophrenia (K-SADS) [20] has a good evidence base for use in diagnosing depression in young people. However, K-SADS is labour-intensive and requires training to administer as a clinical tool. There is a growing evidence base for the Development and Well-Being Assessment (DAWBA) [21], although there is a need for significantly more professionals to be trained in the use of these measures before they can be routinely used in community CAMHS [16].

Use of K-SADS alongside other measures has been shown to be effective in identifying cases of depression and suicidality that are often missed in standard clinical assessments [22]; this is of significant concern as effective evidence-based interventions are available, but require appropriate identification of depression to enable timely access to treatment and earlier recovery. The International Consortium for Health Outcomes Measurement recommends the Revised Children's Anxiety and Depression Scale for measuring response to clinical care [23]. The UK Child Outcome Research Consortium website provides helpful updates on tools and recommendations [17].

Aetiology

Familial Risk Factors

An important risk factor for childhood depression is maternal depression; in addition to increasing the risk of depression in offspring, maternal depression also increases risk of exposure to other risk factors such as partner cruelty, substance use and inadequate living conditions [24] – each additional risk factor increases the risk of mental health problems in the child by 20% [24].

The UK Avon Longitudinal Study of Parents and Children collected data on maternal and paternal depression at 18 weeks gestation and 8 weeks postpartum [25]. The highest risk exposure for adolescent depression was the combination of maternal antenatal depression (ANTD) and maternal postnatal depression (PNTD), although both independently increased risk [25]. Exposure to both paternal ANTD and paternal PNTD also increased the risk of adolescent depression but paternal ANTD alone or paternal PNTD alone did not [25].

Another UK population-based cohort study found that paternal depressive symptoms during childhood predicted depressive symptoms in adolescence in offspring, independent of maternal depression [26]. Research into the association between paternal mental health and adolescent depression is predominantly in the form of cross-sectional studies, which do indicate an association, but further longitudinal research is needed [27].

However, depression in the offspring of depressed parents is not inevitable [28]. Protective factors, such as the parent expressing positive emotion, support from co-parents, good quality social relationships, youth self-efficacy, regular physical exercise, low levels of perceived maternal psychological control and high child IQ have been shown to reduce the risk of developing depression, with a cumulative effect [28,29].

Treating maternal depression can improve the mental health outcomes for their children [30], including reduced rates of offspring diagnosis of depression and increased rates of offspring remission [31]. One study found an improvement in maternal mental health and the mental health of their child, both diagnosed with depression, following a brief psychotherapeutic intervention for the mother [32].

Biological Risk Factors

Biological theories of depression include the role of serotonin in neuroplasticity (particularly during the early years of life) and endocrine alterations, including cortisol, growth hormone, thyroid stimulating hormone, melatonin and prolactin [33]. Increased inflammation and hyperactivity of the hypothalamic–pituitary–adrenal axis has been linked to chronic stress and depression, and excessive glutamatergic neurotransmission has been linked to child and adolescent depression [33]. Early puberty in girls is associated with an increased risk of depressive disorder [34]. Lower IQ at 8 years and higher interleukin-6 levels at the age of 9 are both associated with the risk of persistent depressive symptoms from 10 to 19 years [35].

Sleep disturbance is seen in most young people with depression [14], and is a predictor of subsequent depression severity [36,37] and poorer response to treatment with fluoxetine [38]. Other suggested risk factors include traumatic brain injury [39], obesity [40] and Western dietary patterns [41]. Potential mechanisms for the association between obesity and depression include hypothalamic-pituitary axis dysregulation, metabolic disturbance, lack of physical exercise and maternal depression, which is associated with both obesity and depression in offspring [40].

Developmental and Psychological Risk Factors

Emotional competence is rapidly acquired during the pre-school years [42], and factors that disrupt normative development in this period are likely to be associated with the early-onset of mood abnormalities in infants and toddlers [8]. Early puberty has been linked to depression, and psychosocial acceleration theory suggests that young people growing up in an unstable environment will reach hormonal maturation more quickly than peers in a stable environment [43]. Atypical brain maturation and disparities in the timing or rate of synapse formation in combination with other risk factors have been proposed as predisposing factors for depression [43].

Specific deficits in the emotional recognition of others have been associated with adolescent depression: over-perceiving anger, sensitivity to sad facial affect and under-perceiving of happy affect [44]. Lower emotional awareness is a predictor of depression onset and is significantly related to higher depression symptoms and MDD diagnosis among adolescents [44].

Attachment-informed theories suggest that vulnerability to depression stems from early experiences of caregiver attachment, which contributes to schemas about relationships with others [33]. Insecure attachments, feelings of loneliness, abandonment, failure and worthlessness have all been associated with adolescent depression [33]. Peer attachments in adolescence have been shown to reduce the risk of depression in at-risk adolescents [45].

Cognitive theories of depression state that depression is linked to negative views about oneself, the world and the future (Beck's cognitive triad) [33]; however, there is limited evidence that altering cognitions is the mechanism of action for CBT [46]. Other components of CBT such as behavioural activation, non-specific treatment effects, interpersonal skills training, problem solving and third-wave components have been identified as potentially beneficial [46].

Environmental Risk Factors

Multiple environmental risk factors during pregnancy and childhood have been linked to mental health problems and these risk factors are often interrelated [47,48]. Experiencing poverty, particularly persistent poverty, has marked effects on a child's mental health [49]. UK population data of cohorts of 11-year-old children assessed in 1999, 2004 and 2012 showed substantial income inequalities in child mental health, which increased between 1999 and 2012 [50].

Longitudinal research has shown that childhood trauma, particularly complex trauma such as abuse, bullying or neighbourhood violence, increases the risk of psychopathology, including MDD, and cognitive deficits at the age of 18 [51]. In contrast to earlier research that demonstrated a cumulative risk of adverse childhood experiences, more recent research has found that subjective reports of childhood maltreatment more accurately predict the risk of psychopathology [52,53].

LGBTQ youth are at higher risk of depression and suicidality and have a higher prevalence of health-risk behaviours [54]. One study found that in a community sample of LGBTQ youth, 15% met criteria for depression and 31% had attempted suicide [55]. Unique risk factors for depression in LGBTQ youth include internalised stigma, discrimination, family rejections, homelessness and hostile school environments [56].

Young people of black ethnicity are at increased risk of developing depression, partly due to the health consequences of prejudice and racism [57]. Racial inequalities have also been found in youth mental health services in the UK including discriminatory racist treatment, lack of culturally appropriate care, language barriers and a lack of trust in mental health services resulting in delays in treatment for people of ethnic minorities [58].

In recent years, there has been increasing attention paid to the impact of technology on mental health. While there are many positive benefits of technology, and evidence for causal links remain limited, there is emerging evidence from longitudinal studies that digital technology and social media can affect mood and increase the risk of developing mental health problems in adolescence [59]. Specific content with themes of adolescent suicide have also been found to increase risk of suicide in adolescent audiences [60].

The effects of the Covid-19 pandemic and associated containment measures disproportionately affected young people and low-income families [6,61] and improvement in mental health services for young people has been identified as a key priority to reduce health inequality [62]. There was a significant increase in symptoms of depression (median 28% increase) in adolescents following the onset of the Covid-19 pandemic, particularly for young people living under lockdown restrictions [63]. The Mental Health of Children and Young People Survey found that young people with a probable mental health disorder were more likely to have experienced loneliness during the Covid-19 pandemic and more likely to report anxiety about Covid-19 [6]. More specifically, the pandemic resulted in a 25.4–29.2% increase in the prevalence of MDD in the UK, with young people, women and girls disproportionately affected [64]. In addition to the detrimental impact of the Covid-19 pandemic on children and young people's mental health [65], there is growing evidence that the effects of climate change will also disproportionately impact the most vulnerable children and young people, both directly and indirectly, and increase the risk of developing mental health problems including depression [66].

Management: Prevention

In the light of the impacts of parental depression on children and young people, pregnancy and infancy are key times for preventative interventions. In addition to the potential for intervention described above (see aetiology) this should also include access to good maternal care and promotion of parent–infant bonding [47]. Other important considerations for a universal prevention strategy are supportive school environments, prevention of substance abuse and good nutrition and exercise [47].

However, although a Cochrane review of CBT and IPT prevention programmes for adolescent depression found small positive short-term benefits for self-rated depressive symptoms and depression diagnoses, the effects did not persist at 12-months follow-up and the evidence was not sufficient to support the implementation of CBT or IPT depression prevention programmes [67]. Anti-bullying programmes have been described as cost-effective interventions for promoting good mental health in young people [68], although no statistically significant effect has been seen on depression scores [69].

Management: Treatment

A range of evidence-based treatment options are available and it is important that the risks and benefits of each are discussed with the young person and their family [70]. All clinicians working in CAMHS should receive training in values-based practice and should work collaboratively with young people and their families to deliver an evidence and values-based approach [71]. For example, families and clinicians may have differing perspectives on different types of treatments, which may be based on personal experiences, and will require a collaborative dialogue.

The NICE guidelines recommend a stepped care model, guided by age and severity of depression [15]. This model recommends watchful waiting, digital CBT, group CBT, group Interpersonal Psychotherapy (IPT) or group non-directive supportive therapy for mild depression [15]. For moderate to severe depression, NICE recommends family-based IPT, family therapy, psychodynamic psychotherapy, or individual CBT, with or without fluoxetine for 5–11-year-olds [15]. For 12–18-year-olds with moderate to severe depression, NICE recommends individual CBT with or without fluoxetine or, if CBT would not be clinically appropriate, IPT for adolescents, family therapy, brief psychosocial intervention (see below – psychological therapy) or psychodynamic psychotherapy, with or without Fluoxetine [15]. For young people that do not respond to the recommended treatment, experience recurrent depression or have psychotic depression, NICE recommends intensive psychological therapy with or without a Selective Serotonin Reuptake Inhibitor (SSRI – fluoxetine, sertraline or citalopram) plus augmentation with an antipsychotic if indicated [15].

It is important to note that systematic reviews and guidelines for the management of adolescent depression are often based on the results of randomised controlled trials that would have excluded the majority of young people that present to CAMHS in the UK [72]. Trials have most commonly excluded young people on the basis of comorbidity and risk of self-harm and suicide meaning that the results are not necessarily generalisable to the clinical population in CAMHS [72].

School-Based Interventions

A review of 45 trials of school-based interventions for depression and anxiety found a small effect on reducing depression symptoms immediately after the intervention, but this improvement was not maintained at follow-up [73]. Most of the studies recruited based on a symptom score rather than a clinical diagnosis and most of the interventions were CBT based [73]. There is evidence for improvements in mental health (as measured on the Strengths and Difficulties Questionnaire) at 2-year follow-up after school-based counselling, although this is not specific to depression [74]. Targeted classroom-based CBT for adolescents deemed to be at high risk of depression has not been found to be effective [75].

The UK-based MYRIAD trial showed no benefit of school-based mindfulness training (SBMT) over treatment as usual in promoting adolescent mental health [76]. SBMT also resulted in worse outcomes, in terms of risk of depression and well-being, in young people at risk of depression and is therefore not indicated as a universal intervention [77].

Psychological Therapy

There are no current validated psychotherapeutic strategies that target depressive syndromes arising in the early years [8]. Recognition of the risks to infant mental health associated with untreated maternal depression has led to a focus on developing toddler–parent psychotherapy as a preventative intervention [8].

In evaluating treatment responses in a large community sample of 7–14-year-olds, one study found that family-focused treatment was associated with an accelerated resolution in depressive symptoms following 16 weeks of treatment, when compared with an individual supportive psychotherapy approach [78]. There were also significantly fewer suicidal acts and mental-health related hospital attendances recorded in the group receiving the family-based strategy [78]. At 1-year follow-up, response to treatment was similar in both groups [79].

CBT is the most studied therapy modality in adolescent depression [80]. While earlier studies suggested large effect sizes, more recent studies with improved methodology suggest much smaller effects for adolescents with a diagnosis of depression (standardised mean difference of 0.11 for studies with active control groups or placebo control) [81]. Modular CBT, including flexible use of CBT for depression, CBT for comorbid anxiety and behavioural parent training for comorbid conduct problems, has been shown to be more effective than standard manualised CBT and usual care [82].

The large UK IMPACT trial [14] found that a brief psychosocial intervention (BPI) was equally effective as CBT and short-term psychoanalytic therapy at reducing depression symptoms at 12 months post-treatment. In IMPACT, BPI consisted of 12 sessions over 20 weeks including up to 4 family sessions. The focus is on psychoeducation and 'action-oriented, goal-focused, and interpersonal activities as therapeutic strategies'; clinicians with some expertise in CAMHS and knowledge of depression management can carry out the intervention following two days of training.

There is evidence in support of IPT (effect size of 0.51 at 16-week follow-up compared to an active control group) with greater improvements in moderate, compared to mild depression [83]. However, the evidence base is currently very small and further research is required [80]. There is limited evidence in support of family therapy for adolescent depression, despite its inclusion in NICE guidelines, it has not been found to be more effective than TAU [80,84]. There is not enough evidence at present to determine whether CBT or IPT are more effective in the individual or group format [84].

Digital health interventions are now widely available, in part due to changes in regulation and increased demand during the Covid-19 pandemic, and have the potential to improve access to treatment for young people, particularly hard-to-reach populations and those who may not meet the threshold for mental health services [85]. There is some evidence to suggest that computerised CBT can be effective for mild depression in older adolescents [86]. However, the research remains limited particularly for non-CBT interventions, severe depression, children and younger adolescents [86,87]. Information on the evidence base for the interventions, safety and cost-effectiveness is often lacking [85,86,87].

There has been research into single session interventions that have been found to be promising for anxiety and conduct problems, but the effect size for young people with depression was nonsignificant [88].

Iatrogenic Effects

The potential adverse effects of medication are often emphasised [89], but the potential harms of psychological therapy, including from ineffective engagement, ineffective practice or adverse effects, are rarely considered [90,91]. Adverse effects of psychological treatments can be difficult to assess, and there is a need for better reporting of untoward events [92].

Medication

NICE guidelines [15] recommend the use of fluoxetine for moderate to severe depression in 12–18-year-olds if the young person has not responded to psychological therapy or in combination with psychological therapy as initial treatment. NICE guidelines do allow for cautious consideration of fluoxetine in 5–11-year-olds, but only if unresponsive to psychological therapy. The evidence base is limited in this age group. Fluoxetine is considered as off-label use both for children under 8 years old and as initial treatment for those over 8 years old.

NICE guidelines [15] also outline several recommendations around the use of medication for adolescent depression including assessment by a child and adolescent psychiatrist, comprehensive information (including written information) about the rationale for treatment and potential adverse effects, regular monitoring and review of mental state and monitoring for emergence of suicidal ideation, self-harm or hostility.

The starting dose for fluoxetine is 10mg and higher doses should only be used after one week if clinically indicated and tolerated by the young person. Fluoxetine is only licensed up to 20mg once daily for adolescents [93]. Higher doses are sometimes used in clinical practice although the evidence base for the use of higher doses in adolescent depression is limited.

NICE guidelines [15] recommend that if fluoxetine in combination with psychological therapy is ineffective and the young person presents with depression that is 'sufficiently severe and/or causing sufficiently serious symptoms', then a trial of sertraline or citalopram can be considered following reassessment and with advice from a senior child and adolescent psychiatrist. Both sertraline and citalopram are currently used off-label in adolescent depression. Tricyclic antidepressants should not be used [15] and a Cochrane review concluded that the small potential benefit was not outweighed by the risk of toxicity at both therapeutic doses and in overdose [94].

Common side effects (affecting 1:100 to 1:10 people) of SSRIs, such as sertraline, fluoxetine and citalopram include headache, abdominal pain, nausea, constipation, diarrhoea, vomiting, changes in appetite, dizziness and QT prolongation [95]. Most side effects will resolve within the first week but may last longer in some young people [96]. Sexual side effects may also occur and may persist after treatment has stopped [95]. There is a risk of serotonin syndrome with antidepressant medication following initiation, dose increase, switching from one antidepressant to another or overdose [97]. Incidence rates are difficult to calculate due to underreporting of milder cases of serotonin syndrome, lack of recognition and misattribution of the symptoms as psychopathology [98]. The symptoms can vary from mild to life-threatening and include neuromuscular hyperactivity, autonomic dysfunction and altered mental state [97].

There has been a tendency in both academic literature and the media to under-report the positive effects of medication for adolescent depression and over-report the risks. A large network meta-analysis [99] gave a limited recommendation for fluoxetine despite a moderate effect size of 0.51, which is greater than the effect size for psychological therapies found in meta-analyses. A meta-analysis of 50 years of psychological therapy trials in children and adolescents found a small effect size of 0.32 by youth report and 0.15 by parent report for interventions for depression [100], considerably smaller than that reported for fluoxetine, and for anxiety. When measured by teacher report, psychological interventions for depression were less effective than controls (ES-0.41) [100].

The FDA 'Black Box' warning on suicidality (suicidal ideation, attempts and non-suicidal self-harm) associated with the use of SSRIs in adolescent depression resulted in a decline in the use of antidepressants and a subsequent increase in suicidality [89]. While the FDA's meta-analysis [101] showed a modest increase in suicidality with no deaths by suicide, a more recent meta-analysis [102] using individual-level data has shown that suicidality reduced in both the fluoxetine and placebo groups. There is also evidence that the risk of suicide attempt is highest prior to initiation of an antidepressant [103]. In addition, nearly all young people who have died by suicide did not receive antidepressant treatment at the time of their death [104], indicating that lack of treatment may have been implicated in their deaths, rather than an adverse response to antidepressants. Therefore, when discussing the potential risks of antidepressants, this should always be weighed up against the severity of the depressive disorder, and impact of depressive symptoms on the young person's life, including life-threatening symptoms.

Combination Treatment

The US Treatment for Adolescents with Depression Study (TADS) is one of the largest randomised controlled trials for adolescent depression and compared fluoxetine, CBT, placebo and combination treatment (fluoxetine and CBT) [105]. After 12 weeks of treatment, combination treatment and fluoxetine alone were more effective than CBT or placebo in treating depression (rated on Children's Depression Rating Scale-Revised) [106]. There was no benefit of CBT over placebo at 12 weeks [106]. However, for the second primary outcome measure, overall improvement (measured by Clinical Global Impressions improvement score), there was no significant advantage of combined treatment over fluoxetine alone [106]. By 36 weeks there was no difference between the three treatment options [106].

In the UK-based ADAPT trial there was no benefit at any time point from the addition of CBT to treatment with an SSRI on any measures of impairment, depression or improvement [106]. There was also no protective effect of CBT on suicidal ideation [106]. This is consistent with other trials of sertraline and CBT, in which combination treatment did not produce better outcomes [107,108]. However, the addition of CBT to medication does seem to be more beneficial for adolescents with comorbid anxiety than those without [109].

In contrast, an Australian RCT did not find any benefit of adding fluoxetine to CBT, compared to CBT plus placebo, for depressed adolescents and young adults, but found that combination treatment may be beneficial for adolescents with comorbid anxiety [110].

Additional Treatment Options

Exercise programmes may be beneficial in reducing symptoms of depression, but the evidence is very limited and there is a need for more data [111]. There is also some limited evidence for music therapy [112]. There is emerging evidence for nature-based interventions in improving mental health in adults, including those with pre-existing mental health problems, but further research is needed in children and young people [113]. There is also evidence to support a significant relationship between reduced depressive symptoms in adolescents and the amount of green space in their neighbourhood [114].

Predictors of Outcome

There are high rates of non-response to treatment for adolescent depression [109]. Early referral to CAMHS is associated with improved outcomes; young people with depressive symptoms who do not receive any contact with CAMHS in early adolescence are 7 times more likely to report depressive symptoms in older adolescence [115]. Poorer treatment outcomes are also associated with increasing severity and chronicity [109]. Older age at the start of treatment, increased severity of depression, suicidal ideation, parent–child conflict, hopelessness and functional impairment are all predictors of poorer treatment outcome [116]. Young people with a history of trauma are less likely to respond, or likely to respond more slowly to a range of treatments [116].

Treatment Resistant Depression

MDD is regularly characterised as treatment resistant depression (TRD) in cases where a young person's symptoms have not responded to two successive and adequate trials of different SSRIs [117]. This descriptor is largely borrowed from a parallel concept applied to adult populations, as there is no current universally accepted definition for TRD in adolescence [117,118].

The understanding of TRD as a definable concept is subject to much semantic debate [117]. There is growing consensus that this terminology fails to reflect the reality of treating depressive illness, with its complex aetiology, as well as its often chronic, relapsing-remitting course with fluctuating symptom severity [117,118,119]. Evaluation of pharmacotherapy alone neglects the impact of variables, such as medication adherence and social circumstances on treatment response [117,118,119]. Many past definitions of TRD have taken no account of non-pharmacological interventions [117].

An alternative framework for approaching 'difficult-to-treat depression', or DTD, has been proposed [119]. This heuristic approach emphasises the importance of regular reassessment and case formulation, as well as recognition of any modifiable barriers to treatment; categorising these as patient-, illness- and treatment-related factors [119].

Residual symptoms of MDD that respond poorly to first-line psychotherapy and SSRI treatment may be maintained by predisposing, precipitating and perpetuating aetiological factors, which can be viewed as risk factors for DTD [118]. Assessing for these risk factors, both at the outset and during treatment, may assist clinicians in anticipating obstacles to symptomatic remission, and identifying areas for focussed intervention [118,119]. NICE guidelines recommend a multidisciplinary review of young people who do not respond to first line treatment options, which should consider maintaining factors, including parental mental health problems [15].

Significant overlap in symptomatology between MDD and other common comorbid mental disorders presents another clinical challenge; both in diagnosis and in evaluating a patient's response to treatment, which may be suboptimal where comorbidity has been missed [118].

Diagnostic assessment should in all cases include efforts to screen for differential diagnoses including bipolar depression, anxiety disorders, PTSD, substance misuse and psychotic disorders [118,119]. Consideration should also be given to non-psychiatric causes of depressed mood, including thyroid dysfunction and pain [118,119].

A consensus statement on the management of DTD proposes a shift in therapeutic goal setting, away from full remission and towards a paradigm that aims to reduce the negative impact of relapse, while optimising symptom control and psychosocial functioning [119].

The US Treatment of Resistant Depression in Adolescents (TORDIA) study [120] evaluated treatment of adolescents (aged 12-18) who had not responded to a 2-month initial treatment with an SSRI. The treatment arms were [a] switch to a different SSRI (paroxetine, citalopram or fluoxetine); [b] switch to a different SSRI plus CBT; [c] switch to venlafaxine; and [d] switch to venlafaxine plus CBT [120]. The study found that a switch to either another SRRI or venlafaxine plus CBT was more effective than a medication switch alone, and SSRIs were associated with fewer adverse effects than venlafaxine [120].

Experimental treatment options include repetitive Transcranial Magnetic Stimulation; although research into its use in children and adolescents remains very limited [121], data suggest that it appears to be safe and tolerable [122]. As yet, there is no evidence for its use as a stand-alone treatment for TRD but initial evidence suggests it is effective as an add-on treatment [122]. Ketamine is emerging as a treatment option for depression, the evidence remains limited in all age groups but there is some limited evidence that Ketamine is safe, tolerable and effective for depressive symptoms in adolescents [123].

ECT can be used for young people aged 11-18 with life-threatening depression or severe treatment-resistant depression [124]. In England, formal approval must be obtained from a Second Opinion Appointed Doctor prior to treatment with ECT even if the young person has the capacity to consent [125].

Inpatient Admission

Admission is sometimes required for young people with complex presentations and/or risk that is unmanageable in the community. However, inpatient admission should be a last resort because it is associated with disruption of relationships with family and friends, disruption of access to education, negative impacts on the young person's sense of identity, stigma and a potential for mimicking of harmful behaviours from peers [126].

Prognosis

All of the treatment arms (fluoxetine versus CBT versus combination) of the TADS study resulted in improved functioning but those in the placebo arm declined, emphasising the importance of active treatment; those with multiple comorbidities were functioning poorly at long-term follow-up compared to those with one comorbidity or no comorbidities [127]. The IMPACT trial (CBT versus short-term psychoanalytical psychotherapy versus a BPI) showed continued improvement in depression symptoms at 86 weeks in all three arms of the study [14] with no significant differences in depressive symptoms between young people who dropped out of treatment and those who completed the intervention [128]; these findings question whether full courses of therapy are always needed. Fluoxetine and CBT have both been shown to prevent relapse [129].

In the TADS study the overall remission rate was 27% at week 12, 40% at week 18 and 60% at 9 months [130]. In IMPACT 48% of participants were in remission at week 12 and 77% at week 86 [14]. In the TORDIA trial, 55% of adolescents treated with CBT plus a medication switch, and 41% treated with just a medication switch, showed an adequate clinical response at 12 weeks [120]. At 6 months around 40% achieved remission in all treatment arms; greater depression severity predicted poorer response and an increased risk of relapse [131].

Longer-term follow-up demonstrates associations between adolescent depression and mental health problems, illicit substance dependence and intimate partner violence [132]. Adolescent depression is also linked to poorer educational attainment [133].

Despite increasing evidence for the treatment of adolescent depression, a significant number of young people fail to respond to either first- or second-line treatments, and there is an urgent need to continue to improve treatment outcomes. Many unanswered questions, remain, for example a considerable number of children and adolescents improve without treatment and the reasons for this are not currently understood [134]. The heterogeneity of depression, the number of different outcome measures used in trials, and the lack of evidence in early-onset depression all contribute to a continued need to find out what works for whom [134].

Bipolar Disorder

A substantial body of research has validated the diagnosis of bipolar disorder (BD), which was historically a controversial diagnosis in children and adolescents [135]. Some of this controversy resulted from the varying operational definitions of a 'broad phenotype' (elated mood or irritability) versus a 'narrow phenotype' (discrete periods of elated mood only) [136]. The prevalence of BD in children and adolescents is 1.8%, with similar mean rates in US and non-US studies; however, there is more variability in the prevalence rates within US studies, mostly due to differences in diagnostic criteria [137].

The only data on incidence of first-time diagnosis of narrow phenotype bipolar I disorder in those under 16 years of age across the UK and the Republic of Ireland reported 0.59/100 000 (95% CI 0.41–0.84) [138]. Within clinical practice, there is evidence to suggest that clinicians in the USA are significantly more likely to diagnose mania than UK clinicians, based on the same clinical information [139]. Furthermore, the discharge rates for BD per 100 000 population ranged from 95.6 (USA) to 0.9 for England [140].

Aetiology

Heritability for BD is estimated at 58% and there is considerable correlation with other psychiatric disorders, particularly depression and schizophrenia [141]. Having at least one parent with BD is associated with a 9-fold increased risk of developing BD and a 2.5-fold increased risk of developing another affective disorder [142].

Family history of affective illness or substance abuse among first-degree relatives is more prevalent in childhood onset (83%) than adolescent onset (61%) [143]. There are a small number of genetic studies identifying genes that may be associated with BD in children and young people but the studies involve small sample sizes and the results have not yet been replicated [144].

Longitudinal studies of the offspring of bipolar parents (OBP) have shown prevalence rates of BD of around 10% [145]. The majority of OBP present with recurrent depressive episodes followed, on average, 5 years later by a hypomanic or manic episode [135]. Depressive episodes preceded by substance abuse, recurrent depressive episodes and psychotic symptoms increased the risk of developing BD in high-risk young people [135].

Experiences of childhood trauma are common in people with BD, with one study finding that 40% of adults with BD had a history of assaultive trauma (rape, physical attack or physical threats), mostly occurring before the age of 16 [146]. Emotional maltreatment is significantly associated with the development of mood disorders in OBP [147]. A history of verbal, physical or sexual abuse is also associated with earlier onset of BD [148].

Classification

Historically there has been controversy over descriptions of BD in children characterised by chronic irritability and explosive temper versus descriptions of discrete episodes of depressed or elated mood, more consistent with adult presentations [135]. Longitudinal studies of the children of parents with BD have shown two different trajectories: anxiety and sleep problems in early childhood, followed by episodic depressive disorder and hypomanic symptoms in adolescence leading to BD in early adulthood. Due to concerns regarding the overdiagnosis of BD, the diagnosis of disruptive mood dysregulation disorder (DMDD) was developed in the USA to differentiate children who show a trajectory of developmental disorders and ADHD in childhood, followed by chronic mood dysregulation in adolescence and persisting into early adulthood [135]. There is however no comparable diagnosis in the ICD-11 (Table 13.2).

Table 13.2 Bipolar and Cyclothymia Disorder in ICD-11 and DSM-5

ICD-11 [12]	DSM-5 [13]
Bipolar type 1 • episodic mood disorder • one or more manic or mixed episodes • Manic episode must last at least 1 week, and mixed episode at least 2 weeks, unless shortened by treatment • Depressive episode is not essential for diagnosis	Bipolar I disorder • At least one manic episode • Major depressive episodes and hypomanic episodes are common but are not required for the diagnosis
Bipolar type 2 • episodic mood disorder • one or more hypomanic episodes and at least one depressive episode • Hypomanic episode must last at least a few days and depressive episode must last at least 2 weeks • No history of manic or mixed episodes	Bipolar II disorder • One or more major depressive episodes • One of more hypomanic episodes • No history of manic or mixed episodes
Cyclothymic disorder • Persistent instability of mood over at least 2 years • Numerous periods of hypomanic and depressive symptoms • Hypomanic symptoms may meet criteria for hypomanic episode, but depressive symptoms have never been sufficiently severe or prolonged to meet requirements for diagnosis of depressive episode • Significant distress or significant impairment in functioning	Cyclothymia • Hypomanic and depressive symptoms that do not meet criteria for bipolar II disorder • No episodes meeting diagnostic criteria for manic, hypomanic or depressives • Symptoms present for at least 2 years

There was a 40-fold increase in BD clinical diagnoses between 1994 and 2003 in the USA [149], which has not been replicated in other countries [135]. However, since the addition of DMDD to DSM-5 in 2013 there has been a rapid uptake of the use of the diagnosis of DMDD in clinical practice in the USA, and young people with a diagnosis of DMDD are more likely to be prescribed antipsychotics and more likely to be admitted to hospital than those with a diagnosis of BD [150]. It appears that many of these young people would have previously been diagnosed with BD and as such the rates of BD diagnosis have decreased over the same time period [150].

Important differential diagnoses include schizophrenia, schizoaffective disorder, adverse effects of medication (e.g. steroids and antidepressants can induce mania), substance abuse (including intoxication and withdrawal) and ADHD [151]. There are also a number of medical conditions that can cause symptoms imitating mania, including meningitis, head injury, thyroid disease, SLE and Wilson's disease [151].

There is overlap between the affective instability seen in personality disorder and rapid mood switching seen in BD, which may suggest a similar underlying aetiology [152], and is associated with the misdiagnosis of BD in people with personality disorder [153]. A history of sexual abuse is common in people with BD, but may also result in sexualised behaviour that is not consistent with the young person's age and therefore misinterpreted as the disinhibition associated with mania [151].

Severe ADHD with dysregulated mood also needs to be differentiated from hypomanic or manic presentations [154]. Comorbid diagnoses of ADHD are however very common and the reported rates of comorbidity vary widely due to methodological issues [154]. Longitudinal studies of people with ADHD do not demonstrate higher than average rates of BD in adulthood [154].

Assessment

An assessment should cover the longitudinal course of symptoms, including the nature of any episodes of mood changes and baseline functioning [136]. It is important to take a family history, not just of BD diagnosis within the family, but also of symptoms of mania because family members may not have been diagnosed or may have received an incorrect diagnosis [136]. Children whose parents have BD are at risk of early-onset BD and 75% of those who do go on to develop BD will have their first episode of mood disorder before the age of 12 [145]. Collateral history is important [136] and caregiver reports have been found to be more accurate than reports from the young person or their teacher in identifying BD [155]. In young people presenting with mania, caregivers are more likely than the young person to report irritability whereas young people are more likely than their caregiver to report increased energy and hyperactivity [156].

Youngstorm et al [157] suggested cues for detailed assessment of potential BD:
- episodes of aggressive behaviour (particularly in the context of other manic symptoms)
- early age of onset for depression
- mood disorder with psychotic features
- recurrent depressive episodes that are resistant to treatment
- episodic presentation of symptoms otherwise appearing similar to ADHD
- mood destabilisation secondary to trials of stimulant or antidepressant medications

A meta-analysis found that increased energy (weighted rate 89%), distractibility (84%) and pressured speech (82%) were the most common symptoms of mania in young people with BD [158]. There was significant heterogeneity in the rates of reported irritability and elation; flight of ideas and hypersexuality were the least common symptoms of mania in young people [158].

Comorbidity is common in BD, particularly ADHD (48–53%), anxiety (23–54%), disruptive behaviour disorders (31%) and substance use disorder (9–31%) [159,160]. Comorbid ADHD is associated with greater severity of manic symptoms and a tendency to present with irritable rather than elated mood [160]. Comorbid disruptive behaviour disorders are associated with increased rate of hospital admissions and poorer response to treatment [160]. Comorbid anxiety is associated with more affective episodes, increased severity of depressive episodes and greater impairment [160].

The Child Behaviour Checklist has been used in the assessment of BD in young people and a subscale, termed the CBCL-Pediatric Bipolar Disorder phenotype, was commonly seen in children with BD [161]. However, longitudinal studies have shown that, while this phenotype does predict significant psychiatric morbidity, it is not specific to BD [161]. The Parent Version of the Young Mania Rating Scale (P-YMRS) has shown acceptable internal consistency ($\alpha = .75$) [162]. Logistic regressions have shown that the P-YMRS has the ability to differentiate BD from depression and other diagnoses [162].

The Child Mania Rating Scale-Parent version is a 21-item measure [163]. The authors have reported that on an exploratory and confirmatory factor analysis the scale was unidimensional with its internal consistency and retest reliability both reported at 0.96 [163]. Furthermore, its convergence with the Washington University K-SADS mania module, the Schedule for Affective Disorders and Schizophrenia Mania Rating Scale, and the P-YMRS was reported as excellent (.78–.83) [163]. NICE guidelines advise against the use of screening questionnaires to aid in the diagnosis of BD in under-18s [164].

Treatment

Children and young people with BD should be managed in specialist mental health services, either Early Intervention in Psychosis services or CAMHS, and should have access to a multidisciplinary team who have experience of treating BD in young people [164]. A comprehensive risk management and recovery plan should be developed jointly with the young person and their parent or guardian, covering any triggers, early warning signs, coping strategies, management plan for primary and secondary care, identified professional contacts and crisis service contact details [164]. Inpatient admission may need to be considered if a young person is presenting with high-risk behaviours.

The potential adverse effects of medication need to be fully discussed with young people and their carers, as well as the risks of untreated episodes. Potential side effects from antipsychotic medication [164] include sedation, extra pyramidal and metabolic side effects [165]. NICE guidelines state that antipsychotic treatment should not routinely continue past 12 weeks [164] but effective timely treatment is important to facilitate a return to normal functioning with a focus on ensuring maintenance of euthymia. As atypical antipsychotics have the best evidence to both treat mania and maintain euthymia, treatment with psychotropic agents, and in particular atypical antipsychotics, may need to be in excess of the NICE-recommended 12-week period.

Evidence for the use of psychosocial interventions is promising but remains limited; interventions that involve families, psychoeducation and skill-building may be beneficial [166]. Psychosocial interventions are an important adjunct to pharmacological treatment of BD, but there is no evidence to date of a psychosocial intervention that is comparable in efficacy to pharmacotherapy. Further details of interventions specific to under-18s are described in the relapse prevention section.

Treating Depression in BD

For bipolar depression, NICE recommends individual CBT or IPT for at least 3 months, with an MDT review after 4–6 weeks if there has been limited or no response [164]. If the depression is moderate to severe, NICE recommends following adult BD guidance and using fluoxetine with olanzapine or quetiapine first line depending on patient preference.

However, more recent evidence for adolescents shows that olanzapine and fluoxetine in combination or lurasidone monotherapy are effective [136,167,168] but quetiapine is not [168]. The olanzapine and fluoxetine combination, however, may result in significant weight gain, which needs careful monitoring. Lurasidone was also associated with fewer side effects (specifically with regard to weight gain and raised cholesterol and triglycerides) compared to olanzapine and fluoxetine in combination [168]. Monotherapy with quetiapine, aripiprazole, risperidone, valproate or lithium have been found to be ineffective for bipolar depression in children and adolescents [167].

Treating Mania in BD

For moderate to severe manic episodes, aripiprazole may be used for up to 12 weeks in adolescents aged 13 and older and is deemed to be as effective as other antipsychotics with a comparable and acceptable adverse reaction profile [169]. Extrapyramidal symptoms, somnolence and akathisia are more common with aripiprazole than placebo but there is not known to be an associated increase in weight or BMI [169]. There is also evidence for the use of lithium or other antipsychotics, including risperidone, olanzapine, quetiapine, ziprasidone and asenapine [136]. If a young person is presenting with a manic episode, antidepressants should be discontinued immediately. In severe presentations, additional medication may be required for rapid tranquillisation. The use of short acting benzodiazepines may result in paradoxical disinhibition, so their use particularly in the community must be carefully considered.

Treating Mixed Episodes in BD

For BD with mixed episodes there is evidence for the use of high dose quetiapine (600 mg/day) [167]. Treatment with both antimanic and antidepressant treatment may be warranted but this requires careful monitoring.

Treating Comorbid ADHD

There is increasing evidence to support the treatment of comorbid ADHD with stimulant medication with or without mood stabilisation [154]. The available data does not suggest any increased mood symptoms associated with stimulant medication [154].

Relapse Prevention

Most trial data for pharmacological treatment of BD is based on acute treatment with less data available on longer term management [136]. NICE guidelines recommend a structured individual or family psychological intervention for longer-term treatment [164]. Structured approaches developed in the USA include Family Focused Treatment for Early Onset and Youth [170] and child and family-focused cognitive-behavioural therapy [171]. The only UK data are based on a feasibility study reporting that Family Focused Treatment for Adolescents is an acceptable treatment for families of adolescents with BD in remission, but RCT data on clinical- and cost-effectiveness is not yet available [172]. Aripiprazole can be useful for relapse prevention but the data remains limited [173]. Lamotrigine has been shown to be beneficial in preventing relapse in adolescents aged 13–17 but not in younger children [136].

Lithium

Lithium has long been used for the treatment of BD in adults and with weight-related dosing and monitoring of serum levels, it is a viable treatment option in adolescents [174]. It is an effective treatment for manic or mixed states and has a proven effect in reducing suicide over the lifespan [174]. Further research is required into the use of lithium for BD depression in young people [174]. Lithium is generally well tolerated but has been found to cause side effects in young people, including nausea, abdominal pain, vomiting, headache, tremors and dizziness [174].

Valproate

The UK Medicines and Healthcare Products Regulatory Agency states that valproate should not be prescribed to women and girls of childbearing age without a pregnancy prevention programme in place and should never be used in pregnancy to treat BD unless there is no other effective treatment available [175]. This is due to the risk of serious congenital malformations and neurodevelopmental disorders in children exposed to valproate in utero [175].

Prognosis

Most young people recover from the index episode (81.5% after 2 years); however, relapse is common (62.5%) and many experience mood symptoms between episodes [176]. One follow-up study found four different mood trajectories over 8 years of follow-up, on a spectrum from 24.0% who were euthymic 84% of the time to 22.3% of the sample who were only euthymic 11.5% of the time [177].

In the same study, higher age at onset of mood symptoms, less severe depression, less severe manic or hypomanic symptoms, fewer subsyndromal episodes, fewer suicide attempts, less history of sexual abuse and less family history of BD or substance use disorders were all significantly associated with better outcomes [177]. Another study with a large multinational sample found that childhood onset predicted worse functional outcomes and higher rates of comorbidity (91% versus 54%) than adolescent or adult onset but did not predict higher severity of symptoms [143].

The risk of attempted suicide is high, with nearly one-third of people with adolescent onset BD attempting suicide in their lifetime [178]. A history of mixed episodes, psychosis, hospitalisation, comorbid panic disorder, self-harm and comorbid substance use disorder predict higher risk of attempted suicide [178].

Deficits in cognitive flexibility in childhood-onset BD – type 1 persist into adulthood and are associated with increased depression and suicidal ideation [179]. A history of childhood trauma is associated with a poorer prognosis, including increased risk of rapid cycling, more frequent episodes of depression and attempted suicide [146,180].

Longitudinal studies suggest that there may be less stability in the DSM diagnoses of BD type II and BD-not otherwise specified (BD-NOS) with 25% of young people with BD-II and 19.9% of young people with BD-NOS converting to BD-I over a 2.5-year follow-up period [176].

References

1. World Health Organisation. *Adolescent Mental Health* [Internet]. World Health Organisation, November 2021. Available from: https://www.who.int/news-room/fact-sheets/detail/adolescent-mental-health (cited 17 January 2022).
2. Avenevoli S, Swendsen J, He JP, Burstein M, Merikangas K. Major Depression in the National Comorbidity Survey- Adolescent Supplement: Prevalence, Correlates, and Treatment. J Am Acad Child Adolesc Psychiatry. 2015 Jan;**54**(1):37–44.
3. Clayborne ZM, Varin M, Colman I. Systematic Review and Meta-Analysis: Adolescent Depression and Long-Term Psychosocial Outcomes. J Am Acad Child Adolesc Psychiatry. 2019 Jan;**58**(1):72–79.
4. Wickersham A, Sugg HVR, Epstein S, Stewart R, Ford T, Downs J. Systematic Review and Meta-analysis: The Association Between Child and Adolescent Depression and Later Educational Attainment. J Am Acad Child Adolesc Psychiatry. 2021 Jan 1;**60**(1):105–18.
5. World HealthOrganisation. *10 Facts on Mental Health* [Internet]. World Health Organisation, 2019. Available from: https://www.who.int/news-room/facts-in-pictures/detail/mental-health (cited 17 January 2022).
6. Vizard T, Sadler K, Ford T, et al. *Mental Health of Children and Young People in England, 2020*. NHS Digital, 2022 Oct. Available from: https://www.infocoponline.es/pdf/mhcyp_2020_rep.pdf.
7. Sadler K, Vizard T, Ford T, et al. *Mental Health of Children and Young People in England, 2017* [Internet]. NHS Digital, 2018. Available from: https://digital.nhs.uk/data-and-information/publications/statistical/mental-health-of-children-and-young-people-in-england/2017/2017 (cited 27 March 2019).
8. Luby J, Whalen D. Depression in Early Childhood. In CH Zeanah Jr. (ed.), *Handbook of Infant Mental Health*. 4th ed. New York: The Guilford Press, 2019, 426–37.
9. Egger H, Angold A. Common Emotional and Behavioral Disorders in Preschool Children: Presentation, Nosology, and Epidemiology. J Child Psychol Psychiatry. 2006;**47**(3–4):313–37.
10. Merikangas KR, He J-Ping, et al. Lifetime Prevalence of Mental Disorders in US Adolescents: Results from the National Comorbidity Study-Adolescent Supplement (NCS-A). J Am Acad Child Adolesc Psychiatry. 2010 Oct;**49**(10):980–89.
11. Yorbik O, Birmaher B, Axelson D, Williamson D, Ryan ND. Clinical Characteristics of Depressive Symptoms in Children and Adolescents with Major Depressive Disorder. J Clin Psychiatry. 2004 Dec;**65**(12):1654–59.
12. World Health Organisation. *ICD-11. International Statistical Classification of Diseases*. 11th ed. [Internet]. World Health Organisation, 2019. Available from https://icd.who.int/en/ (cited 17 January 2022).
13. American Psychiatric Association. Diagnostic and Statistical Manual of Mental Disorders. 5th ed. Washington, DC: American Psychiatric Publishing, 2013.
14. Goodyer IM, Reynolds S, Barrett B, et al. Cognitive Behavioural Therapy and Short-Term Psychoanalytical Psychotherapy Versus a Brief Psychosocial Intervention in Adolescents with Unipolar Major Depressive Disorder (IMPACT): A Multicentre, Pragmatic,

15. NICE. *Depression in Children and Young People: Identification and Management*. NICE Guideline [NG134] [Internet]. NICE, 2019 Jun. Available from: https://www.nice.org.uk/guidance/ng134 (cited 23 January 2022).

16. Simmons M, Wilkinson P, Dubicka B. Measurement Issues: Depression Measures in Children and Adolescents. Child Adolesc Ment Health. 2015 Nov;20(4):230–41.

17. Anna Freud Centre. CORC Website [Internet]. Available from: https://www.corc.uk.net/ (cited 24 January 2022).

18. Beck AT. An Inventory for Measuring Depression. Arch Gen Psychiatry. 1961 Jun 1;4(6):561.

19. Lee A, Park J. Diagnostic Test Accuracy of the Beck Depression Inventory for Detecting Major Depression in Adolescents: A Systematic Review and Meta-Analysis. Clin Nurs Res. 2021 Dec 27;31(8);1481–1490 https://doi.org/10.1177/10547738211065105.

20. Kaufman J, Birmaher B, Brent D, et al. Schedule for Affective Disorders and Schizophrenia for School-Age Children-Present and Lifetime Version (K-SADS-PL): Initial Reliability and Validity Data. J Am Acad Child Adolesc Psychiatry. 1997 Jul;36(7):980–88.

21. Aebi M, Kuhn C, Metzke CW, Stringaris A, Goodman R, Steinhausen HC. The Use of the Development and Well-Being Assessment (DAWBA) in Clinical Practice: A Randomized Trial. Eur Child Adolesc Psychiatry. 2012 Oct;21(10):559–67.

22. Fitzpatrick C, Abayomi NN, Kehoe A, et al. Do We Miss Depressive Disorders and Suicidal Behaviours in Clinical Practice? Clin Child Psychol Psychiatry. 2012 Jul 1;17(3):449–58.

23. Krause KR, Chung S, Adewuya AO, et al. International Consensus on a Standard Set of Outcome Measures for Child and Youth Anxiety, Depression, Obsessive-Compulsive Disorder, and Post-traumatic Stress Disorder. Lancet Psychiatry. 2021 Jan 1;8(1):76–86.

24. Barker ED, Copeland W, Maughan B, Jaffee SR, Uher R. Relative Impact of Maternal Depression and Associated Risk Factors on Offspring Psychopathology. Br J Psychiatry. 2012 Feb;200(2):124–29.

25. Rajyaguru P, Kwong ASF, Braithwaite E, Pearson RM. Maternal and Paternal Depression and Child Mental Health Trajectories: Evidence from the Avon Longitudinal Study of Parents and Children. BJPsych Open. 2021 Sep 24;7(5):e166.

26. Lewis G, Neary M, Polek E, Flouri E, Lewis G. The Association Between Paternal and Adolescent Depressive Symptoms: Evidence from Two Population-Based Cohorts. Lancet Psychiatry. 2017 Dec;4(12):920–26.

27. Wickersham A, Leightley D, Archer M, Fear NT. The Association Between Paternal Psychopathology and Adolescent Depression and Anxiety: A Systematic Review. J Adolesc. 2020 Feb;79(1):232–46.

28. Collishaw S, Hammerton G, Mahedy L, et al. Mental Health Resilience in the Adolescent Offspring of Parents with Depression: A Prospective Longitudinal Study. Lancet Psychiatry. 2016 Jan;3(1):49–57.

29. Pargas RCM, Brennan PA, Hammen C, Le Brocque R. Resilience to Maternal Depression in Young Adulthood. Dev Psychol. 2010 Jul;46(4):805–14.

30. Cuijpers P, Weitz E, Karyotaki E, Garber J, Andersson G. The Effects of Psychological Treatment of Maternal Depression on Children and Parental Functioning: A Meta-analysis. Eur Child Adolesc Psychiatry. 2015 Feb;24(2):237–45.

31. Weissman MM, Pilowsky DJ, Wickramaratne PJ, et al. Remissions in Maternal Depression and Child Psychopathology A STAR*D-Child Report. JAMA. 2006 Mar 22;295(12):1389–98.

32. Swartz HA, Cyranowski JM, Cheng Y, et al. Brief Psychotherapy for Maternal Depression: Impact on Mothers and Children. J Am Acad Child Adolesc Psychiatry. 2016 Jun;55(6):495–503.e2.

33. Bernaras E, Jaureguizar J, Garaigordobil M. Child and Adolescent Depression: A Review of Theories, Evaluation Instruments, Prevention Programs, and Treatments. Front Psychol. 2019 Mar 20;10. https://doi.org/10.3389/fpsyg.2019.00543.

34. Graber JA. Pubertal Timing and the Development of Psychopathology in Adolescence and Beyond. Horm Behav. 2013 Jul;64(2):262–69.

35. Khandaker GM, Stochl J, Zammit S, Goodyer I, Lewis G, Jones PB. Childhood Inflammatory Markers and Intelligence as Predictors of Subsequent Persistent Depressive Symptoms: A Longitudinal Cohort Study. Psychol Med. 2018 Jul;48(9):1514–22.

36. Orchard F, Gregory AM, Gradisar M, Reynolds S. Self-Reported Sleep Patterns and Quality Amongst Adolescents: Cross-Sectional and Prospective Associations with Anxiety and Depression. J Child Psychol Psychiatry. 2020 Oct;61(10):1126–37.

37. Shanahan L, Copeland WE, Angold A, Bondy CL, Costello EJ. Sleep Problems Predict and Are Predicted by Generalized Anxiety/Depression and Oppositional Defiant Disorder. J Am Acad Child Adolesc Psychiatry. 2014 May 1;53(5):550–58.

38. Emslie GJ, Kennard BD, Mayes TL, et al. Insomnia Moderates Outcome of Serotonin-Selective Reuptake Inhibitor Treatment in Depressed Youth. J Child Adolesc Psychopharmacol. 2012 Feb;22(1):21–28.

39. Ryttersgaard TO, Johnsen SP, Riis JØ, Mogensen PH, Bjarkam CR. Prevalence of Depression After Moderate to Severe Traumatic Brain Injury Among Adolescents and Young Adults: A Systematic Review. Scand J Psychol. 2020 Apr;61(2):297–306.

40. Rao WW, Zong QQ, Zhang JW, et al. Obesity Increases the Risk of Depression in Children and Adolescents: Results from a Systematic Review and Meta-analysis. J Affect Disord. 2020 Apr;267:78–85.

41. Chopra C, Mandalika S, Kinger N. Does Diet Play a Role in the Prevention and Management of Depression Among Adolescents? A Narrative Review. Nutr Health. 2021 Jun 1;27(2):243–63.

42. Denham S. *Emotional Development in Young Children*. New York: Guilford Press, 1998.

43. Hagan CC, Graham JME, Wilkinson PO, et al. Neurodevelopment and Ages of Onset in Depressive Disorders. Lancet Psychiatry. 2015 Dec;2(12):1112–26.

44. Nyquist AC, Luebbe AM. An Emotion Recognition-Awareness Vulnerability Hypothesis for Depression in Adolescence: A Systematic Review. Clin Child Fam Psychol Rev. 2020 Mar;23(1):27–53.

45. Ju S, Lee Y. Developmental Trajectories and Longitudinal Mediation Effects of Self-Esteem, Peer Attachment, Child Maltreatment and Depression on Early Adolescents. Child Abuse Negl. 2018 Feb;76:353–63.

46. Furukawa TA, Suganuma A, Ostinelli EG, et al. Dismantling, Optimising, and Personalising Internet Cognitive Behavioural Therapy for Depression: A Systematic Review and Component Network Meta-analysis Using Individual Participant Data. Lancet Psychiatry. 2021 Jun;8(6):500–11.

47. Arango C, Díaz-Caneja CM, McGorry PD, et al. Preventive Strategies for Mental Health. Lancet Psychiatry. 2018 Jul;5(7):591–604.

48. Thapar A, Collishaw S, Pine DS, Thapar AK. Depression in Adolescence. Lancet. 2012 Mar 17;379(9820):1056–67.

49. Michael Marmot, Jessica Allen, Tammy Boyce, Peter Goldblatt, Joana Morrison. *Health Equity in England: The Marmot Review Ten Years On* [Internet]. London: Institute of Health Equity, 2020. Available from: https://www.health.org.uk/sites/default/files/2020-03/Health%20Equity%20in%20England_The%20Marmot%20Review%2010%20Years%20On_executive%20summary_web.pdf (cited 1 May 2022).

50. Collishaw S, Furzer E, Thapar AK, Sellers R. Brief Report: A Comparison of Child Mental Health Inequalities in Three UK Population Cohorts. Eur Child Adolesc Psychiatry. 2019 Nov;**28**(11):1547–49.

51. Lewis SJ, Koenen KC, Ambler A, et al. Unravelling the Contribution of Complex Trauma to Psychopathology and Cognitive Deficits: A Cohort Study. Br J Psychiatry. 2021 Aug;**219**(2):448–55.

52. Danese A, Lewis SJ. New Directions in Research on Childhood Adversity. Br J Psychiatry. 2022 Mar;**220**(3):107–108.

53. Danese A, Widom CS. Objective and Subjective Experiences of Child Maltreatment and Their Relationships with Psychopathology. Nat Hum Behav. 2020 Aug;**4**(8):811–18.

54. Kann L, Olsen EO, McManus T, et al. Sexual Identity, Sex of Sexual Contacts, and Health-Related Behaviors Among Students in Grades 9-12 – United States and Selected Sites, 2015. Morb Mortal Wkly Rep Surveill Summ. 2016 Aug 12;**65**(9):1–202.

55. Brian S. Mustanski, Robert Garofalo, Erin M. Emerson. Mental Health Disorders, Psychological Distress, and Suicidality in a Diverse Sample of Lesbian, Gay, Bisexual, and Transgender Youths. Am J Public Health. 2010 Dec;**100**(12):465–87.

56. Johnson B, Leibowitz S, Chavez A, Herbert SE. Risk Versus Resiliency. Child Adolesc Psychiatr Clin N Am. 2019 Jul;**28**(3):509–21.

57. Landim JMM, Rolim Neto ML, Christofolini DM. Psychic Suffering and Depression in Black Children and Adolescents: Systematic Review and Meta-analysis. Braz J Med Biol Res Rev Bras Pesqui Medicas E Biol. 2021 Jul 16;**54**(10). https://doi.org/10.1590/1414-431X2020e10380.

58. Kapadia D, Zhang J, Salway S, Nazroo J, Booth A. *Ethnic Inequalities in Healthcare: A Rapid Evidence Review*. NHS Race and Health Observatory, 2022. Available from: https://www.nhsrho.org/wp-content/uploads/2023/05/RHO-Rapid-Review-Final-Report_.pdf.

59. Dubicka B, Theodosiou L. *Technology Use and the Mental Health of Children and Young People [CR225]* [Internet]. RCPsych, 2020 Jan. Available from: https://www.rcpsych.ac.uk/docs/default-source/improving-care/better-mh-policy/college-reports/college-report-cr225.pdf (cited 3 February 2022).

60. Niederkrotenthaler T, Stack S, Till B, et al. Association of Increased Youth Suicides in the United States with the Release of *13 Reasons Why*. JAMA Psychiatry. 2019 Sep 1;**76**(9):933–40.

61. Marmot Michael, Allen Jessica, Goldblatt Peter, Herd Eleanor, Morrison Joana. *Build Back Fairer: The COVID-19 Marmot Review. The Pandemic, Socioeconomic and Health Inequalities in England* [Internet]. London: Institute of Health Equity, 2020. Available from: https://www.health.org.uk/publications/build-back-fairer-the-covid-19-marmot-review.

62. Marmot Michael, Allen Jessica, Boyce Tommy, Goldblatt Peter, Morrison Joana. *Building Back Fairer in Greater Manchester: Health Equity and Dignified Lives* [Internet]. London: Institute of Health Equity, 2021. Available from: https://www.instituteofhealthequity.org/resources-reports/build-back-fairer-in-greater-manchester-health-equity-and-dignified-lives/build-back-fairer-in-greater-manchester-main-report.pdf (cited 2 May 2022).

63. Barendse M, Flannery J, Cavanagh C, et al. *Longitudinal Change in Adolescent Depression and Anxiety Symptoms from Before to During the COVID-19 Pandemic: A Collaborative of 12 Samples from 3 Countries* [Internet]. PsyArXiv, 2021. Available from: https://doi.org/10.1111/jora.12781 (cited 27 April 2022).

64. Santomauro DF, Mantilla Herrera AM, Shadid J, et al. Global Prevalence and Burden of Depressive and Anxiety Disorders in 204 Countries and Territories in 2020 Due to the COVID-19 Pandemic. The Lancet. 2021 Nov;**398**(10312):1700–12.

65. Creswell C, Shum A, Pearcey S, Skripkauskaite S, Patalay P, Waite P.

Young People's Mental Health During the COVID-19 Pandemic. Lancet Child Adolesc Health. 2021 Aug;**5**(8):535–37.

66. Burke SEL, Sanson AV, Van Hoorn J. The Psychological Effects of Climate Change on Children. Curr Psychiatry Rep. 2018 May;**20**(5):35. https://doi.org/10.1007/s11920-018-0896-9.

67. Hetrick SE, Cox GR, Witt KG, Bir JJ, Merry SN. *Cognitive Behavioural Therapy (CBT), Third-Wave CBT and Interpersonal Therapy (IPT) Based Interventions for Preventing Depression in Children and Adolescents.* [Internet]. Cochrane Database Syst Rev, 2016. Available from: https://www.cochranelibrary.com/cdsr/doi/10.1002/14651858.CD003380.pub4/full (cited 18 November 2021).

68. Burstow P, Newbigging K, Tew J, Costello B. *Investing in a Resilient Generation: Keys to a Mentally Prosperous Nation. Executive Summary and Call to Action* [Internet]. Birmingham: University of Birmingham, 2018. Available from: https://www.birmingham.ac.uk/Documents/research/policycommission/Investing-in-a-Resilient-Generation-Executive-Summary-and-Call-to-Action.pdf (cited 23 February 2022).

69. Williford A, Boulton A, Noland B, Little TD, Kärnä A, Salmivalli C. Effects of the KiVa Anti-bullying Program on Adolescents' Depression, Anxiety, and Perception of Peers. J Abnorm Child Psychol. 2012 Feb;**40**(2):289–300.

70. Dubicka B, Wilkinson PO. Latest Thinking on Antidepressants in Children and Young People. Arch Dis Child. 2018 Aug 1;**103**(8):720–21.

71. The Royal College of Psychiatrists. *The Values-Based Child and Adolescent Mental Health System Commission. What Really Matters in Children and Young People's Mental Health. Summary Document.* The Royal College of Psychiatrists, 2016. Available from: https://valuesbasedpractice.org/wp-content/uploads/2015/04/Values-Based-summary.pdf.

72. McCulloch A, Kroll L, Glass J, Dubicka B. A Systematic Review of the Characteristics of Adolescents with Major Depressive Disorder in Randomised Controlled Treatment Trials. Eur J Psychiatry. 2022 Jan 1;**36**(1):1–10.

73. Gee B, Reynolds S, Carroll B, et al. Practitioner Review: Effectiveness of Indicated School-Based Interventions for Adolescent Depression and Anxiety – A Meta-analytic Review. J Child Psychol Psychiatry. 2020 Jul;**61**(7):739–56.

74. Finning K, White J, Toth K, Golden S, Melendez-Torres GJ, Ford T. Longer-Term Effects of School-Based Counselling in UK Primary Schools. Eur Child Adolesc Psychiatry. 2022 Oct;**31**(10):1591–99. Available from: https://link.springer.com/10.1007/s00787-021-01802-w (cited 3 March 2022).

75. Stallard P, Sayal K, Phillips R, et al. Classroom Based Cognitive Behavioural Therapy in Reducing Symptoms of Depression in High Risk Adolescents: Pragmatic Cluster Randomised Controlled Trial. BMJ. 2012 Oct 5;**345**. https://doi.org/10.1136/bmj.e6058.

76. Kuyken W, Ball S, Crane C, et al. Effectiveness and Cost-Effectiveness of Universal School-Based Mindfulness Training Compared with Normal School Provision in Reducing Risk of Mental Health Problems and Promoting Well-Being in Adolescence: The MYRIAD Cluster Randomised Controlled Trial. Evid Based Ment Health. 2022 Jul 12;**25**(3):99–109. https://doi.org/10.1136/ebmental-2021-300396. Epub ahead of print. PMID: 35820992; PMCID: PMC9340028. Available from: https://ore.exeter.ac.uk/repository/handle/10871/129085 (cited 28 June 2022).

77. Montero-Marin J, Allwood M, Ball S, et al. School-Based Mindfulness Training in Early Adolescence: What Works, for Whom and How in the MYRIAD Trial? Evid Based Ment Health. 2022 Jul 12. https://doi.org/10.1136/ebmental-2021-300396.

78. Tompson M, Sugar C, Langer D, Asarnow J. A Randomized Clinical Trial Comparing Family-Focused Treatment and Individual Supportive Therapy for Depression in Childhood and Early Adolescence. J Am Acad Child Adolesc Psychiatry. 2017 Jun;**56**(6):515–23.

79. Asarnow JR, Tompson MC, Klomhaus AM, Babeva K, Langer DA, Sugar CA. Randomized Controlled Trial of Family-Focused Treatment for Child Depression Compared to Individual Psychotherapy: One-Year Outcomes. J Child Psychol Psychiatry. 2020 Jun;**61**(6):662–71.

80. Hussain H, Dubicka B, Wilkinson P. Recent Developments in the Treatment of Major Depressive Disorder in Children and Adolescents. Evid Based Ment Health. 2018 Aug;**21**(3):101–106.

81. Klein JB, Jacobs RH, Reinecke MA. Cognitive-Behavioral Therapy for Adolescent Depression: A Meta-Analytic Investigation of Changes in Effect-Size Estimates. J Am Acad Child Adolesc Psychiatry. 2007 Nov;**46**(11):1403–13.

82. Weisz JR, Chorpita BF, Palinkas LA, et al. Testing Standard and Modular Designs for Psychotherapy Treating Depression, Anxiety, and Conduct Problems in Youth: A Randomized Effectiveness Trial. Arch Gen Psychiatry. 2012 Mar 1;**69**(3):274–82.

83. Mufson L, Dorta KP, Wickramaratne P, Nomura Y, Olfson M, Weissman MM. A Randomized Effectiveness Trial of Interpersonal Psychotherapy for Depressed Adolescents. Arch Gen Psychiatry. 2004 Jun 1;**61**(6):577–84.

84. Méndez J, Sánchez-Hernández Ó, Garber J, Espada JP, Orgilés M. Psychological Treatments for Depression in Adolescents: More Than Three Decades Later. Int J Environ Res Public Health. 2021 Apr 26;**18**(9). https://doi.org/10.3390/ijerph18094600.

85. Torous J, Bucci S, Bell IH, et al. The Growing Field of Digital Psychiatry: Current Evidence and the Future of Apps, Social Media, Chatbots, and Virtual Reality. World Psychiatry. 2021;**20**(3):318–35.

86. Hollis C, Falconer CJ, Martin JL, et al. Annual Research Review: Digital Health Interventions for Children and Young People with Mental Health Problems – A Systematic and Meta-review. J Child Psychol Psychiatry. 2017 Apr;**58**(4):474–503.

87. Grist R, Porter J, Stallard P. Mental Health Mobile Apps for Preadolescents and Adolescents: A Systematic Review. J Med Internet Res. 2017 May 25;**19**(5):e176.

88. Schleider JL, Weisz JR. Little Treatments, Promising Effects? Meta-Analysis of Single-Session Interventions for Youth Psychiatric Problems. J Am Acad Child Adolesc Psychiatry. 2017 Feb;**56**(2):107–15.

89. Dubicka B, Brent D. Editorial: Pharmacotherapy and Adolescent Depression – An Important Treatment Option. Child Adolesc Ment Health. 2017 May;**22**(2):59–60.

90. Nutt DJ, Sharpe M. Uncritical Positive Regard? Issues in the Efficacy and Safety of Psychotherapy. J Psychopharmacol (Oxf). 2008 Jan;**22**(1):3–6.

91. Wolpert M, Deighton J, Fleming I, Lachman P. Considering Harm and Safety in Youth Mental Health: A Call for Attention and Action. Adm Policy Ment Health. 2015;**42**(1):6–9.

92. Dimidjian S, Hollon SD. How Would We Know If Psychotherapy Were Harmful? Am Psychol. 2010 Jan;**65**(1):21–33.

93. Paediatric Formulary Committee. *BNF for Children (online): Fluoxetine* [Internet]. BMJ Group. Available from: https://bnfc.nice.org.uk/drug/fluoxetine.html#indicationsAndDoses (cited 14 February 2022).

94. Hazell P, Mirzaie M. *Tricyclic Drugs for Depression in Children and Adolescents* [Internet]. Cochrane Common Mental Disorders Group, editor. Cochrane Database Syst Rev, 2013 Jun 18. Available from: http://doi.wiley.com/10.1002/14651858.CD002317.pub2 (cited 14 December 2020).

95. Paediatric Formulary Committee. BNF for Children (online): Sertraline [Internet]. BMJ Group, Pharmaceutical Press, and RCPCH Publications. Available from: https://bnfc.nice.org.uk/drug/sertraline.html#sideEffects (cited 14 May 2022).

96. Medicines for Children. *Sertraline for Obsessive Compulsive Disorder (OCD) and Depression* [Internet]. BMJ Group, Pharmaceutical Press, and RCPCH

Publications. Available from: https://www.medicinesforchildren.org.uk/medicines/sertraline-for-obsessive-compulsive-disorder-ocd-and-depression/#possible-side-effects (cited 14 May 2022).

97. Joint Formulary Committee. *British National Formulary (online): Antidepressant Drugs* [Internet]. BMJ Group and Pharmaceutical Press. Available from: https://bnf.nice.org.uk/treatment-summary/antidepressant-drugs.html (cited 15 May 2022).

98. Boyer EW, Shannon M. Current Concepts: The Serotonin Syndrome. N Engl J Med. 2005 Mar 17;**352**(11):1112–20.

99. Cipriani A, Zhou X, Giovane CD, et al. Comparative Efficacy and Tolerability of Antidepressants for Major Depressive Disorder in Children and Adolescents: A Network Meta-analysis. The Lancet. 2016 Aug 27;**388**(10047):881–90.

100. Weisz JR, Mei Yi Ng, Ugueto AM, et al. What Five Decades of Research Tells Us About the Effects of Youth Psychological Therapy: A Multilevel Meta-Analysis and Implications for Science and Practice. Am Psychol. 2017 Mar 2;**72**(2):79–117.

101. Hammad TA, Laughren T, Racoosin J. Suicidality in Pediatric Patients Treated with Antidepressant Drugs. Arch Gen Psychiatry. 2006 Mar;**63**(3):332–39.

102. Gibbons RD, Brown CH, Hur K, Davis JM, Mann JJ. Suicidal Thoughts and Behavior with Antidepressant Treatment: Reanalysis of the Randomized Placebo-Controlled Studies of Fluoxetine and Venlafaxine. Arch Gen Psychiatry. 2012 Jun 1;**69**(6):580–87.

103. Simon GE, Savarino J. Suicide Attempts Among Patients Starting Depression Treatment with Medications or Psychotherapy. Am J Psychiatry. 2007;**164**(7):1029–34. https://doi.org/10.1176/ajp.2007.164.7.1029.

104. Dudley M, Goldney R, Hadzi-Pavlovic D. Are Adolescents Dying by Suicide Taking SSRI Antidepressants? A Review of Observational Studies. Australas Psychiatry. 2010 Jun;**18**(3):242–45.

105. March J, Silva S, Petrycki S, et al. Fluoxetine, Cognitive-Behavioral Therapy, and Their Combination for Adolescents with Depression: Treatment for Adolescents with Depression Study (TADS) Randomized Controlled Trial. JAMA. 2004 Aug 18;**292**(7):807–20.

106. Dubicka B, Brent D. Combined Therapy in Adolescent Depression. Int J Cogn Ther. 2014 Jun;**7**(2):136–48.

107. Melvin GA, Tonge BJ, King NJ, et al. A Comparison of Cognitive-Behavioral Therapy, Sertraline, and Their Combination for Adolescent Depression. J Am Acad Child Adolesc Psychiatry. 2006 Oct;**45**(10):1151–61.

108. Iftene F, Predescu E, Stefan S, David D. Rational-Emotive and Cognitive-Behavior Therapy (REBT/CBT) Versus Pharmacotherapy Versus REBT/CBT Plus Pharmacotherapy in the Treatment of Major Depressive Disorder in Youth: A Randomized Clinical Trial. Psychiatry Res. 2015 Feb 28;**225**(3):687–94.

109. Asarnow JR, Emslie G, Clarke G, et al. Treatment of Selective Serotonin Reuptake Inhibitor-Resistant Depression in Adolescents: Predictors and Moderators of Treatment Response. J Am Acad Child Adolesc Psychiatry. 2009 Mar;**48**(3):330–39.

110. Davey CG, Chanen AM, Hetrick SE, et al. The Addition of Fluoxetine to Cognitive Behavioural Therapy for Youth Depression (YoDA-C): A Randomised, Double-Blind, Placebo-Controlled, Multicentre Clinical Trial. Lancet Psychiatry. 2019 Sep;**6**(9):735–44.

111. Wegner M, Amatriain-Fernández S, Kaulitzky A, Murillo-Rodriguez E, Machado S, Budde H. Systematic Review of Meta-analyses: Exercise Effects on Depression in Children and Adolescents. Front Psychiatry. 2020 Mar 6;**11**:81. https://doi.org/10.3389/fpsyt.2020.00081. PMID: 32210847; PMCID: PMC7068196.

112. Belski N, Abdul-Rahman Z, Youn E, Balasundaram V, Diep D. Review: The Effectiveness of Musical Therapy in Improving Depression and Anxiety

113. Coventry PA, Brown Jennifer VE, Pervin J, et al. Nature-Based Outdoor Activities for Mental and Physical Health: Systematic Review and Meta-analysis. SSM – Popul Health. 2021 Dec 1;**16**. https://doi.org/10.1016/j.ssmph.2021.100934.

114. Mavoa S, Lucassen M, Denny S, Utter J, Clark T, Smith M. Natural Neighbourhood Environments and the Emotional Health of Urban New Zealand Adolescents. Landsc Urban Plan. 2019 Nov 1;**191**. https://doi.org/10.1016/j.landurbplan.2019.103638.

115. Neufeld SAS, Dunn VJ, Jones PB, Croudace TJ, Goodyer IM. Reduction in Adolescent Depression After Contact with Mental Health Services: A Longitudinal Cohort Study in the UK. Lancet Psychiatry. 2017 Feb;**4**(2):120–27.

116. Courtney DB, Watson P, Krause KR, et al. Predictors, Moderators, and Mediators Associated with Treatment Outcome in Randomized Clinical Trials Among Adolescents with Depression: A Scoping Review. JAMA Netw Open. 2022 Feb 1;**5**(2). https://doi.org/10.1001/jamanetworkopen.2021.46331.

117. McAllister-Williams RH. When Depression Is Difficult to Treat. Eur Neuropsychopharmacol J Eur Coll Neuropsychopharmacol. 2022 Mar;**56**:89–91.

118. Dwyer JB, Stringaris A, Brent DA, Bloch MH. Annual Research Review: Defining and Treating Pediatric Treatment-Resistant Depression. J Child Psychol Psychiatry. 2020 Mar;**61**(3):312–32.

119. McAllister-Williams RH, Arango C, Blier P, et al. The Identification, Assessment and Management of Difficult-to-Treat Depression: An International Consensus Statement. J Affect Disord. 2020 Apr;**267**:264–82.

120. Brent D, Emslie G, Clarke G, et al. Switching to Another SSRI or to Venlafaxine with or Without Cognitive Behavioral Therapy for Adolescents With SSRI-Resistant Depression. JAMA J Am Med Assoc. 2008 Feb 27;**299**(8):901–13.

121. Oberman LM, Hynd M, Nielson DM, Towbin KE, Lisanby SH, Stringaris A. Repetitive Transcranial Magnetic Stimulation for Adolescent Major Depressive Disorder: A Focus on Neurodevelopment. Front Psychiatry. 2021 Apr 13;**12**. https://doi.org/10.3389/fpsyt.2021.642847.

122. Majumder P, Balan S, Gupta V, Wadhwa R, Perera TD. The Safety and Efficacy of Repetitive Transcranial Magnetic Stimulation in the Treatment of Major Depression Among Children and Adolescents: A Systematic Review. Cureus. 2021 Apr 19;**13**(4). Available from: https://www.cureus.com/articles/56400-the-safety-and-efficacy-of-repetitive-transcranial-magnetic-stimulation-in-the-treatment-of-major-depression-among-children-and-adolescents-a-systematic-review (cited 10 January 2022).

123. Di Vincenzo JD, Siegel A, Lipsitz O, et al. The Effectiveness, Safety and Tolerability of Ketamine for Depression in Adolescents and Older Adults: A Systematic Review. J Psychiatr Res. 2021 May;**137**:232–41.

124. Royal College of Psychiatrists. *Electroconvulsive Therapy (ECT)* [Internet]. Royal College of Psychiatrists, 2020. Available from: https://www.rcpsych.ac.uk/mental-health/treatments-and-wellbeing/ect (cited 20 February 2022).

125. ECT Accreditation Service (ECTAS). *Standards for the Administration of ECT* [Internet]. ECT Accreditation Service (ECTAS), 2019 Jan. Report No.: CCQI28. Available from: https://web.archive.org/web/20220224211107/https://www.rcpsych.ac.uk/docs/default-source/improving-care/ccqi/quality-networks/electro-convulsive-therapy-clinics-(ectas)/ectas-14th-edition-standards.pdf?sfvrsn=932fa3b4_2 (cited 20 February 2022).

126. Edwards D, Evans N, Gillen E, et al. What Do We Know About the Risks for Young People Moving Into, Through and Out of Inpatient Mental Health Care? Findings from an Evidence Synthesis. Child Adolesc Psychiatry Ment Health. 2015 Dec 23;9(1):55. https://doi.org/10.1186/s13034-015-0087-y. PMID: 26702297; PMCID: PMC4689041.

127. Peters AT, Jacobs RH, Feldhaus C, et al. Trajectories of Functioning into Emerging Adulthood Following Treatment for Adolescent Depression. J Adolesc Health. 2016 Mar;58(3):253–59.

128. O'Keeffe S, Martin P, Goodyer IM, Kelvin R, Dubicka B. Prognostic Implications for Adolescents with Depression Who Drop Out of Psychological Treatment During a Randomized Controlled Trial. J Am Acad Child Adolesc Psychiatry. 2019 Oct;58(10):983–92.

129. Kennard BD, Emslie GJ, Mayes TL, et al. Sequential Treatment with Fluoxetine and Relapse Prevention CBT to Improve Outcomes in Pediatric Depression. Am J Psychiatry. 2014 Oct 1;171(10):1083–90.

130. Kennard BD, Silva SG, Tonev S, et al. Remission and Recovery in the Treatment for Adolescents with Depression Study (TADS): Acute and Long-term Outcomes. J Am Acad Child Adolesc Psychiatry. 2009 Feb;48(2):186–95.

131. Emslie GJ, Mayes T, Porta G, et al. Treatment of Resistant Depression in Adolescents (TORDIA): Week 24 Outcomes. Am J Psychiatry. 2010 Jul;167(7):782–91.

132. McLeod GFH, Horwood LJ, Fergusson DM. Adolescent Depression, Adult Mental Health and Psychosocial Outcomes at 30 and 35 Years. Psychol Med. 2016 May;46(7):1401–12.

133. Wickersham A, Dickson H, Jones R, et al. Educational Attainment Trajectories Among Children and Adolescents with Depression, and the Role of Sociodemographic Characteristics: Longitudinal Data-Linkage Study. Br J Psychiatry. 2021 Mar;218(3):151–57.

134. Cuijpers P, Stringaris A, Wolpert M. Treatment Outcomes for Depression: Challenges and Opportunities. Lancet Psychiatry. 2020 Nov;7(11):925–27.

135. Duffy A, Carlson G, Dubicka B, Hillegers MHJ. Pre-Pubertal Bipolar Disorder: Origins and Current Status of the Controversy. Int J Bipolar Disord. 2020 Dec;8(1):18. https://doi.org/10.1186/s40345-020-00185-2. PMID: 32307651; PMCID: PMC7167382.

136. Findling RL, Stepanova E, Youngstrom EA, Young AS. Progress in Diagnosis and Treatment of Bipolar Disorder Among Children and Adolescents: An International Perspective. Evid Based Ment Health. 2018 Nov;21(4):177–81.

137. Meter ARV, Moreira ALR, Youngstrom EA. Meta-Analysis of Epidemiologic Studies of Pediatric Bipolar Disorder. J Clin Psychiatry. 2011 May 31;72(9). https://doi.org/10.4088/JCP.10m06290.

138. Sharma A, Neely J, Camilleri N, James A, Grunze H, Le Couteur A. Incidence, Characteristics and Course of Narrow Phenotype Paediatric Bipolar I Disorder in the British Isles. Acta Psychiatr Scand. 2016;134(6):522–32.

139. Dubicka B, Carlson GA, Vail A, Harrington R. Prepubertal Mania: Diagnostic Differences Between US and UK Clinicians. Eur Child Adolesc Psychiatry. 2008 Apr;17(3):153–61.

140. Clacey J, Goldacre M, James A. Paediatric Bipolar Disorder: International Comparisons of Hospital Discharge Rates 2000–2010. BJPsych Open. 2015 Oct;1(2):166–71.

141. Song J, Bergen SE, Kuja-Halkola R, Larsson H, Landén M, Lichtenstein P. Bipolar Disorder and Its Relation to Major Psychiatric Disorders: A Family-Based Study in the Swedish Population. Bipolar Disord. 2015;17(2):184–93.

142. Lau P, Hawes DJ, Hunt C, Frankland A, Roberts G, Mitchell PB. Prevalence of Psychopathology in Bipolar High-Risk

Offspring and Siblings: A Meta-Analysis. Eur Child Adolesc Psychiatry. 2018 Jul 1;**27**(7):823–37.

143. Baldessarini RJ, Tondo L, Vazquez GH, et al. Age at Onset Versus Family History and Clinical Outcomes in 1,665 International Bipolar-I Disorder Patients. World Psychiatry. 2012;**11**(1):40–46.

144. Mick E, Faraone SV. Family and Genetic Association Studies of Bipolar Disorder in Children. Child Adolesc Psychiatr Clin N Am. 2009 Apr;**18**(2):441–53.

145. Birmaher B, Axelson D, Monk K, et al. Lifetime Psychiatric Disorders in School-aged Offspring of Parents with Bipolar Disorder. Arch Gen Psychiatry. 2009 Mar;**66**(3):287–96.

146. Neria Y, Bromet EJ, Carlson GA, Naz B. Assaultive Trauma and Illness Course in Psychotic Bipolar Disorder: Findings from the Suffolk County Mental Health Project. Acta Psychiatr Scand. 2005;(111):380–83.

147. Koenders MA, Mesman E, Giltay EJ, Elzinga BM, Hillegers MHJ. Traumatic Experiences, Family Functioning, and Mood Disorder Development in Bipolar Offspring. Br J Clin Psychol. 2020 Sep;**59**(3):277–89.

148. Post RM, Altshuler LL, Kupka R, et al. Verbal Abuse, Like Physical and Sexual Abuse, in Childhood Is Associated with an Earlier Onset and More Difficult Course of Bipolar Disorder. Bipolar Disord. 2015 May;**17**(3):323–30.

149. Moreno C, Laje G, Blanco C, Jiang H, Schmidt AB, Olfson M. National Trends in the Outpatient Diagnosis and Treatment of Bipolar Disorder in Youth. Arch Gen Psychiatry. 2007 Sep;**64**(9):1032–39.

150. Findling RL, Zhou X, George P, Chappell PB. Diagnostic Trends and Prescription Patterns in Disruptive Mood Dysregulation Disorder and Bipolar Disorder. J Am Acad Child Adolesc Psychiatry. 2022 Mar;**61**(3):434–45.

151. Dubicka B, Kowatch RA. *BMJ Best Practice: Bipolar Disorder in Children UK* [Internet]. BMJ Best Practice. Available from: bestpractice.bmj.com/info.

152. MacKinnon DF, Pies R. Affective Instability as Rapid Cycling: Theoretical and Clinical Implications for Borderline Personality and Bipolar Spectrum Disorders. Bipolar Disord. 2006;**8**(1):1–14.

153. Ruggero CJ, Zimmerman M, Chelminski I, Young D. Borderline Personality Disorder and the Misdiagnosis of Bipolar Disorder. J Psychiatr Res. 2010 Apr;**44**(6):405–408.

154. Pataki C, Carlson GA. The Comorbidity of ADHD and Bipolar Disorder: Any Less Confusion? Curr Psychiatry Rep. 2013;7. https://doi.org/10.1007/s11920-013-0372-5. PMID: 23712723.

155. Youngstrom EA, Genzlinger JE, Egerton GA, Van Meter AR. Multivariate Meta-analysis of the Discriminative Validity of Caregiver, Youth, and Teacher Rating Scales for Pediatric Bipolar Disorder: Mother Knows Best about Mania. Arch Sci Psychol. 2015;**3**(1):112–37.

156. Freeman AJ, Youngstrom EA, Freeman MJ, Youngstrom JK, Findling RL. Is Caregiver-Adolescent Disagreement Due to Differences in Thresholds for Reporting Manic Symptoms? J Child Adolesc Psychopharmacol. 2011 Oct;**21**(5):425–32.

157. Youngstrom EA, Birmaher B, Findling RL. Pediatric Bipolar Disorder: Validity, Phenomenology, and Recommendations for Diagnosis. Bipolar Disord. 2008 Feb;**10**(1 Pt 2):194–214.

158. Kowatch RA, Youngstrom EA, Danielyan A, Findling RL. Review and Meta-analysis of the Phenomenology and Clinical Characteristics of Mania in Children and Adolescents. Bipolar Disord. 2005;**7**(6):483–96.

159. Van Meter AR, Burke C, Kowatch RA, Findling RL, Youngstrom EA. Ten-Year Updated Meta-analysis of the Clinical Characteristics of Pediatric Mania and Hypomania. Bipolar Disord. 2016 Feb;**18**(1):19–32.

160. Frías Á, Palma C, Farriols N. Comorbidity in Pediatric Bipolar

Disorder: Prevalence, Clinical Impact, Etiology and Treatment. J Affect Disord. 2015 Mar;**174**:378–89.

161. Meyer SE, Carlson GA, Youngstrom E, et al. Long-Term Outcomes of Youth Who Manifested the CBCL-Pediatric Bipolar Disorder Phenotype During Childhood and/or Adolescence. J Affect Disord. 2009 Mar;**113**(3):227–35.

162. Gracious BL, Youngstrom EA, Findling RL, Calabrese JR. Discriminative Validity of a Parent Version of the Young Mania Rating Scale. J Am Acad Child Adolesc Psychiatry. 2002 Nov 1;**41**(11):1350–59.

163. Pavuluri MN, Henry DB, Devineni B, Carbray JA, Birmaher B. Child Mania Rating Scale: Development, Reliability, and Validity. J Am Acad Child Adolesc Psychiatry. 2006 May 1;**45**(5):550–60.

164. NICE. *Bipolar Disorder: Assessment and Management [CG185]* [Internet]. NICE, 2020 Feb. Available from: https://www.nice.org.uk/guidance/cg185/chapter/1-Recommendations#recognising-diagnosing-and-managing-bipolar-disorder-in-children-and-young-people-2 (cited 16 March 2022).

165. Cohen D, Bonnot O, Bodeau N, Consoli A, Laurent C. Adverse Effects of Second-Generation Antipsychotics in Children and Adolescents: A Bayesian Meta-analysis. J Clin Psychopharmacol. 2012 Jun;**32**(3):309–16.

166. Fristad MA, MacPherson HA. Evidence-Based Psychosocial Treatments for Child and Adolescent Bipolar Spectrum Disorders. J Clin Child Adolesc Psychol Off J Soc Clin Child Adolesc Psychol Am Psychol Assoc Div 53. 2014;**43**(3):339–55.

167. Atkin T, Nuñez N, Gobbi G. Practitioner Review: The Effects of Atypical Antipsychotics and Mood Stabilisers in the Treatment of Depressive Symptoms in Paediatric Bipolar Disorder. J Child Psychol Psychiatry. 2017 Aug;**58**(8):865–79.

168. DelBello MP, Kadakia A, Heller V, et al. Systematic Review and Network Meta-analysis: Efficacy and Safety of Second-Generation Antipsychotics in Youths with Bipolar Depression. J Am Acad Child Adolesc Psychiatry. 2022 Feb;**61**(2):243–54.

169. NICE. *Aripiprazole for Treating Moderate to Severe Manic Episodes in Adolescents with Bipolar I Disorder Technology Appraisal Guidance [TA292]* [Internet]. NICE, 2013 Jul. Available from: https://www.nice.org.uk/guidance/ta292/chapter/4-Consideration-of-the-evidence (cited 19 March 2022).

170. Miklowitz DJ, Axelson DA, Birmaher B, et al. Family-Focused Treatment for Adolescents with Bipolar Disorder: Results of a 2-Year Randomized Trial. Arch Gen Psychiatry. 2008 Sep;**65**(9):1053–61.

171. West AE, Weinstein SM, Peters AT, et al. Child- and Family-Focused Cognitive-Behavioral Therapy for Pediatric Bipolar Disorder: A Randomized Clinical Trial. J Am Acad Child Adolesc Psychiatry. 2014 Nov;**53**(11):1168-1178.e1.

172. Sharma A, Glod M, Forster T, et al. FAB: First UK Feasibility Trial of a Future Randomised Controlled Trial of Family Focused Treatment for Adolescents with Bipolar Ddisorder. Int J Bipolar Disord. 2020 Dec;**8**(1):24. https://doi.org/10.1186/s40345-020-00189-y.

173. Díaz-Caneja CM, Moreno C, Llorente C, Espliego A, Arango C, Moreno D. Practitioner Review: Long-Term Pharmacological Treatment of Pediatric Bipolar Disorder. J Child Psychol Psychiatry. 2014 Sep;**55**(9):959–80.

174. Grant B, Salpekar JA. Using Lithium in Children and Adolescents with Bipolar Disorder: Efficacy, Tolerability, and Practical Considerations. Paediatr Drugs. 2018 Aug;**20**(4):303–14.

175. Medicines and Healthcare Products Regulatory Agency. *Valproate Use by Women and Girls* [Internet]. GOV.UK, 2018. Available from: https://www.gov.uk/guidance/valproate-use-by-women-and-girls (cited 19 March 2022).

176. Birmaher B, Axelson D, Goldstein B, et al. Four-Year Longitudinal Course of

Children and Adolescents with Bipolar Spectrum Disorder. Am J Psychiatry. 2009 Jul;**166**(7):795–804.

177. Birmaher B, Gill MK, Axelson DA, et al. Longitudinal Trajectories and Associated Baseline Predictors in Youths with Bipolar Spectrum Disorders. Am J Psychiatry. 2014 Sep 1;**171**(9):990–99.

178. Goldstein TR, Birmaher B, Axelson D, et al. History of Suicide Attempts in Pediatric Bipolar Disorder: Factors Associated with Increased Risk. Bipolar Disord. 2005;**7**(6):525–35.

179. MacPherson HA, Kudinova AY, Schettini E, et al. Relationship Between Cognitive Flexibility and Subsequent Course of Mood Symptoms and Suicidal Ideation in Young Adults with Childhood-Onset Bipolar Disorder. Eur Child Adolesc Psychiatry. 2022 Feb;**31**(2):299–312.

180. Garno JL, Goldberg JF, Ramirez PM, Ritzler BA. Impact of Childhood Abuse on the Clinical Course of Bipolar Disorder. Br J Psychiatry. 2005 Feb;**186**(2):121–25.

Chapter 14
Psychosis in Children and Adolescents

Sofia Manolesou and Marinos Kyriakopoulos

Introduction

The terms psychosis and psychotic disorder are used to characterise clinical presentations associated with impairment in reality testing, including hallucinations and delusions, disorganised thinking or behaviour, negative or catatonic symptoms and functional impairment. These conditions have been classified as primary, when they do not arise as part of another mental health, organic or substance misuse disorder, or secondary, when they do [1,2]. Schizophrenia and other primary psychotic disorders are serious and frequently long-term or recurrent mental health conditions, commonly co-occurring with a degree of cognitive decline and social communication deficits [3]. However, psychotic symptoms in keeping with a psychotic disorder may also be seen in mood disorders [4,5,6], ASD [3], personality disorders [7,8], substance misuse [6,9] and in neurological and endocrine conditions [3]. Most research on psychosis in children and young people has been conducted in relation to schizophrenia spectrum disorders.

Early-onset psychosis (EOP), at least in its primary form, is conceptualised as a condition with neurodevelopmental origins, with the first non-specific signs of aberrant development frequently being present before the overt manifestations of the clinical syndrome. Several lines of evidence suggest that the interaction between genetic and environmental factors lead to its emergence. The final pathophysiological outcome seems to be a brain disorder where cerebral integration is compromised giving rise to its phenomenological characteristics.

Epidemiology

Most studies on the epidemiology of EOP are related to schizophrenia spectrum disorders. The prevalence of such cases presenting before the age of 18 years is not totally clear with reported rates varying considerably in the literature. A total of 8.2% of all schizophrenia cases and 12.3% of all schizophrenia spectrum disorders present before the age of 18 years [10]. There has been variation between studies; Cannon and colleagues (1999), estimated 4.7% of all cases of schizophrenia experiencing the onset of the disorder before adulthood in probably the most robust study in this area [11] while higher rates of EOP among first-episode patients have also been reported, reaching 12% [12]. The 3-year prevalence of EOP has been estimated at 5.9/100 000 in a study conducted in Scotland [13]. Childhood onset schizophrenia is much rarer with its incidence being accepted to be around 0.04% [14]. A more recent surveillance study across the UK identified the 1-year incidence of these disorders under the age of 14 years to be 0.21/100 000 [15]. When these figures are compared to the estimated 1-year incidence of schizophrenia across all ages at 0.2/1000 [16], the relative rarity of EOP becomes clear.

On the other hand, psychotic symptoms both in adulthood and in childhood and adolescence are relatively common. In population samples, the median prevalence of psychotic symptoms in childhood was found to be 17% and in adolescence 7.5% [17]. In clinical community clinic samples this seems to be even higher. Depending on the inclusion criteria and the setting, rates of such symptoms vary from 43% to 97.7% [18,19,20,21]. Importantly, high rates of psychotic symptoms in clinical samples with associated distress or adverse functional impact have been reported, reaching 60% in the study by Gin and colleagues [21]. The relatively high prevalence of these symptoms both in epidemiological and in clinical samples would suggest a lack of specificity in terms of risk for psychosis.

Aetiology

Despite the significant progress in understanding the factors affecting the development of psychosis, its aetiology remains to a large extent elusive. Twin and family studies have identified that schizophrenia is a heritable condition, with its heritability being in the region of 80% [22,23]. Genetic factors, such as single nucleotide polymorphisms (SNPs) and copy number variants (CNVs) in several genes, for example, the DISC1, DRD2, NRXN1, and neuregulin 1, and chromosome regions, for example, 22q11.2 and 16p11.2, have shown associations with the disorder [24,25]. However, no single gene or genetic variant has been identified as necessary and sufficient, and their effects are typically small. More sophisticated approaches have employed genome-wide association studies, screening up to millions of common genetic variants, and the calculation of a polygenic risk score as a sum of alleles associated with the disorder, which also cannot fully account for it. It seems that the disorder is a result of combined small effects of hundreds to thousands of variants across the genome.

In addition, environmental factors are also conferring small effects towards the emergence of psychotic conditions. These include poor maternal health and infections during pregnancy, preterm birth, obstetric complications, winter or early spring birth, urban living, low socio-economic status, minority status, low income, migration, childhood trauma, maltreatment and bullying, and misuse of substances like methamphetamine, cannabis and tobacco [26,27]. Some of these effects may be conferred through epigenetic processes, that is, alterations in gene expression, without modification of the underlying DNA sequence. Studies of gene-environment interaction, that is, of the environmental effects depending on the genetic profile of the individual, have been promising but progress in this field has been relatively slow [25].

Psychosis has been conceptualised as a condition with neurodevelopmental origins. Evidence of aberrant neurodevelopment in children who will later develop psychosis include delays in motor and language development, social adjustment deficits and deviant cognitive development [22,23]. However, this trajectory does not seem to be specific to psychosis and neurodevelopmental deviance has been observed in a large number of other mental health and neurodevelopmental disorders. Risk factors affecting specifically earlier onset of these disorders are not totally clear, but this has been associated with genetic factors, such as familial loading [28,29] and also environmental factors, such as head injury before the age of 10 [30].

Course and Prognosis

EOP is generally considered as a more severe variant of the adult-onset form of the disorder. Most children and young people are likely to have several episodes and long-term difficulties, including educational and occupational impairment and social disability [22]. Recovery from the acute episode is possible with functional outcomes being similar to other severe conditions requiring hospitalisation [31]. Some studies have also reported promising outcomes with up to around 60% of children and young people with schizophrenia showing significant improvement at follow-up [32,33,34]. However, repeated hospitalisations are not unlikely, with up to 83% of adolescents having at least one further episode requiring hospitalisation over a 10-year period after their first one [35]. In addition, the majority of follow-up studies have found most adolescents with schizophrenia being chronically ill, with functional impairment and active symptoms [22]. Poor premorbid function, younger age at onset, more insidious onset, longer duration of untreated psychosis (DUP), more severe psychopathology, longer stay in hospital, residual and negative symptoms and repeated hospitalisations are predictors of poorer outcome [22,36,37]. Age at first hospitalisation has been associated with differential outcomes in terms of length of first admission, more than one hospital admission, average number of days in hospital and number of admissions per year in an Israeli national population-based cohort from 1978 to 1992 [38]. The authors used recursive partitioning to empirically determine cut-off points for age groups showing the greatest difference on these variables and demonstrated that the ages of 17 years and 12 years seem to mark cut-off points in that respect with the earlier the onset the worse the prognosis [38]. More specifically, across the lifespan, age at first admission seemed to significantly affect the number of days at first hospitalisation (with children under the age of 11 years spending on average more than 1200 days in hospital versus young people and adults over 17 years spending less than 200 days) and the average number of days per year in hospital (from more than 150 days in children under 12 years gradually reducing to less than 50 days in the age group of 27–48-year-old patients). Of patients with age of first admission below 17 years, 82.5% had more than one admission decreasing for subsequent age groups to 73.54% (18–28 years), 69.36% (29–31 years), 62.88% (32–45 years) and 50.77% (over 45 years). Within EOP, negative symptoms, ASD, older age at first presentation, black ethnicity and family history of psychosis have been also associated with multiple treatment failure, defined as the initiation of the third novel antipsychotic due to prior insufficient response, intolerable adverse-effects or non-adherence [39].

Clinical Symptomatology

EOP is manifesting with the same types of symptoms with the adult-onset form of the disorder, but their relative prevalence and characteristics may differ. In addition, psychotic symptoms may more likely point towards other diagnoses given their high prevalence in clinical samples combined with the relative rarity of psychosis in this age range. In general, EOP is associated with a more insidious onset in comparison to adult psychotic disorders and alternative explanations for symptomatology may be mistakenly but understandably employed for longer. Auditory hallucinations are a prominent feature in such cases but their combination with other types of hallucinations including visual, tactile, and olfactory is also likely [40]. Delusions are very common but, depending on the age of the child or young person, are probably less well formed compared to adult psychosis. Negative symptoms including flattened or inappropriate affect have also been consistently reported in younger patients. Catatonic symptoms and bizarre behaviour may be less frequent. Given the comorbidity with other neurodevelopmental disorders, it can be hard to establish a speech and language baseline and differentiate formal thought disorder associated with a psychotic episode to premorbid developmental language abnormalities [22]. It may also be hard to evaluate, especially in younger neurodiverse patients, treatment outcomes related to return to their communication baseline [3]. The phenomenology of EOP to a large extent depends on the age at onset, neurodevelopmental profile, comorbid conditions and cognitive abilities of the child or adolescent and a number of environmental factors that may affect its clinical picture.

Diagnostic Assessment and Differential Diagnosis

All children and young people who present with psychotic symptoms or suspected psychotic disorder would require a comprehensive, multidisciplinary diagnostic assessment [41]. Differential diagnosis should consider medical causes of psychotic symptoms including epilepsy and other neurological conditions, infectious diseases, malignancies, genetic syndromes, inborn errors of metabolism, autoimmune and endocrine disorders and side effects of medication or substance intoxication [3,42,43,44]. Secondary psychosis due to organic causes may vary from atypical psychotic conditions to more typical presentations. With the exception of psychotic symptoms emerging in the context of substance use and intoxication, most medical aetiologies of psychotic symptoms are rare [44]. A careful medical history, physical examination and investigations can identify possible organic causes of secondary psychosis and their treatment may resolve the psychotic symptoms [42,43]. The age at onset is likely to determine the extent of these investigations; psychosis in children would normally require a more detailed physical workup as its rarity would mandate the exclusion of other equally rare organic conditions presenting with psychotic symptoms. A detailed evaluation by a paediatric neurologist is likely to be required and investigations such as a brain MRI, an electroencephalogram and genetic testing with array comparative genomic hybridisation may be warranted [3]. For older adolescents, the extent of the investigations will need to be decided depending on the young person's history and clinical presentation. Although no clear guidelines exist on how such a decision can be made for new cases of psychosis at that age, the absence of systemic or neurological signs and symptoms, a family history of psychosis, characteristic presentation with unusual experiences and beliefs without apparent confusional state, potential temporally associated environmental stressors or risk factors, including substance misuse and overall grossly neurotypical premorbid development, may all point towards the disorder not being organic in nature. In general, immunologic investigations, like N-methyl-D-aspartate receptor antibodies, may be clinically advisable in addition to the standard baseline blood tests in all young people presenting with psychosis. A list of all potential investigations for psychosis can be found in the paper by Pina Camacho and colleagues [3].

EOP should also be differentiated from difficulties on the background of neurodevelopmental disorders such as ASD. ASD and psychotic disorders share genetic risk factors and often present concurrently. In children presenting with psychosis in particular, premorbid ASD seems to be identifiable in 30–50% of cases [24]. The negative symptoms of social withdrawal and flattened affect need to be distinguished from deficits in executive functioning, social interaction and emotional reciprocity, which are characteristic of ASD [45]. Overvalued and idiosyncratic beliefs, bizarre ideas and language and cognitive impairments, which are common in ASD, must be differentiated from thought disorders in schizophrenia and other psychoses [44]. Other mental health problems such as anxiety, acute distress and traumatic reactions either in the acute phase or as part of a post-traumatic stress manifestation can also cause hallucinations or distorted thinking [44]. Among psychotic disorders, and especially during an acute onset of psychotic symptoms, it is often a challenge to establish a definite diagnosis and to distinguish between psychotic affective disorder and schizophrenia; it might take some time before the disorder is fully manifested and an accurate diagnosis is confirmed [44].

Comorbidities are also not uncommon in children and young people with psychosis. These include depression and anxiety, pre-existing neurodevelopmental difficulties and substance misuse [41]. The use of illicit drugs is increased among individuals with psychosis, and it can precede, co-occur, or follow the psychotic symptoms; there are bidirectional causal and complex interactions between the substance misuse and mental health problems [46]. Such substances have been found to include cannabis, stimulants, hallucinogens and more recently inhalants, nitrous oxide and ketamine [46,47]. Cannabis is the most frequently used illicit drug [48]. There is evidence that the adolescent brain is more susceptible to its effects, which also seem to be dose related [49,50]. There is strong evidence that cannabis use is often associated with adolescent psychosis either as a possible risk factor or as a comorbidity [47,50].

Given the significant burden and multiple negative outcomes on the individual and the society associated with established psychosis, there has been a focus in identifying people at risk of developing psychosis and to prevent its onset. The construct of the 'At Risk Mental State' (ARMS) or 'Clinical/Ultra High Risk for Psychosis' (CHR-P) has been developed for over two decades and has informed the service provision in adults [51]. CHR-P prevention, a primary indicated prevention, involves identifying individuals with subtle psychotic symptoms and signs and offering targeted specialised intervention in order to prevent the full transition to the disorder [52,53]. Naturally, there has been a lot of interest in applying the same methodology to children and young people showing subtle symptoms of psychosis in order to prevent its full manifestation. Even though there are some indications that the CHR-P methodology could be relevant to young people, there is no evidence of increased risk of transition to psychosis among those characterised as high-risk adolescents [54], nor evidence of effective intervention that can prevent psychosis in this age group [52]. It is recommended therefore that there is caution when using the ARMS methodology for children and adolescents [54]. The guidelines from the UK's National Institute for Health and Care Excellence UK (NICE) clearly state that it is not recommended to prescribe antipsychotic medication when the diagnostic criteria of a psychotic disorder are not met with the aim to 'prevent' psychosis [41].

Treatment

Once the diagnosis of a psychotic disorder has been confirmed, the treatment should start as soon as possible in an outpatient or inpatient setting. The care pathways might include multiple care providers and transitions and there are different models of care in different countries [55]. Long DUP, the period between the emergence of symptoms and the initiation of treatment, has been associated with negative outcomes in regard to both symptoms severity and overall functionality and prognosis [56,57,58]. The principles of treating psychosis in children and adolescents have derived from the relevant research and clinical practice in adults. Given however the atypicality of symptoms, the frequent comorbidities, the developmental vulnerabilities and the unique social, cognitive and psychological aspects of this age, the treatment of psychosis in this group may present with additional challenges.

Medication

Currently, the cornerstone of treatment for psychotic disorders in children and young people is pharmacological with antipsychotic medications in an inpatient or outpatient setting, preferably alongside psychosocial interventions [41]. Antipsychotic medications appear to have similar efficacy in both adults and younger people, but there is higher prevalence of side effects in the latter group and higher rates of discontinuation of treatment [59]. There is no clear evidence suggesting that Second Generation Antipsychotics (SGA) are more effective than typical antipsychotics. However, they are preferred for children and adolescents because of their more tolerable side effect profile [60].

Among SGAs, with the exception of clozapine, there do not seem to be significant differences in efficacy and effectiveness. Olanzapine and risperidone have some indications of being more effective while lurasidone and aripiprazole are better tolerated [61,62]. There is no clear evidence of efficacy for ziprasidone and asenapine [63,64]. Clozapine appears to be distinctly more effective in overall symptom reduction, relapse rates and treatment resistant psychosis; however, it is underused across the lifespan resulting in polypharmacy [65]. This is due to the possible severe side effects that require specialised monitoring and is even more evident in children and adolescents where there may be an even bigger delay and hesitation by clinicians to initiate clozapine treatment. Given its effectiveness though, clozapine should be considered as an option for older children and adolescents with psychosis who do not show good response to adequate trials of SGAs [37,66].

The therapeutic doses of antipsychotic medication in adolescents seem to be similar to those for adults. Treatment is usually initiated at a lower dose and is titrated more slowly. In clinical practice, lower doses for children are normally used. There is some indication that aripiprazole can be effective in lower doses [60]. In any case of prescribing antipsychotics, there should be careful baseline physical evaluation, monitoring and recording of the response and possible side effects of treatment [41].

With regard to long-term treatment with antipsychotics, there is almost non-existing randomised controlled trial evidence with the only such data showing some efficacy for aripiprazole for maintenance treatment with this indication beyond 8 weeks [67]. Furthermore, when prescribing medication for psychosis, one should always consider the possible comorbid conditions, which might require additional treatments such as mood stabilisers for bipolar disorder symptoms, selective serotonin reuptake inhibitors for anxiety and depression or benzodiazepines for short-term treatment of anxiety, insomnia, agitation or catatonia [37,44].

Antipsychotic side effects are an important factor in the choice of treatment. Common side effects include sedation, hyperprolactinaemia, which can in turn impact on growth, menstruation and sexual function and maturation, cardiovascular side effects, movement side effects, and metabolic changes including weight gain, dyslipidaemia and diabetes [64,66]. The metabolic side effects contribute to chronic poor physical health outcomes and reduce life expectancy [68,69]. Antipsychotics vary with regard to their side effects: olanzapine and clozapine seem to affect weight gain and metabolic parameters more compared with other SGAs, while aripiprazole and lurasidone seem to have less side effects of that kind [62,63,64]. Among SGAs, risperidone, paliperidone and, to a lesser extent, olanzapine can increase prolactin [63]. Signs of tardive dyskinesia need to be regularly and specifically monitored as this serious movement side effect is not very uncommon even with SGAs and is potentially irreversible [70,71]. Adjunct medication might moderate side effects for example anticholinergic medication for extrapyramidal side effects, beta-blockers for akathisia and metformin for antipsychotic-induced weight gain [44,72,73,74]. Antipsychotic medication may also result in rarer serious side effects. At present, clozapine treatment is usually initiated in inpatient settings in this age range in the UK due to the monitoring requirements necessary for its use. As in the case of adults, regular blood investigations are necessary to identify potential neutropenia early, due to the risk of agranulocytosis. Other serious side effects that need to be specifically monitored include cardiac complications, severe constipation potentially leading to paralytic ileus and seizures [75].

The choice of antipsychotic medication should be jointly made with the young person and their carers, taking into account the individual circumstances, preferences and clinical needs [41].

Psychosocial Interventions

Psychosocial interventions also have a significant place in the care of children and young people with psychotic disorders. NICE recommends that if psychotherapy is provided, this should happen alongside pharmacological treatment [41]. Unfortunately, there is paucity of good quality research on psychological interventions for psychosis in this age group and it is a high priority to build the evidence base for these treatments before implementing them [59,76,77].

With regard to specific psychosocial interventions, in the existing limited literature there is some evidence that family therapy in combination with individual CBT can have a beneficial effect [59]. Cognitive remediation therapy (CRT) has been shown to be beneficial for cognitive functioning, and CBT and CRT seem to have a positive effect in psychosocial functioning for adolescents with psychosis [78]. There is not strong evidence that psychosocial interventions can improve or alter the course of psychotic symptoms in this age group [78]. It is acknowledged that psychotherapeutic interventions in children and adolescents should differ from the ones in adults and respond to their unique developmental and psychosocial needs [79].

Early Intervention Services

Over the last two decades, the Early Intervention in Psychosis Services (EIP) have been widely developed, accumulating evidence of effectiveness in multiple domains, and are considered the treatment of choice for the first psychotic episode in adults [56,80,81]. These services are founded on two principles: first, the delivery of a timely intervention that aims at reducing the DUP, and secondly, the provision of a multimodal evidence-based treatment during the critical period of 2 to 5 years after the onset of psychosis when the intervention can be most effective [57,81]. Their ultimate aim is to improve the clinical course and functional outcomes for people with these disorders. For adolescent patients in the UK, it is recommended that a referral to an EIP should be made if there is a diagnosis of a first psychotic episode [82]. Usually, a child and adolescent psychiatrist offers input to an EIP team based within adult mental health services. There is evidence that specialist EIP for this age group can be effective in all domains and that there is scope for further shaping developmentally adjusted specialist services for young people experiencing psychosis [83].

Conclusions

Psychosis is a severe mental disorder with developmental risk factors that needs comprehensive assessment and physical evaluation in children and adolescents. Treatment strategies are mostly pharmacological with SGAs and should involve extensive monitoring of response and side effects. Given the comparable effectiveness of most SGAs, their side-effect profile and patient preference commonly influence the choice of treatment. Early intervention is likely to improve the course and outcome of children and young people with the disorder. All available strategies including the use of clozapine should be considered in treatment resistant cases.

References

1. World Health Organisation. *International Statistical Classification of Diseases and Related Health Problems*. 11th ed. World Health Organisation, 2019. https://icd.who.int.

2. American Psychiatric Association. *Diagnostic and Statistical Manual of Mental Disorders*. 5th ed. Washington, DC: American Psychiatric Association, 2013.

3. Pina-Camacho L, Parellada M, Kyriakopoulos M. Autism Spectrum Disorder and Schizophrenia: Boundaries and Uncertainties. BJPsych Advances. 2016;**22**:316–24.

4. Jääskeläinen E, Juola T, Korpela H, et al. Epidemiology of Psychotic Depression: Systematic Review and Meta-analysis. Psychol Med. 2018;**48**:905–18.

5. Smith LM, Johns LC, Mitchell RLC. Characterizing the Experience of Auditory Verbal Hallucinations and Accompanying Delusions in Individuals with a Diagnosis of Bipolar Disorder: A Systematic Review. Bipolar Disord. 2017;**19**:417–33.

6. van Nierop M, van Os J, Gunther N, et al. Phenotypically Continuous with Clinical Psychosis, Discontinuous in Need for Care: Evidence for an Extended Psychosis Phenotype. Schizophr Bull. 2012;**38**:231–38.

7. Balaratnasingama S, Janca A. Normal Personality, Personality Disorder and Psychosis: Current Views and Future Perspectives. Curr Opin Psychiatry. 2015;**28**: 30–34.

8. Bebbington P, Freeman D. Transdiagnostic Extension of Delusions: Schizophrenia and Beyond. Schizophr Bull. 2017;**43**:273–82.

9. Rössler W, Hengartner MP, Angst J, Ajdacic-Gross V. Linking Substance Use with Symptoms of Subclinical Psychosis in a Community Cohort over 30 Years. Addiction. 2012;**107**:1174–84.

10. Solmi M, Radua J, Olivola M, et al. Age at Onset of Mental Disorders Worldwide: Large-Scale Meta-analysis of 192 Epidemiological Studies. Mol Psychiatry. 2022;**27**:281–95.

11. Cannon M, Jones P, Huttunen MO, et al. School Performance in Finnish Children and Later Development of Schizophrenia: A Population-Based Longitudinal Study. Arch Gen Psychiatry. 1999;**56**:457–63.

12. Amminger GP, Henry LP, Harrigan SM, et al. Outcome in Early-Onset Schizophrenia Revisited: Findings from the Early Psychosis Prevention and Intervention Centre Long-Term Follow-Up Study. Schizophr Res. 2011;**131**:112–19.

13. Boeing L, Murray V, Pelosi A, McCabe R, Blackwood D, Wrate R. Adolescent-Onset Psychosis: Prevalence, Needs and Service Provision. Br J Psychiatry. 2007;**190**:18–26.

14. Driver DI, Thomas S, Gogtay N, Rapoport JL. Childhood-Onset Schizophrenia and Early-Onset

Schizophrenia Spectrum Disorders: An Update. Child Adolesc Psychiatr Clin N Am. 2020;29:71–90.

15. Tiffin PA, Kitchen CEW. Incidence and 12-Month Outcome of Childhood Non-Affective Psychoses: British National Surveillance Study. Br J Psychiatry. 2015;206:517–18.

16. Messias EL, Chen CY, Eaton WW. Epidemiology of Schizophrenia: Review of Findings and Myths. Psychiatr Clin North Am. 2007;30:323–38.

17. Kelleher I, Connor D, Clarke MC, Devlin N, Harley M, Cannon M. Prevalence of Psychotic Symptoms in Childhood and Adolescence: A Systematic Review and Meta-analysis of Population-Based Studies. Psychol Med. 2012;42:1857–63.

18. Kelleher I, Devlin N, Wigman JTW, et al. Psychotic Experiences in a Mental Health Clinic Sample: Implications for Suicidality, Multimorbidity and Functioning. Psychol Med. 2014; 44:1615–24.

19. Pontillo M, de Luca M, Pucciarini ML, Vicari S, Armando M. All That Glitters Is not Gold: Prevalence and Relevance of Psychotic-Like Experiences in Clinical Sample of Children and Adolescents Aged 8–17 Years Old. Early Interv Psychiatry. 2018;12:702–07.

20. Brandizzi M, Schultze-Lutter F, Masillo A, et al. Self-Reported Attenuated Psychotic-Like Experiences in Help-Seeking Adolescents and their Association with Age, Functioning and Psychopathology. Schizophr Res. 2014;160:110–17.

21. Gin K, Banerjea P, Abbott C, et al. Childhood Unusual Experiences in Community Child and Adolescent Mental Health Services in South East London: Prevalence and Impact. Schizophr Res. 2018;195:93–96.

22. Kyriakopoulos M, Frangou S. Pathophysiology of Early Onset Schizophrenia. Int Rev Psychiatry. 2007;19:315–24.

23. Jaaro-Peled H, Sawa A. Neurodevelopmental Factors in Schizophrenia. Psychiatr Clin North Am. 2020;43:263–74.

24. Rapoport J, Chavez A, Greenstein D, Addington A, Gogtay N. Autism Spectrum Disorders and Childhood-Onset Schizophrenia: Clinical and Biological Contributions to a Relation Revisited. J Am Acad Child Adolesc Psychiatry. 2009;48:10–18.

25. Zwicker A, Denovan-Wright EM, Uher R. Gene-Environment Interplay in the Etiology of Psychosis. Psychol Med. 2018;48:1925–36.

26. Davies C, Segre G, Estradé A, et al. Prenatal and Perinatal Risk and Protective Factors for Psychosis: A Systematic Review and Meta-analysis. Lancet Psychiatry. 2020;7:399–410.

27. Beckmann D, Lowman KL, Nargiso J, McKowen J, Watt L, Yule AM. Substance-Induced Psychosis in Youth. Child Adolesc Psychiatr Clin N Am. 2020;29:131–43.

28. Byrne M, Agerbo E, Mortensen PB. Family History of Psychiatric Disorders and Age at First Contact in Schizophrenia: An Epidemiological Study. Br J Psychiatry. 2002;181(suppl43):S19–S25.

29. Suvisaari JM, Haukka J, Tanskanen A, Lönnqvist JK. Age at Onset and Outcome in Schizophrenia Are Related to the Degree of Familial Loading. Br J Psychiatry. 1998;173:494–500.

30. AbdelMalik P, Husted J, Chow EWC, Bassett AS. Childhood Head Injury and Expression of Schizophrenia in Multiply Affected Families. Arch Gen Psychiatry. 2003;60:231–36.

31. Galitzer H, Anagnostopoulou N, Alba A, Gaete J, Dima D, Kyriakopoulos M. Functional Outcomes and Patient Satisfaction Following Inpatient Treatment for Childhood-Onset Schizophrenia Spectrum Disorders vs Non-psychotic Disorders in Children in the United Kingdom. Early Interv Psychiatry. 2021; 15: 412–19.

32. Asarnow JR, Tompson MC, Goldstein MJ. Childhood-Onset Schizophrenia: A Followup Study. Schizophr Bull. 1994;20:599–617.

33. Pencer A, Addington J, Addington D. Outcome of a First Episode of Psychosis in Adolescence: A 2-Year Follow-Up. Psychiatry Res. 2005;**133**:35–43.
34. Russell AT. The Clinical Presentation of Childhood-Onset Schizophrenia. Schizophr Bull. 1994;**20**:631–46.
35. Lay B, Blanz B, Hartmann M, Schmidt MH. The Psychosocial Outcome of Adolescent-Onset Schizophrenia: A 12-Year Followup. Schizophr Bull. 2000;**26**:801–16.
36. Clemmensen L, Vernal DL, Steinhausen HC. A Systematic Review of the Long-Term Outcome of Early Onset Schizophrenia. BMC Psychiatry. 2012; **12**:150.
37. Hayes D, Kyriakopoulos M. Dilemmas in the Treatment of Early-Onset First-Episode Psychosis. Ther Adv Psychopharmacol. 2018;**8**:231–39.
38. Rabinowitz J, Levine SZ, Häfner H. A Population Based Elaboration of the Role of Age of Onset on the Course of Schizophrenia. Schizophr Res. 2006;**88**:96–101.
39. Downs J, Dean H, Lechler S, et al. Negative Symptoms in Early-Onset Psychosis and Their Association with Antipsychotic Treatment Failure. Schizophr Bull. 2019;**45**:69–79.
40. David CN, Greenstein D, Clasen L, et al. Childhood Onset Schizophrenia: High Rate of Visual Hallucinations. J Am Acad Child Adolesc Psychiatry. 2011;**50**:681–86.
41. National Institute for Health and Care Excellence. *Psychosis and Schizophrenia in Children and Young People: Recognition and Management: Clinical Guideline CG155*. NICE, 2013; updated: 2016. Available from: https://www.nice.org.uk/guidance/cg155.
42. Giannitelli M, Consoli A, Raffin M, et al. An Overview of Medical Risk Factors for Childhood Psychosis: Implications for Research and Treatment. Schizophr Res. 2018;**192**:39–49.
43. Merritt J, Tanguturi Y, Fuchs C, Cundiff AW. Medical Etiologies of Secondary Psychosis in Children and Adolescents. Child Adolesc Psychiatr Clin N Am. 2020;**29**:29–42.
44. McClellan J. Psychosis in Children and Adolescents. J Am Acad Child Adolesc Psychiatry. 2018;**57**:308–12.
45. Chandrasekhar T, Copeland JN, Spanos M, Sikich L. Autism, Psychosis, or Both? Unraveling Complex Patient Presentations. Child Adolesc Psychiatr Clin N Am. 2020;**29**:103–13.
46. Nathan R, Lewis E. Assessment of Coexisting Psychosis and Substance Misuse: Complexities, Challenges and Causality. BJPsych Adv. 2021;**27**:38–48.
47. Mustonen A, Niemelä S, Nordström T, et al. Adolescent Cannabis Use, Baseline Prodromal Symptoms and the Risk of Psychosis. Br J Psychiatry. 2018;**212**:227–33.
48. Peacock A, Leung J, Larney S, et al. Global Statistics on Alcohol, Tobacco and Illicit Drug Use: 2017 Status Report. Addiction. 2018;**113**:1905–26.
49. Abush H, Ghose S, van Enkevort EA, et al. Associations Between Adolescent Cannabis Use and Brain Structure in Psychosis. Psychiatry Res. Neuroimaging. 2018;**276**:53–64.
50. Gage SH, Hickman M, Zammit S. Association Between Cannabis and Psychosis: Epidemiologic Evidence. Biol Psychiatry. 2016;**79**:549–56.
51. Fusar-Poli P. The Clinical High-Risk State for Psychosis (CHR-P), Version II. Schizophr Bull. 2017;**43**:44–47.
52. Catalan A, Salazar de Pablo G, Vaquerizo Serrano J, et al. Annual Research Review: Prevention of Psychosis in Adolescents – Systematic Review and Meta-analysis of Advances in Detection, Prognosis and Intervention. J Child Psychol Psychiatry. 2021;**62**:657–73.
53. Arango C, Díaz-Caneja CM, McGorry PD, et al. Preventive Strategies for Mental Health. Lancet Psychiatry. 2018;**5**:591–604.
54. Lång U, Yates K, Leacy FP, et al. Systematic Review and Meta-analysis: Psychosis Risk in Children and Adolescents with an

At-Risk Mental State. J Am Acad Child Adolesc Psychiatry. 2022;**61**:615–25.

55. Simon GE, Stewart C, Hunkeler EM, et al. Care Pathways Before First Diagnosis of a Psychotic Disorder in Adolescents and Young Adults. Am J Psychiatry. 2018;**175**:434–42.

56. McGorry PD. Early Intervention in Psychosis: Obvious, Effective, Overdue. J Nerv Ment Dis. 2015;**203**:310–18.

57. Penttilä M, Jääskeläinen E, Hirvonen N, Isohanni M, Miettunen J. Duration of Untreated Psychosis as Predictor of Long-Term Outcome in Schizophrenia: Systematic Review and Meta-analysis. Br J Psychiatry. 2014;**205**:88–94.

58. Stentebjerg-Olesen M, Pagsberg AK, Fink-Jensen A, Correll CU, Jeppesen P. Clinical Characteristics and Predictors of Outcome of Schizophrenia-Spectrum Psychosis in Children and Adolescents: A Systematic Review. J Child Adolesc Psychopharmacol. 2016;**26**:410–27.

59. Stafford MR, Mayo-Wilson E, Loucas CE, et al. Efficacy and Safety of Pharmacological and Psychological Interventions for the Treatment of Psychosis and Schizophrenia in Children, Adolescents and Young Adults: A Systematic Review and Meta-analysis. PLoS One. 2015;**10**:e0117166.

60. Kumar A, Datta SS, Wright SD, Furtado VA, Russell PS. Atypical Antipsychotics for Psychosis in Adolescents. *Cochrane Database Syst Rev.* 2013:CD009582.

61. Correll CU, Cortese S, Croatto G, et al. Efficacy and Acceptability of Pharmacological, Psychosocial, and Brain Stimulation Interventions in Children and Adolescents with Mental Disorders: An Umbrella Review. World Psychiatry. 2021;**20**: 244–75.

62. Arango C, Ng-Mak D, Finn E, Byrne A, Loebel A. Lurasidone Compared to Other Atypical Antipsychotic Monotherapies for Adolescent Schizophrenia: A Systematic Literature Review and Network Meta-analysis. Eur Child Adolesc Psychiatry. 2020;**29**:1195–205.

63. Krause M, Zhu Y, Huhn M, Schneider-Thoma J, Bighelli I, Chaimani A, et al. Efficacy, Acceptability, and Tolerability of Antipsychotics in Children and Adolescents with Schizophrenia: A Network Meta-analysis. Eur Neuropsychopharmacol. 2018;**28**:6596–74.

64. Pagsberg AK, Tarp S, Glintborg D, et al. Acute Antipsychotic Treatment of Children and Adolescents with Schizophrenia-Spectrum Disorders: A Systematic Review and Network Meta-Analysis. J Am Acad Child Adolesc Psychiatry. 2017;**56**:191–202.

65. Wagner E, Siafis S, Fernando P, et al. Efficacy and Safety of Clozapine in Psychotic Disorders: A Systematic Quantitative Meta-review. Transl Psychiatry. 2021;**11**:487.

66. Schneider C, Taylor D, Zalsman G, Frangou S, Kyriakopoulos M. Antipsychotics Use in Children and Adolescents: An On-going Challenge in Clinical Practice. J Psychopharmacol. 2014;**28**:615–23.

67. Singappuli P, Sonuga-Barke E, Kyriakopoulos M. Antipsychotic Long-Term Treatment in Children and Young People: A Systematic Review and Meta-Analysis of Efficacy and Tolerability Across Mental Health and Neurodevelopmental Conditions. CNS Spectr. 2022;**27**:570–87.

68. Hjorthøj C, Stürup AE, McGrath JJ, Nordentoft M. Years of Potential Life Lost and Life Expectancy in Schizophrenia: A Systematic Review and Meta-analysis. Lancet Psychiatry. 2017;**4**:295–301.

69. Walker ER, McGee RE, Druss BG. Mortality in Mental Disorders and Global Disease Burden Implications: A Systematic Review and Meta-analysis. JAMA Psychiatry. 2015;**72**:334–41.

70. Garcia-Amador M, Merchán-Naranjo J, Tapia C, et al. Neurological Adverse Effects of Antipsychotics in Children and Adolescents. J Clin Psychopharmacol. 2015;**35**:686–93.

71. Wonodi I, Reeves G, Carmichael D, et al. Tardive Dyskinesia in Children Treated

with Atypical Antipsychotic Medications. Mov Disord. 2007;**22**:1777–82.

72. Correll CU, Sikich L, Reeves G, et al. Metformin Add-on vs. Antipsychotic Switch vs. Continued Antipsychotic Treatment Plus Healthy Lifestyle Education in Overweight or Obese Youth with Severe Mental Illness: Results from the IMPACT Trial. World Psychiatry. 2020; **19**:69–80.

73. de Silva VA, Suraweera C, Ratnatunga SS, et al. Metformin in Prevention and Treatment of Antipsychotic Induced Weight Gain: A Systematic Review and Meta-analysis. BMC Psychiatry. 2016;**16**:1–10.

74. Stroup TS, Gray N. Management of Common Adverse Effects of Antipsychotic Medications. World Psychiatry. 2018;**17**:341–56.

75. Schneider C, Corrigall R, Hayes D, Kyriakopoulos M, Frangou S. Systematic Review of the Efficacy and Tolerability of Clozapine in the Treatment of Youth with Early Onset Schizophrenia. Eur Psychiatry. 2014;**29**:1–10.

76. Calvo A, Moreno M, Ruiz-Sancho A, et al. Intervention for Adolescents with Early-Onset Psychosis and Their Families: A Randomized Controlled Trial. J Am Acad Child Adolesc Psychiatry. 2014;**53**:688–96.

77. Datta SS, Daruvala R, Kumar A. Psychological Interventions for Psychosis in Adolescents. Cochrane Database Syst Rev. 2020;7:CD009533.

78. Anagnostopoulou N, Kyriakopoulos M, Alba A. Psychological Interventions in Psychosis in Children and Adolescents: A Systematic Review. Eur Child Adolesc Psychiatry. 2019;**28**:735–46.

79. Browning S, Corrigall R, Garety P, Emsley R, Jolley S. Psychological Interventions for Adolescent Psychosis: A Pilot Controlled Trial in Routine Care. Eur Psychiatry. 2013;**28**:423–26.

80. Correll CU, Galling B, Pawar A, Krivko A, Bonetto C, Ruggeri M, et al. Comparison of Early Intervention Services vs Treatment as Usual for Early-Phase Psychosis: A Systematic Review, Meta-analysis, and Meta-regression. JAMA Psychiatry. 2018;**75**:555–65.

81. Malla A, McGorry P. Early Intervention in Psychosis in Young People: A Population and Public Health Perspective. Am J Public Health. 2019;**109**:S181–84.

82. Kendall T, Hollis C, Stafford M, Taylor C. Recognition and Management of Psychosis and Schizophrenia in Children and Young People: Summary of NICE Guidance. BMJ. 2013;**346**:f150.

83. Thomson A, Griffiths H, Fisher R, McCabe R, Abbott-Smith S, Schwannauer M. Treatment Outcomes and Associations in an Adolescent-Specific Early Intervention for Psychosis Service. Early Interv Psychiatry. 2019;**13**:707–14.

Chapter 15

Substance Misuse in Young People

Paul McArdle and Eilish Gilvarry

Introduction

Substance misuse by young people is one of a range of health-related behaviours that threaten the long-term health and potentially the lives of young people. This is especially true where young people have disposable income, now including large regions in Asia. However, this chapter focuses mainly on experiences in the UK, Europe and the Anglosphere.

Substance misuse tends to emerge from a complex interplay of personal characteristics, social disruption and availability of substances and can fluctuate in prevalence. Chronic use can have serious consequences, even in youth. Evidence based interventions developed over the past two decades or so have not yet yielded substantial breakthroughs. What to do for those with intractable difficulties remains a substantial challenge.

Prevalence

The NHS Digital Smoking Drinking and Drug Use survey is conducted every two years in representative schools in England. This shows that the percentage of pupils who had used any drugs in the past month declined from 12% in the early years of this millennium to 6% in 2011–14, but then increased again, 11% in 2016 and 10% in 2018. The 8% in 2020 and 6% in 2021 may have been suppressed by the Covid pandemic (https://digital.nhs.uk/data-and-information/publications/statistical/smoking-drinking-and-drug-use-among-young-people-in-england/2021).

UK-published literature may refer to 'misuse', but the more common international term is 'substance use disorder' [1]. Considering its role in tracking internationally the misuse of substances [2] the ICD-11 tends to focus on individual substances and related harmful use [3]. All are concerned with frequent use associated with social, occupational, or physical harm. Unusual in adolescence, substance dependence is 'a psychobiological driving force to consume the substance' [1].

The US National Comorbidity Study – Adolescent Supplement (NCS-A) – holds data on a large (10 123) nationally representative sample of adolescents of 13–18 years, mean age 15.2 years. Based on systematic interview data, an estimated 6.5% of the total youth population suffered DSM-IV alcohol use disorder and 8.9% drug use disorders [4]. Also, 7% of a representative Australian cohort, 13% of those who had 'ever used' and 1:3 of weekly users were reported to have become cannabis dependent by young adulthood [5]. Further, a follow-up study based on the US Monitoring the Future school survey data, reported that of all US 18-year-olds surveyed, 11.5% reported more than 6 dependence symptoms ('severe') (Table 15.1) [6].

Table 15.1 Substance use disorder including dependence symptoms (adapted from DSM-5, APA 2013)

1	Using more substance than intended
2	Being unable to cut down
3	Intense cravings to use
4	Needing more to obtain desired effect – tolerance
5	Withdrawal symptoms
6	Spending more time getting, using and recovering from substance
7	Neglecting responsibilities at home, school or work
8	Continuing to use even when it causes relationship problems
9	Giving up desirable social and recreational activities due to substance use
10	Using in risky settings that put you in danger
11	Continuing to use despite physical and mental health problems

Hence, substantial numbers of young people have a substance use disorder (SUD) and ultimately many become dependent.

In a recent Global Burden of Disease Study, young people in the UK reported the highest prevalence of combined severe mental and drug use disorders [7]. According to this study, the Socio-Demographic-Index (SDI), a composite of income per capita, mean education for the population over 15 years and total fertility rate for women under 25 years (lower fertility rated positively), correlates positively with life expectancy (www.thelancet.com/pb-assets/Lancet/infographics/gbd-2019/catch-up-development.pdf). However, among young people, the SDI correlates in the opposite direction, with increasing self-harm, increasing SUDs and increasing mental disorders.

A striking implication is that, at least as measured by the SDI, economic growth and development are not contributing as expected to youth well-being. This finding needs replication and better understanding, but it may be a warning sign that, at the least, societies require to add youth well-being indicators to development measures. Some indeed argue that analogous with Type 2 diabetes, youth substance misuse should be considered as a 'disease' of modernity [8], a controversial but interesting view.

Origins of Substance Use Disorders

Family Environment

Maternal smoking during pregnancy, socio-economic adversity, parental substance misuse and criminality, family instability, sexual and physical abuse and interparental violence correlate with youth SUDs [9,10]. However, as these risk factors are also intercorrelated, longitudinal studies that account for confounding variables are crucial to quantification of discrete risks.

Early Behaviour Problems

The Christchurch Health and Development Study (CHDS) followed 1000 children from early childhood to middle age and reported on early risk factors and later outcomes. Controlling for parental education, socio-economic status and other potential confounders, analyses demonstrated that those assessed as having early conduct problems (fighting, aggression, defiance) compared to children without those problems, are at increased risk of later substance misuse during adolescence [9].

Similarly, an adoption study demonstrated that, compared to matched adolescent adoptee controls whose biological parents were healthy, there was a higher rate of substance misuse among adoptees with either substance misuse or antisocial biological parents [11]. As the adoptees had been removed shortly after birth, they concluded that this relationship reflected genetic transmission, and this link with substance misuse was mediated by childhood irritability and aggression.

Using different terminology for an overlapping concept, another genetically informed study evaluated the role of childhood 'neurobehavioral disinhibition (ND) ... a deficient capacity to control behavior and regulate emotion commensurate with situational demands' [12]. ND is characterised by ' ... impulsivity, reactive aggression, sensation seeking, and excessive risk-taking (as well as) irritability (and) negative affect'. Such 'high-risk youth more frequently qualify for conduct disorder, attention deficit hyperactivity disorder (ADHD), oppositional defiant disorder (and) ... behavioral and affective dysregulation'. They demonstrated that identified at 13 years, ND independently predicted SUD at 19, whereas IQ and socio-economic status did not. They argued that ND was 'consistent with the pattern of disturbances concomitant to a prefrontal cortex dysfunction', and attributable to a developmental lag. A similar term, 'psychological dysregulation' was also used to describe this phenomenon emerging in early childhood, characterised by 'interacting genetic liability and environmental influences' [13].

The US National Comorbidity Study – Adolescent Supplement reported on the prevalence of alcohol and drug abuse and dependence among those with prior behaviour disorders such as ADHD and conduct disorder [14]. NCS-A interviewers reported that by the age of 14.0 years, 15% of this population warranted alcohol abuse and 24% drug abuse diagnoses.

Mood Disorder, Trauma, Alcohol and Harm

A related question concerns links between substances, harms and mood. For instance, in a latent class analysis of 7 600 Swedish alcohol misusing adoptees, researchers described a predominantly female group with low rates of conduct problems and late onset alcohol misuse among whom over 50% had a mood disorder [15]. Major depression in adolescent females is associated with a 3-fold increase in rates of SUD [16]. Clinicians certainly encounter depressed young people who report self-treatment with substances. However, the direction of causation is sometimes unclear: substances may also lead to depression, or both may arise due to third factors such as those identified by the CHDS [9]. Nevertheless, according to the US NCS-A the rate of alcohol use or drug use disorders among 14-year-old adolescents reporting prior mood (13.9% for alcohol and 19.3% for drug use) or anxiety disorders (20%) is markedly elevated.

Exposure to sexual trauma, especially penetrative sex before 16 years, independently predicted a 3-fold increase in anxiety and depression, and a 7-fold increase in conduct disorder and substance misuse [17]. Contact abuse short of intercourse, perhaps including the sort allegedly common in schools (www.gov.uk/government/publications/review-of-sexual-abuse-in-schools-and-colleges/review-of-sexual-abuse-in-schools-and-colleges#what-did-we-find-out-about-the-scale-and-nature-of-sexual-abuse-in-schools) was linked with increased anxiety, depression, and substance misuse. However, when confounders were accounted for, only an increase in anxiety survived.

The CHD-A also examined the predictive ability of individual mental disorders independent of other mental disorders, as well as controlling for demographics [14]: of all the mood and anxiety disorders, post-traumatic stress disorder was the most potent predictor of alcohol use disorder that the authors considered was due to the pharmacological effects of alcohol 'assuaging' symptoms of distress. The authors concluded that, 'the burden of SUDs in adolescence is disproportionately concentrated among youth with prior mental disorders' [14].

Deviant Peers

In further analyses[18,19], the CHDS explored the influence of 'delinquent or substance using . . . deviant peers' (DPs) on adolescent substance misuse. They concluded that indices of low socio-economic status, family dysfunction, abuse and, as referenced in the Early Behaviour Problems section, the young person's conduct problems at 10 years of age, independently predicted such DP 'affiliation'. Low social status alone proved a weak independent predictor. Another longitudinal study reported that being actively liked or disliked (i.e. 'respected') in middle school, having conduct problems and poor school grades, independently predicted association with DPs and coalescing groups of DPs forming gangs [20]. They concluded 'through a process of selective reinforcement ("shopping") young adolescents end up interacting with individuals who support their attitudes, values and behaviours'.

The CHDS also reported that once DP affiliation was established, it then independently predicted a range of antisocial adolescent behaviours including substance misuse [19]. The effect appeared to peak in early- to mid-adolescence (DPs were associated with an 8-fold increase in mid-adolescent substance misuse risk but a 1.6-fold increase in substance misuse for 20–21-year-olds). Via access to charismatic role models, and substance availability, unsupervised DP affiliation may be a necessary intermediate step for the emergence of adolescent substance misuse.

Others suggest that via affiliation, or 'attachment' to DPs, troubled youth also strive to meet unmet emotional needs [21]. There appears to be an interactive effect identified as early as kindergarten: 26% of those with a conduct problem profile (hyperactivity, fearless and not prosocial), but 55% of those with the same profile, plus family adversity, followed an early adolescence DP trajectory. Interestingly, family adversity alone did not have a main effect on outcome. In a UK study that did not report childhood ND-like variables, the key early predictive factor was low infant maternal attachment [22]. Emotional neediness alone is not a sufficient condition for poor outcomes though combined with impaired early attachment (compromising early distress regulation) amplifies the disinhibition profile and its negative effects that manifest in poor outcomes.

Trends

Cohorts born in the 1950s, so-called 'baby-boomers' were much more likely to have used illicit drugs than earlier generations [23]. Consumption of alcohol and drugs by young people fluctuated until the 1990s 'relapse' (https://monitoringthefuture.org/wp-content/

uploads/2022/12/mtf2022.pdf) across Western type nations. Writing in 2000, Fukuyama attributed the rise in 'psychosocial disorders' in general to 'The Great Disruption' of social ties and traditional norms that had marked Western societies from the late 1950s, although this phenomenon only partially mapped onto substance misuse [24].

Using crime and substance misuse as proxies for wider difficulties, potential influences such as the removal of lead from petrol, changes in policing, even preferential abortion of those most predisposed to behavioural issues, have been ultimately unconvincing (www.economist.com/the-economist-explains/2013/07/23/why-is-crime-falling). More recently, an analysis of the US Monitoring the Future Study reported a systematic and marked decline in personal contact between peers, which included exposure to the so-called DPs described so far in this chapter. The authors attributed it to the 'immersive online activities' of generation Z [25] that could explain the decline in disruptive behaviour including substance misuse. Fukuyama's 'Disruption' did not change direction and, conceivably, the processes he described may now be beginning to reassert themselves, overwhelming this novel and unexpected social effect of technology.

Harm

A peak age for experimentation, adolescence is associated with initiation of the use of tobacco, drugs and alcohol. However, an early systematic review of longitudinal studies concluded that associations between adolescent cannabis and other substance use and psychosocial harms were not necessarily causal [26].

Analyses from a longitudinal study of adolescent drinkers, recruited from accident and emergency, and followed up after a year addressed this question. Self-reported indices of disinhibition, and not alcohol use itself, independently predicted subsequent psychosocial harms [27]. This suggested that underlying ND-like characteristics and not alcohol, were responsible in mid adolescence for behaviours harmful to self and others.

However, longer term follow-up studies do tend to show that substance-related harm accumulates over time. A sample of 3 762 twins of whom 2 410 were monozygotic were followed into adulthood [28]. The study compared those monozygotic twins, where only one but not the other had been exposed to cannabis. Findings suggested that cannabis use independently predicts poorer education, occupation and income, arguing that cannabis-impacted educational engagement and motivation during adolescence contributed to these outcomes.

Others reported significant differences in the development of adolescent brain myelination between those adolescents reported as binge drinkers and those whose intake was low or zero [29]. This could be consistent with the differential myelination reported among those known to be at risk for substance misuse, for example, with ADHD [30]. However, diminished myelination was also detectable among young people transitioning from no- or low- to high-intake patterns, suggesting a dose–response relationship between alcohol misuse and 'attenuated development of major white matter tracts in early adolescence'. The same group also reported altered myelination at lower alcohol doses among females than among males [31].

Others have also reported significant differences both in myelination and in a range of neuropsychological functions between regular cannabis users and non-users that were not apparent at baseline, were dose-related and emerged during a 3-year follow up [32]. A meta-analysis of longitudinal studies reported 'pervasive deterioration' in cognitive functioning and white matter that showed little recovery after 80 days of abstinence [33]. The authors concluded that once the adolescent period of maximum neural plasticity had passed, full recovery might take months or years, and that educational decline and psychosis associated with cannabis and other substance misuse has a neurological basis. These studies converge in their argument for a causal relationship between persistent substance misuse and neurological harm.

It seems possible that around a tenth of all our youth have significant and chronic misuse problems that have very early developmental roots and that once established may persist for years, leaving them with subtle neurological dysfunction. This is of remarkable concern not only for them and their families but potentially for health care demands, broad economic well-being (lost productivity and innovation), crime and parenting (www.unodc.org/pdf/technical_series_1998-01-01_1.pdf).

Mortality

UK Office of National Statistics data show a considerable decline in overall 'avoidable mortality' among young people aged 0–19 between 2001 and 2020, from 19.4:100 000 to 9:100 000. The most dramatic fall occurred in infectious disease, but other causes also dropped substantially. The same pattern was evident for 'alcohol related and drug-related' avoidable deaths, from a total of 176 in 2001 to 49 in 2012 but, quite unlike other causes of avoidable mortality, the number climbed again, in parallel with the misuse statistics, reaching 85:100 000 in 2020, the most recent year for which data are available (www.ons.gov.uk/peoplepopulationandcommunity/healthandsocialcare/causesofdeath/datasets/avoidablemortalityintheukchildrenandyoungpeople). Rates of youth suicide in England and Wales have also increased from a low of 3.1:100 000 (2010), more than doubling to 6.4:100,000 (2021) in the past 10 years (www.ons.gov.uk/peoplepopulationandcommunity/birthsdeathsandmarriages/deaths/bulletins/suicidesintheunitedkingdom/2021registrations). It is unclear whether the correlation with substances is causal. However, a review of psychological post-mortem studies reported the presence of substance misuse in a substantial number of completed adolescent suicides, 35% in the largest study cited, 'especially in older adolescent males when comorbid with mood disorder or disruptive disorders' [10].

Assessment

Basic principles of assessment have been outlined in the Royal College of Psychiatrists Practice Standards (www.rcpsych.ac.uk/docs/default-source/improving-care/ccqi/quality-networks/child-and-adolescent-community-teams-cahms/practice-standards-for-young-people-with-substance-misuse-problems.pdf?sfvrsn=1f333692_2). Clinical examination should aim to uncover often previously unsuspected complexities, potential underlying drivers of misuse. The developmentally most superficial layer is the substance misuse itself, which requires evaluation concerning its nature and extent, facilitators and the presence of abuse or dependence characteristics. A second layer may be mood, the use of substances to manage depression or symptoms of trauma. Neurodevelopmental disorders will often include ADHD, perhaps obscured by school non-attendance or a more pervasive conduct disorder, school failure due to unsuspected learning difficulties or intellectual disability. Many will have suffered the loss or compromise of close attachments related to family breakdown, abuse or illness and are simultaneously emotionally at a loss, uncaring about their own fate and suspicious of adults. The clinical picture of emotional instability, self-harm, poly-substance use, a sort of reckless emotional life and few ties, may resemble a personality disorder and may prompt discussion of interventions, such as safeguarding and interagency intervention in addition to addressing substance use itself.

Intervention

Secondary Prevention

An intervention study compared three brief interventions for alcohol-using adolescents who had attended accident and emergency departments [34]. The interventions included (a) assessment only, (b) an electronic brief intervention and (c) personalised feedback and brief advice [34]. In all three groups, alcohol consumption decreased by approximately 50% at 6 months follow up, remaining lower than T1 at 12 months follow up. However, there were no differences between intervention groups at 6 and 12 months. Although the null hypothesis was rejected, the decline in alcohol use is notable.

Single Modality Intervention

In addition to generic skills, certain specific interventions are regularly mentioned in relation to substance misuse. The Cannabis Youth Treatment Study was a landmark attempt to compare what are often termed 'evidence-based' interventions for adolescent substance misusers [35]. The interventions of the study included cognitive behaviour therapy, multidimensional family therapy, motivation enhancement therapy and another less well-known intervention, a community networking approach. Participants were mostly male (81%), almost half had other SUDs besides cannabis use disorders as well as multiple other comorbidities. The study interviewed 94% of the participants 12-months post-treatment. They reported an overall decline in substance misuse of 30% and that on average 24% were 'in recovery' post-treatment, sustained over follow up, but 76% were not in recovery. There were no differences between interventions.

A multisite European study compared individual counselling (treatment as usual) to multidimensional family therapy delivered twice weekly over a period of up to 6 months [36]. Participants were recruited based on a cannabis use disorder (abuse or dependence). The authors reported that, overall, the percentage of those with cannabis use disorder reduced to 71% after 12 months with no difference between treatments.

Another treatment trial for a group of adolescents with complex difficulties including substance misuse [37] described another relatively high recovery rate (approximately 50%). Once again, the trial reported no differences between different therapies adapted for borderline personality disorder (including a family therapy component) or individual drug counselling. However, a subgroup analysis appeared to show that those with more psychiatric comorbidity reduced substance misuse in the more comprehensive borderline PD therapy.

This may tally with the reported effect on two latent classes, one with higher psychiatric comorbidity and substance misuse and the other with lower rates of both [38], comparing two interventions conducted over 6 months. Randomisation included 284 eligible youth of which 87 completed the interventions reflecting a common problem of drop out from therapy in this group. Nevertheless, multidimensional family therapy was associated with faster and more substantial reduction in substance misuse problem severity (but not frequency of use) compared to services as usual, but only in the higher use/more comorbid group. Possibly more skilled and committed therapists can yield greater dividends or may be more likely to engage the more distressed young people.

More Complex Interventions

Among depressed adolescents with SUDS, compared to placebo and CBT, the addition of fluoxetine to CBT resulted in statistically significant improvement in mood and more negative urines [39]. The same group compared the effect on substance misuse of atomoxetine, a non-stimulant treatment for ADHD, commonly comorbid with substance misuse [40]. No differential effect on ADHD or on substance misuse between those receiving CBT and placebo and those receiving CBT and atomoxetine was observed. However, a large Swedish observational study of an adult population showed that treating ADHD with medication was associated with subsequent significant declines in crime, including substance-related crime [41]. A metanalysis suggested that among adults with comorbid ADHD and SUD, pharmacological treatment of ADHD resulted in reduction in both ADHD and SUD severity. The authors suggested that, taking care to ensure the medications themselves are not abused, for those with ADHD and SUD comorbidity, pharmacological treatment is 'the groundwork for treatment and risk mitigation' [42].

It is possible that the helpfulness of ADHD treatment with medication is maximised when a young person has constructive activities requiring active attention such as schoolwork, training or employment – if they are only hanging out or playing computer games, benefit may be hard to detect. Enabling a user to improve focus so that they can effectively deal drugs may be regarded as counterproductive. Hence, NICE recommends medication as part of 'a comprehensive, holistic shared treatment plan' (www.nice.org.uk/guidance/ng87/chapter/recommendations#medication).

A Cochrane Review reported, 'no conclusions can be made about the efficacy of psychological interventions (delivered alone or in combination with pharmacotherapy) for the treatment of comorbid depression and SUDS, as they are yet to be compared with no treatment, treatment as usual or delayed interventions in this population' [43]. Similarly, another complex therapy, Multisystemic Therapy (MST), did not differ in outcome compared to usual services [44]. A further study of MST reached the same conclusion [45]. This is not to say that MST is ineffective, but that control conditions, multi-component treatment as usual, may have been equally effective [46].

Hence, a parsimonious estimate is that most organised interventions conducted by competent and trained workers in a well-governed system (all the published evidence regards 'well supervised' as at least trainee professionals such as social workers and psychologists) are likely to be helpful. If, as in the CYT they achieve a 30% reduction in use, that is an important achievement. One caveat drawn from adult research however, is that improvement in alcohol consumption was only somewhat better among those who attended treatment compared to dropouts [47]. The pre-intervention motivation of those who enter trials may drive some of the change observed.

Substances and Complex Psychopathology

How to treat the substantial group for whom conventional treatments are unsuccessful is not yet clear. One suggestion is that the answer must be primary prevention, such as ensuring that children have at least a minimum amount of success in school [17]. Indeed, adolescents in severe difficulty who may have embedded pathology, are often mistrustful

Table 15.2 European Monitoring Centre for Drugs and Drug Abuse Quality Standards for drug prevention intervention among young people in contact with criminal justice systems (CJS). [www.emcdda.europa.eu/drugs-library/handbook-quality-standards-interventions-aimed-drug-experienced-young-people-contact-criminal-justice-systems-eppic_en]

1	Interventions targeting drug use among young people in contact with criminal justice are evidence informed and assessed for effectiveness
2	Governing structures and processes are in place to ensure delivery of high-quality interventions
3	Screening and assessment for drug use among young people in contact with CJS is undertaken as part of a comprehensive assessment
4	Young people's multiple vulnerabilities and compelling needs are at the centre of interventions and are effectively addressed
5	An appropriate bundle of intervention options is provided
6	Continuity of care within and between services and community interventions is ensured
7	Young people's participation in designing and implementing and intervention is promoted and ensured as far as possible at every stage of intervention
8	Equity and non-discrimination are ensured within interventions targeting drug use among young people in contact with CJS
9	Practitioners demonstrate professional competence
10	Practitioners respect ethical principles and professional codes of practice

and suspicious of yet another intrusive adult. They may superficially or fleetingly engage, concealing layers of distress [48]. With histories of trauma and sustained adversity, some of these young people suffer psychopathology not dissimilar to those on personality disorder type trajectories. It may take months to engage their trust or to convince a young person that the therapist has something new to offer. Indeed, some young people may not regard their choices as problematic, rather 'alternative', and may be sceptical in principle towards the adults whom they blame for their predicament in the first place. Nevertheless, their needs are often profound, and we need to connect.

Fundamental and individual competence is required to overcome barriers (www.rcpsych.ac.uk/docs/default-source/improving-care/ccqi/quality-networks/child-and-adolescent-community-teams-cahms/practice-standards-for-young-people-with-substance-misuse-problems.pdf?sfvrsn=1f333692_2): appropriate interpersonal skills to establish suitable rapport; understanding the legal frameworks surrounding young people; the safeguarding role of a range of agencies; a capacity for outreach for engaging parents and boundaries. These principles are consistent with common factors found efficacious across types of youth and adult psychotherapy [49]. The European Monitoring Centre for Drugs and Drug Addiction publishes reports and data relevant to youth. This includes guidance on working with young users in contact with the criminal justice system [50]. Standards 8 and 9 in Table 15.2 expect that, 'In addition to their professional training and experience, practitioners need knowledge, skills and training specific to working with young people.' Also, 'Practitioners have a duty of care ... underpinned by ethical and professional codes of practice. Adherence to ethical and professional principles and codes of practice supports equity and probity in developing and delivering interventions and in all interaction with young people.'

Organisational competence requires aligned, shared goals and values between therapists and organisation, quality supervision and teamwork and continuity so that young people 'should experience care as seamless ... and should have regular contact with the same worker/therapist' (www.rcpsych.ac.uk/docs/default-source/improving-care/ccqi/quality-networks/child-and-adolescent-community-teams-cahms/practice-standards-for-young-people-with-substance-misuse-problems.pdf?sfvrsn=1f333692_2) and interagency competence: although as a colleague commented, 'it can be harder to engage the (interagency) professionals than the young people', intervention will often require coordination 'across professional and agency boundaries' [50], safeguarding, youth offending services, and education. If we get any of this wrong, there is also the capacity to do harm.

In the search for therapeutic synergy, a practitioner may support a parent to, for example, leverage available community resources, work to re-engage a young person in some form of modified education that will offer structure, sustainable relationships with helpful adults and non-using peers and purposefulness. It may be supported by medication, for example, for ADHD to sustain the educational placement. These tailored interventions represent what the Medical Research Council terms 'complex' [51]. They are difficult and expensive to evaluate and as a result struggle to appear in academic research.

Conclusion

Adolescent substance misuse appears to arise because of personal characteristics, interacting with family adversity, painful trauma and loss, thus separating a child from benign adults and peers, school and conventional/constructive aspirations and forming potentially an alternative dysfunctional community. Some argue that such disruption is a function of a certain type of western modernity. Ready availability, which correlates with economic development, is a necessary condition.

Particular therapies (e.g. CBT) appear to offer no distinct advantage in treatment of substance misuse. However, they may directly facilitate the therapist's own persistence, hope and direction, thereby indirectly sustaining the young person. More complex, sustained interventions may achieve much for those with complex psychopathology, but we don't know for sure what components or combinations are active. Acknowledgement of the young person's adversity and struggle, of the camouflaged pain, and thus even engagement alone, may facilitate change; services may offer a safe space to facilitate maturation. Hence, there is hope but we have a lot to learn.

References

1. American Psychiatric Association. *Diagnostic and Statistical Manual of Mental Disorders.* 5th ed. American Psychiatric Association, 2013. Available at: https://psychiatryonline.org/doi/book/10.1176/appi.books.9780890425596.

2. Saunders J. Substance Use and Addictive Disorders in DSM-5 and ICD 10 and the Draft ICD 11. Curr Opin Psychiatry. 2017;30(4):227–37. https://doi.org/10.1097/YCO.0000000000000332.

3. World Health Organisation. *International Statistical Classification of Diseases and Related Health Problems.* 11th ed. World Health Organisation, 2019. Available at: https://www.who.int/standards/classifications/classification-of-diseases.

4. Swendsen J, Burstein M, Case B, et al. Use and Abuse of Alcohol and Illicit Drugs in U.S. Adolescents: Results of the National

Comorbidity Survey– Adolescent Supplement. Archives of General Psychiatry. 2012;**69**:390–98.

5. Coffey C, Carlin J, Lynskey M, Ning L, Patton G. Adolescent Precursors of Cannabis Dependence: Findings from the Victorian Adolescent Health Cohort Study. British Journal of Psychiatry. 2003;**182**: 330–36.

6. McCabe S, Schulenberg J, Schepis T, McCabe V, Veliz P. Longitudinal Analysis of Substance Use Disorder Symptom Severity at Age 18 Years and Substance Use Disorder in Adulthood. JAMA Netw Open. 2022;**5**(4): e225324. https://doi.org/10.1001/ jamanetworkopen.2022.5324.

7. Castelpietra G, Knudsen A, Agardh E, et al. The Burden of Mental Disorders, Substance Use Disorders and Self-Harm Among Young People in Europe, 1999-2019: Findings from the Global Burden of Disease Study 2019. The Lancet Regional Health Europe. 2022;**16**:1–18.

8. Levy, S. The Role of Addiction-Medicine Specialists in the Global Fight Against Addiction. Nature Medicine. 2020;**26**(456). https://doi.org/10.1038/s41591-020-0830-7.

9. Lynskey M, Fergusson D. Childhood Conduct Problems, Attentional Behaviours and Adolescent Alcohol, Tobacco and Illicit Drug Use. Journal of Abnormal Child Psychology. 1995;**23**:281–302. https://doi.org/10.1007/BF01447558.

10. Bridge J, Goldstein T, Brent D. Adolescent Suicide and Suicidal Behaviour. J Child Psychol Psychiatry. 2006;**47**:372–94.

11. Cadoret RJ, Yates WR, Ed T, Woodworth G, Stewart MA. Adoption Study Demonstrating Two Genetic Pathways to Drug Abuse. Arch Gen Psychiatry. 1995;**52**(1):42–52. https://doi.org/10.1001/ archpsyc.1995.03950130042005.

12. Tarter RE, Kirisci L, Mezzich A, et al. Neurobehavioral Disinhibition in Childhood Predicts Early Age At Onset of Substance Use Disorder. American Journal of Psychiatry. 160(6):1078–85.

13. Clark D. The Natural History of Adolescent Alcohol Use Disorders. Addiction. 2004;**99**: 5–22.

14. Conway K, Swendsen K, Husky M, He J, Merkikangas K. Association of Lifetime Mental Disorders and Subsequent Alcohol and Illicit Drug Use: Results from the National Comorbidity Survey- Adolescent Supplement. Journal of the American Academy of Child and Adolescent Psychiatry. 2016;**55**:280–88.

15. Kendler K., Ji J., Edwards A, Ohlsson H, Sundquist J, Sundquist K. An Extended Swedish National Adoption Study of Alcohol Use Disorder. JAMA Psychiatry. 2015;**72**:211–18. https://doi.org/10.1001/ jamapsychiatry.2014.2138.

16. Avenevoli S, Swenson J, Jian-Ping H, Burstein M, Merikangas M. Major Depression in the National Comorbidity Survey – Adolescent Supplement. Journal of the American Academy of Child and Adolescent Psychiatry. 2015;**54**:37–44e2.

17. Fergusson D, Horwood LJ, Lynskey M. Childhood Sexual Abuse and Psychiatric Disorder in Young Adulthood II Psychiatric Outcomes. Journal of the American Academy of Child and Adolescent Psychiatry. 1996; **35**:1365–74.

18. Fergusson D, Horwood L. Prospective Childhood Predictors of Deviant Peer Affiliations in Adolescence. Journal of Child Psychology and Psychiatry. 1999;**40**:581–92. https://doi.org/10.1111/ 1469-7610.00475.

19. Fergusson D, Swain-Campbell NR, Horwood LJ. Deviant Peer Affiliations, Crime and Substance Use: A Fixed Effects Regression Analysis. Journal of Abnormal Child Psychology. 2002;**30**(4):419–30.

20. Dishion T, Nelson S, Yasui M. Predicting Early Adolescent Gang Involvement from Middle School Adaptation. Journal of Clinical Child Psychology. 2005;**34**:62–73.

21. Lacourse E, Nagin DS, Vitaro F, Côté S, Arseneault L, Tremblay RE. Prediction of Early-Onset Deviant Peer Group Affiliation: A 12-Year Longitudinal Study. Archives of General Psychiatry. 2006;**63**(5):562–68. https://doi.org/10.1001/archpsyc.63.5.562.

22. Reyes, B, Hargreaves D, Creese H. Early-Life Maternal Attachment and Risky

Health Behaviours in Adolescence: Findings from the United Kingdom Millennium Cohort Study. BMC Public Health. 2021;**21**:2039. https://doi.org/10.1186/s12889-021-12141-5.

23. Silbereisen R, Robins L, Rutter M. Secular Trends in Substance Use: Concepts and Data on the Impact of Social Change on Alcohol and Drug Abuse. In D Smith & M Rutter (eds.), *Psychosocial Disorders in Young People: Time Trends and Their Cause*. London: Wiley, 1995, 490–543.

24. Fukuyama F. *The Great Disruption Human Nature and the Reconstitution of Social Order*. London: Simon and Schuster, 2000.

25. Borodovsky J, Krueger R, Agrawal A, Elbanna B, de Looze M, Grucza R. U.S. Trends in Adolescent Substance Use and Conduct Problems and Their Relation to Trends in Unstructured In-person Socializing with Peers. J Adolesc Health. 2021;**69**(3):432–39. https://doi.org/10.1016/j.jadohealth.2020.12.144.

26. Macleod J, Oakes R, Chrome I, et al. Psychological and Social Sequelae of Cannabis and Other Illicit Drug Use by Young People: A Systematic Review of Longitudinal, General Population Studies. Lancet. 2004;**3633**:1579–88.

27. McArdle P, Coulton S, Kaner E, Gilvarry E, Drummond C. Alcohol Misuse among English Youth, Are Harms Attributable to Alcohol or to Underlying Disinhibitory Characteristics? Alcohol and Alcoholism. 2022;**57**(3):372–77. https://doi.org/10.1093/alcalc/agab077. PMID: 34875694.

28. Schaefer J, Hamdi N, Malone S, et al. Associations Between Adolescent Cannabis Use and Young Adult Functioning in Three Longitudinal Twin Studies. Proceedings of the National Academy of Sciences. 2013;**118**:e2013180118. https://doi.org/10.1073/pnas.2013180118.

29. Zhao Q, Sullivan E, Honnorat N, et al. Association of Heavy Drinking With Deviant Fiber Tract Development in Frontal Brain Systems in Adolescents. JAMA Psychiatry. 2021;**78**:407–15.

30. Shaw P, Eckstrand K, Sharp W, Rapoport J. Attention-Deficit/Hyperactivity Disorder Is Characterized by a Delay in Cortical Maturation. Proceedings of the National Academy of Sciences. 2007;**104**:19649–19654.

31. Zhao Q, Sullivan E, Müller-Oehring M, et al. Adolescent Alcohol Use Disrupts Functional Neurodevelopment in Sensation Seeking Girls. Addiction Biology. 2021;**26**(2):e12914.

32. Jacobus J, Courtney K, Hodgdon E, Baca R. Cannabis and the Developing Brain: What Does the Evidence Say? Birth Defects Research. 2019;**111**(17):1302–07. https://doi.org/10.1002/bdr2.1572. Epub 2019 Aug 5. PMID: 31385460; PMCID: PMC7239321.

33. Debenham J, Birrell L, Champion K, Lee B, Murat Y, Newton N. Neuropsychological and Neurophysiological Predictors and Consequences of Cannabis and Illicit Substance Use During Neurodevelopment: A Systematic Review of Longitudinal Studies. Lancet Child and Adolescent Health. 2021;**5**:589–604. https://doi.org/10.1016/S2352-4642(21)00051-1.

34. Deluca P, Coulton S, Alam M, et al. Effectiveness and Cost-Effectiveness of Face-to-Face and Electronic Brief Interventions Versus Screening Alone to Reduce Alcohol Consumption Among High-Risk Adolescents Presenting to Emergency Departments: Three-Arm Pragmatic Randomized Trial (SIPS Junior high risk trial). Addiction. 2022;**117**:2200–14.

35. Dennis M, Godley S, Diamond G, et al. The Cannabis Youth Treatment Study. Journal of Substance Misuse Treatment. 2004;**27**:197–213.

36. Rigter H, Henderson C, Pelc I, Tossmann P, Phan O, Hendricks V, Schaub M, Rowe C. Multidimensional Family Therapy Lowers the Rate of Cannabis Dependence in Adolescents: A Randomised Controlled Trial in European Outpatient Settings. Drug and Alcohol Dependence. 2013;**130**:85–93.

37. Santisteban D, Mena M, Muir J, McCabe B, Abalo C, Cummings A. The Efficacy of Two Adolescent Substance Abuse Treatments and the Impact of

Comorbid Depression: Results of a Small Randomized Controlled Trial. Journal of Psychiatric Rehabilitation. 2015;38:55–64. https://doi.org/10.1037/prj0000106. PMID: 25799306; PMCID: PMC5021542.

38. Henderson CE, Dakof GA, Greenbaum PE, Liddle HA. Effectiveness of Multidimensional Family Therapy with Higher Severity Substance-Abusing Adolescents: Report from Two Randomized Controlled Trials. Journal of Consulting and Clinical Psychology. 2010;78(6):885–97. https://doi.org/10.1037/a0020620. PMID: 20873891; PMCID: PMC4892370.

39. Riggs P, Mikulich-Gilbertson S, Davies R, Lohman M, Klein C, Stover S. A Randomized Controlled Trial of Fluoxetine and Cognitive Behavioral Therapy in Adolescents with Major Depression, Behavior Problems and Substance Use Disorders. Archives of Pediatric and Adolescent Medicine. 2007;161:1026–34.

40. Thurstone C, Riggs P, Salomonsel-Sautel S, Mikulich-Gilbertson S. Randomized, Controlled Trial of Atomoxetine for Attention-Deficit/Hyperactivity Disorder in Adolescents with Substance Use Disorder. Journal of the American Academy of Child and Adolescent Psychiatry. 2010;49:573–82.

41. Lichtenstein P, Halldner L, Zetterqvist J, et al. Medication for Attention Deficit-Hyperactivity Disorder and Criminality. New England Journal of Medicine. 2012;367(21):2006–14. https://doi.org/10.1056/NEJMoa1203241. PMID: 23171097; PMCID: PMC3664186.

42. Fluyau D, Revadigar N, Pierre CG. Systematic Review and Meta-Analysis: Treatment of Substance Use Disorder in Attention Deficit Hyperactivity Disorder. American Journal on Addictions. 2021;30:110–21. https://doi.org/10.1111/ajad.13133.

43. Hides L, Quinn C, Stoyanov S, Kavanagh D, Baker A. Psychological Interventions for Co-occurring Depression and Substance Use Disorders. Cochrane Database Systematic Review. 2019;26(11):CD009501. https://doi.org/10.1002/14651858.CD009501.pub2. PMID: 31769015; PMCID: PMC6953216.

44. Littell J, Campbell M, Green S, Toews B. Multisystemic Therapy for Social, Emotional and Behavioural Problems in Youth Aged 10-17. Cochrane Database of Systematic Reviews. 2005;4. https://doi.org/10.1002/14651858.CD004797.pub4. Art. No.:CD004797.

45. Fonagy P, Butler T, Cottrell D, et al. Multisystemic Therapy Versus Management As Usual in the Treatment of Adolescent Antisocial Behaviour (START): A Pragmatic, Randomised Controlled, Superiority Trial. Lancet Psychiatry. 2018;5:119–33. https://doi.org/10.1016/S2215-0366(18)30001-4.

46. Mustafa F. Randomised Controlled Trials for Multisystemic Therapy: When Is Enough Enough? Lancet Psychiatry. 2018;5:390.

47. Cutler RB, Fishbain DA. Are Alcoholism Treatments Effective? The Project MATCH Data. BMC Public Health. 2005;5(75). https://doi.org/10.1186/1471-2458-5-75.

48. Rasmussen L, Moffitt T, Arsenault L, et al. Association of Adverse Experiences and Exposure to Violence in Childhood and Adolescence With Inflammatory Burden in Young People. JAMA Pediatrics. 2020;174:38–47.

49. Peterson B. Editorial: Common Factors in the Art of Healing. Journal of Child Psychology and Psychiatry. 2019;60:927–29. https://doi.org/10.1111/jcpp.13108.

50. Graf N, Moazen B, Stöver H. *Handbook on Quality Standards for Interventions Aimed at Drug Experienced Young People in Contact with Criminal Justice Systems*. Frankfurt: Frankfurt University of Applied Sciences, 2019. www.emcdda.europa.eu/drugs-library/handbook-quality-standards-interventions-aimed-drug-experienced-young-people-contact-criminal-justice-systems-eppic_en.

51. Castle DD, Hawke L, Henderson J, et al. Complex Interventions for Youth Mental Health: A Way Forward. The Canadian Journal of Psychiatry. 2022;67(10):755–57. https://doi.org/10.1177/07067437221093396.

Chapter 16

Evolving Perspectives on Eating Disorders: From Diagnosis to Digital Therapies

Cecily M. Donnelly and Dasha Nicholls

Eating disorders (ED) have historically been dogged by pervasive myths, often affecting the support offered. The stereotype of underweight white teenage girls and a diet gone wrong has prevented people from seeking help for themselves, and parents from seeking help for their children. There are many reports of children and their families being turned away from primary and secondary health care services by clinicians who have not recognised the signs and symptoms of an eating disorder. ED are incredibly distressing for both sufferers and their families, and research has demonstrated that early intervention for ED improves the likelihood of recovery, although recovery is still possible after many years of illness [1]. With high mortality and morbidity rates, it is vital that clinicians have as much understanding as possible about how to quickly recognise and treat ED in children and adolescents.

Since the last edition of this book was published, there have been changes to the diagnostic criteria used for assessing ED included in DSM-5 [2] and ICD-11 [3]. In addition, new research has been conducted into the best treatments to be offered to young people and their families, and national guidance has been updated to reflect this research evidence. This chapter will touch on these changes and how they can be used by clinicians to serve the needs of their patients.

The chapter will also shed some light on the issues that surround more complex ED presentations. Increasing numbers of clinicians are reporting a rise in patients presenting with disordered eating behaviours and traits associated with a neurodevelopmental disorder and personality disorder. Differential treatment options should be considered with these clients, and a multiservice approach should not be ruled out.

Finally, a negative side to a digital world is the impact of social media on young people's eating behaviours. Alongside the impact on self-esteem and body image that has been demonstrated by excessive use of mainstream sites, there has been concern about how to protect young people from media that potentially promotes ED, including pro-anorexia forums. This chapter will give an overview of the thin line that clinicians need to tread between providing useful online resources and exposing young people to dangerous influences. With increased referrals to children and young people's (CYP) mental health services, there is a need for a wide range of accessible resources. Digital therapies, including family therapy, have started to take centre stage, particularly during the Covid-19 pandemic, when non-urgent services were closed.

Classification of ED

To treat an eating disorder, one must understand the current consensus on when an eating disorder reaches clinical threshold. The two major systems used for mental health diagnosis are DSM-5, published in 2013, and ICD-11, published in 2019. There are small but noticeable differences between the systems, and clinicians should be encouraged to use a combination of both when assessing CYP presenting at services. The academic literature on ED has historically predominantly used the North American DSM system, but this may change as the two systems more closely align. This section gives an overview of changes that were made in the most up-to-date editions of each manual. The disorders covered here are Anorexia Nervosa, Bulimia Nervosa, Binge Eating Disorder, Other Specified Feeding and Eating Disorders and Avoidant Restrictive Food Intake Disorder.

Anorexia Nervosa

Possibly the most widely known eating disorder is Anorexia Nervosa (AN), partly due to the risks and visible clinical impact it is associated with, and partly because of its potential for glamourisation. AN has one of the highest mortality rates of any mental health condition, at roughly 6% [4]. Death by suicide, pulmonary problems like pneumonia, endocrine diseases and organ failure appear to account for this elevated mortality rate [5]. Even if AN does not lead to death there are potentially irreversible long-term physical effects of untreated AN, including fertility problems, weakened immune systems and osteoporosis [6]. Full recovery is very possible for the majority of sufferers, but recovery can take time, with many struggling for many years [7]. One recent surveillance study of secondary care suggests an incident rate (new cases) of 13.68 per 100 000 population, with peak incidence at 15-years-old for girls and 16-years-old for boys [8].

The term Anorexia Nervosa was coined in 1873 by English doctor Sir William Gull [9], but the diagnostic criteria have been revised multiple times. Key criteria for the diagnosis are [2]:

(1) *Restriction of energy intake relative to nutritional requirements, leading to a significantly low body weight for age, sex, developmental trajectory, or with impacts on physical health.*

Note that in the ICD-11 criteria, rapid weight loss (e.g. more than 20% of total body weight within 6 months) may replace the low body weight guideline as long as other diagnostic requirements are met. Thus in ICD-11, AN can be diagnosed at any weight. The same is not true in DSM-5; a diagnosis of atypical AN is made in DSM-5 when all other criteria are met but body weight is not low.

(2) *Intense fear of gaining weight or of becoming fat, or persistent behaviour that interferes with weight gain, such as behaviour to increase energy expenditure (e.g. excessive exercise) or reduce energy intake (restriction of intake, self-induced vomiting), even though weight is low.*

(3) *Low body weight or shape is central to the person's self-evaluation or is inaccurately perceived to be normal or even high. The seriousness of low body weight is minimised.*

DSM-5 distinguishes *restricting type* and *binge-eating/purging type* [2], a distinction that has some validity in terms of differences in course, treatment response and outcome [10]. Current criteria reflect changes in the language to focus on behaviour as well as cognitions, and the word 'refusal' has been removed around weight maintenance, as it is difficult to assess and ascribes a degree of blame to the patient [11]. Importantly, although menses are important for physical health, *amenorrhea* was removed from both DSM-5 and ICD-11, as this was seen as preventing several groups of people from receiving a diagnosis, including male patients, patients taking contraceptives and those who have not yet reached puberty [11].

Both DSM-5 and ICD-11 offer ratings for severity of AN that are based on Body Mass Index (BMI). 'Extreme' severity of BMI <15 aligns with the thresholds used in the Medical Emergencies in Eating Disorders (MEED) guidance [12] for when medical intervention may be required. The evidence supporting these severity ratings is not strong. In addition, for patients under 18, ICD-11 recommends the use of BMI-for-age and sex rather than BMI, with the threshold for diagnosis as under the 5th percentile [13].

Alongside the more classic signs of weight loss and amenorrhea, physical signs can include tiredness, stomach pains, bloating and constipation, lanugo, poor circulation and low blood pressure and oedema [6]. Patients and parents report behavioural symptoms, such as avoidance of family meals, food rituals and changes in behaviour (e.g. chewing very slowly, cutting food into very small pieces), excessive exercise, refusal to eat once-enjoyed foods (particularly high calorie foods), fasting, purging and social withdrawal [14]. Common psychological symptoms include fear of fatness, excessive focus on calories, distorted body perception, struggling to concentrate, perfectionism and underestimating the seriousness of the problem [15,16]. Some recent research reports that younger adolescents presenting at eating disorder clinics show a preoccupation with obesity and the health consequences of unhealthy eating as well as a focus on vegetarianism and veganism (often attributed by the patient to climate change concerns) [17]. Initial physical health screening should exclude differential diagnoses such as inflammatory bowel disease, Addison's disease, thyroid disease.

Treatment and Management

The UK's National Institute for Health and Care Excellence UK (NICE) guidelines state that treatment for AN should be multidisciplinary and actively involve family members; monitoring physical health and supporting people to achieve weight restoration is essential, as it is key in supporting psychological changes that are needed for recovery [18]. The recommended treatment for AN in CYP is Family Therapy for Anorexia Nervosa (FT-AN). FT-AN is a manualised approach to treating ED, which can be delivered to individual families or in a group setting (known as Multi-Family Therapy) [19], and in a conjoint (whole family) or separated (parent only) format. Online-therapist-delivered and self-care versions have also been developed in order to increase access [20,21], especially during the Covid-19 pandemic when demand for ED care increased significantly [22]. FT-AN focuses on working with the family to assist recovery, externalisation of the eating disorder and building self-efficacy in parents to take the lead in management of their child's eating; the therapist establishes and builds on family strengths and resources, acknowledging how the eating disorder may have disrupted family dynamics [19].

If FT-AN is not possible or is ineffective, young people should be offered individual therapies in the form of Cognitive Behavioural Therapy for Eating Disorders (CBT-ED) or adolescent-focused psychotherapy for AN (AFP-AN). CBT-ED for AN usually consists of up to 40 sessions, with more frequent sessions at the start of treatment [18]. Treatment should cover nutrition, emotion regulation, self-esteem and body image concerns; self-monitoring of dietary intake and connected cognitions and emotions is recommended as part of the homework, alongside other CBT techniques like behavioural experiments [23]. AFP-AN usually consists of up to 40 individual sessions, and is often more appropriate for older, less severely unwell young people [24]. The approach uses several therapeutic techniques including CBT and dynamic approaches; focus is on empowering young people to manage life without AN behaviours, improving self-esteem and externalising the eating disorder [24]. Developing a formulation of the young person's psychological issues allows the therapist and the client to assess how AN behaviours are used as coping strategies. In clinical trials, CBT-ED and AFP-AN have comparable longer-term outcomes to Family Based Treatment (FBT). However, FBT tends to result in more rapid remission and have greater benefit on eating-related obsessionality and eating-disorder-specific psychopathology, and patients with binge-eating/purging type responded less well to FBT than those with restricting type [25,26].

Alongside psychological treatment and physical monitoring, dietary counselling should be available to young people and their families if needed as part of a multidisciplinary approach to re-establishing regular, appropriate nutrition [18]. In the early stages of weight gain, a regularly assessed meal plan can prevent refeeding syndrome if the patient is medically unstable [27]. There are different approaches to meal plan usage through AN treatment, but the general principles include making the plan flexible and individualised, incorporate feared foods early, and being aware of the role of 'diet' foods [28].

The NICE guidelines are clear that medication should not be offered as the sole treatment for AN; however some research suggests that medication such as the atypical antipsychotic medication olanzapine may be helpful for adolescents for supporting management of emotions (extreme distress and anxiety) and has the side effect of increasing appetite which supports weight gain [29]. However, the evidence supporting this practice remains sparse [30].

Bulimia Nervosa

Many celebrities have opened up about their struggle with Bulimia Nervosa (BN) over the last few decades, including Lady GaGa, Princess Diana and Elton John. BN is characterised by a vicious cycle of binge eating and compensatory behaviours [2]. The compensatory behaviours associated with BN can have very serious physical consequences. For example, vomiting can cause permanent damage to teeth, vocal chords and throat, and the use of laxatives can cause damage to internal organs [6]. Fewer studies have examined the prevalence of BN in adolescence, compared to AN, but some research suggests that the lifetime prevalence rate of BN is over 2% [31].

The diagnostic criteria for BN are similar in DSM-5 and ICD-11 and include the following features:

(1) *Recurrent episodes of binge eating at least once a week for a sustained period (usually three months). Binge eating behaviours has two main characteristics:*

   (a) *Eating large amount of food in a discrete period of time (e.g. any 2-hour period). The amount of food should be more than most individuals would eat in similar circumstances.*

   (b) *The experience of lack of control overeating during the binge. This feeling of being unable to stop eating (sometimes until vomiting) and being out of control is crucial, since it associated with feelings of distress.*

(2) *Recurrent compensatory behaviours in order to prevent weight gain as a result of binge eating. Compensatory behaviours can be purging in nature (e.g. self-induced vomiting; misuse of laxatives, diuretics, or other medications such as insulin in people with Type 1 diabetes (see below)) or restrictive (fasting or excessive exercise).*

(3) *As for AN, self-evaluation is heavily influenced by body shape and weight.*

Little has changed in the criteria for BN other than a reduction in the frequency of binges and compensatory behaviours required for diagnosis from twice to once a week in the DSM-5 [11]. ICD-11 criteria are more flexible in relation to binge-eating frequency; in addition, episodes of bingeing are defined more by the feeling of loss of control and distress, rather than by the objective amount of food consumed [32]. BN can be diagnosed regardless of the person's weight, assuming weight is not so low or weight loss so extreme that it fits the criteria for binge-eating/purging type AN [32].

Common physical symptoms associated with frequent vomiting include swelling of salivary glands, callouses on the back of the hands, teeth enamel erosion and swelling of extremities [6]. Other physical signs including stomach problems, bloating and constipation, irregular periods and weight fluctuation. Young people with BN may show behavioural and psychological signs before physical signs, however. These may include hoarding food, excessive exercise, secrecy around mealtimes (such as disappearing after meals), feelings of shame, guilt and loss of control, loss of confidence and self-esteem, and excessive focus on food and weight [33]. Substance misuse and self-harm are often comorbid with BN [34,35].

Treatment and Management

The NICE guidelines recommend family therapy for BN for CYP [18]. Like FT-AN, treatment should provide psychoeducation about BN and what causes and maintains it, alongside the consequences of BN; there should be a focus on the family's role in improving eating patterns and breaking the binge-eating/purge cycle [36]. The therapist assumes that BN is having a negative effect on the family and endeavours to separate the young person from the condition [36].

Where family therapy is not possible, CBT-ED should be offered [18]. Individuals are encouraged to monitor thoughts, feelings and behaviours; to set goals and challenge problematic thoughts and behaviours; and to recognise and manage triggers to prevent relapse [37,38].

A Note on Diabetes

Another very serious compensatory behaviour associated with BN is the omission of insulin by those with Type 1 diabetes mellitus (DM) in order to lose weight – this is sometimes referred to as *diabulimia* [39], although most such patients meet criteria for BN or purging disorder depending on whether binge-eating behaviour is present. While this behaviour is incredibly dangerous, disordered eating in the context of Type 1 DM is not unusual, with some research suggesting that over 30% of young people with Type 1 DM meet the criteria for an ED [40,41]. A diagnosis of DM forces a focus on diet, which can quickly bring a person's attention to body image concerns; furthermore, treating DM naturally equips young people with knowledge about insulin and weight management [42]. It may not be surprising then that adolescents with DM are twice as likely to suffer from an ED as those without [43]. Insulin manipulation can have very severe consequences for people with DM, including kidney disease, stroke, blindness and death [44]. Both the NICE guidelines for ED and the MEED guidance include sections on how to manage and treat patients who restrict their insulin [18], and for managing medical emergencies [27]. The ED and DM teams should collaborate for the entirety of the young persons' ED treatment; it is advised that each team should have sufficient training on the management of comorbid DM and ED [18]. Addressing insulin misuse should form a central part of the ED treatment plan, including in psychological treatment and use of meal plans, and family members should be included to help young people monitor and maintain blood glucose level [18].

Binge Eating Disorder

While binge eating has been included as an eating disorder feature since 1994, Binge Eating Disorder (BED) was only recognised as a distinct diagnosis in 2013, with the publication of DSM-5 [11]. Based on clinical and empirical evidence, BED has now also been included in ICD-11 [32]. BED is characterised by frequent episodes of binge eating that are *not* accompanied by inappropriate, compensatory weight-prevention behaviours.

While AN and BN present more commonly in clinical services, research suggests that BED is equally, if not more, prevalent among children and adolescents in the population, and particularly in CYP at higher weight. A recent systematic review suggested that the prevalence of BED can be up to 6% in community samples, but can reach 16% in samples of children meeting criteria for being overweight or obese [45], and may be even higher in help-seeking populations. This is important as, while treatment of BED does not result in weight loss, it may prevent escalation of weight gain. The average age at the onset of BED is normally stated as *'late adolescence'*, however some research suggests that average age may be as low as 12.6 years old [45]. BED is associated with poor health-related outcomes, like high blood pressure, gall bladder disease and damage to the oesophagus and stomach [46]. Risk factors for the development of BED include weight-related bullying, dieting, childhood food insecurity (as a result of neglect or because of socio-economic status), a history of abuse or neglect and traumatic childhood events [47].

As for BN, CYP with BED experience high levels of shame and guilt, and may hide their struggles, eating and bingeing in secret. Although CYP are often not able to buy and hoard large quantities of food, signs such as eating very rapidly until uncomfortably full or when not hungry and subsequent withdrawal from family or associated distress might suggest the need for further exploration. Physical consequences include stomach pain, constipation, bloating, poor skin condition and difficulty sleeping. BED is associated with other signs of emotional and behavioural dysregulation, such as low mood, self-injury, interpersonal difficulties and substance misuse [47].

Treatment and Management

The NICE guideline recommendations for BED stem from evidence in adults because of the paucity of research evidence in CYP. They advocate that CBT-ED is the best treatment approach, either as guided self-help, individual sessions or in-group format [18]. Treatment should not focus on body weight and weight loss, but on psychoeducation, identifying binge-eating cues, body exposure training and challenging negative beliefs about the body [48]. As part of a multidisciplinary approach, young people should be encouraged to eat regular meals and snacks to avoid feeling hungry as this can be a significant trigger for bingeing [18]. There is a need for more studies into effective treatments for BED in children and adolescents.

Other Specified Feeding and Eating Disorders (OSFED)

OSFED has replaced 'Eating Disorder Not Otherwise Specified' as a diagnostic term for clinically significant ED not reaching the criteria above. A diagnosis of OSFED should always be accompanied by its specified disorder, of which the commonest in CYP are atypical AN, BN or BED and purging disorder. Purging disorder is, as the name suggests, when clinically significant purging occurs in the absence of binge eating, that is, the purging is not compensatory for overeating. Treatment for OSFED should follow the ED it most closely resembles.

Avoidant-Restrictive Food Intake Disorder

In both the DSM-5 and ICD-11, there are a number of conditions that fall under the Feeding Disorder aspect of each publication's Feeding and Eating Disorder chapter. These feeding disorders include PICA, Rumination Disorder and Avoidant-Restrictive Food Intake Disorder (ARFID). While ARFID is sometimes conceptualised as a feeding disorder rather than an eating disorder, we cover this condition in this chapter because it can occur at any age, and more evidence is being accrued on the long-term nature of ARFID and the physical and emotional commonalities between other ED and ARFID.

The classification of ARFID was first included in the DSM-5 and is now ICD-11; however, it is not a 'new' diagnosis. ARFID was an attempt to rationalise several previously described conditions including selective eating, food avoidance emotional disorder, food phobias, infantile anorexia, and post-traumatic feeding disorder, among others [49]. It is thus an umbrella term describing a number of potentially distinct presentations depending on the basis of the restrictive eating. However, these presentations can also co-occur.

There are only a small number of studies that have examined the incidence and prevalence rates of ARFID that were summarised in a systematic review. Estimated prevalence varied widely by setting: specialist feeding clinics showed the highest prevalence rates, ranging from 32% to 64%; specialised ED services prevalence rates were 5%–22.5% and non-clinical samples reported prevalence estimates ranging from 0.3% to 15.5%. Psychiatric comorbidity was common, especially anxiety disorders and ASD [50]. ARFID is most often diagnosed in children, and the average age of diagnosis is around 12-years-old, which is younger than other ED [51].

ARFID is characterised by *avoidance or restriction of food* that does not meet the criteria for another feeding or eating disorder. ICD-11 further elaborates on the DSM-5 criteria by reiterating that '*the pattern of eating behaviour is not motivated by preoccupation with body weight or shape*', to distinguish it from AN [49]. It also makes clear that the disorder can only be diagnosed if there is '*significant impairment in personal, family, social, educational, occupational or other important areas of functioning*'. Many adolescents report that ARFID is affecting their ability to maintain friendships as the fear of unsafe foods makes it impossible to eat around others [52]. Importantly, ARFID can only be diagnosed in the context of other disorders when the symptoms are over and above those expected of the disorder. For example, a child with ASD who eats a good enough range of foods, albeit limited and with high sensory sensitivity, as is common in autistic individuals, would only be diagnosed with ARFID if the eating behaviour is causing significant distress or impairment in its own right.

Possible signs of ARFID include the individual finding eating a chore; finding it difficult to recognise when they are hungry; being sensitive to aspects of some foods (like texture or smell); always eating the same foods and feeling distress when asked to eat anything new; only eating food of a similar colour (typically beige e.g. potatoes or pasta); and heightened anxiety at mealtimes [52]. Some have described ARFID as being extreme 'picky eating' that goes past being a phase and can potentially have severe physical consequences, including growth issues and nutritional deficits. Incorrect diagnosis (i.e. being diagnosed with AN) results in inappropriate treatment that can be distressing and often exacerbates symptoms [53]. When assessing patients, it is important to establish the factors driving behaviours (e.g. sensory-based avoidance, previous trauma around food, etc.), the impact of behaviours (both physical and social or emotional functioning) and whether there are other explanatory causes (including presence of another eating disorder or mental health condition) [54]. ARFID has been associated with many other mental health conditions, particularly ASD, obsessive-compulsive disorder (OCD) and ADHD. ARFID has also been shown to be often comorbid with intellectual disability and medical conditions (e.g. food allergies [55] or gastrointestinal issues [54,56]).

Treatment and Management

In terms of treatment for ARFID, there is currently no randomised controlled trial evidence on which to base treatment decisions. Clinical consensus generally is that treatment should be multidisciplinary to address nutritional, physical and mental health symptoms [13]. The lack of high-quality evidence means that ARFID was not included in the scope of the NICE guidelines for ED. The Canadian Practice Guidelines suggest that there is some evidence from case series for CBT, behavioural approaches and family-based treatment [57]. These guidelines also suggest that medication may be helpful with comorbidities and possibly appetite (e.g. olanzapine) [57]. Psycho-behavioural interventions (e.g. habit-acquisition training), dietetic interventions (including management of nutrient inadequacy, weight restoration and supplement weaning), sensory interventions (e.g. environmental manipulations and sensory processing aids), skills training (e.g. chewing or using cutlery), and medical management (e.g. monitoring physical impact, medication for anxiety) may also be needed on a case-by-case basis [52,58]. It should be noted, however, that there is a need for more evidence of effective interventions, including randomised control trials and longitudinal studies [58,59].

Complex Presentations in CYP with EDs

In recent years, clinicians have reported an increasing number of CYP with ED presenting at services with complex presentations. These patients tend to have increased levels of distress and emotion dysregulation and may not consistently respond well to recommend treatment like family therapy [60,61]. Many display traits and behaviours are characteristic of emerging Personality Disorder (borderline type) such as repeated non-suicidal self-injury (NSSI). Others may struggle with emotion regulation for reasons of diagnosed or unrecognised neurodevelopmental disorders, namely ASD and ADHD. In clinical practice distinguishing emotional dysregulation that is secondary to personality disorder from that due to neurodiversity can be difficult, yet it has significant implications for treatment.

Advances in neuroscience research have led to changes in the way that characteristics of people with ED that were once attributed to personality (e.g. obsessive-compulsive personality disorder) are now understood in terms of neurodevelopmental and neuropsychological diversity. As well as the challenges in recognising and understanding the role these factors play in the context of acute ED symptomatology, there are also complexities in knowing where treatment adaptations are needed. Research suggests that ASD traits influence treatment response, course and outcome [62,63,64], and also increase the likelihood of specific interventions being used such as medication and nasogastric feeding [64,65]. This has resulted in increasing work, often co-produced with people with lived experience of ASD and ED, to adapt ED treatment to better meet the needs of this population [66,67].

Personality disorder is characterised by patterns of instability in self-image, emotion and relationships. Common symptoms include impulsivity, chronic feelings of emptiness, difficulty controlling anger, patterns of suicidal and self-injurious behaviours and severe dissociative symptoms [2]. While it is not usual practice to diagnose those under 18 with personality disorder, multiple studies have suggested that traits begin to emerge in adolescence [68]. One meta-analysis in 2017 that looked at 87 studies from 18 different countries found that more than half of adults with AN or BN have a diagnosis of a personality disorder [69]. Rates of diagnosis of personality disorder are similarly elevated in ED populations (6–11% compared to 2–4% in the general population) [70].

Equally, for adolescents with personality disorder, there is strong evidence to suggest a stable relationship between disordered eating behaviour (DEB) and personality disorder symptomatology [71]. ED symptoms are greatest among CYP reporting feelings of emptiness, inappropriate anger and identity disturbance (often defined as an uncertainty about one's own self) [72]. Inappropriate anger and impulsivity show stronger relationships with BN than AN, while identity disturbance and feelings of emptiness are more strongly related to AN [60,72].

There are a number of transdiagnostic elements between ED and personality disorders, including emotion dysregulation, interpersonal sensitivity and impulse dysregulation (for patients with binge-eating or purging behaviours) [73]. Understanding these elements can help clinicians to understand the purpose served by disordered behaviours: self-injury, starvation, bingeing and purging can all serve as mechanisms with which to achieve feelings of control, indirectly communicate negative affect to others and regulate mood [74]. Clinicians caring for CYP with comorbid ED and personality disorders should therefore be aware of the potential for symptom crossover: for example, self-harm may increase when young people are prevented from restricting or purging in hospital [73]. Identifying these elements form part of a comprehensive biopsychosocial formulation that is unique to each patient.

Comorbidity between personality disorder and ED is often associated with increased levels of distress, NSSI and suicide attempts [73,75] and can negatively impact on treatment outcomes [60]. For example, for CYP with high levels of emotion dysregulation or who are exhibiting personality disorder traits, Family Therapy is not always successful. There has been a move to see if Dialectical Behaviour Therapy (DBT) can be integrated with Family Therapy when treating CYP with these comorbidities, particular for binge-eating and purging behaviours [61].

DBT [76] uses a mixture of cognitive behavioural therapy, distress tolerance techniques, acceptance ideas and mindfulness. DBT views eating disorder behaviours as an attempt to escape from distressing feelings and the related physiological responses [77]. A cycle of dependence can manifest: the relief felt from escaping these feelings motivates the behaviour; the distress that is felt when the behaviour is not used becomes increasingly worse, making the behaviour difficult to challenge and change. Multiple studies have looked at the effectiveness of using DBT for eating behaviours in children. A 10-week DBT skills group resulted in a reduction of emotional eating and binge-eating behaviours, and the adolescent participants (aged 14 to 18) mostly reported that the therapy was useful for them [78]. Other results from services trying to integrate DBT and family therapy suggest a decrease in binge-purge behaviours, increased weight and fewer re-admissions to intensive treatment, compared to services using family therapy alone [61].

Most of the research on ED and DBT have looked at binge-eating and purging behaviours, but there does appear to be evidence that integrating DBT with family therapy can be effective for adolescents struggling with restrictive ED too [79]. Sometimes known as radically open DBT the focus is on over rather than under-controlled behaviours [80]. Adolescent girls, aged 13 to 18, with restrictive ED attended weekly DBT skills sessions for 6 months, alongside Family Therapy. The intervention improved appropriate coping skills, increased body weight and reduced eating psychopathology [79]. Integrating Family Therapy and DBT potentially has long-term effects: adolescents who completed an intensive outpatient programme showed a significant decrease in eating disorder psychopathology up to 1 year after treatment, with 64% of underweight female patients achieving weight restoration and normal menstruation [81].

ASD and personality are just two of the common comorbidities with ED and those most often those found in complex cases where treatment response, severity or complexity is heightened. However, comorbidities, such as depression, anxiety, OCD and ADHD, are the norms rather than the exceptions. In some situations, it can be difficult to determine the most appropriate treatment approach for this reason. The NICE guidelines advocate shared decision-making and a pragmatic approach based on risk, functional impairment and choice.

Living in a Digital World
The Effects of Social Media

Celebrities, from Marilyn Monroe to the Kardashian family, have had an influence on body ideals and what society deems attractive. These body ideals can have a negative effect on young people: a recent systematic review demonstrated that exposure and comparison to celebrities, through traditional and digital media, is associated with poor body image [82]. There is a strong relationship between poor body image and ED symptoms, and it has been identified as an important risk factor for ED to be addressed in health promotion strategies and forms the basis for most ED prevention approaches[83,84].

Multiple meta-analyses have demonstrated that social media use has a long-term negative relationship with body image; more frequent use of social media is associated with poor body satisfaction [85]. In particular, social media images that promote the idea of an ideal appearance have a negative impact on body image [86]. More frequent use of social media with a visual focus (like Instagram) is associated with higher exposure to 'thinspiration' and 'fitspiration' [87]. Thinspiration encompasses social media content that is designed to encourage viewers to be thin. Fitspiration is content that attempts to motivate people to sustain or improve health and fitness. Fitspiration and thinspiration are very similar, with a focus on thinness and eating behaviours that are considered disordered by most clinicians and academics [88]. Often the content promotes extreme weight loss, through images of very thin people or 'inspirational' quotes [89]. Promotion of thinspiration and fitspiration is on the rise: in just one week, over 200 posts promoting weight loss, food guilt and body guilt were uploaded on Tumblr, a UK website frequented mostly by young people [89]. Exposure to thinspiration or fitspiration was indirectly associated with greater severity of eating disorder symptoms, in a sample of adolescents [87]. Thinspiration has a stronger relationship with symptom severity than fitspiration, but fitspiration content exposure is more common [87]. The effects of this were exacerbated during the Covid-19 pandemic, when exposure to social media content was heighted and often coupled with encouragement to exercise and lose weight, due to the risks the virus posed to those at higher weights. These factors, together with lack of social connection, are thought to be important in the rise in ED incidence seen worldwide during the pandemic [90,91].

How people use social networking sites is important, not just how much time is spent using sites. Use of image-based social media like Instagram or Snapchat has a stronger relationship with negative body image than social media that is more textual, like Facebook [92]. Reassurance-seeking through social networking sites, where individuals actively look for validation from others, predicts body dissatisfaction and DEBs, for both black and white women [85]. In a sample of over 4 000 Australian adolescents, appearance-related social media behaviours predicted the risk of meeting the criteria for an eating disorder [93]. These behaviours included avoidance of posting selfies to social media, degree of photo investment (the effort put into choosing a selfie and monitoring the response), photo manipulation (extent of editing of selfie prior to posting) and investment in other people's selfies (how much participants scrutinised selfies posted by others). Each behaviour was associated with high odds of meeting the criteria for an eating disorder, although which eating disorder each behaviour was associated with varied. For example, increased photo investment was the only behaviour that was associated with increased odds of meeting the diagnostic criteria for *all* EDs [93]. Other research suggests that the process of taking and editing selfies appeared to be more harmful to body image than actually posting selfies [92].

There have been some commentators, particularly in the body-positivity movement, who suggest that social media can be used to promote positive body image, and recent studies support this. However, a recent mega-review of meta-analyses, systematic reviews and narrative reviews suggests that the relationship between social media and adolescent mental health is mixed [94]. Social media content that portrays diverse bodies that do not fit society's conception of ideal appearance had a positive effect on body image [95]. Other attempts at positive content however, such as fitspiration, can in fact have a negative effect on body image [92]. Additionally, body acceptance related text, such as inspirational quotes, do not appear to have a helpful effect on body image [95].

There are many websites and social media profiles that promote health and wellness. However, these sites often still promote the idea of a perfect body that can be achieved through diet and exercise [96]. The promotion of weight management through often extreme measures (like juice cleanses or very low-calorie intake) can result in poor lifestyle choices, including yo-yo dieting and exercise avoidance [96]. Thus, young people at higher weights are particularly vulnerable to exposure to diet promoting material in combination with media likely to trigger negative body image.

While much research has looked at the effect of social media on children's body image and DEBs, attention has moved towards examining the efficacy of interventions that could mediate any negative relationships [97]. A recent meta-analysis examined the effectiveness of school-based interventions that aim to promote positive body image, in children aged 10–15-years-old [98]. It found that media literacy interventions have the potential to reduce body dissatisfaction, with interventions based on cognitive dissonance being the most effective. Unfortunately, school resources are often stretched, and many teachers do not have the time to implement multi-week interventions. Therefore, single session interventions are often preferred. One such intervention is Digital Bodies [99]. It focuses on deconstructing myths around the perfect body, critiquing socially constructed body ideals and examining the adolescent's roles in reinforcing these ideals. Evidence from a randomised control trial in the UK suggests that this intervention can have a positive effect on body satisfaction and reduces thin ideal internalisation in girls [99].

Explicitly Pro-eating Disorder Websites

The previous paragraphs described the effects of mainstream social media on body image and EDs. However, there is a much more hidden area of the internet that has long concerned eating disorder clinicians: pro-anorexia and pro-bulimia websites. These websites actively promote the development of an eating disorder, including providing tips on how to lose weight more effectively and hide symptoms from others, particularly clinicians [100]. Many users of pro-eating disorder community sites actively pursue dangerously low body weight goals [101]. Almost all pro-eating disorder sites are open to the public and often include interactive elements; 60–80% contain content that encourages AN and BN [100]. The number of sites has risen rapidly with the growth of the internet and the use of smartphones and so has the number of children and adolescents exposed to pro-eating disorder content [102]. This is incredibly worrying: high usage of pro-eating disorder community sites longitudinally predicts both greater levels of weight loss and greater reduction in desired body weight [101]. Almost all surveyed users of pro-anorexia websites report that they have learned new techniques, including purging behaviours [103]. Use of these websites lowers self-esteem, reinforces self-identity with being an eating disorder patient, prevents help-seeking behaviours and may even elongate the duration of illness [95,101,104,105,106]. Pro-eating disorder sites are notoriously hard to track, with most parents reporting that they are not aware that their child is using specific sites, and that they would not recognise the content of the sites as being particularly pro-eating disorder [102,107]. Academics and clinicians urge close monitoring of pro-eating disorder websites and have urged social media companies to take strong action at shutting pages down. However, some have suggested that monitoring and reporting content is getting increasingly more difficult with the advent of temporary social media (e.g. Snapchat or Instagram stories), and content is often coded [107,108]. Interventions such as checking the users' intent to view the content have been suggested as strategies to reduce harmful use.

Digital Therapies

The world is becoming increasingly digitalised. While this can cause significant issues with exposure to ED content, digitalisation can also be used positively. In fact, the use of, and research into, digital therapy for ED in children and adolescents have been significantly increasing, thanks to the worldwide Covid-19 lockdowns. There was an urgent need to move online, in order for young people to receive support consistently.

Many types of therapy, including art therapy, group CBT and other one-to-one therapies, have been delivered online, with family-based therapy being the most frequently used [109,110,111]. Most online therapies are delivered through live videos, though some are delivered using apps or other online platforms. Most of the studies have supported the feasibility of online therapies, with improvements in different therapeutic targets (including physical health, eating disorder symptoms and anxiety) [112]. Experience of therapeutic alliance, recruitment and retention rates of participants and treatment outcomes were all found to be comparable to in-person therapies [109,110]. The characteristic of the therapist who is delivering the therapy, including appropriate eye-gaze and attention, was found to be an important factor in treatment outcome [111,113]. From the patient's perspective, advantages of online therapies include increased accessibility and flexibility, decreased commute cost and ease for all family members to attend the therapy at the same time, especially when the patient is separated from other family members [114,115]. Patients who started therapy online rated the effectiveness of online therapies higher than those who transitioned from face-to-face therapies.

Online therapy is not without its negatives however: patients worry about feeling less connected with their therapist, technological and connection issues disrupt the flow of a session and therapists have noted less engagement from patients [111,116]. Additionally, unequal accessibility to digital resources may result in some patients being disadvantaged and having reduced access to support [114]. This may mean some groups will have better outcomes than others. From the clinician's perspective, it is important to balance the time and effort that is needed for training with treatment efficacy, as well as with accessibility for clients and therapeutic engagement when adopting a new digital therapy [114,116]. The technology also needs to be advanced enough to provide a stable portal to deliver the therapy online effectively [114].

Clinical Implications and Future Directions

The prevalence of ED in the population of CYP, when BED, OSFED and ARFID are included, now approaches 2.6–12.5%, depending on whether symptoms are reported by parents or self-reported [117]. Considered relatively rare less than 20 years ago, with no specialist service provision outside certain countries and a heavy reliance on inpatient care, there has been a shift to ED community care provision with increasing calls for a more active public health approach worldwide [118]. While the prevalence of AN has probably not changed significantly overall except in younger age groups [8], the rise in ED associated with normal or higher weight has been linked to the worldwide increase in obesity [119]. Although research addressing the overlap between ED and obesity in CYP remains relatively limited, efforts to explore the areas of tension in clinical and public health approaches are gaining traction [120,121,122].

Consequently, embedding clinical services in every region that are trained in the delivery of evidence-based interventions that can interface with schools, primary care and other community providers to reach CYP as early as possible in the pathway has become a priority in the UK, as in many countries. However, this has highlighted the historical relative underfunding of ED research and therefore a lack of evidence to support clinical practice [123]. For example, there are currently no psychopharmacological clinical trials involving adolescents with BN and no clinical interventions trials for ARFID [30].

In summary, there has been huge progress in understanding the risk and maintaining factors in ED, the value of early intervention and models of service delivery that best support CYP with ED. But much remains to be done. EDs have been shrouded in myths and struggled with visibility in the mental health landscape – a trend that needs to be reversed now that it is clear how many CYP and their families are affected. ED present across the health care system as well as in community settings – identification and early intervention is everybody's business.

References

1. Allen KL, Mountford VA, Elwyn R, et al. A Framework for Conceptualising Early Intervention for Eating Disorders. Eur. Eat. Disord. Rev. 2023;**31**(2):320–34.
2. American Psychiatric Association. *Diagnostic and Statistical Manual of Mental Disorders: DSM-5.* Arlington, VA: American Psychiatric Association, 2013. Available from: www.psychiatry.org/News-room/News-Releases/APA-Releases-Diagnostic-and-Statistical-Manual-of.
3. World Health Organisation. *ICD-11: International Statistical Classification of Diseases and Related Health Problems.* 11th ed. World Health Organisation: 2022. Available from: https://icd.who.int/en.
4. Arcelus J, et al. Mortality Rates in Patients with Anorexia Nervosa and Other Eating Disorders: A Meta-analysis of 36 Studies. Arch Gen Psychiatry. 2011;**68**(7):724–31.
5. Auger N, et al. Anorexia Nervosa and the Long-Term Risk of Mortality in Women. World J Psychiatry. 2021;**20**(3):448–49.
6. Westmoreland P, Krantz MJ, Mehler PS. Medical Complications of Anorexia Nervosa and Bulimia. Am J Med. 2016;**129**(1):30–37.
7. Dobrescu SR, et al. Anorexia Nervosa: 30-Year Outcome. BJ Psych. 2020;**216**(2):97–104.
8. Petkova H, et al. Incidence of Anorexia Nervosa in Young People in the UK and Ireland: A National Surveillance Study. BMJ Open. 2019;**9**(10):e027339.
9. Gull WW. V.-Anorexia Nervosa (Apepsia Hysterica, Anorexia Hysterica). Obes Res. 1997;**5**(5):498–502.
10. Le Grange D, et al. Moderators and Mediators of Remission in Family-Based Treatment and Adolescent Focused Therapy for Anorexia Nervosa. Beh Res Ther. 2012;**50**(2):85–92.
11. American Psychiatric Association Division of Research. Highlights of Changes from DSM-IV to DSM-5: Feeding and Eating Disorders. Focus. 2014;**12**(4):414–15. Available from: https://psychiatryonline.org/doi/full/10.1176/appi.focus.11.4.525.
12. Royal College of Psychiatrists. *Medical Emergencies in Eating Disorders (MEED): Guidance on Recognition and Management.* Royal College of Psychiatrists: 2022.
13. Hay P. Current Approach to Eating Disorders: A Clinical Update. Intern Med J. 2020;**50**(1):24–29.
14. Rosello R, Gledhill J, Yi I, et al. Recognition and Duration of Illness in Adolescent Eating Disorders: Parental Perceptions of Symptom Onset. Early Interv Psychia. 2021;**16**(8):854–61.
15. Dahlenburg SC, Gleaves DH, Hutchinson AD. Anorexia Nervosa and Perfectionism: A Meta-analysis. Int J Eat Disord. 2019;**52**(3):219–29.
16. Walker DC, White EK, Srinivasan VJ. A Meta-analysis of the Relationships Between Body Checking, Body Image Avoidance, Body Image Dissatisfaction, Mood, and Disordered Eating. Int J Eat Disord. 2018;**51**(8):745–70.
17. Herpertz-Dahlmann B, Dahmen B. Children in Need – Diagnostics, Epidemiology, Treatment and Outcome of Early Onset Anorexia Nervosa. Nutrients. 2019;**11**(8):1932.
18. National Institute of Health and Care Excellence. *Eating Disorders: Recognition and Treatment.* National Institute of Health and Care Excellence, 2017. www.ni

ce.org.uk/guidance/ng69 (accessed 9 May 2025).
19. Simic M, Eisler I. Maudsley Family Therapy for Eating Disorders. In J Lebow, A Chambers, D Breunlin (ed.), *Encyclopedia of Couple and Family Therapy*. Cham: Springer, 2018. https://doi.org/10.1007/978-3-319-15877-8_168-1.
20. Couturier J, et al. Applying Online Parental Guided Self-Help Family-Based Treatment for Adolescent Anorexia Nervosa: A Comparison to Family-Based Treatment Delivered by Videoconferencing. Clin Child Psychol Psychiatry. 2022;**27**(3):538–48.
21. Wade T, et al. Is Guided Self-Help Family-Based Treatment for Parents of Adolescents with Anorexia Nervosa on Treatment Waitlists Feasible? A Pilot Trial. Int J Eat Disord. 2022;**55**(6):832–37.
22. Madigan S, Vaillancourt T, Dimitropoulos G, et al. A Systematic Review and Meta-Analysis: Child and Adolescent Healthcare Utilization for Eating Disorders During the COVID-19 Pandemic. J Am Acad Child Adolesc Psychiatry. 2024;**64**(2):158–71.
23. Dalle Grave R, et al. A Conceptual Comparison of Family-Based Treatment and Enhanced Cognitive Behavior Therapy in the Treatment of Adolescents with Eating Disorders. J. Eat Disord. 2019;**7**(1):1–9.
24. Lock J. *Adolescent-Focused Therapy for Anorexia Nervosa: A Developmental Approach*. New York: Guilford Publications, 2020.
25. Lock J, et al. Randomized Clinical Trial Comparing Family-Based Treatment with Adolescent-Focused Individual Therapy for Adolescents with Anorexia Nervosa. Arch Gen Psychiatry. 2010;**67**(10):1025–32.
26. Gowers, S., et al., A Randomised Controlled Multicentre Trial of Treatments for Adolescent Anorexia Nervosa Including Assessment of Cost-Effectiveness and Patient Acceptability-the TOuCAN Trial. HTA. 2010;**14**(15):1–98.
27. Royal College of Psychiatrists. *Medical Emergencies in Eating Disorders: Guidance on Recognition and Management (CR233)*. Royal College of Psychiatrists, 2022. Available from: www.rcpsych.ac.uk/improving-care/campaigning-for-better-mental-health-policy/college-reports/2022-college-reports/cr233 (accessed 9 May 2025).
28. O'Connor G, Oliver A, Corbett J, Fuller S. Developing Clinical Guidelines for Dietitians Treating Young People with Anorexia Nervosa-Family Focused Approach Working Alongside Family Therapists. Ann Nutr Disord Ther. 2019;**6**(1):1056.
29. Han R Bian Q, Chen H. Effectiveness of Olanzapine in the Treatment of Anorexia Nervosa: A Systematic review and meta-analysis. Brain Behav. 2022;**12**(2):e2498.
30. Himmerich H, Lewis YD, Conti C, et al. World Federation of Societies of Biological Psychiatry (WFSBP) Guidelines Update 2023 on the Pharmacological Treatment of Eating Disorders. World J Biol Psychiatry. 2023:1–64. https://doi.org/10.1080/15622975.2023.2179663. Epub ahead of print. PMID: 37350265.
31. Glazer KB, et al. The Course of Eating Disorders Involving Bingeing and Purging Among Adolescent Girls: Prevalence, Stability, and Transitions. J Adolesc Health. 2019;**64**(2):165–71.
32. Reed GM, et al. Innovations and Changes in the ICD-11 Classification of Mental, Behavioural and Neurodevelopmental Disorders. World Psychiatry. 2019;**18**(1):3–19.
33. Ciao AC, et al. Predictors and Moderators of Psychological Changes During the Treatment of Adolescent Bulimia Nervosa. Behav Res Ther. 2015;**69**:48–53.
34. Peterson CM, Fischer S. A Prospective Study of the Influence of the UPPS Model of Impulsivity on the Co-occurrence of Bulimic Symptoms and Non-suicidal Self-Injury. Eat Behav. 2012;**13**(4):335–41.
35. Bahji A, et al. Prevalence of Substance Use Disorder Comorbidity Among Individuals with Eating Disorders: A Systematic

Review and Meta-analysis. Psychiatry Res. 2019;273:58–66.
36. Hail L, Le Grange D. Bulimia Nervosa in Adolescents: Prevalence and Treatment Challenges. Adolesc Health, Med Ther. 2018;9:11–16.
37. Craig M, et al. Optimizing Treatment Outcomes in Adolescents with Eating Disorders: The Potential Role of Cognitive Behavioral Therapy. International Journal of Eating Disorders. 2019;52(5):538–42.
38. Le Grange D, et al. Randomized Clinical Trial of Family-Based Treatment and Cognitive-Behavioral Therapy for Adolescent Bulimia Nervosa. JAACAP. 2015;54(11):886–94.
39. Coleman SE, Caswell N. Diabetes and Eating Disorders: An Exploration of 'Diabulimia'. BMC Psychology. 2020;8(1):101.
40. Colton PA, et al. Eating Disorders in Girls and Women with Type 1 Diabetes: A Longitudinal Study of Prevalence, onset, remission, and recurrence. Diabetes Care. 2015;38(7):1212–17.
41. Jones JM, et al. Eating Disorders in Adolescent Females with and Without Type 1 Diabetes: Cross Sectional Study. Bmj. 2000;320(7249):1563–66.
42. Torjesen I. Diabulimia: The World's Most Dangerous Eating Disorder. BMJ. 2019;364:l982.
43. Gagnon C, Aimé A, Bélanger C. Predictors of Comorbid Eating Disorders and Diabetes in People with Type 1 and Type 2 Diabetes. Can J Diabetes. 2017;41(1):52–57.
44. Corbett T, Smith J. Disordered Eating and Body Image in Adolescents with Type 1 Diabetes. Diabetes Care for Children & Young People. 2020;9(3):49–55.
45. Kjeldbjerg ML, Clausen L. Prevalence of Binge-Eating Disorder Among Children and Adolescents: A Systematic Review and Meta-analysis. European Child & Adolescent Psychiatry. Eur Child Adolesc Psychiatry. 2023 Apr;32(4):549–74.
46. Nitsch A, et al. Medical Complications of Bulimia Nervosa. Cleveland Clinic J Med. 2021;88(6):333–43.
47. Keski-Rahkonen A. Epidemiology of Binge Eating Disorder: Prevalence, Course, Comorbidity, and Risk Factors. Curr Opin Psychiatry. 2021;34(6).
48. Schmidt R, Hilbert A. Predictors of Symptom Trajectories After Cognitive-Behavioral Therapy in Adolescents with an Age-Adapted Diagnosis of Binge-Eating Disorder. Behav Ther. 2022;53(1):137–49.
49. Claudino AM, Pike KM, Hay P, et al. The Classification of Feeding and Eating Disorders in the ICD-11: Results of a Field Study Comparing Proposed ICD-11 Guidelines with Existing ICD-10 Guidelines. BMC Med. 2019;17(1):93.
50. Sanchez-Cerezo J, et al. What Do We Know About the Epidemiology of Avoidant/Restrictive Food Intake Disorder in Children and Adolescents? A Systematic Review of the Literature. Eur Eat Disord Rev. 2023;31(2):226–46.
51. Duncombe Lowe K, Barnes TL, Martell C, et al. Youth with Avoidant/Restrictive Food Intake Disorder: Examining Differences by Age, Weight Status, and Symptom Duration. Nutrients. 2019;11(8):1955.
52. Bryant-Waugh R, et al. Towards an Evidence-Based Out-Patient Care Pathway for Children and Young People with Avoidant Restrictive Food Intake Disorder. JBCT. 2021;31(1):15–26.
53. Davis E, Stone EL. Avoidant Restrictive Food Intake Disorder – More Than Just Picky Eating: A Case Discussion and Literature Review. JNP. 2020;16(10):713–17.
54. Dinkler L, Bryant-Waugh R. Assessment of Avoidant Restrictive Food Intake Disorder, Pica and Rumination Disorder: Interview and Questionnaire Measures. Curr Opin Psychiatry. 2021;34(6):532–42.
55. Patrawala MM, et al. Avoidant-Restrictive Food Intake Disorder (ARFID): A Treatable Complication of Food Allergy. JAACI: In Practice. 2022;10(1):326–28.

56. Nicholas JK. et al. The Diagnosis of Avoidant Restrictive Food Intake Disorder in the Presence of Gastrointestinal Disorders: Opportunities to Define Shared Mechanisms of Symptom Expression. Int J Eat Disord. 2021;54(6):995–1008.

57. Couturier, J., et al., Canadian practice guidelines for the treatment of children and adolescents with eating disorders. J Eat Disord, 2020. 8(1):4.

58. Thomas JJ, et al. Cognitive-Behavioral Therapy for Avoidant/Restrictive Food Intake Disorder: Feasibility, Acceptability, and Proof-of-Concept for Children and Adolescents. Int J Eat Disord. 2020;53(10):1636–46.

59. Lock J, Sadeh-Sharvit S, L'Insalata A. Feasibility of Conducting a Randomized Clinical Trial Using Family-Based Treatment for Avoidant/Restrictive Food Intake Disorder. Int J Eat Disord. 2019;52(6):746–51.

60. Lekgabe E, et al. Borderline Personality Disorder Traits in Adolescents with Anorexia Nervosa. Brain Behav. 2021;11(12):e2443.

61. Pennell A, Webb C, Agar P, Federici A, Couturier J. Implementation of Dialectical Behavior Therapy in a Day Hospital Setting for Adolescents with Eating Disorders. J Can Acad Child Adolesc Psychiatry. 2019;28(1):21–29.

62. Nielsen S, Dobrescu SR, Dinkler L, et al. Effects of Autism on 30-Year Outcome of Anorexia Nervosa. J Eat Disord. 2022;10(1):4.

63. Zhang R, et al. Association of Autism Diagnosis and Polygenic Scores with Eating Disorder Severity. Eur Eat Disord Rev. 2022;30(5):442–58.

64. Stewart CS, et al. Impact of ASD Traits on Treatment Outcomes of Eating Disorders in Girls. Eur Eat Disord Rev. 2017;25(2):123–28.

65. Fuller S, Sheridan E, Hudson LD, Nicholls D. Nasogastric Tube Feeding Under Physical Restraint of Children and Young People with Mental Disorders: A Comprehensive Audit and Case Series Across Paediatric Wards in England. Arch Dis Child. 2024;109(8):649–53.

66. Loomes R, Bryant-Waugh R. Widening the Reach of Family-Based Interventions for Anorexia Nervosa: Autism-Adaptations for Children and Adolescents. J Eat Disord. 2021;9:1–11.

67. Li Z, et al. Autistic Characteristics in Eating Disorders: Treatment Adaptations and Impact on Clinical Outcomes. Eur Eat Disord Rev. 2022;30(5):671–90.

68. Bozzatello P, Bellino S, Bosia M, Rocca P. Early Detection and Outcome in Borderline Personality Disorder. Front Psychiatry. 2019;10:710

69. Martinussen M, et al. The Comorbidity of Personality Disorders in Eating Disorders: A Meta-analysis. Eat Weight Disord- Studies on Anorexia, Bulimia and Obesity. 2017;22(2):201–209.

70. Zanarini MC, et al. The Course of Eating Disorders in Patients with Borderline Personality Disorder: A 10-Year Follow-Up Study. Int J Eat Disord. 2010;43(3):226–32.

71. Farstad SM, McGeown LM, von Ranson KM. Eating Disorders and Personality, 2004–2016: A Systematic Review and Meta-analysis. Clin Psychol Rev. 2016;46:91–105.

72. Miller AE, Racine SE, Klonsky ED. Symptoms of Anorexia Nervosa and Bulimia Nervosa Have Differential Relationships to Borderline Personality Disorder Symptoms. Eat Disord. 2021;29(2):161–74.

73. Brown A. The Management of Eating Disorders Where There Is a Comorbid Personality Disorder. In J Morris, A McKinlay (eds), *Multidisciplinary Management of Eating Disorders*. Cham: Springer, 2018, 159–75.

74. Newton JR. Borderline Personality Disorder and Eating Disorders: A Trans-diagnostic Approach to Unravelling Diagnostic Complexity. Australas Psychiatry. 2019;27(6):556–58.

75. Cliffe C, et al. Suicide Attempts Requiring Hospitalization in Patients with Eating

Disorders: A Retrospective Cohort Study. Int J Eat Disord. 2020;53(5):728-35.

76. Linehan M. *Skills Training Manual for Treating Borderline Personality Disorder.* Vol. 29. New York: Guilford Press, 1993.

77. Chen EY, et al. Dialectical Behavior Therapy for Clients with Binge-Eating Disorder or Bulimia Nervosa and Borderline Personality Disorder. Int J Eat Disord. 2008;41(6):505-12.

78. Kamody RC, et al. Implementing A Condensed Dialectical Behavior Therapy Skills Group for Binge-Eating Behaviors in Adolescents. Eat Weight Disord-Studies on Anorexia, Bulimia and Obesity. 2019;24(2):367-72.

79. Peterson CM, et al. Dialectical Behavioral Therapy Skills Group as an Adjunct to Family-Based Therapy in Adolescents with Restrictive Eating Disorders. Eat Disord. 2020;28(1):67-79.

80. Isaksson M, et al. Radically Open Dialectical Behavior Therapy for Anorexia Nervosa: A Multiple Baseline Single-Case Experimental Design Study Across 13 Cases. J Behav Ther Exp Psychiatry. 2021;71:101637.

81. Johnston JA, et al. A Pilot Study of Maudsley Family Therapy with Group Dialectical Behavior Therapy Skills Training in an Intensive Outpatient Program for Adolescent Eating Disorders. J Clin Psychol. 2015;71(6):527-43.

82. Brown Z, Tiggemann M. Celebrity Influence on Body Image and Eating disorders: A Review. J Health Psychol. 2021;27(5):1233-51. https://doi.org/10.1177/1359105320988312.

83. Fatt SJ, et al. Seeing Yourself Clearly: Self-Identification of a Body Image Problem in Adolescents with an Eating Disorder. J Early Interv. 2021;15(3):577-84.

84. Le LK, et al. Prevention of Eating Disorders: A Systematic Review and Meta-analysis. Clin Psychol Rev. 2017;53:46-58.

85. Howard LM, et al. Is Use of Social Networking Sites Associated with Young Women's Body Dissatisfaction and Disordered Eating? A Look at Black–White Racial Differences. Body Image. 2017;23:109-13.

86. de Valle MK, et al. Social Media, Body Image, and the Question of Causation: Meta-analyses of Experimental and Longitudinal Evidence. Body Image. 2021;39:276-92.

87. Griffiths S, et al. How Does Exposure to Thinspiration and Fitspiration Relate to Symptom Severity Among Individuals with Eating Disorders? Evaluation of a Proposed Model. Body Image. 2018;27:187-95.

88. Dignard NA, Jarry JL. The 'Little Red Riding Hood effect': Fitspiration Is Just as Bad as Thinspiration for Women's Body Satisfaction. Body Image. 2021;36:201-13.

89. Wick MR, Harriger JA. A Content Analysis of Thinspiration Images and Text Posts on Tumblr. Body Image. 2018;24:13-16.

90. Devoe, JD, Han A, Anderson A, et al. The Impact of the Covid-19 Pandemic on Eating Disorders: A Systematic Review. Int J Eat Disord. 2023;56(1):5-25.

91. Paraskeva N, et al. An Exploration of Having Social Media Influencers Deliver a First-Line Digital Intervention to Improve Body Image Among Adolescent Girls: A Qualitative Study. Body Image. 2024;51:101753.

92. Vandenbosch L, Fardouly J, Tiggemann M. Social Media and Body Image: Recent Trends and Future Directions. Curr Opin Psychol. 2021;45:101289.

93. Lonergan AR, et al. Protect Me from my Selfie: Examining the Association Between Photo-Based Social Media Behaviors and Self-Reported Eating Disorders in Adolescence. Int J Eat Disord. 2020;53(5):755-66.

94. Valkenburg PM, Meier A, Beyens I. Social Media Use and Its Impact on Adolescent Mental Health: An Umbrella Review of the Evidence. Curr Opin Psychol. 2022;44:58-68.

95. Rodgers RF, Paxton SJ, Wertheim EH. # Take Idealized Bodies Out of the Picture: A Scoping Review of Social Media Content

Aiming to Protect and Promote Positive Body Image. Body Image. 2021;**38**:10–36.

96. Marks RJ, De Foe A, Collett J. The Pursuit of Wellness: Social Media, Body Image and Eating Disorders. Child Youth Serv Rev. 2020;**119**:105659.

97. Gordon CS, Jarman HK, Rodgers RF, et al. Outcomes of a Cluster Randomized Controlled Trial of the SoMe Social Media Literacy Program for Improving Body Image-Related Outcomes in Adolescent Boys and Girls. Nutrients. 2021;**13**(11):3825.

98. Kurz M. Rosendahl J, Rodeck J, Muehleck J, Berger U. School-Based Interventions Improve Body Image and Media Literacy in Youth: A Systematic Review and Meta-analysis. J Prim Prev. 2021;**43**(1):5–23.

99. Bell BT, Taylor C, Paddock D, Bates A. Digital Bodies: A Controlled Evaluation of a Brief Classroom-Based Intervention for Reducing Negative Body Image Among Adolescents in the Digital Age. Br J Educ Psychol. 2021;**92**(1):280–98.

100. Borzekowski DL, et al. e-Ana and e-Mia: A Content Analysis of Pro–eating Disorder Web Sites. Am J Public Health. 2010;**100**(8):1526–34.

101. Feldhege J, Moessner M, Bauer S. Detrimental Effects of Online Pro–Eating Disorder Communities on Weight Loss and Desired Weight: Longitudinal Observational Study. JMIR. 2021;**23**(10):e27153.

102. Custers, K., The Urgent Matter of Online Pro-eating Disorder Content and Children: Clinical Practice. Eur J Pediatr. 2015;**174**(4):429–33.

103. Jett S, LaPorte DJ, Wanchisn J. Impact of Exposure to Pro-eating Disorder Websites on Eating Behaviour in College Women. Eur Eat Disord Rev. 2010;**18**(5):410–16.

104. Rodgers RF, et al. A Meta-analysis Examining the Influence of Pro-eating Disorder Websites on Body Image and Eating Pathology. Eur Eat Disord Rev. 2016;**24**(1):3–8.

105. Turja T, et al. Proeating Disorder Websites and Subjective Well-being: A Four-Country Study on Young People. Int J Eat Disord. 2017;**50**(1):50–57.

106. Mento C, Silvestri MC, Muscatello MRA. Psychological Impact of Pro-Anorexia and Pro-Eating Disorder Websites on Adolescent Females: A Systematic Review. IJERPH. 2021;**18**(4):2186.

107. Arseniev-Koehler A, et al. # Proana: Pro-eating Disorder Socialization on Twitter. J Adolesc Health. 2016;**58**(6):659–64.

108. Branley DB, Covey J. Pro-ana Versus Pro-recovery: A Content Analytic Comparison of Social Media Users' Communication About Eating Disorders on Twitter and Tumblr. Front Psychiatry. 2017;**8**:1356.

109. Anderson KE, et al. Utilizing Telehealth to Deliver Family-Based Treatment for Adolescent Anorexia Nervosa. Int J Eat Disord. 2017;**50**(10):1235–38.

110. Anderson KE, et al. Telemedicine of Family-Based Treatment for Adolescent Anorexia Nervosa: A Protocol of a Treatment Development Study. J Eat Disord. 2015;**3**(1):1–7.

111. Shaw L. 'Don't look!' An Online Art Therapy Group for Adolescents with Anorexia Nervosa. Int. J. Art Ther. 2020;**25**(4):211–17.

112. Lock J, et al. Feasibility of Conducting a Randomized Controlled Trial Comparing Family-Based Treatment via Videoconferencing and Online Guided Self-Help Family-Based Treatment for Adolescent Anorexia Nervosa. Int J Eat Disord. 2021;**54**(11):1998–2008.

113. Albano G, et al. The Relationship Between Working Alliance with Peer Mentors and Eating Psychopathology in a Digital 6-Week Guided Self-Help Intervention for Anorexia Nervosa. Int J Eat Disord. 2021;**54**(8):1519–26.

114. Stewart C, Konstantellou A, Kassamali F, et al. Is This the 'new normal'? A Mixed Method Investigation of Young Person, Parent and Clinician Experience of Online Eating Disorder Treatment

During the Covid-19 Pandemic. J Eat Disord. 2021;**9**(1):78.

115. Brothwood PL, Baudinet J, Stewart CS, et al. Moving Online: Young People and Parents' Experiences of Adolescent Eating Disorder Day Programme Treatment During the Covid-19 Pandemic. J Eat Disord. 2021;**9**(1):62.

116. Lindgreen P, Clausen L, Lomborg K. Clinicians' Perspective on an App for Patient Self-Monitoring in Eating Disorder Treatment. Int J Eat Disord. 2018;**51**(4):314–21.

117. Newlove-Delgado T, Marcheselli F, Williams T, et al. *Mental Health of Children and Young People in England, 2023*. Leeds: NHS England, 2023. Available from: https://digital.nhs.uk/data-and-information/publications/statistical/mental-health-of-children-and-young-people-in-england/2023-wave-4-follow-up#.

118. Ford T. Worrying Post-pandemic Trends in Eating Disorders and Self-Harm in Adolescents. Lancet Child Adolesc Health. 2023;**7**(8):521–23.

119. Hay P, Mitchison D. Eating Disorders and Obesity: The Challenge for Our Times. Nutrients. 2019;**11**(5):1055.

120. Lister NB, et al. Eating Disorders in weight-Related Therapy (EDIT) Collaboration: Rationale and Study Design. Nutr Res Rev. 2024;**37**(1):32–42.

121. Silén Y, et al. DSM-5 Eating Disorders Among Adolescents and Young Adults in Finland: A Public Health Concern. Int J Eat Disord. 2020;**53**(5):790–801.

122. Le LK, Tan EJ, Hay P, Ananthapavan J, Lee YY, Mihalopoulos C. The Modeled Cost-Effectiveness of a Prevention Program Targeting Both Eating Disorders and High BMI. Int J Eat Disord. 2024;**57**(9):1945–58.

123. Solmi F, et al. The Shrouded Visibility of Eating Disorders Research. Lancet Psychiatry. 2021;**8**(2):91–92.

Chapter 17

Benefits and Risks of the Digital World

Alka S. Ahuja MBE and Gemma Johns

Introduction

This chapter will look at using internet-based technology (IBT) within the context of mental health and children and young people (CYP).

The following acronyms will be used throughout the chapter:

IBT – Internet-based technology

CYP – children and young people

Background

Back in the early 1990s, when the internet first arrived, it was referred to as *'Athens without slaves'* [1] in that the internet would provide society with an abundance of information, and a platform for them to openly express themselves. As the digital revolution took hold, so did the condemnation of the internet and its associations with social ills and threats, specifically to poor mental health [2,3].

Fast forward 30 years, and the Covid-19 pandemic hits, and as a result, society witness significant transformations to the digital landscape once again [4]. The speed and adoption of digital technologies during this time increased considerably, which was particularly evident in health care and education settings, where much of traditional in-person delivery was replaced with IBT [5]. Again, this fast-paced transformation was condemned and widely associated with its potential threats to society, with particular concern regarding a 'digital divide' [6]. However, despite many of the pandemic-specific measures now returning to normal, some of the lessons learned during this time, particularly ones that resulted in successful digital transformations and improvement, are being held onto, and considered a change for the better [7,8], with additional reassurance that the digital divide isn't that much of a problem either [9]. It is therefore important to understand these ongoing digital changes, and to become better familiar with both the benefits and risks of using IBT for the delivery of care and education.

Understanding Internet-Based Technology

The increasing emergence of IBT has transformed the way that people of all ages communicate with each other, particularly among CYP [10].

CYP's use of IBT is increasing. The UK Council for Child Internet Safety state that now 94% of CYP aged 5 to 16 use IBT for a range of activities, many use it on a daily basis [11].

These activities may include searching the internet for homework/school project; reading a book/magazine on an e-Reader; online browsing or shopping; watching TV or online subscriptions, for example, Netflix, Disney Plus, YouTube; using social media platforms, for example, TikTok, Snapchat, Instagram, Twitter; and playing games interactively with peers via consoles, for example, Xbox or PlayStation or mobile devices or PCs and the use of 'multi-playing' for gaming and interacting with other players.

While the majority of CYP are using similar types of IBT for similar purposes, CYP can still have vastly different experiences and outcomes depending on the use, duration of use, content and impact of the IBT. Therefore, when considering the benefits and risks of IBT use, a good clinical knowledge base and understanding of its content, and impact specific to CYP is essential.

As a clinician, it is important to consider the benefits and risks of IBT in relation to both the 'CYP' and to your clinical role for the CYP. As a clinician, it is important that you:

(a) Have a good understanding and evidence base of IBT.
(b) Have a good understanding and evidence base of how IBT suits CYP.
(c) Understand how IBT fits into your clinical role.
(d) Base your clinical judgements and decisions on what the CYP want and need, rather than personal preference.

To do this, you will need to ensure that you understand:

(a) CYP preferences, attitudes, and purpose/use of IBT to understand what the CYP will want from IBT.
(b) Time spent on IBT.
(c) Websites and apps used.
(d) Impact of IBT on their sleep, mood, appetite, concentration, day-to-day life and schoolwork.

Understanding the Benefits and Risks of IBT

Benefits

IBT is an integral part of CYP lives, and for many, it can provide numerous benefits. For example:

Socialisation
- It offers immediate contact and communication with family and friends.
- It can be accessed at any time of the day, and any day of the year – making access/socialising a 24/7 space if needed.
- It allows for CYP to develop and enhance social relationships.
- It allows for CYP to socialise in a range of different environments, which extends their skills sets and encourages them to learn new cultures.
- For some CYP with high levels of anxiety or poor social skills it can support socialisation.
- During the Covid-19 pandemic, it helped reduced isolation for many CYP.

Development
- It presents the space to learn and play.
- A space to express individuality and creativity.
- A space to be more independent and objective.

Education and Knowledge
- It presents unlimited access to high-quality information, which can lead to increased knowledge and improved educational outcomes.
- Increase reading ability, due to fast access of eBooks.
- It lends itself well to extending educational and occupational opportunities far and wide, for example, remote learning and remote working.
- Linking with educational and occupational opportunities across the world.

Access to Health Care Services
- It offers access to various online support for a range of health and well-being concerns, for example, online CBT, mindfulness and counselling.
- It also presents the ability to obtain information and understand some common health care concerns, such as the RCPsych website or Mind website [12,13].

Remember: Some websites can provide unhelpful information or be harmful to a CYP, so carefully, and regularly, research and recommend trusted sites.

- Websites can reduce anxiety and stress in some people, for example, virtual consultations may help some CYP with high levels of anxiety by providing a virtual platform, reducing the need for in-person contact, waiting rooms, travel and missed school/work.
- Websites can sometimes be more accessible and potentially reduce waiting times, as virtual appointments are more readily available, which can impact positively on CYP clinical outcomes.
- Online mental well-being communities can provide free, safe and anonymous support, for example, Kooth.

Risks
However, there is similar evidence to suggest that IBT may impact adversely on comparable themes for the CYP. For example:

Socialisation
- The reliance of online socialisation may isolate or institutionalise CYP from in-person contact.
- CYP may become lonely due to peers' reliance on IBT.
- Online bullying can be 24/7.
- There is potential for exploitation/grooming in vulnerable CYP.
- Online socialisation may reinforce anxiety/lack of socialisation in some CYP.

Development
- Excessive use of IBT may impact on child development.

Education and Knowledge
- Excessive use of IBT may distract CYP from doing homework and impact on educational outcomes.
- Fast-access internet browsing may impact on other forms of obtaining knowledge and education, that is, reading books.

Health Care Access
- Impact on sleep, mood and so on.
- Online support and consultations may not be suitable in some CYP, for example, safeguarding concerns, high-risk behaviours and digital poverty.

Take-Home Message
Based on the comparable evidence, it is unclear as to whether IBT benefits a CYP any more than it can put a CYP at risk. But after 30 years of controversy, all we can do as clinicians is to better understand IBT use in CYP so we can provide our patients with the best possible clinical advice that best suit them and their current IBT use.

Understanding Your Clinical Role in IBT

Digital History Taking
The evidence surrounding IBT is in its infancy and therefore we are still unable to reach a definitive conclusion on IBT and its contribution to mental health disorders and addictions. It is therefore, recommended that, when assessing a CYP, a **digital history** is included as part of history taking in every CYP seen in-clinic.

Digital History Screening
Using digital screening questions, the clinician can learn more about the CYP individual use of IBT, with specific targeting/individualised questions towards more relatable content and impacts specific to the CYP.

Remember: Keep digital history screening questions 'balanced' and refrain from assuming any causal direction of IBT and health outcomes.

Rather, seek to explore areas such as the use and purpose of the IBT used by the CYP, the duration of each use, preferences and interests, satisfaction level (e.g., an unhealthy habit versus a happy place), perceived attitudes on IBT (CYP and their peers/parents) and impacts on sleep, eating habits, well-being and so on.

It can also be helpful to engage the CYP in a more relatable discussion, utilising language and understanding that CYP are more familiar with. With the support of a Young Person Representative Group, Box 17.1 provides simple questions to help approach these areas of discussion.

Box 17.1 Questions to Ask CYP

If trying to establish a **social media** or **Internet** usage, you could ask the CYP:
  Do you use social media platforms, such as TikTok, Snapchat, Instagram or Twitter?
Or
  Do you have a YouTube channel?
And if so,
  Do you make online content, or are you just a viewer?
  What content do you make/view, e.g., images or videos?
  Do you think your content builds a positive atmosphere?
  Do you feel comfortable in the comments section of the content you share or view?

If trying to understand a **privacy** or **risk** concern, you could ask the CYP:

Do you have privacy options enabled on your social media/online account?
Do you have an extensive online following?
How much information do you generally share online?
Do you speak personally with your followers?

If trying to establish a **gaming** or **gambling** presence, you could ask the CYP:

Do you play video games?

If so,

What console do you use? Or do you play via mobile or PC?
Do you play multiplayer games?
How often do you play alone or with others?
Do you feel reliant on playing video games?
Do you buy in-game purchases or have gaming subscriptions? Who pays for these?
What games do you play?

Additional Assessment: If any problematic behaviour is identified at digital screening, it is important to understand and consider some following areas of assessment. Seek to understand the impact of presenting difficulties, such as:
- family and friend relationships
- intimate relationships/relationship status
- identity and value systems of CYP and others around them
- school attendance or educational performance
- other responsibilities, for example, paid job, voluntary and caring role, chores
- home life, home set-up and safeguarding implications
- impact on sleep, eating, schoolwork and emotional well-being

Role of Parents/Guardians

Also, talk to parents/guardians about how they can safeguard CYP when using IBT, by:
(a) Engaging in relatable and balanced discussions with their CYP, taking about both the benefits and risks of IBT.
(b) Focusing on the positive impacts of IBT, for example, having a healthy routine rather than any negative concerns.
(c) Encouraging discussions on IBT content that is viewed online, and how this makes them feel.
(d) Having discussions early in child development as healthy IBT habits are easier to establish when children are younger.
(e) Setting appropriate and balanced screentime boundaries and model this approach with all family members. In other words, be a good role model.
(f) Safeguarding CYP by setting/reviewing privacy and location settings [14].

Understanding Social Media

Social media is defined as a *'website and applications (apps) that enable users to create and share content or to participate in social networking'* [15].

It is reported that 70% of 12–15-year-olds have a social media account, and 95% of CYP over 15-years-old use social media regularly in the UK [16].

To understand a CYP use of social media, it is important to keep on top of 'current' and 'popular' social media sites. These may include TikTok, Instagram, Snapchat, Twitter, Facebook, WhatsApp and other messaging services.

The rise in social media use, particularly among CYP has changed the way they communicate with friends and family, and how they showcase themselves as individuals.

Social media is now also used as a platform for immediate notifications and updates, such as daily news and public issues.

The benefits of social media for CYP can include its ability to motivate them to action; its ability to influence social, political and economic thinking and change; provide a platform for CYP to voice their opinions, and to be heard; and enables CYP voices to come together, providing a sense of shared identity and empowerment [17].

For example, climate activist Greta Thunberg has achieved significant social media following and positive reinforcement, impact and change due to her online ability to influence and lead.

In addition, social media enables CYP to communicate and socialise with friends and family across the world; find new friends and communities and network with people that share their own interests; join and promote groups and causes; raise awareness; seek or offer emotional support; seek out social connections when living in isolated or rural settings or marginalised groups; improve social anxiety in some CYP; improve creativity and self-expression; discover sources of information, support and learning; and seek out new opportunities, such as job adverts, educational sponsorships and more.

However, social media can also result in challenges and clinical risks for some CYP. For example, the immediate and ongoing notifications of social media, and the normalisation of sharing a filtered sense of their lives (showing only what the content sharer wants to share) can have significant implications on CYP mental health. These may include:

- difficulties with development and identity formation
- false sense of reality
- unhealthy balance between real life and virtual reality and connections
- self-esteem and worth issues
- body image problems

As a CYP clinician, there are some things to look out for, such as:

- low self-esteem and worth
- low mood when viewing content
- envy and comparison of others
- excessive or compulsive social media viewing or content sharing
- fear of missing out (FOMO)/not knowing about something 'immediately'
- avoidance of in-person contact
- becoming self-absorbed or obsessed with content sharing
- type of content being viewed or shared, for example, violent, sexual or graphic
- cyberbullying
- grooming and sexual exposure

Understanding Compulsive Use, Gaming, Gambling, Cyber Bullying and Grooming

Compulsive Use and Addiction

Compulsive use or addition has been associated with the use of many types of IBT in CYP, but two areas of particular interest tend to be in relation to social media use and gaming.

In social media, compulsion or addiction is often associated with the notification aspects of the platforms, such as the need for a post to receive a strong reaction of 'likes' or 'shares' to validate its public recognition. In gaming, competition, goal attainment and social gratification are common goals, but when used in excess, can lead to compulsive use and addictive behaviours in pursuit of winning.

For CYP, this behaviour can impact on restlessness, low mood, low self-esteem, depression, anxiety, impacts on sleep, body image, weight and diet, socialisation and interaction, academic, physical and social performance and self-harm and suicidal thoughts/actions.

What Does the Evidence Say?

IBT and compulsive behaviours and addictions are often associated [10]. However, the evidence of positive and negative associations is mixed.

Positive Associations

Research demonstrates that IBT provide positive associations with the mental health of CYP. For example, IBT is a means of creating connections with other individuals, which can reduce loneliness. A second benefit that was acknowledged included the improved self-esteem of CYP in that it is 'boosted' from presenting a positive version of themselves to the world and their networks [18].

Please note: It is unknown whether this improvement is sustained over time, or if there are differing impacts associated with vulnerability or additive behaviours.

Furthermore, IBT can encourage social connections with others and the ability to share experiences. This is particularly important for CYP suffering from poor mental health whereby online engagement is a critical tool [18].

Negative Associations

The compulsive use of IBT has negative associations with mental health. For example, its associations between screen-time duration. Cross-sectional and longitudinal studies have documented negative associations of excessive screen-time with increased anxiety and depressive symptoms. There is also an association with screen-time and internalising problems, which is a common symptom of both anxiety and depression [19].

When Gaming Becomes a Disorder

Gaming Disorder

Gaming disorder is now considered a mental health condition and is part of ICD-11. Gaming disorder is defined by the WHO as a pattern of gaming behavior ('digital-gaming' or 'video-gaming') characterized by impaired control over gaming, increasing priority given to gaming over other activities to the extent that gaming takes precedence over other interests and daily activities, and continuation or escalation of gaming despite the occurrence of negative consequences [20].

However, for gaming disorder to be diagnosed, the behaviour pattern must be:

(a) Of sufficient severity to result in significant impairment in personal, family, social, educational/occupational areas of functioning.
(b) Typically evident for at least 12 months [20].

When attempting to understand the disorders associated with gaming, it is essential to understand where the problem stems from.

Think of it like this . . .

Online gaming is associated to the notion that players create and build relationships with online characters or other online players that ultimately develop into **virtual relationships** and social interactions, similar to real life [21]. If, however, these relationships break down, or present a negative connotation, reactions may become apparent, such as aggression, irritability and restlessness.

For example, if a CYP in real life was 'denied or unable to play' with a friend, there would be a negative reaction felt to that CYP, such as social exclusion or loneliness. It is just as important to consider this feeling online as you would do in real life. Nevertheless, other studies investigating gaming addiction and mental health highlight a direct relationship with negative symptoms of depression, anxiety and stress [22].

Please note: It is therefore important to encourage a balance of gaming behaviours to CYP, by keeping an open mind to the benefits, but also weighing up the risks when used in excess.

Online Gaming to Online Gambling

According to the National Audit Office, there are 55 000 problem gamblers aged 11–16 in the UK [23]. For CYP, online gambling and gaming disorder are often closely linked, in that online gaming can encourage gambling or 'gambling-like' behaviour, for example, in-game incentives and additional in-play purchases.

The clinical concern is that by the time a CYP reaches the legal gambling area, they may have **'normalised'** their gambling behaviour (as part of the gaming experience) and may fail to see the risks at later life. There are however clinics and interventions (both in-person and virtual) available to support CYP with this condition.

An additional concern is that CYP are more susceptible to online gambling as access to the internet increases the convenience of doing so. It is therefore recommended to ensure **'gambling blocks'** are activated on IBT devices that are used by CYP.

What Does the Evidence Say?

The mental health association with online gambling can be problematic for CYP. For example, the number of CYP internet gamblers increased greatly during the Covid-19 pandemic lockdowns, which in turn matched the higher rates of mental health problems reported during this time, such as an increase in depression and stress [24], which is a common association with online gambling [25].

While multifaceted, the association between online gambling and mental health can be explained by either **neurological factors** associated with brain activation and structural changes or explained by **social factors,** such as financial hardship from monetary losses often leading to poor mental health conditions, such as depression and stress. A systematic literature review of neuroimaging studies identified that areas of the brain associated with reward, addiction, craving and emotion are increasingly activated when individuals are playing games, and even more prominent in individuals who are addicted to the internet [26].

Neuroimaging research highlighted how structural changes are often observed in the brains of those who are online gamers. Changes in the brain are regularly seen in the mesocorticolimbic system, which is the part of the brain associated with **reward and addiction.** This evidence supports the claim that online gaming and gambling can be addictive and associated to the neurological factors of the CYP. The meso-corticolimbic system **mediates depression-like symptoms** and therefore, changes that can occur in the brains of gaming addicts are linked to mental health disorders such as depression [27].

Gaming addicts have been found to have **decreased gray matter** in areas of the brain that are associated with motor control, cognition, motivation and processing emotion, such as the inferior parietal cortex convexity [26]. Reduced gray matter is commonly observed in patients with **major depressive disorder** [28].

Cyberbullying

Cyberbullying is a form of bullying and harassment that is conducted using digital forums and mediums.

It is therefore important to remember that anyone with an online presence is vulnerable to cyberbullying.

Traditional Bullying Versus Cyberbullying

Research by Landstedt and Persson [29] explored the mental health impacts of traditional in-person bullying and cyberbullying. Interestingly, both present similar outcomes. However, a combination of the two at the same time lead to much poorer mental health, such as depression. This study also discovered that both types of bullying can contribute to psychosomatic problems in females (more than males).

Despite the commonalities of the two, cyberbullying can present additional challenges to the CYP [30,31,32]. For example, cyberbullying can:

(a) Extend traditional bullying, for example, in-person at school, and continues to follow CYP into their home, often invading their safe space.
(b) Present an opportunity to save and store content, and therefore a single cyber-bullying episode can be permanently recorded.
(c) Present an opportunity to use content such as social media feeds, pictures or videos to target victims, such as name calling, insults and threats.
(d) Present an opportunity for 'anonymity' thus protecting the bully from disclosing themselves, and therefore increasing the chances and capacity to do so.

Cyberbullying and Mental Health

Although there are many ways in which IBT can be used for good, there are many negative influences such as cyberbullying [33].

Cyberbullying can have a significant impact on CYP and their mental health. There are strong links reported between cyberbullying and mental health. For example, a systematic mapping review investigated the association between cyberbullying and mental health in CYP [34]. This review concluded that cyberbullying is only increasing as the availability, accessibility and functionality of internet-enabled technologies continue to develop and expand [34].

With this, the expansion of IBT and accessibility of cyberbullying is an increase in the negative impact on CYP's mental health [34].

The review additionally identified the negative outcomes that have been found to accompany cyberbullying such as depression, suicidality, anxiety, hostility/aggression, substance misuse/use, self-harm, ADHD/hyperactivity, low self-esteem, peer problems, stress/distress, loneliness and life dissatisfaction.

However, it was acknowledged that none of the 19 reviews included longitudinal evidence therefore, it is difficult to establish to what extent these poor mental health outcomes are a result of cyberbullying [34].

Cyberbullying and Trauma/PTSD

In some cases, the CYP may become traumatised by cyberbullying which may cause physiological stress responses and for some, PTSD. This is often caused when the CYP relives the stressful event over and over, and the CYP has trouble dealing with the negative thoughts and difficulty controlling emotions.

Cyberbullying, Self-Harm and Suicidal Thoughts/Actions

Self-harm or suicidal thoughts can sometimes be experienced by CYP who are cyberbullied, where the CYP starts to think about physically harming themselves.

Grooming Risks

In addition to the increase of IBT, CYP are now more vulnerable to online grooming and sexual exploitation as a result [33].

Grooming has been universally defined as *'a technique to help turn a sex offender's fantasy into reality, whether online of offline'* [35].

IBT is rapidly developing and expanding, therefore, the opportunity for sexual offenders to access and build relationships with CYP online is on the rise [35]. For example, in the UK there were 5 441 Sexual Communication with a Child offences recorded between April 2021 and March 2021, which depicted a 70% increase from previous years [36]. Online groomers are increasing using social media sites to groom CYP. It is reported to have increased significantly in recent years, with the National Society for the Prevention of Cruelty to Children reporting that 34% of sexual grooming offences involve social media sites such as Facebook-owned apps such as Messenger, Instagram and WhatsApp, with Instagram being the most commonly reported [36].

There is work currently being done by the UK government, to introduce Artificial Intelligence technology that can identify and block grooming conversations, which therefore places a legal duty of care on social media companies. However, in the meantime, it is therefore important to 'educate' CYP about these risks.

Online Copycat Behaviour in CYP

CYP can have enormously different experiences of IBT depending on what content they are utilising and accessing [14].

For example, video sharing sites such as YouTube score highly in self-expression, awareness, self-identity and community building measures, which has contributed to high scores in positive impacts on mental health and well-being. On the other hand, social media sites such as Instagram have high scores in negative impacts on mental health and well-being due to scoring highly on body image, FOMO and bullying measures [18].

In a similar way, IBT can encourage a wide range of 'learning' opportunities. However, in the same way that a CYP can share and learn a positive experience online, they can do so with a negative one.

Negative experiences and lessons learned can often be encouraged by poor online messages or trends.

Clinical areas to look out for are body image, disordered eating, low self-esteem, self-harm, suicide and/or involuntary body movements, such as tics.

For example, it is important to be made aware of social media and internet sites that promote terms such as 'Thinspiration' and 'Fitspiration', and even illegal sites such as Pro-Anorexia (Pro-Ana) content [37,38].

There are many social media sites where this content is available such as, Instagram (where images are depicted) or Facebook and Twitter (where written content is favoured), however, TikTok utilises short duration videos [39].

Another clinical concern with social media sites is the 'algorithm of the app' that creates a personalised page for each user that suggests content and videos that the user may be interested in. However, for themes such as eating disorders and self-harming behaviour, the poor content filtering and privacy protection can lead to an overload of content delivered to the CYP.

For example, if a user views one video with Pro-Ana content and searches for similar content, the algorithm will keep suggesting similar content that contributes to the obsessive behaviour that is regularly seen in eating disorders [39].

Harmful content on social media and the internet does not just extend to eating disorders or self-harm, it can impact all types of mental illnesses [40]. There have been many attempts to normalise mental health disorders and spread awareness in the last decade. However, this openness on social media has contributed to the glamorisation of mental health disorders and as a result have led to more complex disorders [40]. A prominent example of this was in 2019 when the streaming service Netflix was forced to delete a graphic suicide scene from the 2017 show *13 Reasons Why*. Although the aim of this scene was to capture the horrific consequences of suicide, others saw this concept as a 'revenge fantasy' and made it seem like it is something that is methodical and premediated, which it rarely is in real life [41]. Furthermore, *Euphoria* a 2019 TV series addresses many issues such as mental health, sex and drug use. Experts believe this show additionally affects CYP due to how it glamorises problematic behaviour such as drug use, physical violence and promiscuity [41].

Previous research has investigated young adults whose mental health issues as teenagers were exacerbated by social media. A 19-year-old who was clinically diagnosed with depression at the age of 15 highlighted how pictures that depicted depression and self-harm drove him to suicidal thoughts and aggravated his mental health problem [40]. Therefore, many CYP are predisposed to thinking that they may be suffering a mental health disorder due to how relatable, normal and desirable they are seen to be online [40].

Conclusion

Since its inception in the 1990s, IBT has often been associated with mental health and well-being outcomes. However, as research and clinical evaluation has demonstrated over the past 30 years, there is very little evidence to suggest a definitive association or direction between IBT and mental health and well-being outcomes. In other words, the positive and negative association between IBT and mental health tend to be comparable.

This chapter highlights that for CYP in particular, IBT offers many benefits for their mental health and well-being, and therefore this should be considered thoroughly when weighing up CYPs 'wants and needs'. However, it is important to also consider the potential risks and challenges that IBT can present for some CYP. It is however recommended that, as a clinician, it is of good practice to better understand IBT in the context of CYP, and to keep updated on the ever-changing landscape of digital transformation. It is also essential that a clinician keeps a balanced clinical opinion on IBT and its associations with mental health among CYP, as at present, the evidence is not strong enough to support either direction (positive or negative impacts), and therefore no clinical decision should be made without clear and consistent evidence.

References

1. Robins K, Webster F. Athens Without Slaves … or Slaves Without Athens? The Neurosis of Technology. Sci Cult. 1998;1(3):7–53. https://doi.org/10.1080/09505438809526211.
2. Kiger M. The Digital Individual. TIS. 1994;10(2):73–76. https://doi.org/10.1080/01972243.1994.9960159.
3. Young KS. Internet Addiction and Mental Health. BMJ. 1999;319:9910351. https://doi.org/10.1136/sbmj.9910351.
4. De' Rahul, Pandey N, Pal A. Impact of Digital Surge During Covid-19 Pandemic: A Viewpoint on Research and Practice. Int J Inf Manage. 2020;55:102171. https://doi.org/10.1016/j.ijinfomgt.2020.102171.
5. Feger H., Crump B., Scott P. Editorial: UK Learning About Digital Health and Covid-19. BMJ Health Care Inform. 2021;28(1). http://dx.doi.org/10.1136/bmjhci-2021-100376.
6. Baker C, Hutton G, Christie L, Wright S. *COVID-19 and the Digital Divide*. UK Parliament, 2020. Available from: https://post.parliament.uk/covid-19-and-the-digital-divide/.
7. Johns G, Burhouse A, Tan J, John O, et al. Remote Mental Health Services: A Mixed Methods Survey and Interview Study on the Use, Value, Benefits and Challenges of a National Video Consulting Service in NHS Wales, UK. BMJ Open. 2021a;11(9):e053014. https://doi.org/10.1136/bmjopen-2021-053014.
8. Johns G, Khalil S, Ogonosky M, et al. Early Evidence and Lessons Learnt from an NHS Wales Video Consulting Service. Health Informatics J. 2022;28(1). https://doi.org/10.1177/14604582211069030.
9. Johns G, Khalil S, Ogonosky M, Ahuja A. Access to the Digital NHS Is Not Much of a Problem in Wales. BMJ (Clinical Research Ed). 2021b;374:n2212. https://doi.org/10.1136/bmj.n2212.
10. Kutty NA, Sreeramareddy CT. A Cross-Sectional Online Survey of Compulsive Internet Use and Mental Health of Young Adults in Malaysia. J. Family Community Med. 2014;21(1):23–28.
11. UK Government. *UK Council for Child Internet Safety (UKCCIS)*. UK Government, 2022. Cited at: https://www.gov.uk/government/groups/uk-council-for-child-internet-safety-ukccis.
12. Royal College of Psychiatrists. 2022. Cited at https://www.rcpsych.ac.uk.
13. Mind. 2022. Cited at https://www.mind.org.uk.

14. Dubicka B, Theodosiou L. *College Report on Technology Use and the Health of Children and Young People*. Royal College of Psychiatrists, 2020. Available from: https://www.rcpsych.ac.uk/docs/default-source/improving-care/better-mh-policy/college-reports/college-report-cr225.pdf.

15. Chandler D, Munday RA. *Dictionary of Social Media*. Oxford University Press, 2022. Cited at: https://www.oxfordreference.com/view/10.1093/acref/9780191803093.001.0001/acref-9780191803093 (accessed 22 April 2025).

16. House of Commons. *Impact of Social Media and Screen-Use on Young People's Health. Fourteenth Report of Session 2017–2019*. House of Commons, 2019. Available from: https://publications.parliament.uk/pa/cm201719/cmselect/cmstech/822/822.pdf.

17. Mental Health Foundation. *Social Media and Young People's Mental Health 2016*. Mental Health Foundation, 2016. Cited at: https://www.mentalhealth.org.uk/explore-mental-health/blogs/social-media-and-young-peoples-mental-health.

18. Stephen R, Edmonds R. *Social Media, Young People and Mental Health*. Centre for Mental Health, 2018:53. Retrieved from https://www.consaludmental.org/publicaciones/Social-media-young-people-mental-health.pdf.

19. Stiglic N, Viner RM. Effects of screentime on the health and well-being of children and adolescents: a systematic review of reviews. BMJ Open. 2019;**9**(1): e023191.

20. World Health Organisation. *Addictive Behaviours: Gaming Disorders*. World Health Organisation, 2020. Cited at: https://www.who.int/news-room/questions-and-answers/item/addictive-behaviours-gaming-disorder.

21. Singh M. Compulsive Digital Gaming: An Emerging Mental Health Disorder in Children. Indian J. Pediatr. 2019;**86**(2):171–73.

22. Loton D, Borkoles E, Lubman D, Polman R. Video Game Addiction, Engagement and Symptoms of Stress, Depression and Anxiety: The Mediating Role of Coping. Int J Ment Health Addict. 2016;**14**(4): 565–78.

23. National Audit Office. *Gambling Regulation: Problem Gambling and Protecting Vulnerable People*. National Audit Office, 2020. Cited at: https://www.nao.org.uk/press-release/gambling-regulation-problem-gambling-and-protecting-vulnerable-people/.

24. Emond A, Nairn A, Collard S, Hollén L. Gambling by Young Adults in the UK During Covid-19 Lockdown. J Gambl Stud. 2022;**38**(1):1–13.

25. Benson V, Hand C, Hartshorne R. How Compulsive Use of Social Media Affects Performance: Insights from the UK by Purpose of Use. Behav. Inform. Technol. 2019;**38**(6), 549–63.

26. Kuss DJ, Griffiths MD. Internet and Gaming Addiction: A Systematic Literature Review of Neuroimaging Studies. Brain Sci. 2012;**2**(3):347–74.

27. Nestler EJ, Carlezon Jr WA. The Mesolimbic Dopamine Reward Circuit in Depression. Biol Psychiatry. 2006;**59**(12):1151–59.

28. Webb CA, Weber M, Mundy EA, Killgore WD. Reduced Gray Matter Volume in the Anterior Cingulate, Orbitofrontal Cortex and Thalamus As a Function of Mild Depressive Symptoms: A Voxel-Based Morphometric Analysis. Psychol. Med. 2014;**44**(13):2833–43.

29. Landstedt E, Persson S. Bullying, Cyberbullying, and Mental Health in Young People. Scand J Public Health. 2014;**42**(4):393–99.

30. Betts LR, Spenser KA. 'People think it's a harmless joke': Young People's Understanding of the Impact of Technology, Digital Vulnerability and Cyberbullying in the United Kingdom. J Child Media. 2017;**11**(1):20–35.

31. Slonje R, Smith PK. Cyberbullying: Another Main Type of Bullying? Scand J Psychol. 2008;**49**:147–54. https://doi.org/10.1111/j.1467-9450.2007.00611.x.

32. Vandebosch H, Van Cleemput K. Cyberbullying Among Youngsters: Profiles

33. of Bullies and Victims. New Media Soc. 2009;**11**:1349–71. https://doi.org/10.1177/1461444809341263.
34. House of Commons. *Impact of Social Media and Screen-Use on Young People's Health. Fourteenth Report of Session 2017-2019*. House of Commons, 2019. Available from: https://publications.parliament.uk/pa/cm201719/cmselect/cmsctech/822/822.pdf.
35. Kwan I, Dickson K, Richardson M, et al. Cyberbullying and Children and Young People's Mental Health: A Systematic Map of Systematic Reviews. Cyberpsychol Behav Soc Netw. 2020;**23**(2):72–82.
36. Whittle H, Hamilton-Giachritsis C, Beech A, Collings G. A Review of Online Grooming: Characteristics and Concerns. Aggress Violent Behav. 2013;**18**(1):62–70.
37. NSPCC. *Record High Number of Recorded Grooming Crimes Lead to Calls for Stronger Online Safety Legislation*. NSPCC, 2024. Available from: https://www.nspcc.org.uk/about-us/news-opinion/2024/online-grooming-crimes-increase/.
38. Turner PG, Lefevre CE. Instagram Use Is Linked to Increased Symptoms of Orthorexia Nervosa. Eat Weight Disord. 2017;**22**(2):277–84.
39. Jennings AF, LeBlanc H, Kisch K, Lancaster S, Allen J. Blurred Boundaries Between Pro-Anorexia and Fitspiration Media? Diverging Cognitive and Emotional Effects. Eat Disord. 2021;**29**(6):580–90.
40. Logrieco G, Marchili MR, Roversi M, Villani A. The Paradox of Tik Tok Anti-pro-anorexia Videos: How Social Media Can Promote Non-suicidal Self-Injury and Anorexia. Int J Environ Res Public Health. 2021;**18**(3):1041.
41. Jadayel R, Medlej K, Jadayel JJ. Mental Disorders: A Glamorous Attraction on Social Media. J Teach Educ. 2017;**7**(1):465–76.
42. Cabral, S. *Op-Ed: From Stigmatized to Glamourized: Mental Illness in the Media*. The Upstream, 2021. Available from: https://cvhsnews.org/7373/opinion/op-ed-from-stigmatized-to-glamorized-mental-illness-in-media/ (accessed 7 April 2025).

Chapter 18

Bodily Distress Disorder and Dissociative Disorders

Charlotte Ulrikka Rask and Karen Hansen Kallesøe

Introduction

Bodily Distress Disorder (BDD) and Dissociative Disorders (DD), which are characterised by the presence of distressing persistent bodily symptoms in combination with excessive attention directed towards the symptoms, are common causes of morbidity in children and adolescents. In young children different pain complaints are prominent, whereas chronic fatigue, neurological symptoms such as gait or sensory disorders and non-epileptic seizures (NES) are rarer presentations but more frequently seen in adolescents. The disorders are associated with impaired functioning in multiple domains and high health care utilisation and costs. Their complex nature with medical and psychiatric comorbidities, diverse symptomatology, and often waxing and waning course can make them difficult to study and treat. The first part of this chapter will address current definitions and diagnostic classification in ICD-11. Next, prevalence and aetiology will be covered, followed by a presentation of principles for assessment and treatment. Finally, organisational aspects and future directions are discussed.

Diagnostic Classification and Clinical Presentation

Depending on symptom pattern and level of severity, various terminologies and diagnoses are used in both clinical practice and research [1].

The most common terminologies and diagnoses include:

- Non-diagnostic descriptors such as functional somatic symptoms and medically unexplained symptoms (MUS) and the relatively recent transdiagnostic term persistent physical symptoms, spanning both medical and psychological conditions [2]. These symptoms are often transient or intermittent and, therefore, not classified as a disease. However, the symptoms can be burdensome, and the health care system is often contacted.
- Defined clusters of somatic symptoms described under the overarching term functional somatic syndromes (FSS), e.g. juvenile fibromyalgia, tension type headache, functional gastrointestinal disorders, chronic fatigue and chronic widespread pain. The symptoms are present over an extended period of time and cause impairment. The patients are often evaluated by paediatricians either in the hospital system or in private clinics.
- Disorders where somatic symptoms co-exist with psycho-behavioural features (e.g. excessive attention towards symptoms and frequent contacts to the health care system) as seen in the ICD-11 diagnoses BDD and DD as well as in the DSM-5 diagnoses Somatic Symptom Disorder and Functional Neurological (Symptom) Disorder (Conversion Disorder) [3,4]. The disorders cause significant impairment in daily life. The young patients are often referred to mental health care due to complexity caused by the interaction of somatic, psychological and behavioural features.

> **Box 18.1** Diagnostic overview of Bodily Distress Disorder (ICD-11)
>
> **Bodily Distress Disorder (6C20)**
>
> **Mild bodily distress disorder (6C20.0)**
> - Excessive attention to distressing symptoms and their consequences, but the person is not preoccupied with the symptoms (e.g. spends less than an hour per day focusing on them)
> - Frequent medical visits
> - No substantial impairment
>
> **Moderate bodily distress disorder (6C20.1)**
> - Persistent preoccupation with the distressing symptoms and their consequences (e.g. spends more than an hour a day thinking about them)
> - Frequent medical visits
> - Moderate impairment
>
> **Severe bodily distress disorder (6C20.2)**
> - Pervasive and persistent preoccupation with the symptoms and their consequences to the extent that these may become the focal point of the person's life
> - Extensive interactions with the health care system
> - Serious impairment

This chapter will focus on the severely affected young people fulfilling the diagnostic criteria for the ICD-11 diagnoses BDD and DD.

Bodily Distress Disorder

BDD is characterised by the presence of distressing somatic symptoms and excessive thoughts and behaviours in relation to the symptoms. BDD can be categorised according to symptom severity and impairment as seen in Box 18.1. The somatic symptoms are persistent and present on most days for several months, and cause impairment of functioning (e.g. absence from school, social withdrawal and cessation of leisure-time activities). The most common symptoms in young people are abdominal pain, constipation, nausea, headache and fatigue as well as limb and muscle pain [5,6]. Younger children commonly present with one or two main symptoms whereas involvement of multiple somatic symptoms is more likely to emerge in early adolescence. The BDD diagnosis does not necessitate absence of a somatic disorder, but the degree of attention directed towards the symptoms is clearly excessive when taking the usual symptom presentation, severity and progression of the somatic disorder into account [4].

When applying the BDD diagnosis to young people, it is important to take into consideration that the diagnosis is based on adult symptomatology and does not take the developmental perspective on cognition and behaviour into account. Especially in young children the clinical manifestations may differ, as they seldom have excessive thoughts directed towards symptoms as the majority are not likely to have yet developed the cognitive skills to process and articulate specific symptom beliefs. Furthermore, as seeking medical help is a parental responsibility, the often-repeated contacts with health care providers are initiated by parents. Hence, parental beliefs and attention towards symptoms play a key role, and the psycho-behavioural features required for the BDD diagnosis may be fulfilled in a combination between symptoms presented by the child and the symptom-related beliefs and behaviours of the parents.

Common comorbidities include emotional disorders, with up to one-third having comorbid anxiety or depression [7], and underlying neurodevelopmental disorders such as autism, ADHD or learning disabilities [8,9]. Concurrent somatic disorders are also frequent with amplification and expansion of the somatic symptoms, for example, chronic pain in children with an inactive rheumatic disorder. Comorbidities add to the complexity of BDD with a need for more specialised interventions and a higher risk of persistence of symptoms [10].

> **Case story 18.1**
>
> *Oliver is a 10-year-old boy who has experienced abdominal pain on and off since he was 6 years old. Over the past year, the abdominal pain has worsened, and other symptoms have started to emerge, including constipation, headaches and tiredness. The symptoms are now affecting his everyday life with school absence exceeding 50% during the last two months. Oliver has also stopped playing soccer and is reluctant to visit friends or participate in birthday parties as he is trying to avoid situations where symptoms may be triggered or exacerbated. Oliver and his parents are very attentive towards the symptoms, and Oliver's parents support him in staying home from school so they can keep an eye on him to ensure that the symptoms do not worsen.*
>
> *Several medical evaluations have been done with blood samples and ultrasound of abdomen with no clear organic explanation. Oliver has been on restricted diets and has also tried different types of alternative treatment with only short-term effect. Oliver has always struggled in school, especially with reading and is now scheduled for a dyslexia test.*
>
> **Diagnosis: Bodily Distress Disorder, moderate**

Dissociative Disorders

The diagnostic category of DD encompasses a range of diagnoses (see Box 18.2). The most common dissociative symptoms experienced in young people are paralysis, seizures, localised weakness, dizziness, tremors and visual disturbances/blindness [6,11]. These symptoms all belong to the diagnostic category of dissociative neurological symptom disorder (DNSD). DNSD is characterised by the presentation of motor, sensory or cognitive symptoms that imply an involuntary discontinuity in the normal integration of motor, sensory or cognitive functions [12]. The symptoms may vary in frequency and intensity from intermittent to persistent, and all result in significant impairment in personal, family, social and/or educational functioning. Due to the often-sudden onset of symptoms and the serious somatic differential diagnoses demanding immediate medical attention such as epilepsy, the patients are often evaluated at the emergency departments with a high risk of medication errors (e.g. antiepileptic medication for non-epileptic seizures). The previous requirement for a temporal association with a traumatic experience (ICD-10 DF44) has been dropped, as many young people do not report an immediate identifiable stressor though this may become more evident over time.

Psychiatric disorders are common comorbidities with a range of disorders displaying elevated risk, including emotional disorders, adjustment disorder and neurodevelopmental disorders [13]. Also, somatic comorbidity is common as 14% of young patients with NES have comorbid epilepsy [14].

Box 18.2 Diagnostic overview of Dissociative Disorders (ICD-11)

Dissociative disorders

Dissociative disorders:

Dissociative Neurological Symptom Disorder (6B60), Dissociative Amnesia (6B61), Trance Disorder (6B62), Possession Trance Disorder (6B63), Dissociative Identity Disorder (6B64), Partial Dissociative Identity Disorder (6B65) and Depersonalisation-derealisation Disorder (6B66)

Dissociative neurological symptom disorder (6B60)

For all dissociative neurological symptoms:

Not consistent with a recognised disease of the nervous system, other mental, behavioural or neurodevelopmental disorder, or other medical condition.

Specific dissociative neurological symptom disorders:

- Visual disturbance (6B60.0): Blindness, tunnel vision, diplopia, visual distortions or hallucinations
- Auditory disturbance (6B60.1): Loss of hearing or auditory hallucinations
- Vertigo or dizziness (6B60.2): A sensation of spinning while stationary (vertigo) or dizziness
- Other sensory disturbance (6B60.3): Numbness, tightness, tingling, burning, pain, or other symptoms related to touch, smell, taste, balance, proprioception, kinaesthesia or thermoception
- Non-epileptic seizures (6B60.4): Seizures or convulsions
- Speech disturbance (6B60.5): Difficulty with speaking (dysphonia), loss of the ability to speak (aphonia) or difficult or unclear articulation of speech (dysarthria)
- Paresis or weakness (6B60.6): Difficulty or inability to intentionally move parts of the body or to coordinate movements
- Gait disturbance (6B60.7): Symptoms involving the individual's ability or manner of walking, including ataxia and the inability to stand unaided
- Movement disturbance (6B60.8): Symptoms such as chorea, myoclonus, tremor, dystonia, facial spasm, parkinsonism or dyskinesia
- Cognitive symptoms (6B60.9): Impaired cognitive performance in memory, language or other cognitive domains that is internally inconsistent

Case story 18.2

Emily is a 14-year-old girl with repeated emergency department visits over the last 6 months due to seizures. The seizures only appear when Emily is in school and often starts with a tingling sensation in her whole body followed by her body collapsing onto the floor. During most seizures Emily experiences spasms in both arms and legs and twisting of her head. She has a blurry awareness of what is happening around her and she can hear people talking to her but cannot respond.

> *A year ago, Emily's parents divorced. Emily has since lived with her mom who struggles to make ends meet. After Emily's recent visit to the emergency department, a long-term video EEG monitoring was scheduled, which did not reveal any pathological findings.*
> ***Diagnosis: Non-epileptic seizures (6B60.4)***
> *Over time it becomes evident that Emily has been exposed to cyberbullying. A classmate has shared an intimidating video of Emily online and from there on constant negative comments about Emily were posted in chat forums. Emily has been reluctant to share her problems, as she is embarrassed and ashamed.*

Differential Diagnoses

Anxiety and Depression

In addition to occurring as comorbid disorders, anxiety and depression are also common differential diagnoses to especially BDD. The presence of somatic symptoms are key features of both anxiety and depression, which complicates the diagnostic evaluation. As regards anxiety, muscular tension, motor restlessness and sympathetic autonomic overactivity, they are included in the diagnostic criteria whereas psychomotor agitation or retardation, and reduced energy or fatigue, are included in the diagnostic criteria for depression. Therefore, it is important to perform a thorough psychiatric assessment to ensure identification of the primary disorder and based on this a treatment plan with the right focus (see Assessment).

Factitious Disorder

Factitious disorder (imposed on self or another (ICD-11 6D50 and 6D51)) [4] is an important but rare differential diagnosis to BDD and DD. The disorder is characterised by feigning, falsifying or inducing signs and symptoms in self or others, and is associated with identified deception. In the paediatric population it is mainly signs and symptoms imposed by parents. The disorder is difficult to diagnose due to the deceptive nature. However, when suspected, the most important role of the health professional is to protect the child against receiving unnecessary or even harmful medical care as a result of the parental behaviour.

Epidemiology and Aetiology

Most research regarding epidemiology and aetiology in young people is based on the non-diagnostic descriptive terminologies or FSS diagnoses. However, a large overlap of the different disorders has been seen in adults [15], hence the following will report on literature across terminologies and diagnoses.

Epidemiology of Bodily Distress Disorder

Studies in some Western countries indicate an increase in daily somatic symptoms in young people in the general population [16] and a growing corresponding number of adolescents presenting with non-specific somatic symptoms in the hospital system [17], which could suggest a general increase in BDD. Prevalence estimates of impairing and persistent somatic symptoms are 3–10% in youths depending on classification and study population [18,19]. There are contradictory results on prepuberty sex distribution ranging from no difference

[20] to a higher prevalence in females as also seen in adolescence and adulthood [5]. Factors related to a poorer prognosis include multi-symptomatic presentation and family predisposition [10,21]. Without relevant treatment, continuity of symptoms into adulthood is common and associated with high personal and societal consequences including development of emotional disorders, lower probability of earning a college degree and high health care use [21,22].

Epidemiology of Dissociative Disorder

As there are few population-based data on DD in youths, more exact prevalence and incidence estimates are difficult to establish. Most studies report that dissociative symptoms are rarely seen before the age of 5, and that the incidence increases with age [23]. In a large German epidemiologic sample of adolescents, the prevalence estimate of dissociative disorder was 0.8% [24]. A recent study points towards a potential increase in NES in youths [14]. In general, both pre- and post-pubertal sex distribution show female predominance, but with some studies pointing towards a more equal sex distribution in children [23]. Few studies have explored long-term outcome, and most studies represent small clinical samples from tertiary hospital care. One study found that childhood DDs were associated with a high risk of continuity of symptoms and development of mood and personality disorders [25].

Cultural Aspects

Cultural effects are inconsistent in the literature. Although some studies find a globally constant prevalence, others highlight differences in frequency, intensity or presentation noting that non-white adolescents are more likely to report multiple, high frequency somatic symptoms compared to their white peers [26,27]. Specifically for functional gastrointestinal disorders, geographical differences have been reported with higher pooled prevalence rates in South America and Asia compared to North America and Europe [27,28].

The semiology of the disorders can also vary by country of origin, for example, in Japan, 71% of paediatric patients with bodily-distress-related disorders report orthostatic intolerance, which is a much higher percentage than in other countries [29]. With regard to DD the most common presentation in the United Kingdom, Ireland and Australia has been reported to be mixed sensory motor changes (e.g. weakness and paraesthesia) contrasting epidemiologic data from other nationalities with paralysis in Singapore, NES in Turkey and syncope in India [30]. Migratory status appears to be an independent risk for developing these disorders likely associated with acculturative stress as well as experiences with discrimination [27].

Aetiology: The Biopsychosocial Explanatory Model

There is a broad consensus that the development and maintenance of BDD and DD are best understood within the multifactorial framework of the biopsychosocial model with interacting biological, psychological and social/environmental factors [18,31]. These factors come into play at different stages as predisposing, precipitating and/or perpetuating (see Figure 18.1). In most cases it is impossible to pinpoint a single determining factor for development and perpetuation of symptoms, which is why the biopsychosocial factors should be evaluated

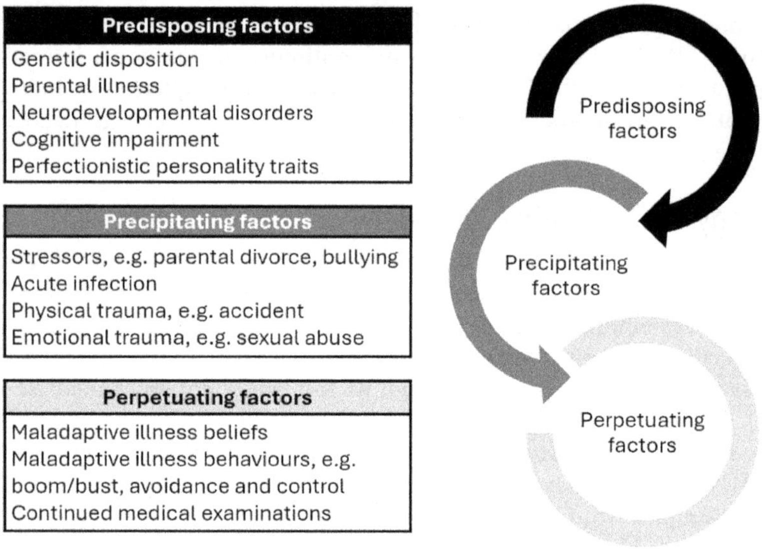

Predisposing factors
- Genetic disposition
- Parental illness
- Neurodevelopmental disorders
- Cognitive impairment
- Perfectionistic personality traits

Precipitating factors
- Stressors, e.g. parental divorce, bullying
- Acute infection
- Physical trauma, e.g. accident
- Emotional trauma, e.g. sexual abuse

Perpetuating factors
- Maladaptive illness beliefs
- Maladaptive illness behaviours, e.g. boom/bust, avoidance and control
- Continued medical examinations

Figure 18.1 Predisposing, precipitating and perpetuating factors of BDD and DD

within an integrated understanding where multiple factors may be of importance. The more recent theory of predictive processing combines potential neurobiological and psychosocial factors in the understanding of BDD and DD. The theory proposes that the development and perpetuation of symptoms should be understood as a complex interplay between central top-down brain-derived predictions (e.g. influenced by thoughts, feelings and behaviours based on previous symptom experiences) and bottom-up peripheral somatic input (e.g. the autonomic nervous system) resulting in an overall perceptual dysregulation [32,33].

Predisposing factors comprise a range of innate or acquired vulnerabilities. The innate vulnerabilities include genetic predisposition with a family history of BDD/DD or when the child has a neurodevelopmental disorder. Hypersensitivity to sensory stimuli in infancy has also been shown to constitute a vulnerability factor [34], as well as specific child personality traits such as perfectionism, or difficulties with emotion regulation [35]. Acquired vulnerabilities in early childhood include exposure to adverse childhood experiences, such as having parents who suffer from severe somatic or psychiatric disorders.

Precipitating factors comprise a broad range of physical and emotional stressors and adverse events that acutely or continuously increases the level of overall bodily distress. Physical stressors may be well-defined somatic disorders such as acute infections or sudden physical injuries. The most common and often longstanding stressors are bullying, family conflicts and continued academic pressure [36]. More rarely, trauma such as physical and sexual abuse may have occurred [37].

Perpetuating factors encompass negative illness beliefs and maladaptive illness behaviours both in the child, the parents and the close environment. Examples of negative beliefs can be catastrophising that one cannot control the symptoms, that the symptoms will persist or that they are signs of serious bodily damage.

Maladaptive behaviours are often triggered by negative illness beliefs. The fearful or inflexible symptom beliefs are typically associated with an increased focus on bodily sensations and withdrawal from activities due to fear of provoking symptoms (avoidance behaviour) or excessive rest (limiting behaviour) [38]. Other maladaptive behaviours may be the opposite, for example, exertion ('pushing through symptoms') or oscillations between periods with very low and very high levels of physical and mental activity, often referred to as 'all-or-nothing' behaviour. These may all be regarded as behavioural attempts to reduce symptoms while actually maintaining the symptoms as vicious circles may develop. For example, excessive rest may lead to reduced physical and mental stamina so that less and less activity may trigger symptoms that may again lead to more rest.

It is well-known that having a child with BDD/DD often inflicts parental concern and distress, and parents often report insecurities on how to help their child [39]. Parents as well as others in the close network may unintentionally support the maladaptive behaviours by encouraging inactivity and withdrawal from normal activities/social events and absence from school to protect the child from exacerbation of symptoms, or in contrast pushing the child to do too much so they overstrain and need to rest excessively. In an urge to act and help the child, and especially in families with a continuous biomedical understanding and worry about symptoms despite negative findings, parents may seek continued medical examinations with the risk of iatrogenic harm from unnecessary invasive procedures or operations. Many parents also seek alternative treatment for their child, which may prolong or worsen the disorder. Hence, addressing illness beliefs and behaviours in the family and close network is an essential part of treating young people with BDD and DD. This is further supported by a recent study where complete recovery was highly correlated with full acceptance of the diagnosis in the family [40]. For some parents the cause of continued examinations is rooted in their own excessive and distressing worries about their child's health, which in recent literature is named health anxiety by proxy [41]. In these cases, the parents may need treatment specifically aimed at their own health-related anxiety.

Assessment

Children and adolescents with clinical presentation of transient or mild to moderate symptoms will primarily be assessed by their family doctor or a paediatrician. In the majority of these cases, a symptom screening followed by an appropriate physical examination to exclude a treatable medical condition, in parallel with the consideration of potential psychosocial contributors and vulnerabilities, will be sufficient to clarify the nature of the problem and lead to fast improvement or a resolution [42].

Young people with more severe and disabling symptoms, who are likely to fulfil the diagnostic criteria for either BDD or DD, frequently present a longer medical history with multiple health care contacts and medical investigations as well as several failed treatment attempts. These young patients will often be in need of interdisciplinary assessment and care provided by both paediatric and child psychiatry specialities [43]. At this point the majority would already have a complete and comprehensive medical workup to rule out serious medical illness, but it is important to emphasise that BDD and DD are not simply diagnoses of exclusion (see Box 18.3).

Although no single element in the psychiatric assessment is conclusive, the presence of psycho-behavioural factors may increase the likelihood of meeting the diagnostic criteria for BDD/DD. A typical assessment should include a thorough illness history screening for

> **Box 18.3** Psychiatric assessment of children and adolescents with BDD/DD
>
> **Review hospital records/illness history with emphasis on medical findings suggesting BDD/DD:**
> - negative findings despite thorough medical workup
> - inconsistent findings on clinical examinations, for example, sensory changes inconsistent with anatomical distribution, periods of normal function when distracted
> - onset of symptoms coincides with psychosocial stressors
>
> **Perform a systematic and detailed somatic symptom interview with emphasis on:**
> - types, patterns and severity of symptoms
> - associated impact: emotional distress, family (e.g. disruption of work schedule, marital relationship, family conflicts), social and peer relationships, academic performance including school absence
>
> **Obtain a biopsychosocial history focusing on potential predisposing, precipitating and perpetuating factors:**
> - family history of persistent somatic symptoms
> - previous and/or current strain and stressors
> - psychiatric comorbidity, including anxiety/depression and underlying neurodevelopmental disorders/cognitive disabilities
> - maladaptive illness beliefs and behaviours in the family (e.g. somatic attribution, catastrophising, parental overprotection and over-involvement)
> - patterns of reinforcement of symptoms in close environment (e.g. increased attention in school, by friends/other family/medical providers)
>
> **Perform a focused physical assessment to:**
> - identify potential excessive fear regarding certain movements (kinesiophobia)
> - judge whether further medical evaluation is needed

typical somatic symptom patterns for BDD or DD, the presence of psychosocial stressors, familiar predisposition and the presence of maladaptive illness beliefs or reinforcing behaviours in close environment. The possibility of sexual or physical abuse must be carefully explored [37]. The physical examination may reveal that symptoms do not follow known physiological principles or anatomical patterns and may be relieved or disappear under distraction. Also, phenomena such as catastrophic thinking about bodily functions and kinesiophobia, that is, fear of pain due to certain movements, may be observed. Finally, any comorbid psychiatric disorders must be assessed and diagnosed when suspected.

> Four important questions that are important to answer at the primary psychiatric assessment are:
> (1) Are there red flags associated with the presenting symptoms which are suggestive of an underlying organic pathology?
> (2) Could there be an underlying undiagnosed psychiatric disorder?
> (3) Are there any current factors at home, school or in the peer group that could contribute to the presentation and be remedied?
> (4) Is the child/adolescent at risk of harm?

It follows that the psychiatric assessment requires specialised skills in medical/psychiatric differential diagnoses and skills to help move the families from a purely physical to a biopsychosocial framework while at the same time avoiding the pitfall of presenting the somatic symptoms in a reductive psychological context. It is crucial that this is done at a pace that is appropriate and acceptable for the individual family to support a shift of their focus from medical investigations to active management and symptom control. The medical and psychosocial findings should be presented to the child and the family in a supportive and non-judgemental manner, and it may also be important to allow room for prior frustrating experiences with the health care system. If they feel understood and met with empathy with regard to the degree of distress the somatic symptoms have produced, they are more likely to be motivated and actively involved in further treatment. Poor communication at this point risks destroying the alliance and may cause the child/adolescent and their family to lose trust in a whole system approach [39]. This may alienate the child/adolescent, exacerbate their symptoms and lead to renewed search for help, diagnosis and a cure in the somatic setting or outside the health care system by alternative therapists.

Treatment

Basic Treatment Strategies

Basic treatment strategies such as education about the symptoms and the introduction of general health promoting strategies can be effective as a first step in treatment regardless of symptom presentation and whether the child or adolescent has received a specific diagnosis for BDD or DD. It is essential to take the developmental aspects into account, which means that the younger the patient, the more it will require the involvement of parents/carers and extended network (e.g. school and social services) in the treatment early on.

Education About Symptoms

Supporting the child and family in making individual sense of the symptoms based on the biopsychosocial explanatory model plays a central therapeutic role. Step by step, a comprehensible personal explanatory model can be developed, describing experienced psychosocial burdens as well as previous or concomitant somatic illness as potential 'triggers', 'reinforcers' or 'additional problems' avoiding the monocausal explanation with purely psychosocial or somatic attributions. This can be facilitated by a chronological listing of the medical history and psychosocial events on a lifeline starting from birth to present time. This and other simple tools, summarised in Table 18.1, can be used in the communication with the children and their families to obtain a symptom overview and to start identifying potential unhelpful illness perceptions and behaviours that can be replaced with more adaptive coping strategies.

The symptoms can further be explained in lay terminology as physiological expressions (e.g. trembling, pounding heart) of distress (tension, stress, irritability, 'out of balance') by presenting psychophysiological processes with the aid of the vicious circle model on how stress and anxiety can initiate and amplify somatic symptoms. Simplified anatomical illustrations can be used to show how dysregulation of the stress system with an increased bodily stress response and central brain-derived predictions can contribute to the subjective experience of somatic symptoms [44]. Also, information material in the form of leaflets,

Table 18.1 Simple tools to support education

Symptom overview	**Purpose:** Provides an overview when there are several symptoms (e.g. when symptoms are diffuse, fluctuating and moving around in the body). The young person may feel taken seriously when time is invested in obtaining a detailed symptom overview.	**Instruction:** Ask the young person to draw where symptoms have occurred in the body over the past 2 weeks. This can be supplemented with a number from 0–10 or a colour (green (no/mild); yellow (moderate); red (severe)) to indicate the severity of each symptom. Alternatively, the young person can draw a ring around the most severe symptom.
Week schedule 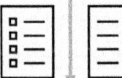	**Purpose:** Helps uncover patterns of potential triggers, perpetuating or reinforcing factors, as well as alleviating factors for the symptoms. These factors are important to consider when empowering the young person and their family to manage the symptoms themselves.	**Instruction:** Ask the young person to register either sum of symptoms or a chosen symptom during a normal week, for example, when doing normal activities. The schedule is filled in during the morning, afternoon and evening with an evaluation of symptom severity marked with a number from 0–10 or by a colour (green (no/mild); yellow (moderate); red (severe)). A few words are noted about what the young person was doing or thinking at the specific time point and who they were with (if any).
Lifeline	**Purpose:** Provides a systematic overview of the entire illness history. If there has been a clear trigger of the symptoms, there is a risk that the family and the health care system may focus solely on this trigger as the cause, potentially overlooking other important factors. The lifeline can help spot correlations between other events and symptom onset or exacerbations, thereby providing a more nuanced understanding of the disorder.	**Instruction:** Family relations (parents and siblings) are noted at the top and whether they have or have had any illnesses. In the middle, a timeline with chronological notion of years is placed. On the left side of the timeline, symptoms, medical investigations, diagnoses, physical injuries and treatments are noted. On the right side, important events such as starting school, the onset of puberty and menarche, major family events. for example, separation/divorce, parental/grandparental illness or death, peer difficulties or trauma are noted. Also, note any involvement with social services, which often relates to psychosocial stressors affecting the entire family unit.

books and webpages developed by experienced health care professionals in the field is an important way to consolidate the information.

General Health Promoting Strategies

More sustained effects can be achieved by learning self-help skills to create a simple management plan and thereby reinforcing the young person and family's empowerment and self-efficacy. These can include general health promoting strategies with a focus on normalising sleep and eating habits, (re)initiating social and physical activity from pleasurable physical activity to more systematic activation programmes and (re)exposure to common daily activities and school attendance in case of avoidance and overprotective parental behaviour.

Specialised Treatment

Specialised treatment should be seen as an extension of the basic treatment principles described above. There is best evidence for psychological interventions with active child and parental involvement as treatment for severe BDD/DD in children and adolescents [45]. The majority of interventions are based on CBT where common elements include further education, identification and problem-solving regarding potential life stressors as well as addressing maladaptive symptom responses. Sessions and homework are used to uncover and explore unhelpful thinking styles in both the child and the family network that may be driving negative feelings, beliefs about the symptoms and associated unhelpful behaviours as illustrated by the cognitive diamond (Figure 18.2) [46].

Accordingly, the main foci for intervention in CBT are both restructuring of negative symptom beliefs and reduction of maladaptive behaviours through gradual exposure to normal activities. As described previously, these factors can be exacerbated by those around the child, for example, the family, the school or the health care system. Working with the wider network and especially the caregivers is therefore often essential. Caregivers can be included as both co-patients and co-therapists depending on the individual family, as perpetuating factors such as within family conflict, parental illness and dysfunctional illness behaviours have to be addressed, while parents are also educated to support and reinforce positive coping behaviour in the child through encouragement, praise and rewards [47]. Parents are also critical treatment partners in order to identify additional environmental factors that may exacerbate symptoms and install preventive measures to mitigate the onset of symptoms [48].

Promising complementary techniques are those that focus on the interaction between the mind and the body with the intent to use the mind to influence physical functions and directly affect health. Young people are very capable of engaging in self-care skills, and there are many body-mind skills that they can learn and apply [49]. Clinical hypnosis, guided imagery, meditation, yoga and biofeedback all embrace this concept where the former has shown good and sustaining results in studies on children with functional abdominal pain [50]. Also, treatment combining classic CBT with methods from the third-wave behaviour therapies such as Acceptance and Commitment Therapy (ACT) with value-based exposure, Mindfulness-Based Therapies (MBT) and emotion-regulation, may be a promising avenue for patients across the age span [51].

With regard to psychopharmacologic interventions, there is no evidence for the use of SSRIs, SNRI and tricyclic antidepressants in the treatment of the BDD/DD themselves in

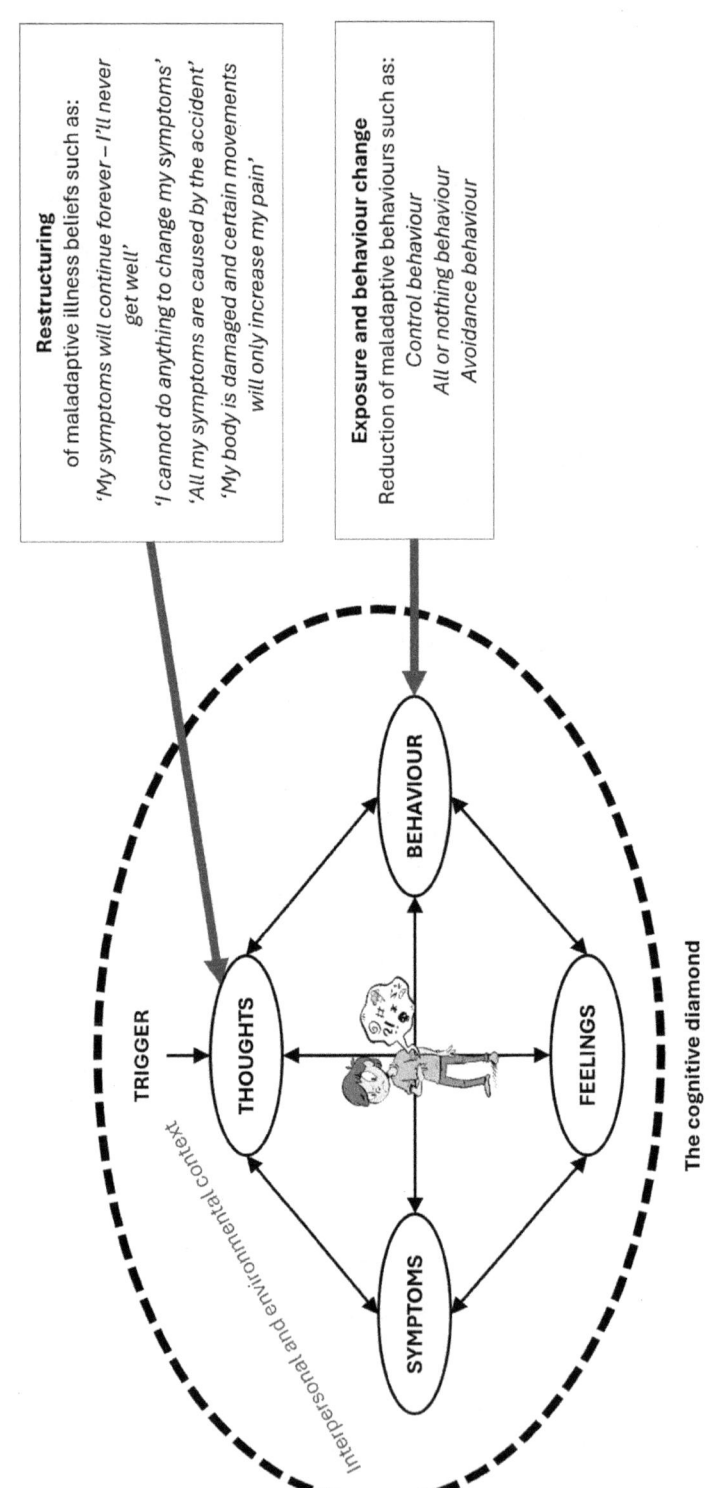

Figure 18.2 Main focus of cognitive behavioural therapy

young people, and drug treatment should therefore be reserved for temporary symptom or pain relief or management of comorbidity like anxiety or depression [52].

Severe cases that do not respond to outpatient treatment, may call for day-hospital or inpatient interdisciplinary rehabilitation, often comprised of physical, occupational and cognitive-behavioural therapies alongside medical and nursing services, in combination with school involvement [53].

Organisational Aspects and the Role of the Child Psychiatrist

The care of these young patients bridges the gap between health care sectors and psychosocial and somatic disciplines and therefore requires close collaboration between general and paediatric practice and child psychiatry. Young people with mild symptoms, not fulfilling the diagnoses for either BDD or DD, are preferably managed in primary care settings in collaboration between primary care health professionals such as general practitioners, specialist community public health nurses and social and school services.

Children and adolescents with more severe, long-lasting and disabling symptoms will often call for further evaluation in the paediatric setting as well as the involvement of child psychiatry [43]. Different scenarios for such an involvement are shown in Figure 18.3.

As previously presented, early consideration of BDD/DD and assessment of potential psychosocial factors alongside medical evaluation can support increased acceptability and decreased stigma of mental health involvement. In this way, psychiatric assessment and treatment avoid being regarded as the last resort when all other medical work-up is negative. Optimally, this would mean collaborative and shared care carried out by the medical and the psychiatric team together, integrating their results and thus obtaining a more complete understanding of the child's problem. Such an approach would ensure ongoing monitoring

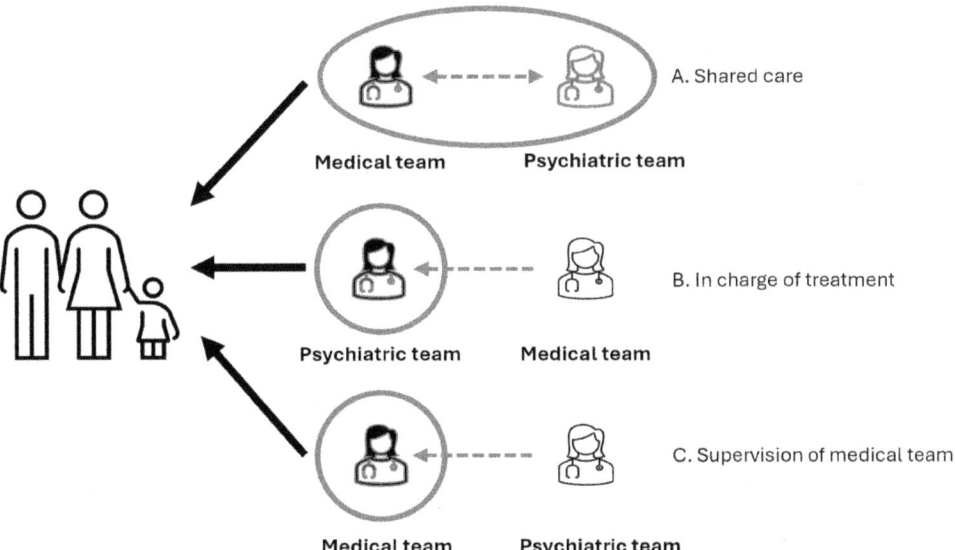

Figure 18.3 Three scenarios for the role of child and adolescent psychiatry in care of young patients with severe symptoms

and treatment for possible somatic illness and relevant medical interventions by the paediatrician (e.g. prevention of muscle contracture in DD or pharmacotherapy for pain when indicated) as well as psychosocial interventions by the psychiatric team (Scenario A, Figure 18.3). In cases dominated by complex family issues or comorbid psychiatric disorders such as depression that need to be treated in their own right, or where more specialised psychological therapy is needed, the primary treatment responsibility may be better placed in the psychiatric setting but still in close collaboration with the paediatric team for consultative purposes in case of the occurrence of alarming symptoms or a change in the illness picture that may call for a new medical evaluation (Scenario B, Figure 18.3). However, the transition from the paediatric department to child psychiatry or involvement of specialist teams with mental health competences can be challenging and difficult for some of the families [54]. Thus, it is not uncommon for some families to remain resistant to mental health interventions. In these situations, the psychiatric team can be helpful to the medical team by advising alternative ways in which they can decrease reinforcement of symptoms and lessen psychosocial stressors (Scenario C, Figure 18.3). The psychiatric team can also help with advice regarding the need for social service intervention in cases of parental or medical neglect, such as seeking unnecessary medical procedures, potential harmful alternative therapies or failing to pursue necessary treatment for additional mental health issues.

Unfortunately, treatment options are commonly lacking within the somatic setting and there are still few paediatric liaison psychiatry services that are able to work jointly together. Furthermore, this field suffers from a general lack of expertise within the child psychiatric setting. As a consequence, many young patients with BDD/DD are offered no or limited specialised assessment and treatment. It follows that a systematised approach to the organisation of evidence-based collaborative care between paediatrics and child psychiatry is needed. This has now been initiated in some countries, for example in the USA [43] and by the Health Care Authorities in Denmark, and could serve as a model in other countries.

Conclusion and Future Perspectives

Young people with BDD or DD are common across different health care settings. The disorders lead to impairment and distress for the young persons and their families as well as high health care costs. The development and maintenance of the disorders may be understood within the biopsychosocial explanatory model with recent research pointing towards an overall perceptual dysregulation. However, more research is needed to understand the developmental trajectories related to BDD/DD, including whether specific early risk factors and gene-environmental interactions determine why some children with early stress reactivity or exposure to negative life events develop BDD/DD, others develop depressive or anxiety disorders, while others remain healthy.

Though psychological interventions can reduce symptom load and disability, there is still room for improvement. Future research could explore whether interventions focusing on emotion regulation, integration of body-mind techniques as well as more family involvement would further increase treatment outcome. Finally, better models for collaborative care across health sectors and the paediatric and child psychiatric specialities are needed to pursue further advancement in the assessment and treatment of these disorders in children and adolescents.

References

1. Roenneberg C, Sattel H, Schaefert R, Henningsen P, Hausteiner-Wiehle C. Functional Somatic Symptoms. Dtsch Arztebl Int. 2019 Jun;**116**(33–34):553–60.
2. Löwe B, Toussaint A, Rosmalen JGM, et al. Persistent Physical Symptoms: Definition, Genesis, and Management. Lancet. 2024;**403**(10444):2649–62.
3. American Psychiatric Association. *Diagnostic and Statistical Manual of Mental Disorders*. 5th ed. 2013. https://doi.org/10.1176/appi.books.9780890425596.
4. World Health Organisation. *International Statistical Classification of Diseases and Related Health Problems: ICD-11*. 11th ed. World Health Organisation, 2019.
5. Rask CU, Olsen EM, Elberling H, et al. Functional Somatic Symptoms and Associated Impairment in 5–7-Year-Old Children: The Copenhagen Child Cohort 2000. Eur J Epidemiol. 2009;**24**(10):625–34.
6. Kallesoe KH, Rimvall MK, Schroder A, Jensen JS, Wicksell RK, Rask CU. Adolescents with Functional Somatic Syndromes: Symptom Profiles, Illness Perception, Illness Worry and Attachment Orientation. J Psychosom Res. 2021;**145**:110430.
7. Campo JV. Annual Research Review: Functional Somatic Symptoms and Associated Anxiety and Depression – Developmental Psychopathology in Pediatric Practice. J Child Psychol Psychiatry. 2012;**53**(5):575–92.
8. McWilliams A, Reilly C, Gupta J, Hadji-Michael M, Srinivasan R, Heyman I. Autism Spectrum Disorder in Children and Young People with Non-epileptic Seizures. Seizure. 2019;**73**:51–55.
9. Lipsker CW, Bölte S, Hirvikoski T, Lekander M, Holmström L, Wicksell RK. Prevalence of Autism Traits and Attention-Deficit Hyperactivity Disorder Symptoms in a Clinical Sample of Children and Adolescents with Chronic pain. J Pain Res. 2018;**11**:2827–36.
10. Janssens KA, Klis S, Kingma EM, Oldehinkel AJ, Rosmalen JG. Predictors for Persistence of Functional Somatic Symptoms in Adolescents. J Pediatr. 2014;**164**(4):900–905 e2.
11. Kozlowska K. The Developmental Origins of Conversion Disorders. Clin Child Psychol Psychiatry. 2007;**12**(4):487–510.
12. World Health Organisation. *International Statistical Classification of Diseases and Related Health Problems. ICD-11. Dissociative Disorders*. 11th ed. World Health Organisation, 2019.
13. Hansen AS, Rask CU, Christensen A-E, Rodrigo-Domingo M, Christensen J, Nielsen RE. Psychiatric Disorders in Children and Adolescents with Psychogenic Nonepileptic Seizures. Neurology. 2021;**97**(5):e464–75.
14. Hansen ASR, Rask CU, Domingo MR, Pristed SG, Christensen J, Nielsen RE. Incidence Rates and Characteristics of Pediatric Onset Psychogenic Nonepileptic Seizures. Pediatr Res. 2020;**88**(5):796–803. https://doi.org/10.1038/s41390-020-0945-z.
15. Petersen MW, Schröder A, Jørgensen T, et al. Irritable Bowel, Chronic Widespread Pain, Chronic Fatigue and Related Syndromes Are Prevalent and Highly Overlapping in the General Population: DanFunD. Sci Rep. 2020;**10**(1):3273.
16. Ottová-Jordan V, Smith OR, Gobina I, et al. Trends in Multiple Recurrent Health Complaints in 15-Year-Olds in 35 Countries in Europe, North America and Israel from 1994 to 2010. Eur J Public Health. 2015;**25** Suppl 2:24–27.
17. Thomsen RW, Öztürk B, Pedersen L, et al. Hospital Records of Pain, Fatigue, or Circulatory Symptoms in Girls Exposed to Human Papillomavirus Vaccination: Cohort, Self-controlled Case Series, and Population Time Trend Studies. Am J Epidemiol. 2020;**189**(4):277–85. https://doi.org/10.1093/aje/kwz284. PMID: 31899791; PMCID: PMC7274189.
18. Rask CU, Bonvanie IJ, Garralda ME. Risk and Protective Factors and Course of Functional Somatic Symptoms in Young People. In M Hodes, S Gau, SG Petrus De Vries (eds), *Understanding Uniqueness and Diversity in*

Child and Adolescent Mental Health. 1st ed. Academic Press, 2018, 77–113.
19. Vesterling C, Schütz-Wilke J, Bäker N, et al. Epidemiology of Somatoform Symptoms and Disorders in Childhood and Adolescence: A Systematic Review and Meta-Analysis. Health & Social Care in the Community. 2023. https://doi.org/10.1155/2023/6242678.
20. Romero-Acosta K, Canals J, Hernández-Martínez C, Penelo E, Zolog TC, Domènech-Llaberia E. Age and Gender Differences of Somatic Symptoms in Children and Adolescents*. J Ment Health. 2013;22(1):33–41. https://doi.org/10.3109/09638237.2012.734655.
21. Horst S, Shelby G, Anderson J, et al. Predicting Persistence of Functional Abdominal Pain from Childhood into Young Adulthood. Clin Gastroenterol Hepatol. 2014;12(12):2026–32.
22. Saunders NR, Gandhi S, Chen S, et al. Health Care Use and Costs of Children, Adolescents, and Young Adults with Somatic Symptom and Related Disorders. JAMA Network Open. 2020;3(7):e2011295-e.
23. Operto FF, Coppola G, Mazza R, et al. Psychogenic Nonepileptic Seizures in Pediatric Population: A Review. Brain Behav. 2019;9(12):e01406.
24. Lieb R, Pfister H, Mastaler M, Wittchen HU. Somatoform Syndromes and Disorders in a Representative Population Sample of Adolescents and Young Adults: Prevalence, Comorbidity and Impairments. Acta Psychiatr Scand. 2000;101(3):194–208.
25. Jans T, Schneck-Seif S, Weigand T, et al. Long-Term Outcome and Prognosis of Dissociative Disorder with Onset in Childhood or Adolescence. Child Adolesc Psychiatry Ment Health. 2008;2(1):19.
26. Kline CL, Shamshair S, Kullgren KA, Leber SM, Malas N. A Review of the Impact of Sociodemographic Factors on the Assessment and Management of Pediatric Somatic Symptom and Related Disorders. J Acad Consult Liaison Psychiatry. 2023;64(1):58–64.
27. Salmon M, Sibeoni J, Harf A, Moro MR, Ludot-Grégoire M. Systematic Review on Somatization in a Transcultural Context Among Teenagers and Young Adults: Focus on the Nosography Blur. Front Psychiatry. 2022;13:897002.
28. Korterink JJ, Diederen K, Benninga MA, Tabbers MM. Epidemiology of Pediatric Functional Abdominal Pain Disorders: A Meta-analysis. PloS One. 2015;10(5):e0126982.
29. Tanaka H, Terashima S, Borres MP, Thulesius O. Psychosomatic Problems and Countermeasures in Japanese Children and Adolescents. Biopsychosoc Med. 2012;6:6.
30. de Gusmão CM, Guerriero RM, Bernson-Leung ME, et al. Functional Neurological Symptom Disorders in a Pediatric Emergency Room: Diagnostic Accuracy, Features, and Outcome. Pediatr Neurol. 2014;51(2):233–38.
31. Walker LS. Commentary: Understanding Somatic Symptoms: From Dualism to Systems, Diagnosis to Dimensions, Clinical Judgement to Clinical Science. J Pediatr Psychol. 2019;44(7):862–67.
32. Henningsen P, Gundel H, Kop WJ, et al. Persistent Physical Symptoms as Perceptual Dysregulation: A Neuropsychobehavioral Model and Its Clinical Implications. Psychosom Med. 2018;80(5):422–31.
33. Kube T, Rozenkrantz L, Rief W, Barsky A. Understanding Persistent Physical Symptoms: Conceptual Integration of Psychological Expectation Models and Predictive Processing Accounts. Clin Psychol Rev. 2020;76:101829.
34. Rask CU, Ornbol E, Olsen EM, Fink P, Skovgaard AM. Infant Behaviors Are Predictive of Functional Somatic Symptoms at Ages 5–7 Years: Results from the Copenhagen Child Cohort CCC2000. J Pediatr. 2013;162(2):335–42.
35. Buchnik-Daniely Y, Vannikov-Lugassi M, Shalev H, Soffer-Dudek N. The Path to Dissociative Experiences: A Direct Comparison of Different Etiological Models. Clin Psychol Psychother. 2021;28(5):1091–102.
36. Ibeziako P, Choi C, Randall E, Bujoreanu S. Bullying Victimization in Medically

37. Bonvanie IJ, van Gils A, Janssens KA, Rosmalen JG. Sexual Abuse Predicts Functional Somatic Symptoms: An Adolescent Population Study. Child Abuse Negl. 2015;**46**:1–7.
38. Brookes M, Sharpe L, Kozlowska K. Attentional and Interpretational Biases Toward Pain-Related Stimuli in Children and Adolescents: A Systematic Review of the Evidence. J Pain. 2018;**19**(10):1091–101.
39. Hulgaard DR, Rask CU, Risør MB, Dehlholm G. 'I Can Hardly Breathe': Exploring the Parental Experience of Having a Child with a Functional Disorder. J Child Health Care. 2019:1367493519864745.
40. Gao X, McSwiney P, Court A, Wiggins A, Sawyer SM. Somatic Symptom Disorders in Adolescent Inpatients. J Adolesc Health. 2018;**63**(6):779–84.
41. Ingeman K, Hulgaard DR, Rask CU. Health Anxiety by Proxy – Through the Eyes of the Parents. J Child Health Care. 2024;**28**(1):22–36.
42. Cottrell DJ. Fifteen-Minute Consultation: Medically Unexplained Symptoms. Arch Dis Child Educ Pract Ed. 2016;**101**(3):114–18.
43. Ibeziako P, Brahmbhatt K, Chapman A, et al. Developing a Clinical Pathway for Somatic Symptom and Related Disorders in Pediatric Hospital Settings. Hosp Pediatr. 2019;**9**(3):147–55.

Hospitalized Patients with Somatic Symptom and Related Disorders: Prevalence and Associated Factors. Hosp Pediatr. 2016;**6**(5):290–96.
44. Kozlowska K. Functional Somatic Symptoms in Childhood and Adolescence. Curr Opin Psychiatry. 2013;**26**(5):485–92.
45. Bonvanie IJ, Kallesoe KH, Janssens KAM, Schroder A, Rosmalen JGM, Rask CU. Psychological Interventions for Children with Functional Somatic Symptoms: A Systematic Review and Meta-Analysis. J Pediatr. 2017;**187**:272–81 e17.
46. Baber K, Rodriguez KAON. Cognitive Behavioral Therapy for Functional Abdominal Pain Disorders. In RD Friedberg, JK Paternostro (eds), *Handbook of Cognitive Behavioral Therapy for Pediatric Medical Conditions*. Cham: Springer International Publishing, 2019, 201–17.
47. Hulgaard D, Dehlholm-Lambertsen G, Rask CU. Family-Based Interventions for Children and Adolescents with Functional Somatic Symptoms: A Systematic Review. J Fam Ther. 2019;**41**(1):4–28.
48. Edwards TM, Wiersma M, Cisneros A, Huth A. Children and Adolescents with Medically Unexplained Symptoms: A Systematic Review of the Literature. Am J Fam Ther. 2019;**47**(3):183–97.
49. American Academy of Pediatrics. Mind-Body Therapies in Children and Youth. Pediatrics. 2016;**138**(3):e20161896. https://doi.org/10.1542/peds.2016-1896.
50. Rutten J, Vlieger AM, Frankenhuis C, et al. Home-Based Hypnotherapy Self-exercises vs Individual Hypnotherapy With a Therapist for Treatment of Pediatric Irritable Bowel Syndrome, Functional Abdominal Pain, or Functional Abdominal Pain Syndrome: A Randomized Clinical Trial. JAMA Pediatr. 2017;**171**(5):470–77.
51. Frostholm L, Rask CU. Third Wave Treatments for Functional Somatic Syndromes and Health Anxiety Across the Age Span: A Narrative Review. CPE. 2019;**1**(1):1–33. https://doi.org/10.32872/cpe.v1i1.32217.
52. Martin AE, Newlove-Delgado TV, Abbott RA, et al. Pharmacological Interventions for Recurrent Abdominal Pain in Childhood. Cochrane Database Syst Rev. 2017;**3**(3):CD010973.
53. Heimann P, Herpertz-Dahlmann B, Buning J, et al. Somatic Symptom and Related Disorders in Children and Adolescents: Evaluation of a Naturalistic Inpatient Multidisciplinary Treatment. Child Adolesc Psychiatry Ment Health. 2018;**12**(34). eCollection 2018. https://doi.org/10.1186/s13034-018-0239-y.
54. Hulgaard DR, Rask CU, Risor MB, Dehlholm G. Illness Perceptions of Youths with Functional Disorders and Their Parents: An Interpretative Phenomenological Analysis Study. Clin Child Psychol Psychiatry. 2020;**25**(1):45–61.

Chapter 19
Psychosocial Approaches in CAMHS

Shaziyah Afzal, Samantha Todd and Paul Wallis

What Do We Mean by Psychosocial Approaches?

Every child and young person seen in CAMHS presents with their own unique narratives, thoughts, ideas and aspirations. For many there may be common features to their presentation, but each will bring their own reasons for reaching this point. They all live within family/care environments that in turn are unique, and all operate in the context of multiple experiences and social environments. The complex interplay between these multiple psychosocial factors presents services with both a richness and challenge in trying to deliver appropriate treatment for mental health need and, through a process of engagement and assessment, practitioners incrementally gain insight into these unique stories.

Psychosocial approaches to treatment are focused on understanding and addressing the psychological and social determinants of behaviour, interaction and psychological processes. Intervention may involve a range of methods including direct therapy with the young person or family/caregiver, providing psychoeducation, enhancing existing strengths and resilience factors, including social prescribing, and working with agencies closely associated with the young person/family.

Psychosocial Factors and Formulation

Understanding the interplay of psychosocial factors unique to each young person we see in CAMHS is assisted by comprehensive assessment, which should take into account the wide range of psychosocial factors at play [1], and lead to the development of a case formulation. A case formulation is a process of linking information gathered over time to produce a tentative explanation for how a set of issues has developed, maintained and fluctuated in the context of predisposing and resilience factors.

Each individual child must be understood individually in the context of their age, stage of development, gender, sexuality, ethnicity, culture and temperament. These factors will also help determine the individual strategies that the young person has employed to manage adversity, challenge and opportunity. Poverty, the built environment, social structures, politics and class will all influence children's development and their experience of adversity, challenge and opportunity. Beyond the immediate context for young people, broader background societal factors including migration, conflict and asylum status will have a profound impact on some of the young people we see in CAMHS.

Family type (birth/care/reconstituted for example), family size, the young person's ordinal position in the family, are all important to consider. Each family adopts its own unique way of functioning as a system and each system in turn manages life events, natural transitions and disruptions across the life-course. Understanding parenting style, parental coping, mental health need, alongside sibling and extended family relationships will also be important. Recent interest in the impact of ACEs has helped to refocus services on the importance of psychosocial determinants of mental health, and led to the development of trauma-aware services and systems [2].

Peer and educational factors will play a significant role in making sense of how the young person's needs have emerged and can be mitigated as well as how they may manage with active intervention. Rapid growth in technology over recent years has led to increased access to information and opportunities for social interaction, via the internet and social media. Although this may have a positive influence for many young people there is evidence of potential detrimental impacts of such ubiquitous access to and excess use including impacts on sleep and affect [3].

Psychosocial Interventions: Shared Elements and Core Principles

All psychosocial interventions share some fundamental common elements but differ in the extent to which these are emphasised across the theoretical base, the aetiological mechanism and therapeutic change elements [4,5]. All psychosocial interventions have an interest in:

- *Behavioural patterns* or the things that happen between people
- *Emotional responses*
- *Thinking patterns* – conscious and unconscious
- *Belief systems* about the self and others, the world, past and future.

There are also well-recognised non-specific treatment effects common to all interventions emphasising the importance of trust, empathy, warmth and genuineness.

In this context it is useful and important to emphasise that the range of psychosocial treatment and conceptual frameworks are not mutually exclusive. Cognitive-Behavioural, Systemic and Dynamic theories for example may be considered descriptive frameworks for understanding the aetiology and maintenance of different but coexisting aspects of human psychosocial experience. As such, despite there being a wide range of therapeutic approaches claiming efficacy and theoretical validity within the landscape of CAMHS, it is evident that there is no one unitary problem it thus follows that there is no one unifying approach to intervention.

This emphasises the necessity of adopting an integrative, multi-modal approach to psychosocial assessment, formulation and intervention. The developing evidence base does clearly highlight that some approaches have demonstrably more effect for certain presentations, but this should not restrict creativity and individually tailored interventions [6].

As seen above the unique profile of all young people seen in CAMHS means that tailoring delivery of psychosocial interventions is maximised by adopting a systematic process beginning with assessment and engagement [7]. Gathering information from a range of sources with a variety of perspectives can allow for a greater depth of understanding of how a young person arrived at the point of seeking support.

All interventions will then attempt to gather this information together, synthesise themes (according to a theoretical understanding/knowledge base) to generate a formulation with a set of hypotheses or a problem description that is used to direct the treatment plan. Developing a treatment plan can enhance client engagement, and provide the therapist, young person, family and other agencies with a clear set of expectations of what treatment will be involved, how long it will last and when it will end. Many psychosocial interventions are offered within a prescribed timeframe, with some evidence that there is an optimum window for the treatment to have a positive impact [8].

Psychosocial interventions all involve a regular element of evaluation, whether this is via client-reported verbal feedback, input from family or other agency sources, or more commonly by self-report routine outcome measures (ROMs) [9]. The use of ROMs is now a regular part of practice in CAMHS and services are expected to submit this data nationally via the Mental Health Minimum Dataset.

Evidence-Based Practice and Psychosocial Interventions in CAMHS

There are a range of meta-reviews of the evidence base for psychosocial interventions in CAMHS, with multi-source evidence for the efficacy of a wide range of treatment approaches [10]. NICE guidance is available in relation to a range of psychosocial interventions, and services and many training courses follow these guidelines. However, the existing and growing evidence base must also be set within the context of complexity. While the evidence base is important in guiding treatment for many defined presentations to CAMHS and helps to define treatment planning in comorbid complex cases, that is, what can you treat, when and where, many young people in CAMHS arrive with presentations that sit outside of the existing diagnostic categories/NICE-approved interventions. Where the evidence base consists of emerging clinical judgement, individual case formulation and theory-based decision-making are also key to effective service delivery [11].

Psychosocial Interventions in CAMHS

Behavioural Approaches: Child-Focused Interventions

Using behavioural change methods can be highly effective for a range of presentations in CAMHS and often may be a first line of intervention. With their origins in behavioural science, conditioning principles and social learning theory these approaches employ a range of techniques to address patterns of functioning that may have been adopted to manage distress or anxiety but have become habitual, maladaptive or avoidant, which in turn can impact on social relationships and opportunities for learning positive outcomes. Some of the presentations in CAMHS where behavioural approaches may form the main focus of treatment include:

- *Anxiety disorders*, especially simple phobias, where a combination of techniques including exposure therapy, systematic desensitisation and flooding aim to enhance habituation to previously feared stimuli or situations [12,13,14].
- *Obsessive Compulsive Disorder* where exposure to anxiety-inducing intrusive thoughts is paired with actively encouraging the client to desist from engaging in previously used neutralising rituals or compulsions. This approach, known as Exposure Response Prevention, can help clients recognise that previously feared outcomes do not occur when they cease their rituals [15].
- *Depression* is often characterised by avoidance, reduced energy and motivation and an associated decline in activity. Behavioural activation recognises that this change in

behaviour pattern in depressed young people significantly impacts on their capacity to gain positive feedback from others or from their relationships, reducing the opportunity to disprove unhelpful beliefs, and reinforcing depressive attributions around self-efficacy, safety and trust, among other factors. Behavioural activation employs techniques such as scheduling to collaboratively develop timetables for clients encouraging engagement in daily activities, along with recording of associated pleasure and mastery. This approach can allow for graduated reintroduction to previously avoided aspects of life, with a focus on amplifying opportunities for positive and realistic feedback [16].

Behavioural Approaches: Parent-Focused Interventions

Psychoeducation

Providing parents and carers with the necessary information to support their child/young person has an indirect positive impact on the child's mental well-being. Formal psychoeducation is recommended by NICE in relation to ADHD [17], and autism [18]. This includes information about the condition as well as signposting to local and national support services, so that parents and carers are enabled to find their way through the network of agencies and processes with whom their child may engage.

Parent Training Approaches

Parent/carer training approaches seek to increase parental skills in order to reduce children's mental health or behavioural difficulties. There are a significant number of well established structured programmes that require training and adherence to the relevant model. Some of these approaches use observation of the parent–child dyad to promote secure attachments, for example Video Interaction Guidance [19]. Others use a group format, grounded in social learning theory, to teach skills around building positive parent–child relationships and positive strategies for behaviour or anxiety (e.g. Timid to Tiger, the Incredible Years Programme, Triple P). Such programmes have good evidence for reducing behavioural and emotional adjustment difficulties in children as well as improving parental psychological well-being [20]. There are also manualised approaches for parents and carers of children with disabilities, or neurodiverse populations. Riding the Rapids is a group-based programme for parents and carers that is based on principles of functional analysis and affirmative support for neurodiverse children and young people and those with significant learning disabilities [21].

Cognitive Behaviour Therapy (CBT) Approaches

CBT combines elements of behavioural theory, recognising that people adopt patterns of functioning based on social learning and environmental conditioning, but also make attributions about the world, themselves and the future. Cognitive theory states that it is not simply events that influence emotions, but rather the way in which we interpret those events. We don't passively receive or respond to our environment but rather actively construct information by selecting, encoding and explaining the things that happen to ourselves and others. Changing the way we think about events will lead to changes in how we feel about those events and/or how we interpret and respond to our thoughts [22]:

- CBT uses both behavioural and cognitive techniques to bring about change
- CBT is a collaborative therapy encouraging regular feedback

- CBT is instructive in that it provides people with practical strategies to overcome their difficulties
- CBT is systematic and at its most effective the treatment can follow a clear structure

Clear formulations and protocols exist for many presentations with common techniques including:

- **behavioural change techniques:** the identification of avoidance and safety behaviours, conducting behavioural experiments, behavioural activation/activity scheduling, self-instructional techniques
- **cognitive change techniques:** diary-keeping/thought-monitoring, laddering, identifying dysfunctional assumptions/cognitive distortions, cognitive restructuring and Socratic questioning

Emphasis is often placed on actively including parents/carers in the intervention to aid generalisation and reinforce change between sessions with regular 'homework'. When working with children, practitioners need to be aware that cognitive development may limit the ability to reflect on one's own thoughts, that is, younger children may be less able to use standard cognitive therapy with better evidence for adolescents. Practitioners may also need to adopt more creative ways of engaging children in process of identifying feelings and thoughts, for example, by using drawing, stories and games [23].

Cognitive Behaviour Therapy has been applied across a wide range of psychological/psychiatric problems with CYP with strong, NICE-approved evidence of effectiveness with *Anxiety disorders* including panic disorder, social phobia, OCD and PTSD, *Depression* and *Eating disorders (CBT-ED)*.

Third-Wave CBT Approaches

In recognition that existing approaches to CBT treatment may have limitations 'third wave' approaches incorporate concepts including metacognition, acceptance, mindfulness and compassion. Traditionally CBT has focused on the content of an individual's person's thoughts and internal experiences, while 'third wave' approaches focus on the context, processes and functions of how a person relates to internal experiences (i.e., thoughts, urges and sensations). Strategies employed in 'third wave' approaches can complement traditional CBT interventions, including exposure therapy and behavioural activation.

Acceptance and commitment therapy (ACT) [24] has its' origins in behavioural and cognitive therapy but is focused on encouraging clients to stop struggling with feelings and thoughts and rather accept that they are appropriate responses to certain situations and that this should not prevent them from progressing with their lives. By learning to accept issues ACT aims to encourage people to commit to making changes in their behaviour, regardless of what is going on in their lives.

Compassion-focused therapy (CFT) [25] focuses on encouraging people to be compassionate towards themselves and other people. In recognition that people with emotional health issues have a tendency towards self-criticism and negative evaluation CFT actively promotes compassion, both towards the self and towards others, as an essential aspect of well-being.

Family and Systemic Approaches

NICE guidelines indicate that systemic approaches can work effectively for a number of different presentations in CAMHS including **Conduct Disorder, Self-harm, ED** and **Depression** [7]. Systemic approaches focus on moving away from a one-person blame narrative, which can be viewed as pathologising, to understanding presenting difficulties from a more relational perspective and looking at how members of the family/carer system may be contributing towards and maintaining ongoing difficulties in family relationship dynamics. Entrenched and dysfunctional communication patterns within a family system can often present themselves as behavioural difficulties for the child. Viewing client difficulties from a systemic perspective may allow clinicians to open up space and explore difficulties from different perspectives, enabling the presenting difficulties to be viewed in a more holistic manner, adding richness and thicker narratives to the assessment and formulation of difficulties.

In terms of criteria for using a systemic framework many young people who are referred to CAMHS may cite relationship difficulties as being a 'trigger' for the problem behaviour. As part of the assessment with young people who have been referred to CAMHS, the clinician will also gain views from parents/carers about what has initiated and what may be maintaining the difficulties for the referred young person. It may become apparent during this assessment process that particular narratives or family scripts are held by members of the family/carer system. These kinds of presentations within the assessment process would benefit from systemic work/family therapy.

Therapy/Change Techniques

A systemic focus allows time and space to deconstruct difficulties from a more relational perspective and explore in detail the perspectives that family members may be holding and ascertaining whether these 'fit' with members of the family system. Highlighting differences within thinking and communication patterns both by the therapist and family can contribute towards generating change.

Amplifying emergent change involves the process of using intentional systemic techniques to 'shine a light on' changes that have been noticed and identified by the family. These transformations are then magnified in order to help the family to notice and sustain these changes within the family context. Once changes have been identified within the family context, systemic models are used to invite the family to participate in thinking about how the changes can be amplified. This could include inviting the family to 'thicken' the story more in order to continue thinking about how the emergent changes can be extended.

Narrative perspectives recognise people's potential to generate and evolve new stories or 'narratives' about their lived experiences in order to make sense of them in a different way. 'Externalisation' is a well-used process within narrative therapy, which has been largely developed by psychotherapist Michael White [26]. Externalisation focuses on separating the person from the problem, instead of the person being inherently described as the problem. This helps to move away from problem-saturated narratives and from viewing difficulties as 'external' to the person and therefore seek new and different ways of seeing their realities (re-authoring). Systemic concepts such as re-authoring, therapeutic letters, certificates and finding invisible friends and acknowledging witnesses [26,27] are used to generate and amplify change for people that is meaningful and enriching.

Reflexivity in connection to self and relationally are important systemic concepts that remind the clinician to ensure that they are not falling into the traps of using linear thinking around young people's difficulties. By listening to others in a collaborative manner, therapists can demonstrate their own process of change [28]. Burnham [29] describes 'self-reflexivity' as 'a process in which a therapist … grasps an opportunity to observe, listen to, and question the effects of their practice … it emphasizes the internal activity of the therapist'. The aim of listening to this inner dialogue is to help the therapist intentionally position themselves in a helpful direction for the family. Burnham goes on to describe 'relational reflexivity' as 'a process in which therapists and clients explicitly engage one another in coordinating their resources'. This is also known as 'talking about talk' and is an important consideration in the generation and amplification of change. Talking about the talk can be a valuable way of exploring how families communicate and what patterns of communication they bring into the therapy room. For example, ascertaining who tends to make the decisions, which family members tend to agree or disagree the most are all valuable pieces of information that will contribute to the clinician's assessment and formulation.

Family Life Cycle [30] involves exploration of trans-generational family patterns within the family life cycle is a helpful deconstructive method to notice and amplify where parents learn their parenting styles from, and how at times these patterns create meanings that are problematic within their own family life cycles. It also emphasises developmental life cycle transitions (e.g. adolescence, older parenthood) that can contribute to families experiencing difficulties at certain stages in life that can cause distress and lead to difficulties within family dynamics.

Action techniques are also a popular method of using systemic approaches with families. Action techniques such as the use of genograms, timelines and sculpts are well known within the field of systemic therapy. Co-creating genograms with families is a useful and creative tool that can collate information and meanings from family members as it 'can show connections, significant events and help map the larger picture and view problems in their current and historical context' [30]. Genograms can enable discussions to take place around family relationships and dynamics in a non-threatening and non-confrontational manner. They can be used to explore family similarities and differences and consider how these impact on family relationships.

The use of systemic thinking can be used by all clinicians and is a valuable way in which to view difficulties from relational perspectives. Family Therapy within CAMHS is usually delivered by qualified Systemic Psychotherapists, also known as Family Therapists. Family Therapists may work in a range of different ways, including working with families or young people individually using a systemic model. There are also the more well-known Family Therapy models, which include the use of reflecting teams. These can be helpful where there is a complex family dynamic that may include comorbidities, involvement with other agencies such as Social Care and/or historical family trauma.

Non-violent Resistance (NVR)

NVR is a more recent systemic model which focuses on working with parents using a peaceful non-violent parenting approach [31]. The usual age range for the children whose parents attend NVR training ranges from 9- to 17-years-old. NVR can be carried out with parents individually. However, it is usually more effective when delivered as a group intervention. NVR Groups are offered by two qualified Practitioners who have completed training in how to deliver the group. This parenting intervention may differ from other parenting groups as the emphasis throughout is to focus on how parents are embodying their parenting practices, irrespective of the child's behaviour.

There are a range of key concepts within NVR that are taught throughout the programme. Parents who report their struggles to put boundaries in place for their child or may describe themselves as 'walking on eggshells' around their child may be appropriate for the group. It has proven to be effective for parents with children presenting with a range of issues [32,33].

Psychodynamic Approaches

Psychoanalytic psychotherapy with children and young people focuses on enabling the processing of repressed memories of past events that impact on present functioning and developing mastery and insight into how patterns of thinking/behaving may be guided by defensive intra-psychic processes. Psychodynamic approaches recognise that people develop defensive strategies to enable them to negotiate various phases of life, particularly those that are difficult. At times these are relevant but in time may become redundant, and for those who present with emotional distress, interpersonal difficulties and unhelpful patterns of behaviour, psychodynamic approaches seek to understand unconscious communication and interpret this in a meaningful and tolerable way to a person. Over time the therapist works to recognise clues to unconscious conflict, exploring the words and actions, silences and transference/countertransference that may allow memory, thoughts, feelings and behaviours that were previously repressed to enter awareness and become subject to conscious control/adaptation.

In CAMHS Child and Adolescent Psychotherapists (CAPTs) deliver psychodynamic interventions, often working with cases where the patient has not responded to other treatments and may struggle to make use of a more conscious-based and/or cognitive style of therapy. CAPTs are trained to observe the relationship the patient makes with the therapist and the treatment, using this as a source of understanding of the patient's difficulties, drawing on knowledge of the range of developmental disorders that can contribute to developmental delay and the ability to work with their conscious and unconscious meaning for patients.

Techniques in therapy are primarily based on close and detailed observation of the relationship the child or young person makes with their therapist, often via free play, drawing and conversation. The aim is to put into words the therapist's understanding of what the child communicates through play, behaviour and verbal expression. This will include conscious and unconscious thoughts and feelings. A suitable playroom with toys (for younger children) or simple consulting-room (for adolescents) is required. Sessions take place in this same room and at the same time each week for ongoing therapy, and the regularity of the setting is an essential component of the therapeutic process and relationship [34].

Therapy involves a range of 'techniques', including attending to *transference* (where the young person redirects feelings for others onto the therapist) and *countertransference* (when the therapist transfers emotions to the young person), *tolerating silence*, tolerating '*not knowing*', avoiding premature interpretations and adopting a stance of interested observer/ reflective practitioner with periodic questions leading to interpretations of observable behaviour. Taking this stance aims to induce curiosity and insight about why the young person thinks, feels and behaves the way they do.

Psychodynamic approaches are usually applied in relation to complex histories and presentations [35,36] including the following:

- *Attachment difficulties* may arise in the context of early care disruptions, abuse and neglect. Many young people who have experienced such difficulties may struggle to develop their sense of self, capacity to regulate emotions and interpersonal relationships. They may experience extreme psychological states including dissociation and self-harming

behaviours. Psychodynamic approaches aim to provide a stable and secure therapeutic environment for young people to express these extremes of distress with an adult who can tolerate challenging feelings and reflect on psychological processes.
- **Working with parents and carers** can enhance understanding of the young person in their care. For some young people who are placed in care settings this can be extremely important to augment a solution-focused risk management style of intervention.
- **Consultation to networks** both about young people and families but also in relation to inter-agency processes can be instrumental in helping partners to understand their role, the reasons for blockages and challenges. This type of consultation can be offered within CAMHS teams, with acute hospital colleagues or across multi-agency setting.

Other Psychosocial Interventions Offered in CAMHS

Cognitive and Behavioural, systemic and psychodynamic approaches are often viewed as the three main organising frameworks for psychological intervention in CAMHS. As highlighted so far in this chapter these frameworks should not be seen as mutually exclusive, and intervention based on a well-developed case formulation will draw upon many aspects of psychological theory.

There are multiple other approaches that have been developed to address a range of presenting issues in CAMHS. While not exhaustive the following are commonly offered by practitioners in CAMHS:

- *Interpersonal Psychotherapy for Depressed Adolescents (IPT-A)* [37] is a time-limited individual psychotherapy for adolescents ages 12–18 who are suffering from depression. IPT-A was adapted from interpersonal psychotherapy for depressed adults. IPT-A recognises that genetic, biological and personality factors play a role in the development of depression, the focus of IPT-A is on how relationship issues are related to the onset or ongoing occurrence of depressive symptoms. As such it emphasises a number of key goals for treatment, including helping adolescents to recognise their feelings and think about how interpersonal events or conflicts might affect their mood, improve communication and problem-solving skills, enhance social functioning and lessen stress experienced in relationships, and decrease depressive symptoms.
- *Dynamic Developmental Psychotherapy* [38] is most often used for young people in cared-for environments, such as local authority and/or foster placements. DDP aims to build trusting relationships, emotional connections, containment and a sense of security. Techniques such as PACE support parent/carers to adopt particular behaviours amplifying playfulness, acceptance, curiosity and empathy.
- *Eye Movement Desensitisation Re-processing (EMDR)* [39] is increasingly used in CAMHS to treat the effects of trauma including PTSD, and other associated emotional distress. EMDR involves asking the young person to think about distressing and traumatic events while engaging in bilateral/left-right stimulation such as following a therapist's finger, hand tapping or drumming. Left-right eye or bilateral movements may help to process the unconscious material, allowing traumatic memories to become less emotionally charged.
- *Dialectical Behaviour Therapy for Self-Harm (DBT)* [40] is a cognitive-behavioural approach used in CAMHS to treat young people presenting with self-harming behaviours and suicidality, and who may show signs of an emergent emotionally unstable personality style. The intervention can be offered in groups or with individuals and consists of a number of core elements or skills modules – two sets of acceptance-

oriented skills (mindfulness and distress tolerance) and two sets of change-oriented skills (emotion regulation and interpersonal effectiveness). In some areas services are able to offer a comprehensive DBT service that includes skills training groups, individual treatment, DBT phone coaching and a DBT consultation team.
- *Intensive Multi-agency Interventions* may be delivered from CAMHS in partnership with other agencies, notably children's services.
- *Multisystemic Therapy (MST)* [41] is an intensive family and community-based intervention for young people aged 11–17 years, where they are at risk of out-of-home placement in either care or custody due to offending or severe behaviour problems.
- *Functional Family Therapy (FFT)* [42] is a family-based therapy for young people between 11–18 years. The therapy supports the reduction of disruptive communication patterns and focuses on positive interactions, effective supervision and boundary setting.
- *Adolescent Mentalization-Based Integrative Therapy (AMBIT)* [43] is a manualised mentalisation-based approach to working with hard-to-reach young people at risk of a wide range of life adversities that include severe mental illness, substance misuse, family breakdown, school exclusion, offending and homelessness. AMBIT is a systemic intervention requiring attention to four different domains of intervention simultaneously – *working with your client, working with your team, working with your network* and *learning as a team*. Much emphasis is placed on the support systems for workers and thinking together as a system to maintain this balance in what are often chaotic working conditions.

Psychosocial Approaches with Neurodivergent Children and Young People

Children and young people who are Autistic, have Learning Disabilities or ADHD are at increased risk of experiencing additional mental health difficulties [44,45,46], for a range of complex reasons. This is compounded by additional barriers to effective intervention, including a lack of specialist training and 'diagnostic overshadowing', by which all difficulties are attributed to the neurodevelopmental condition [47].

The National Institute for Health and Care Excellence (NICE) provides clear and helpful guidelines on how psychological approaches should be adapted and implemented to meet the needs of children and young people. These guidelines build on a reasonable body of work that explores adaptations to approaches such as Cognitive Behaviour Therapy for neurodivergent young people [48]. The National Autistic Society has also produced the 'Good practice guide for professionals delivering talking therapies for autistic adults and children', which outlines helpful guidelines for all mental health practitioners [49].

When Is Direct Individual Therapy Indicated?

Neurodivergent young people should have equitable access to psychological support for the full range of mental health difficulties. The form that support takes should be made after consideration of the following factors:
- Are there setting/systemic factors that should be addressed first?
- Is the young person able to give informed consent to the intervention?
- Is there a good match between the demands of therapy and the young person's strengths and needs?

While these factors are evidently applicable to all young people, they deserve additional consideration with this group. Neurodivergent young people may face considerable challenges and have unmet needs in their 'settings' – their education provision, access to social and leisure opportunities and others' understanding of their individual needs. It will be more ethical and effective to target these unmet needs instead of, or prior to, implementing direct therapy. For example, if a young person is feeling overwhelmed by the social and academic demands of school without the right support, if their family does not make adjustments related to their needs or if they wish to make friends but lack access to supported/supportive social groups and spaces, individual therapy may not have impact – and worse, may collude with the idea that it is solely down to the neurodivergent young person to make the change, not the world around them.

The first line of psychosocial therapy may therefore not be directly with the young person, but with the system around them. Practitioners in Child and Adolescent Mental Health services should inform themselves of the network that exists to support this group and their families: the charities (for example the National Autistic Society, ADHD Foundation and Mencap); the local authority 'SEND offer' that outlines what is available through statutory and third sector services locally; psycho-educational opportunities for parents and carers; and local specialist health, education and social care services. While it will not be the practitioner's role to make wholesale changes to the young person's support system, they may be key in signposting and joint working with other agencies in order to increase positive mental health and well-being.

As with all psychological therapies, the young person's capacity to consent should be considered. Practitioners should bear in mind how someone's neurodiversity might impact on the young person's ability to give consent. Anxiety about the unknown may reduce an autistic young person's ability to meet a new person to start a new therapy or prevent them from imagining what the therapy might look like and how it may positively benefit them. With this in mind, the referrer and the therapist may need to provide adequate information at the information-giving stage: consider joint meetings, photographs of the therapist, information about how the therapy will proceed and concrete examples of therapy materials like worksheets or goal-based outcomes. This will enable the young person to give more truly informed consent as they will have a clearer idea of what the therapy will be like for them.

The child or young person's strengths and needs will need to be considered when offering individual therapy. Factors that will impact on this include language level, ability to understand concepts and generalise ideas and ability to implement strategies either independently or with support. Many of these factors can be mediated though adaptations to practice, but for some young people, individual therapy will be inappropriate for their developmental stage. For example, young people with severe learning disabilities who are pre-verbal, but experiencing significant anxiety, will be unlikely to benefit from a language-based weekly appointment with a therapist. Their anxiety can still be addressed through a psychosocial approach which explores the reduction of environmental and personal stressors, the building of positive experiences and the implementation of calming/sensory techniques.

Where individual direct therapy is indicated, adaptations to practice will enhance the young person's engagement, understanding and ability to effectively implement strategies to lead to lasting change. Before the therapy gets underway, it is helpful to find out more about the young person to aid the beginning of the therapeutic process and relationship – their communication and sensory needs, special interests and any specific do's and don'ts. This can be achieved either with the young person themselves or (with appropriate consent) their support network.

Language and Communication

The therapist should adapt their language and communication according to the specific strengths and difficulties of the young person. While every child has a different communication profile, the following recommendations are helpful for many neurodivergent children and young people:

- Use neuro-affirmative language, which acknowledges the strengths and challenges of being neurodivergent in a world largely designed for neurotypical people, will be a supportive and empowering tool.
- Keep sentences short and avoid multiple choices within one question – give one or two choices at a time – this will reduce the burden on language processing.
- Use literal language – try to avoid metaphors or irony. The young person may use metaphors, irony or sarcasm themselves, but it is not a given that they will interpret these in the spirit intended by the therapist.
- Make adaptations according to the young person's expressive communication. They may not be 'big talkers' – that's ok. Provide them with alternative means of expressing their experience, for example scaling their moods, giving a thumbs up or down, using visual or written means of expression.
- Don't be concerned about lack of eye contact (unless this is a change in behaviour). Unusual eye contact can be part of their neurodiversity and does not mean the person is not engaged in the interaction. They may in fact find it easier to engage when not distracted by the therapist's face.
- Be aware that some neurodivergent young people will be 'masking', that is, using strategies to hide their distress or their autistic features in an attempt to 'fit in'. This can be draining for the young person, as well as resulting in them saying what they think the therapist wants to hear. If the therapist suspects that masking is occurring, they may choose to carefully discuss this and offer reassurance that distress can be expressed, and the young person's neurodiversity is respected by the therapist.
- Weigh up how much 'small talk' is beneficial. For some young people, small talk places an additional social demand upon the interaction, and leaves them baffled as to why the therapist is asking about their journey or what they want for Christmas.

Visual Supports

Visual supports are particularly helpful for young people who may have additional needs in language processing and working memory, and who have relative strengths in visual processing and reasoning. It is important to target these at the right cognitive/developmental level so that the young person feels both enabled and respected. Visual supports can be used across the board in direct therapy. Some examples are:

- An agenda showing how the session will proceed, either using photographs, drawn pictures, 'Boardmaker' style images or writing. The purpose of a visual agenda is to support the young person to keep in mind the tasks of the session; to keep the session on track; to support transitions between activities and at the end; and to reduce anxiety about what the session will involve.

- Worksheets to support psychological ideas, for example on the fight or flight response or to show a graded hierarchy, which may be modified to increase engagement and understanding, for example by incorporating the young person's special interests.
- A 'take a break' card that the young person can use to indicate to the therapist when they are feeling overwhelmed or want to take some time to process information.

Environmental Adaptations

The practitioner should consider environmental aspects of the therapy setting, and how these may interact with the young person's sensory and cognitive profile. Environmental features such as ticking clocks, voices in the corridor and echoing rooms can all impact on an individual's ability to manage the session. This starts at the waiting room, which can be an overwhelming and aversive experience and then overshadows any positivity from the therapy itself. Therapists can make some adaptations to mediate this, for example, enabling the young person to wait elsewhere, making sure the therapist is on time for appointments, having a silent clock or adding soft furnishings to a room to reduce echo, or choosing a different setting in which to work if necessary.

Sessions with neurodivergent young people may be shorter, in accordance with the young person's attention span and capacity for one-to-one social interaction; or more rarely they may be longer if regular breaks work well within session, or if the young person takes time to settle into the tasks. Sessions may include breaks for other activities, often involving the special interest (for example looking at pug videos on YouTube), calming activities like mindful colouring or alerting activities like playing catch.

Using Special Interests

Special interests and passions, unless inherently harmful, can often aid engagement, understanding and motivation. They can be harnessed in a variety of ways, including:
- as a topic of conversation to settle into the session and build the therapeutic rapport and mutual respect
- as part of visual materials to make them more interesting
- as replenishing activities following a psychologically taxing activity

The therapist does not need to know everything about the young person's special interest, and most young people would not expect them to – however, showing respectful interest in the topic, asking a few questions, and remembering what they have already said about it, are all helpful when incorporating the interest into the work.

Use Concrete Strategies

For many neurodivergent young people, concrete strategies will be more effective than abstract discussions, hypothetical examples or lengthy explorations of cognitive biases, all of which may not play to the strengths of young people with a different thinking style. A young person with significant communication and learning difficulties may not be able to articulate their thoughts around their phobia, but will still benefit from a graded exposure programme for something they wish to work on. In this way, behaviour/action plans are often the starting point for the intervention.

Additional Areas of Focus

Direct therapy with neurodivergent young people may contain elements designed to meet their specific needs associated with their condition. These will be formulation based and may include:

- Sessions on developing understanding of emotions. Tony Attwood [50] has produced a number of tools designed to support young autistic people to recognise and label their emotions, as well as developing a toolkit to support emotional well-being. This toolkit may include neurodiversity positive tools such as sensory strategies and learning about the neurodiversity.
- Additional work on meaningful social contact/peer relationships, which is a mediating factor for anxiety and depression, with loneliness particularly associated with social anxiety [51]. The therapist may support the young person with social problem-solving or bring in the wider network to support this need.
- There has been research interest into the role of tolerance of uncertainty in the maintenance of anxiety [52] for autistic people. Uncertainty about the future, or even whether the therapy will be beneficial, may be so hard to tolerate that the young person withdraws to make the outcome more predictable. Specific discussion on intolerance of uncertainty, and exploring strategies to increase this tolerance, may increase the effectiveness of the therapy.
- Sensory approaches – more traditionally the remit of Occupational Therapists, sensory approaches may support the young person's emotional regulation, both in and out of session.

The Future for Psychosocial Interventions

Managing Demand, Workforce Development and Transforming Models of Care

New prevalence data (especially in the context of Covid-19) indicates an ever-increasing demand for CAMHS year-on-year [53]. There is clear evidence that need and complexity is increasing, and there has been a sharp rise in emergency/crisis intervention work along with a growing population of young people recognised as being autistic or having ADHD. Despite increases in funding for CAMHS there remain significant challenges in recruitment and retention, and ongoing challenges for external services that support/augment the work of CAMHS. There is a risk that services become focused on crisis/risk management, and the provision of high-quality evidence-based psychosocial interventions is diminished. As such there is an ongoing and urgent need to ensure that psychosocial services are maintained and that research continues to demonstrate the effectiveness of a range of interventions delivered by services.

The NHS Long Term Plan has set out clear targets for the number of therapists required to meet the demand for treatment in CAMHS, and alongside innovative ways to approach recruitment, introducing new roles and maintaining and upskilling existing staff, there is a clear need to relook at how services are delivered. In recognition that CAMHS can neither meet all demand nor always be the most appropriate/effective service for intervention to take place, the THRIVE Framework for system change [54] looks to redefine the language used to describe mental health need for children and young people. THRIVE takes an asset-focused approach that encourages early intervention, enhancing shared decision-making and broadening the range of practitioners and services delivering care. This approach requires multi-agency and commissioner commitment to ensure that sufficient resource is available to support training, supervision, consultation and system-wide structural changes.

References

1. Morris T. Psychosocial Factors. In S Gowers (ed.), *Seminars in Child and Adolescent Psychiatry*. 2nd ed. Cambridge: Royal College of Psychiatrists, 2005, 238–53.
2. Bellis MA, Hughes K, Leckenby N, Perkins C, Lowey H. National Household Survey of Adverse Childhood Experiences and Their Relationship with Resilience to Health-Harming Behaviours in England. BMC Medicine. 2014;**12**:72.
3. OECD. *What Do We Know About Children and Technology?* OECD, 2019. Available from: https://www.oecd.org/content/dam/oecd/en/about/projects/edu/21st-century-children/booklet-21st-century-children.pdf (accessed 11 April 2025).
4. Frank JD, Frank JB. Therapeutic Components Shared by All Psychotherapies. In A Freeman, MJ Mahoney, P DeVito, & D Martin (eds.), *Cognition and Psychotherapy*. Springer Publishing Co, 2004, 45–78.
5. Lambert MJ, Bergin AE. The Effectiveness of Psychotherapy. In AE Bergin, S Garfield (eds.), *Handbook of Psychotherapy and Behavior Change*. John Wiley & Sons, 1994, 143–89.
6. Bhide A, Chakraborty K. General Principles for Psychotherapeutic Interventions in Children and Adolescents. Indian J Psychiatry [serial online];2020 Jul 23;**62**(Suppl S2):299–318.
7. Carr A. *The Handbook of Child and Adolescent Clinical Psychology: A Contextual Approach Paperback*. Routledge, 2015.
8. Robinson L, Delgadillo J, Kellett S. The Dose-Response Effect in Routinely Delivered Psychological Therapies: A Systematic Review. Psychother Res. 2019;**30**(1):76–96.
9. Waldron SM, Loades ME, Rogers L. Routine Outcome Monitoring in CAMHS: How Can We Enable Implementation in Practice? CAMHS. 2018;**23**(4):328–33.
10. Roth A, Fonagy P. *What Works for Whom?: A Critical Review of Psychotherapy Research*. Guilford Press, 2006.
11. Pilling S, Fonagy P, Allison E, et al. Long-Term Outcomes of Psychological Interventions on Children and Young People's Mental Health: A Systematic Review and Meta-analysis. PLoS One. 2020;**15**(11):e0236525. https://doi.org/10.1371/journal.pone.0236525. PMID: 33196654; PMCID: PMC7668611.
12. Silverman WK, Pina AA, Viswesvaran C. Evidence-Based Psychosocial Treatments for Phobic and Anxiety Disorders in Children and Adolescents. JCCAP. 2008;**37**:105.
13. Cartwright-Hatton S, McNally D, Field AP, et al. A New Parenting-Based Group Intervention for Young Anxious Children: Results of a Randomized Controlled Trial. J Am Acad Child Adolesc Psychiatry. 2011;**50**:242.
14. Kendall PC. Treating Anxiety Disorders in Children: Results of a Randomized Clinical Trial. J Consult Clin Psychol. 1994;**62**:100.
15. Hezel DM, Simpson HB. Exposure and Response Prevention for Obsessive-Compulsive Disorder: A Review and New Directions. Indian J Psychiatry. 2019;**61**(Suppl 1):85–S92.
16. Shenton N, Redmond T, Kroll L, Parry S. Exploring Behavioural Activation As a Treatment for Low Mood Within CAMHS: An IPA Study of Adolescent Experiences. Clin Child Psychol Psychiatry. 2021;**26**(4):1153–69.
17. National Institute for Health and Care Excellence. *Attention Deficit Hyperactivity*

Disorder: Diagnosis and Management. NICE, 2018. Available from: https://www.nice.org.uk/guidance/ng87 (accessed 10 May 2025).

18. National Institute for Health and Care Excellence. *Autism Spectrum Disorder in Under 19s: Recognition, Referral and Diagnosis Clinical guidelines*. NICE, 2017. Available from: https://www.nice.org.uk/Guidance/CG128 (accessed 10 May 2025).

19. Kennedy H, Landor M, Todd L. Video Interaction Guidance As a Method to Promote Secure Attachment. ECP. 2010;27(3):59–72.

20. Barlow J, Coren E. The Effectiveness of Parenting Programs: A Review of Campbell Reviews. Res Soc Work Prac. 2017;28(1):99–102.

21. Stuttard L, Beresford B, Clarke S, Beecham J, Todd S, Bromley J. Riding the Rapids: Living with Autism or Disability–An Evaluation of a Parenting Support Intervention for Parents of Disabled Children. Res Dev Disabil. 2014;35(10):2371–83.

22. Beck JS. *Cognitive Therapy: Basics and Beyond*. Guilford Press, 1995.

23. Graham P, Reynolds S. (eds). *Cognitive Behaviour Therapy for Children and Families*. [Online]. 3rd ed. Cambridge: Cambridge University Press, 2013.

24. Hayes SC. Acceptance and Commitment Therapy and the New Behavior Therapies: Mindfulness, Acceptance, and Relationship. In SC Hayes, VM Follette, MM Linehan (eds.), *Mindfulness and Acceptance: Expanding the Cognitive-Behavioral Tradition*. Guilford Press, 2004, 1–29.

25. Gilbert P. *The Compassionate Mind: A New Approach to the Challenges of Life*. Constable & Robinson, 2009.

26. White M. *Maps of Narrative Practice*. Norton Professional Books, 2007.

27. Denborough D. *Retelling the Stories of our Lives: Everyday Narrative Therapy to Draw Inspiration and Transform Experience*. W W Norton & Co, 2014.

28. Dallos R, Draper R. *An Introduction to Family Therapy: Systemic Theory and Practice*. Open University Press, 2000.

29. Burnham J. Relational Reflexivity: A Tool for Socially Constructing Therapeutic Relationships. In C Flaskas, B Mason, A Perlesz (eds.), *The Space Between: Experience, Context and Process in the Therapeutic Relationship*. Karnac, 2005.

30. McGoldrick M, Gerson R, Shellenberger S. *Genograms: Assessment and Intervention*. W W Norton & Co, 1999.

31. Omer H. Helping Parents Deal with Children's Acute Disciplinary Problems Without Escalation: The Principle of Nonviolent Resistance. Fam Process. 2001;40(1):53–66.

32. Gleniusz B. Examining the Evidence for the Non-violent Resistance Approach as an Effective Treatment for Adolescents with Conduct Disorder. Context. 2014;132:42–44.

33. Newman M, Fagan C, Webb R. The Efficacy of Non-violent Resistance Groups in Treating Aggressive and Controlling Behaviour in Children and Young People: A Preliminary Analysis of Pilot NVR Groups in Kent. Child and Adolescent Mental Health. 2013;19(2):138–41.

34. Hadley D, Kaushal J, Pick I, Roth T, Shulman, G. *The Competence Framework for Child and Adolescent Psychoanalytic Psychotherapy*. Association of Child Psychotherapists, 2019. Available from: https://childpsychotherapy.org.uk/sites/default/files/documents/Introduction%20to%20the%20Competence%20Framework%20for%20Child%20and%20Adolescent%20Psychoanalytic%20Psychotherapy.pdf (accessed 11 April 2025).

35. Midgley N, O'Keeffe S, French L, Kennedy E. Psychodynamic Psychotherapy for Children and Adolescents: An Updated Narrative Review of the Evidence-Base. J Child Psychother. 2017;43(3):307–29.

36. Midgley N, Mortimer R, Cirasola A, Batra P, Kennedy E. The Evidence-Base for Psychodynamic Psychotherapy with Children and Adolescents: A Narrative Synthesis. Front Psychol. 2021;12:662671.

37. Mufson A, Pollack Dorta K, Moreau D, Weissman M. *Interpersonal Psychotherapy for Depressed Adolescents*. Guildford Press, 2004.

38. Becker-Weidman A, Hughes D. Dyadic Developmental Psychotherapy: An Evidence-Based Treatment for Children with Complex Trauma and Disorders of Attachment. Child Adolesc Soc Work J. 2008;13(3):329–37.

39. Shapiro F. Efficacy of the Eye Movement Desensitization Procedure in the Treatment of Traumatic Memories. J Trauma Stress. 1989;2:199–223.

40. Linehan MM. *DBT Skills Training Manual*. New York: Guilford Press, 2015.

41. Henggeler Scott W, Schaeffer CM. Multisystemic Therapy: Clinical Overview, Outcomes, and Implementation Research. Fam Process. 2016;55(3):514–28.

42. Sexton TF, Alexander JL. *Functional Family Therapy Clinical Training Manual*. WA Anne E. Casey Foundation, 2004.

43. Bevington D, Fuggle P, Cracknell L, Fonagy P. *Adaptive Mentalization Based Integrative Treatment: A Guide for Teams to Develop Systems of Care*. Oxford University Press, 2017.

44. Hudson CC, Hall L, Harkness KL. Prevalence of Depressive Disorders in Individuals with Autism Spectrum Disorder: A Meta-analysis. J Abnorm Child Psychol. 2019;47(1):165–75.

45. Powell V, Riglin L, Hammerton G., Eyre O, Martin J, Anney R, Thapar A, Rice F. What Explains the Link Between Childhood ADHD and Adolescent Depression? Investigating the Role of Peer Relationships and Academic Attainment. Eur Child Adolesc Psychiatry. 2020;29:1581–91.

46. White SW, Oswald D, Ollendick T, Scahill L. Anxiety in Children and Adolescents with Autism Spectrum Disorders. Clin Psychol Rev. 2009;29(3):216–29.

47. Lavis B, Burke C, Hastings R. *Overshadowed: The Mental Health Needs of Children and Young People with Learning Disabilities*. Children and Young People's Mental Health Coalition, 2019.

48. Donaghue K, Stallard P, Kucia J. The Clinical Practice of Cognitive Behavioural Therapy for Children and Young People with a Diagnosis of Asperger's Syndrome. Clinical Child Psychology and Psychiatry. 2011;16(1):89–102.

49. National Autistic Society. *Good Practice Guide for Professionals Delivering Talking Therapies for Autistic Adults and Children*. National Autistic Society, 2021. Available from: https://www.autism.org.uk/shop/products/books-and-resources/good-practice-guide (accessed 11 April 2025).

50. Attwood T. *Exploring Feelings: Anxiety: Cognitive Behaviour Therapy to Manage Anxiety: Cognitive Behavior Therapy to Manage Anxiety*. Future Horizons, 2001.

51. Schiltz HK, McVey AJ, Wozniak BD. The Role of Loneliness as a Mediator Between Autism Features and Mental Health Among Autistic Young Adults. Autism. 2020;25(2):545–55.

52. Jenkinson R, Milne E, Thompson A. The Relationship Between Intolerance of Uncertainty and Anxiety in Autism: A Systematic Review and Meta-analysis. Autism. 2020;24(8):1933–44.

53. NHS Digital. *Mental Health of Children and Young People in England, 2021 – Wave 2 Follow Up to the 2017 Survey*. NHS Digital, 2021. Available for: https://digital.nhs.uk/data-and-information/publications/statistical/mental-health-of-children-and-young-people-in-england/2021-follow-up-to-the-2017-survey (accessed 11 April 2025).

54. Wolpert M, Harris R, Hodges S, et al. *THRIVE Framework for System Change*. CAMHS Press, 2019.

Chapter 20
Gender Diversity and Mental Health in Young People

Akhgar Ghassabian, Melissa Santos and Tonya White

Introduction

There is an increasing number of youth in the USA identifying as either a gender minority (4%) or sexual minority (11%) [1]. Reports in the UK bare very similar numbers [2]. The rates are also similar in reports from other countries, such as Canada, the Netherlands and Germany [3,4,5,6,7]. Sexual and gender minorities refer to those who identify 'as lesbian, gay, bisexual, asexual, transgender, pansexual, Two-Spirit, queer and/or intersex' [1]. Specifically, sexual minorities refer to those youth, who identify as lesbian (sexual or romantic attraction between women), gay (may be used as an umbrella term, but often refers to sexual or romantic attraction between men), bisexual (sexual or romantic attraction towards men and women), asexual (having no sexual or romantic attraction) and pansexual (romantic attraction to all genders). Gender minorities refer to those who are transgender (umbrella term used when the sex assigned at birth does not match their gender identity), Two-Spirit (term often used for Indigenous persons who have both masculine and feminine 'spirits') and intersex (term for someone born with primary sex characteristics that may not match societal standards of male or female) [2,8].

With the increasing population of diverse youth in any clinical setting, providers must be prepared to provide a confidential and competent environment that recognises the vast range of sexual and gender diversity currently seen in youth. Working with gender-diverse youth should be established in a setting that recognises that sexual and gender diversity in youth may evolve and change over time. It speaks to the importance of normalising conversations around sexual and gender identity and creating systems that make providers of information on this topic feel safe. It is critical that providers understand terms often used to describe sexual and gender minority youth [9].

It is also important that providers understand the unique stressors that this population faces. The *gender minority stress framework* is an extension of minority stress theory that suggests that health disparities exist in this group because of the unique stressors they face [10,11]. This becomes even more significant when adding other marginalised identities, such as being a racial minority [12]. The complexity of working with this population of youth requires specialised training of providers working in a safe space where youth need feel no shame for these identities.

The reality is that despite the broader acceptance, transgender and gender-diverse children and adolescents still experience disparity in mental and physical health care that prevent them from getting the care they need [13,14]. Therefore, a comprehensive and supportive model of care for gender-diverse youth is required. This chapter will specifically focus on *gender diversity*, any experience of gender that deviates from the typical masculine and feminine binary, and *gender incongruence*, a marked and persistent difference between a person's gender identity and the sex they were assigned at birth [15]. Gender incongruence of adolescence and adulthood as defined in the ICD-11 [16] is synonymous with gender dysphoria, used in the DSM-5 [17]. Important to note is that ICD-11 includes a change from the previous version that includes moving gender incongruence from disorders of mental health to a chapter on conditions related to sexual health. Here, we provide an overview of epidemiology, mental health problems that youth with gender diversity or gender incongruence might experience, discuss care for gender incongruence and comorbid mental health problems, and present challenges and opportunities to create evidence-based care for transgender and gender-diverse youth.

Epidemiology

The number of youth referred to gender clinics because of gender incongruence has increased over the past several decades, with current reports being between 1 and 2% [18,19,20]. Epidemiological data from the general population are sparse, but estimates suggest that the number of youth who self-identify as gender-diverse are much higher (between 2 and 8%), especially if various dimensions of gender are considered, including felt-gender, gender expression or gender contentedness [6,7]. The trends are on the rise for both transgender identity and gender diversity in children and adolescents [7,21]. This increase in numbers can partly be due to increased awareness, de-stigmatisation, widening of the threshold for what is considered gender diversity, adolescent exploration of various facets of identity that were once considered a taboo and better referrals to specialised clinics. The role of biological and environmental factors has also been suggested as contributors to this increasing trend [20,22,23]. This trend translates into significant public health impacts and potential burden on children, families and health care providers, particularly during the pubertal period.

Current clinical data show that youth who present to clinics specialising in transgender care are mostly those assigned female at birth [24,25]. Adolescents who are assigned female at birth also score higher on continuous scales of gender diversity within the referral setting [26]. This same pattern also extends to the general paediatric population, where gender diversity is more prevalent among youth assigned female at birth outside the referral setting. For example, two community-based studies in the Netherlands of adolescents born during the 1980s, 1990s and early 2000s found the number of adolescents expressing gender diversity changed from higher rates of those assigned male at birth, to being double among those assigned female-at-birth [5,27]. Similar reports exist from community-based studies from Canada and the USA [3,4], confirming similarities across geographical areas, despite potential impacts of societal and cultural factors. This over-representation of youth assigned as female is a shift from trends prior to the early 2000s with the underlying cause of this shift yet to be determined [20].

Gender Incongruence Diagnosis and Differential Diagnosis

Gender diversity reflects variation of identity within the population and is not, in and of itself, a mental health disorder. Gender diversity may reflect typical adolescent exploration with aspects of identity; gender incongruence or gender dysphoria; or in rare cases can involve identity diffusion as can be seen in personality disorders such as borderline personality or dissociative identity disorders. While gender identity characteristics often develop in early childhood, in some individuals gender identity does not become consolidated until adolescence or early adulthood.

Youth might experience considerable distress and impairment that results from a mismatch between their sex assigned at birth and their gender identity. Gender incongruence in the ICD-11 (and gender dysphoria in DSM-5 [17]) may be accompanied with a desire to undergo a transition to align their secondary sex characteristics with their gender identity, which may or may not include undergoing medical and surgical interventions. These interventions have been shown to reduce gender dysphoria; and in many, but not all studies, there is also an improvement in quality of life and a decrease in comorbid mental health symptoms (discussed below under *Gender Affirming Care for Gender Incongruence* and *Mental Health Outcomes Following Gender Affirming Care for Gender Incongruence*). Prior to any medical or surgical interventions, it is important that youth have a comprehensive assessment, including assessing for possible intersex conditions and other medical (including psychiatric) conditions that should be ruled out prior to pursuing non-reversible treatments.

Mental Health Problems in Transgender and Gender-Diverse Youth

Data from clinical referral samples and general population studies consistently show higher rates of mental health problems in transgender and gender-diverse children and adolescents. Transgender high school students have a greater risk of depression, substance use and suicide ideation compared to their non-transgender peers [28,29]. In a group of 12–18-year-old youths referred for gender-affirming care, higher rates of internalising and externalising problems were reported by parents and/or youth [30]. Community-based studies and research within the general population show a relationship between reports of gender-diverse experiences and mental health problem scores, including internalising and externalising problems and suicidality [4,5,27,31,32].

In a community-based study of 16–25-year-olds, the gender-diverse youth in this age group had higher rates of anxiety and depression and lower scores of mental well-being compared to cisgender youth [31]. More than 88% of youth in the gender-diverse group met the criteria for gender dysphoria in this study. In a population-based health survey of 12–17-year old adolescents, gender diversity was associated with self-reported mood and anxiety disorders as well as a risk of suicidality [32]. Two other studies, embedded in large paediatric cohorts, relied on both parent and child report of mental health outcomes to obtain more robust estimates of associations [4,5]. High associations between thought problems and gender diversity [5] and higher risk of psychosis in transgender youth have also been reported [33]. Diagnoses of depression and anxiety disorders are shown to manifest earlier while psychosis-related symptoms are more common in older ages [34]. Transgender and gender-diverse youth are also more likely to report elevated symptoms of eating disorders and/or are diagnosed with an eating disorder [35,36,37]. Interestingly, symptoms of eating disorders were equally elevated in birth-assigned male or female and transgender and gender-diverse youth. The co-occurrence is attributed, to some extent, to the distress associated with gender incongruence that could lead to attempts to prevent further incongruent pubertal development. However, studies within the general population and outside of gender-affirming care clinics for children and adolescents are limited.

There are also reports of co-occurring gender-diversity and autism in both clinical and population-based studies. Clinical data show an overlap between diagnoses of gender incongruence and ASD [38,39]. Autistic children and adolescents are also more likely to identify as transgender or gender-diverse [40] and children referred to gender clinics for gender incongruence have higher rates of autistic traits [41]. The relationship between gender diversity and autistic traits is also present at the level of quantitative traits within the general population [5]. Interestingly, these traits are present even after adjusting for increased rates of other mental health symptoms [5]. Common neurobiological underpinnings are proposed to underlie the occurrence of these two traits, but empirical data are limited [42].

Several studies report differences in mental health risk among children and adolescents assigned male at birth and those assigned as female. One clinical study reported differences in mental health outcomes prior to starting gender-affirming medical treatment, showing higher externalising problems in adolescents assigned female at birth and higher internalising problems among adolescents assigned male at birth [30]. Another study in the general population had similar findings, showing higher internalising problems among adolescents assigned male [27]. However, overall, evidence suggests that children and adolescents assigned male or female at birth are both at greater risk of psychopathology.

Similar to older individuals, transgender and gender-diverse children and adolescents experience distal or proximal stressors, such as violence and discrimination and lack of acceptance from parents or peer victimisation at school [28,32] or at home by siblings that can put them at risk of higher mental health problems [31,43,44]. Importantly, these stressors are associated with poor mental health outcomes, even after controlling for a diagnosis of gender dysphoria (if present) [31]. On the other hand, parental acceptance [43], youth perceptions of school environments [43,45], communicated connectedness [31] and religiosity [46] are considered as resilience factors, associated with better mental health outcomes and overall greater mental well-being in gender-diverse children. As a large number of above-mentioned studies are cross-sectional, directionality of the relationship between risk and resiliency factors and gender-diverse experiences remains unclear, with cognitive and attentional biases explaining the link between stressors and mental health symptoms [47].

Gender Affirming Care for Gender Incongruence

The gender-affirming model of care is grounded in the belief that every person is allowed to live in their most true gender [48]. It is supported by evidence-based guidelines from major professional organisations with the most cited coming from the World Professional Association for Transgender Health (WPATH) and their Standards of Care (SOC) [49]. Support for the gender-affirming model of care for young people is not without controversy. As of the writing of this chapter, several states in the USA have banned youth obtaining gender-affirming care with multiple other states having legislation pending. In the UK, the National Health Service has recently published 'The Cass Review' [50], which was commissioned by NHS England to make recommendations to improve health care for gender-diverse youth. The report stated that 'outside of a research setting, puberty-suppressing hormones should not be routinely commissioned for children and adolescents'. While new service model and training resources are being developed, the outcomes of which will need to be evaluated over time. The care for this group of youth must take into account the additional stressors and subsequent mental health problems that limiting access to care will cause.

The WPATH's SOC details numerous recommendations that should be considered by mental health providers when working with transgender and gender-diverse children and adolescents. These recommendations reflect the need for mental health providers to be trained in the unique needs of children, adolescents and family systems including developmental considerations as well as specific training in gender-specific care. As detailed above, and included in the WPATH's SOC, it is critical for mental health providers working with transgender and gender-diverse youth to have expertise in developmental disorders, specifically ASD. In addition, mental health providers should have the expertise to develop both a differential diagnosis and identification of comorbid conditions in youth who present with gender dysphoria or gender incongruence, including conditions such as personality disorders, eating disorders, psychotic conditions, adolescent exploration and other conditions.

Additional considerations in the assessment and treatment of transgender and gender-diverse youth include assessing the capacity of youth to assent for treatment and supporting any mental health challenges that may interfere with the assenting process. As detailed in recommendations from the American Academy of Pediatrics, when working with older youth, decision-making 'should include, to the greatest extent feasible, the assent of the patient' while supporting them in a developmentally appropriate way in understanding their condition, understanding what they can expect from treatment and supporting factors leading to the adolescent's decisions [51,52]. When working with transgender and gender-diverse youth, it is important to engage in open-ended conversations, not leading the youth in any direction, but being there to explore both intrinsic and extrinsic factors that may interfere with providing optimal care. Families should be included in this process as much as possible, both in the assessment phase and in the discussion of treatment options. It is during this process that it is important for the mental health provider to determine whether mental health treatment is needed. As detailed above, there is significant comorbidity between mental health in transgender and gender-diverse youth, but treatment should not be mandatory (unless in circumstances with serious thoughts of harming self or others), based on a combination of a multidisciplinary assessment of the clinical picture and the standards of care.

There are many more outcome studies in adults with gender dysphoria than in youth [53,54,55], and while these studies measure a number of different outcomes following interventions (i.e. quality of life, mental health, sexual function, etc.), the primary outcome for youth with gender incongruence should be a reduction or elimination of gender dysphoria. Gender-diverse youth are at an increased risk for suicidal ideation and suicidal behaviours, and therefore, the focus of treatment in many cases has been the prevention of suicide. While there is evidence that suicidality continues to be an issue, even following social and medical transition, this should not be used as a case against social, medical or surgical transition for those youth who would benefit from these treatments. Suicidal behaviour is a comorbid condition, emerging from either the experience of gender dysphoria, minority stress, stigma, or other factors, rather than being an integral element of gender dysphoria. As an example, suicidal behaviours are three times more prevalent in those with epilepsy [56]; however, neurologists would not refrain from treating epilepsy because there is no evidence that suicidality improves following anti-epileptic treatments. All comorbid mental health conditions should be treated independently, whether there is an underlying relationship with the gender diversity/incongruence or not.

Mental Health Outcomes Following Gender Affirming Care for Gender Incongruence

Overall, mental outcomes are shown to improve following gender-affirming care. However, there are also heterogeneous outcomes in different mental health domains following various stages of gender-affirming interventions. In addition, limited follow-up periods limit the generalisability of these data. In the short term (around 6 months), adolescents receiving puberty suppression and/or cross-sex hormone therapy had lower depression scores and suicidal ideation and better quality of life scores [57]. In another study of more than one-hundred 13-to-20-year-olds referred for gender-affirming care, moderate to severe depression and suicidality rates were lower after a year of follow-up post-treatment [58]. One of the studies with medium-term follow-up (2 years) reported improved contentment in their appearance, positive affect and life satisfaction increased with gender-affirming hormone treatment in adolescents, and depression and anxiety symptoms decreased. Increases in appearance congruence were associated with concurrent increases in positive affect and life satisfaction and decreases in depression and anxiety symptoms [59]. A cross-sectional study of 530 transgender and gender-diverse adolescents found no difference in anxiety and depression symptoms or in gender dysphoria among those who received menstrual suppression versus those adolescents who did not [60]. Another study with a 2-year follow-up similarly reported decreased behavioural and emotional problems with gender-affirming hormonal therapy but no change in gender dysphoria and body dissatisfaction [61]. A longer follow-up through young adulthood showed that time was a key factor in mitigating gender dysphoria and body image difficulties, but improvement in mental health started at earlier stages of treatment process [62].

Discussion

Gender diversity is relatively common in youth from the general population, involving 2–8% of the population. These rates have recently been increasing. This increase may be related to decreased stigma in gender expression, adolescent experimentation, environmental factors, or due to the recent interest in quantitatively measuring this trait. Gender diversity in and of itself is a not a psychiatric disorder, but rather a spectrum of gender identity that is found within the population. The three domains where those with gender diversity overlap with health care, include: (i) the presence of gender dysphoria with the desire for gender affirming treatment; (ii) assessing and treating psychiatric disorders that are either overlapping or co-occurring with the gender diversity; or (iii) to promote resilience in situations where bullying and stigmatisation are taking place. Clinicians and therapists working in mental health can see youth for any of these three situations. As such, clinicians should be prepared to provide a confidential and competent environment that recognises the vast range of gender-diversity currently seen in youth for a comprehensive care.

While research on mental health in gender-diverse youth has substantially expanded in the past decade, limitations of these data influence interpretation and generalisability. Examples of these limitations are a lack of longitudinal studies with long-term follow-up periods for gender-diverse youth and those who have received gender affirmative care. These studies should assess dynamic trajectories in gender-diversity, factors that predict these trajectories and long-term physical and mental health outcomes, including in those who have undergone differing levels of gender-affirming care. In addition, there is limited work on intersectional identities particularly examining gender-diversity in racial and ethnic minorities who may have different psychiatric presentations. Further, more research is needed to examine the longitudinal stability of gender identity, in particular, a focus on individuals who may 'de-transition' or stop gender-affirming services before or after the typical completion. Specifically, were there factors, such as alternative diagnoses or comorbid mental health symptoms that could have predicted the de-transition? Alternatively, it is possible that the experience of the transition is important for the youth to better understand their identity, and they may not have obtained this perspective without the experience. Well-designed studies will offer the opportunity to better understand the developmental trajectory and stability of gender identity. Finally, given the evolving laws being passed around the world, it is critical to study the resulting mental health implications of these laws, especially since these laws will affect those who have greater health disparities.

Higher rate and burden of mental health problems in transgender and gender-diverse youth suggest that assessment and intervention related to mental health problems (e.g. depression, anxiety, eating disorder, etc.) among transgender and gender-diverse youth is imperative. This is particularly important as these comorbid conditions can be treated during childhood and adolescence and earlier treatment will provide the most optimal outcome. That being said, the choice of treatment should not solely be based on these comorbid conditions.

To conclude, clinicians and researchers should recognise that gender development in children and adolescents can follow diverse paths, with each child going through their individualised path. Gender diversity is not uncommon in a small percentage of the population and, except when associated with gender incongruence with a desire for medical or surgical interventions, does not require treatment. However, youth with gender diversity have higher rates of mental health conditions, which may require treatment. Clinicians should be able to able to address mental health issues in a safe environment without immediately conflating the gender diversity and mental health issues.

References

1. The Sexual & Gender Minority Research Office (SGMRO). *About SGMRO and Strategic Goals.* 2023. Available from: https://web.archive.org/web/20250112055807/https://dpcpsi.nih.gov/sgmro.

2. Office of National Statistics. *Data and Analysis from Census 2021: Cultural Identity.* Office of National Statistics, 2022. Available from: https://www.ons.gov.uk/peoplepopulationandcommunity/culturalidentity.

3. van der Miesen AIR, Nabbijohn AN, Santarossa A, VanderLaan DP. Behavioral and Emotional Problems in Gender-Nonconforming Children: A Canadian Community-Based Study. J Am Acad Child Adolesc Psychiatry. 2018;57(7):491–99.

4. Potter A, Dube S, Allgaier N, et al. Early Adolescent Gender Diversity and Mental Health in the Adolescent Brain Cognitive Development Study. J Child Psychol Psychiatry. 2021;62(2):171–79.

5. Ghassabian A, Suleri A, Blok E, Franch B, Hillegers MHJ, White T. Adolescent Gender Diversity: Sociodemographic Correlates and Mental Health Outcomes in the General Population. J Child Psychol Psychiatry. 2022;63(11):1415–22.

6. Becker I, Ravens-Sieberer U, Ottová-Jordan V, Schulte-Markwort M. Prevalence of Adolescent Gender Experiences and Gender Expression in Germany. J Adolesc Health. 2017;61(1):83–90.

7. Zhang Q, Goodman M, Adams N, et al. Epidemiological Considerations in Transgender Health: A Systematic Review with Focus on Higher Quality Data. Int J Transgend Health. 2020;21(2):125–37.

8. Moreira JD, Haack K, White V, et al. *Importance of Survey Demographic Questions to Foster Inclusion in Medicine and Research and Reduce Health Inequities for LGBTQIA2S+ Individuals*. Rockville, MD: American Physiological Society, 2023, H856–62.

9. Rafferty J. Ensuring Comprehensive Care and Support for Transgender and Gender-Diverse Children and Adolescents. Pediatrics. 2018;142(4).

10. Delozier AM, Kamody RC, Rodgers S, Chen D. Health Disparities in Transgender and Gender Expansive Adolescents: A Topical Review from a Minority Stress Framework. J Pediatr Psychol. 2020;45(8):842–47.

11. Bockting WO, Miner MH, Romine RES, Hamilton A, Coleman E. Stigma, Mental Health, and Resilience in an Online Sample of the US Transgender Population. Am J Public Health. 2013;103(5):943–51.

12. Millar K, Brooks CV. Double Jeopardy: Minority Stress and the Influence of Transgender Identity and Race/Ethnicity. Int J Transgend Health. 2022;23(1–2):133–48.

13. Yee JK, Mao CS. Care of Transgender and Gender-Diverse Children and Adolescents. Adv Pediatr. 2023;70(1):187–98.

14. Liu L, Batomen B, Pollock NJ, et al. Suicidality and Protective Factors Among Sexual and Gender Minority Youth and Adults in Canada: A Cross-Sectional, Population-Based Study. BMC Public Health. 2023;23(1):1469.

15. Claahsen-van der Grinten H, Verhaak C, Steensma T, Middelberg T, Roeffen J, Klink D. Gender Incongruence and Gender Dysphoria in Childhood and Adolescence-Current Insights in Diagnostics, Management, and Follow-Up. Eur J Pediatr. 2021;180(5):1349–57.

16. World Health Organisation. *International Classification of Diseases*. 11th ed. World Health Organisation, 2022. Available from: https://www.psychiatry.org/psychiatrists/practice/dsm.

17. American Psychiatric Association. *Diagnostic and Statistical Manual of Mental Disorders*. 5th ed., Text Revision. American Psychiatric Association, 2022.

18. Wiepjes CM, Nota NM, de Blok CJM, et al. The Amsterdam Cohort of Gender Dysphoria Study (1972–2015): Trends in Prevalence, Treatment, and Regrets. J Sex Med. 2018;15(4):582–90.

19. Skordis N, Kyriakou A, Dror S, Mushailov A, Nicolaides NC. Gender Dysphoria in Children and Adolescents: An Overview. Hormones (Athens). 2020;19(3):267–76.

20. Rosenthal SM. Challenges in the Care of Transgender and Gender-Diverse Youth: An Endocrinologist's View. Nat Rev Endocrinol. 2021;17(10):581–91.

21. Wilson BDM, Meyer IH. *Nonbinary LGBTQ Adults in the United States*. UCLA School of Law: Williams Institute, 2021. Available from: https://williamsinstitute.law.ucla.edu/publications/nonbinary-lgbtq-adults-us/.

22. Polderman TJC, Kreukels BPC, Irwig MS, et al. The Biological Contributions to Gender Identity and Gender Diversity: Bringing Data to the Table. Behav Genet. 2018;48(2):95–108.

23. Pasterski V, Zucker KJ, Hindmarsh PC, et al. Increased Cross-Gender Identification Independent of Gender Role Behavior in Girls with Congenital Adrenal Hyperplasia: Results from a Standardized Assessment of 4- to 11-Year-Old Children. Arch Sex Behav. 2015;44(5):1363–75.

24. Pang KC, de Graaf NM, Chew D, et al. Association of Media Coverage of Transgender and Gender Diverse Issues with Rates of Referral of Transgender Children and Adolescents to Specialist Gender Clinics in the UK and Australia. JAMA Netw Open. 2020;3(7):e2011161.

25. Handler T, Hojilla JC, Varghese R, Wellenstein W, Satre DD, Zaritsky E. Trends in Referrals to a Pediatric Transgender Clinic. Pediatrics. 2019;144(5).

26. Cohen-Kettenis PT, Owen A, Kaijser VG, Bradley SJ, Zucker KJ. Demographic Characteristics, Social Competence, and Behavior Problems in Children with Gender Identity Disorder: A

Cross-National, Cross-Clinic Comparative Analysis. J Abnorm Child Psychol. 2003;31(1):41–53.
27. van Beijsterveldt CE, Hudziak JJ, Boomsma DI. Genetic and Environmental Influences on Cross-Gender Behavior and Relation to Behavior Problems: A Study of Dutch Twins at Ages 7 and 10 Years. Arch Sex Behav. 2006;35(6):647–58.
28. Johns MM, Lowry R, Andrzejewski J, et al. Transgender Identity and Experiences of Violence Victimization, Substance Use, Suicide Risk, and Sexual Risk Behaviors Among High School Students – 19 States and Large Urban School Districts, 2017. MMWR Morbidity and Mortality Weekly Report. 2019;68(3):67–71.
29. Perez-Brumer A, Day JK, Russell ST, Hatzenbuehler ML. Prevalence and Correlates of Suicidal Ideation Among Transgender Youth in California: Findings from a Representative, Population-Based Sample of High School Students. J Am Acad Child Adolesc Psychiatry. 2017;56(9):739–46.
30. Klinger D, Riedl S, Zesch HE, et al. Mental Health of Transgender Youth: A Comparison of Assigned Female at Birth and Assigned Male at Birth Individuals. J Clin Med. 2023;12(14).
31. Hunter J, Butler C, Cooper K. Gender Minority Stress in Trans and Gender Diverse Adolescents and Young People. Clin Child Psychol. 2021;26(4):1182–95.
32. Nilles C, Williams JV, Patten S, Pringsheim T, Orr SL. Association Between Peer Victimization, Gender Diversity, Mental Health, and Recurrent Headaches in Adolescents: A Canadian Population-Based Study. J Neurol. 2023 Oct 24;101(17):e1654–64. https://doi.org/10.1212/WNL.0000000000207738.
33. Termorshuizen F, de Vries ALC, Wiepjes CM, Selten JP. The Risk of Psychosis for Transgender Individuals: A Dutch National Cohort Study. Psychol Med. 2023 Dec;53(16):7923–32.
34. Sorbara JC, Chiniara LN, Thompson S, Palmert MR. Mental Health and Timing of Gender-Affirming Care. Pediatrics. 2020;146(4).
35. Kramer R, Aarnio-Peterson CM, Conard LA, Lenz KR, Matthews A. Eating Disorder Symptoms Among Transgender and Gender Diverse Youth. Clin Child Psychol Psychiatry. 2023 Jan;29(1):30–44.:13591045231184917.
36. Ferrucci KA, Lapane KL, Jesdale BM. Prevalence of Diagnosed Eating Disorders in US Transgender Adults and Youth in Insurance Claims. Int J Eat Disord. 2022;55(6):801–9.
37. Peterson CM, Toland MD, Matthews A, Mathews S, Thompson F, Conard LAE. Exploring the Eating Disorder Examination Questionnaire in Treatment Seeking Transgender Youth. Psychol Sex Orientat Gend Divers. 2020;7(3):304–15.
38. de Vries AL, Noens IL, Cohen-Kettenis PT, van Berckelaer-Onnes IA, Doreleijers TA. Autism Spectrum Disorders in Gender Dysphoric Children and Adolescents. J Autism Dev Disord. 2010;40(8):930–36.
39. Kahn NF, Sequeira GM, Garrison MM, et al. Co-occurring Autism Spectrum Disorder and Gender Dysphoria in Adolescents. Pediatrics. 2023;152(2).
40. Dewinter J, Onaiwu MG, Massolo ML, et al. Short Report: Recommendations for Education, Clinical Practice, Research, and Policy on Promoting Well-Being in Autistic Youth and Adults Through a Positive Focus on Sexuality and Gender Diversity. Autism. 2024 Mar;28(3):770–9. https://doi.org/10.1177/13623613231188349.
41. VanderLaan DP, Leef JH, Wood H, Hughes SK, Zucker KJ. Autism Spectrum Disorder Risk Factors and Autistic Traits in Gender Dysphoric Children. J Autism Dev Disord. 2015;45(6):1742–50.
42. Warrier V, Greenberg DM, Weir E, et al. Elevated Rates of Autism, Other Neurodevelopmental and Psychiatric Diagnoses, and Autistic Traits in Transgender and Gender-Diverse Individuals. Nat Commun. 2020;11(1):3959.
43. Loso H, Chaarani B, Dube SL, et al. Gender Diversity Associated with Patterns of Brain Activation Seen in Populations that

Experience Childhood Stress. Front Integr Neurosci. 2023;17:1084748.
44. Hatzenbuehler ML, Pachankis JE. Stigma and Minority Stress as Social Determinants of Health Among Lesbian, Gay, Bisexual, and Transgender Youth: Research Evidence and Clinical Implications. Pediatr Clin North Am. 2016;63(6):985–97.
45. Semprevivo LK. Protection and Connection: Negating Depression and Suicidality Among Bullied, LGBTQ Youth. Int J Environ Res Public Health. 2023;20(14).
46. Wang JC, McFarland W, Arayasirikul S, Wilson EC. The Association Between Religiosity and Resilience Among Young Trans Women. PloS One. 2023;18(7): e0263492.
47. Everaert J, Koster EHW, Derakshan N. The Combined Cognitive Bias Hypothesis in Depression. Clin Psychol Rev. 2012;32(5):413–24.
48. Lee JY, Rosenthal SM. Gender-Affirming Care of Transgender and Gender-Diverse Youth: Current Concepts. Annu Rev Med. 2023;74:107–16.
49. Coleman E, Radix AE, Bouman WP, et al. Standards of Care for the Health of Transgender and Gender Diverse People, Version 8. Int J Transgend Health. 2022;23 (Suppl 1):S1–S259.
50. Cass H. *Independent Review of Gender Identity Services for Children and Young People*. 2024. Available from: https://webarchive.nationalarchives.gov.uk/ukgwa/20250310143642/https://cass.independent-review.uk/.
51. Bioethics Co. Informed Consent, Parental Permission, and Assent in Pediatric Practice. Pediatrics. 1995;95(2):314–17.
52. Shumer DE, Tishelman AC. The Role of Assent in the Treatment of Transgender Adolescents. Int J Transgend. 2015;16(2):97–102.
53. Park RH, Liu YT, Samuel A, et al. Long-Term Outcomes After Gender-Affirming Surgery: 40-Year Follow-up Study. Ann Plast Surg. 2022;89(4):431–36.
54. Mahfouda S, Moore JK, Siafarikas A, et al. Gender-Affirming Hormones and Surgery in Transgender Children and Adolescents. Lancet Diabetes Endocrinol. 2019;7(6):484–98.
55. Dhejne C, Lichtenstein P, Boman M, Johansson AL, Långström N, Landén M. Long-Term Follow-Up of Transsexual Persons Undergoing Sex Reassignment Surgery: Cohort Study in Sweden. PloS One. 2011;6(2):e16885.
56. Stefanello S, Marín-Léon L, Fernandes PT, Li LM, Botega NJ. Psychiatric Comorbidity and Suicidal Behavior in Epilepsy: A Community-Based Case–Control Study. Epilepsia. 2010;51(7):1120–25.
57. Achille C, Taggart T, Eaton NR, et al. Longitudinal Impact of Gender-Affirming Endocrine Intervention on the Mental Health and Well-Being of Transgender Youths: Preliminary Results. Int J Pediatr Endocrinol. 2020;2020(1):8.
58. Tordoff DM, Wanta JW, Collin A, Stepney C, Inwards-Breland DJ, Ahrens K. Mental Health Outcomes in Transgender and Nonbinary Youths Receiving Gender-Affirming Care. JAMA Netw Open. 2022;5(2):e220978.
59. Chen D, Berona J, Chan Y-M, et al. Psychosocial Functioning in Transgender Youth after 2 Years of Hormones. N Engl J Med. 2023;388(3):240–50.
60. Moussaoui D, O'Connell MA, Elder CV, Grover SR, Pang KC. Characteristics of Menstrual Suppression and Its Association with Mental Health in Transgender Adolescents. Obstet Gynecol. 2023;142(5):1096–104.
61. de Vries AL, Steensma TD, Doreleijers TA, Cohen-Kettenis PT. Puberty Suppression in Adolescents with Gender Identity Disorder: A Prospective Follow-Up Study. J Sex Med. 2011;8(8):2276–83.
62. de Vries ALC, McGuire JK, Steensma TD, Wagenaar ECF, Doreleijers TAH, Cohen-Kettenis PT. Young Adult Psychological Outcome After Puberty Suppression and Gender Reassignment. Pediatrics. 2014;134(4):696–704.

Chapter 21

Mental Health Prevention in Services for Children

Carmen Chan, Matthew Lister and Nick Hindley

Introduction

The maxim 'prevention is better than cure' is much cited but one which belies the complexity of implementation of practical preventative measures in health and welfare. Although the importance of prevention as a concept is undeniable, political and investment support for preventative measures in the application of policy and practice has varied over time. The links between adversity and societal problems and the associated individual impact of poorer health outcomes means that the burden of disease, whether affecting physical or mental health, has huge societal cost and underlies, among others, clear economic arguments for a preventative approach [1].

Prevention and early intervention have recently attracted renewed attention with greater awareness of the long-term physical and mental health impact of early adversity [1]. In 2012 the UK government set up 'Health and Wellbeing Boards' to ensure that the social and emotional well-being of vulnerable children is featured in a locally applicable 'Health and Wellbeing Strategy' as a means of addressing health inequalities. In 2018, the Department of Health and Social Care in the UK published its vision for all services to work together to help everybody to 'live well for longer' [2] by encouraging cooperation and integration between services with the placement of prevention at its heart. In the NHS Long Term Plan [3] further emphasis was put on service developments to address health inequalities and support prevention. More recently, there has been further indication that those already experiencing adversity in their lives developed higher levels of mental health difficulties as a consequence of the Covid-19 pandemic [4]. This has bolstered calls for further emphasis on prevention as a concept within health and welfare policy.

The role of the senior health professional in prevention is important and requires not only consideration of preventative practice in day-to-day clinical work but also consideration of prevention in more strategic developments and decision-making. This chapter will consider the following:

- the meaning of prevention and its relationship with promotion
- the impact of early adversity and other theoretical considerations relating to prevention
- some practical clinical and strategic considerations within services for children
- the role of senior clinicians in children's mental health in supporting the application of prevention within their day-to-day practice

Theoretical Perspectives

Prevention and Promotion

Prevention can be simply defined as the act of stopping something from happening. The reality in health in general and mental health in particular is that causality is complex, frequently multifactorial and either unknown or difficult to establish. This can render prevention far from straightforward. The traditional approach to prevention comprises three levels whereby input can be provided to 'prevent' illness; these are as follows:

- primary prevention – where the focus of efforts is on preventing the occurrence of health problems. The target of primary prevention strategies may be broken down further into:

  - Universal (e.g. applied across an entire population)
  - Selective (e.g. targeted at specific groups who may be at higher risk of developing a condition)
  - Indicative (e.g. targeted at specific individuals who are at particularly high risk of developing a condition)

- secondary prevention – where the focus occurs after a condition has been identified and the aim is prompt treatment and prevention of longer-term consequences and relapse
- tertiary prevention – where the focus occurs after the onset of difficulties that may be long term and concentrates on attenuating negative consequences wherever possible for those affected

Clearly in any condition the best strategy would be to prevent illness occurring in the first place; however, once difficulties arise, there are still a range of options available to reduce the severity, course, duration and the 'knock on' effects of such a condition. This is as true in consideration of young people's mental health as it is elsewhere.

Closely aligned to the concept of prevention is that of promotion. Promotion strategies focus on improving general well-being and quality of life rather than on the prevention or alleviation of specific difficulties. Health promotion thus may include any steps that can be taken to encourage a greater sense of well-being among individuals or across populations; it includes therefore the enhancement of means whereby individuals, families or groups can increase their control over, and improve, their health. Mental health promotion would, among other things, consider how experiences, relationships and the environmental context can affect individuals and groups, including children and their families.

In mental health the distinction between prevention and promotion would be as follows: prevention strategies focus on mitigating vulnerability or risk factors for mental health difficulties, prompt treatment of those difficulties when they occur, prevention of recurrence, and on mitigation of the effects of ongoing symptoms or consequences of a condition. Promotion focuses on bolstering individual and community strengths that underpin psychological well-being. Professionals in children's services need to be mindful of the dynamic interplay between the child, family and social environment [5], ensuring that vulnerability and protective factors are addressed as well as the more traditionally accepted psychological or biological approaches to 'treatment'.

This broad perspective supports a shift from focusing on 'what's wrong' with the child to understanding 'what's happened/what's happening' and to tackle wider contributors to, and maintainers of, mental health difficulties. To do this, it is important to understand the impact of early adversity on cognitive, relational and emotional development. Psychological health should be a clear part of every aspect of children's lives, and thus ideas such as 'trauma informed practice', which have come to prominence recently [6], link well with consideration of prevention within health services. From a pragmatic perspective, many theoretical and practical considerations are considered important and preventative; however, it can be difficult to identify the extent to which they might be considered primary, secondary or tertiary in character. In short, such categories could be seen to frequently overlap.

Impact of Early Adversity and Social Determinants of Health

Childhood and adolescence are key periods of emotional, social and cognitive development the effects of which are evident across the lifespan. There are many differing and nuanced opinions regarding what is needed in childhood to promote physical and mental health later in life. These can be distilled into three broad categories: the meeting of basic needs; the presence of nurturing attachment relationships; and a safe, contained space to guide learning.

Following Maslow (Figure 21.1) [7] it is widely accepted that our basic needs include (but are not limited to) food, warmth, shelter, clothes and sleep. These are the key factors fundamental to human survival. In terms of psychological development, the meeting of such needs is associated with improved concentration and academic achievement as well as greater security in friendships and relationships [8]. Such attributes in turn support the development of nurturing, predictable and supportive attachments fundamental to children's

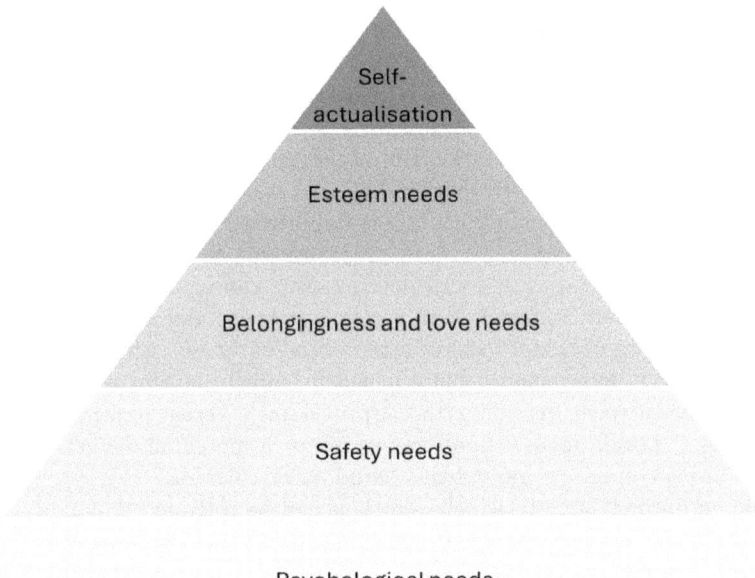

Figure 21.1 Maslow's Hierarchy of Needs

developing sense of self and providing key templates for future relationships [9]; such developmental experience in childhood and adolescence allows for the positive regulation of emotions and negotiation of conflict [9].

When these key factors for healthy childhood development are disrupted or absent then a child's later physical, mental and social well-being may be adversely affected. There is a growing body of evidence suggesting that the presence of ACEs can have a longer-term deleterious biopsychosocial impact [10].

ACEs can be described as extremely distressing and stressful situations that happen in childhood (under 18) that impact upon the family and social environment. The term relates to a study by Felitti and colleagues [11] in which the authors identified ten key childhood experiences which they categorised as:

- abuse (physical, sexual, verbal)
- neglect (physical and emotional)
- household adversity (parental/carer use of drugs/alcohol; mental health problems in parent/carer; domestic violence; parent/carer incarceration; parental separation)

Studies have consistently demonstrated a cumulative effect of ACEs – the greater the number experienced in childhood, the greater the impact [12]. Although it is unwise to adopt a purely numerical approach in clinical situations, it is now widely accepted that the presence of 4 or more ACEs is associated with increased likelihood of adverse consequences: physical and mental health difficulties, poor educational attainment, unemployment in adulthood, health-harming behaviours (e.g. self-harm, alcohol/drug use in adulthood) and premature mortality.

The biopsychosocial impact of ACEs is unlikely to be immediate. McCrory and Viding [13] described the concept of 'latent vulnerability' whereby a child exposed to early maltreatment develops behaviours, feelings and attitudes (such as high emotional expression, hypervigilance and lack of trust in others) that may be protective at the time but which, when adopted in more normative and protected environments (such as school or a caring adoptive home), may appear extreme and be difficult to manage.

The extent to which a child or young person is able to adjust to a safer context will be, in part, exacerbated or mitigated by 'social determinants of health' [8]. The term refers to the conditions and circumstances into which individuals are born, live, learn, work, play and age. Such social determinants include economic stability, access to and quality of education and health care, neighbourhoods and living environments and social/community context and inclusion [14]. Inequalities in social determinants can lead to inequalities in health outcomes, and on general functioning and psychological well-being [8].

Children and young people who have experienced early adversity without the advantages of positive social determinants that might help mitigate its impact can be affected in a number of different ways, including 'threat processing'. Threat processing refers to the process whereby the brain focuses upon and responds to potential dangers. This, in turn, will have an impact upon an individual's 'window of tolerance' [15,16], which can be described as the optimal state in which emotions can be tolerated and experiences integrated. When a child or young person is operating within their window of tolerance, they can engage emotionally and cognitively with their physical and social world. When under stress or when the threat system is activated, a child or young person's ability to tolerate and integrate experience is greatly diminished and they may present in a hyper- or hypo-aroused way. Importantly, a return to functioning within the window of tolerance will not occur until a sense of safety returns. For children and young people living in contexts where adversity is pervasive, basic needs are not met and social determinants exacerbate vulnerability, the possibility of feeling safe and consequently not seeing the world as threatening may thus be significantly reduced.

As noted, this threat-focused mindset will affect a child or young person's perceived and actual social support. Those who have been maltreated are more likely to view others as less trustworthy than those who have not been maltreated [17]. Maltreated children are also more likely to have smaller social networks and receive less social support from friends and family as teenagers and as adults [18,19]. This is unsurprising for children or young people who are consistently operating outside of their window of tolerance because they do not feel safe enough within their environment and within relationships; equally, they are more likely in ambiguous social situations to respond in a way that is considered dangerous and may lead to increased isolation.

The examples in this section highlights the importance of early experience in biopsychosocial development. It is estimated that three-quarters of lifetime mental illnesses arise by the time individuals enter their mid 20s, many of which are reported to have their origins in childhood [20]. A recent survey by NHS Digital in the UK [21], found that 1:6 (16.0%) children aged 5–16 years were identified as having a probable mental disorder (an increase from 1:9 (10.8%) in 2017). Mental health difficulties, however, do not emerge overnight. Understanding key factors across a child's context will help mitigate potential vulnerability and provide professionals with a greater chance of preventing future difficulties. Vulnerability and resilience are not solely located in the child or young person but can also be constructed and determined by their social world and environment. Any preventative or mental health promotion strategies, therefore, must include biologically and socially determined factors as well as considering the interplay between them.

Areas of Focus for Mental Health Prevention

In this section we outline some of the evidence that should require consideration in clinical practice.

Within Education

The prevention agenda (identification, intervention and support, development of positive practice) begins within education settings when a child first attends childcare or nursery settings and this is recognised within NICE guidelines (PH40) [22]. The guidelines acknowledge the crucial importance of nursery education in providing, in many cases, a child's first experience of contact with peers and adults outside the family, experience of a social milieu and the opportunity to explore and learn. Such settings not only provide the opportunity to promote positive interactions and emotional containment but also should be sufficiently able to identify the child who may be struggling in terms of their general conduct or capacity to learn when compared with their peers. Such settings are thus key in identifying children who may demonstrate long-term neurodevelopmental or behavioural difficulties and for whom additional input and support can be provided early.

The recent development within the NHS of 'mental health support teams' in schools specifically aims to improve access to, and provision of, mental health support with a particular focus on emotional difficulties or behavioural disruption for young people within education settings [23]. To date, the level of service provision across the UK varies but the principles are to offer an assessment and intervention if the level of functional disturbance and interference with age-appropriate expectations is significant and to develop 'whole school' approaches to psychological well-being and mental health. The latter are intended to be delivered within and out with the core curriculum and seek to develop within individual young people and their families' awareness of, and specific approaches to problem solving, conflict management, emotional recognition and containment. The approach also emphasises the importance of 'school connectedness' (the extent to which a child or young person identifies positively as part of the school and can develop meaningful relationships with staff and peers [24]). It links with the concept of resilience and can promote this in particular in children who have been described as 'at risk' or 'vulnerable' in terms of their emotional and mental health development.

Peer Relationships

Peers become increasingly important and influential as children reach adolescence, with increased autonomy from parents and carers [25]. Neurologically, teenagers' brains become more sensitive to social input [26], and peers play a crucial role in providing mutual emotional support [27]. Perhaps unsurprisingly, it is the quality rather than the number of these relationships that offers most in the promotion of well-being and prevention of mental health difficulties. Positive peer relationships [28] are characterised by:

- a sense of belonging and acceptance
- a sense of group identity through sharing likes, dislikes, and opinions
- a sense of feeling supported and respected, and with these feelings being reciprocated

Clearly the absence of such factors may also be associated with an increased risk of actual or future emotional or mental health difficulties.

By adolescence, teenagers are most likely to follow the behaviour of their peers and closest friends, irrespective of whether these behaviours are prosocial or risky [29]. For example, in a study where 3 different age-groups – adolescents (aged 13–16), young adults (aged 17–24) and adults (aged 25+) – were asked to play a driving game. In isolation, all demonstrated similar risk-taking behaviours; this state of affairs changed dramatically when friends were allowed to observe: individuals in the younger adolescent group then took 3 times more risks than the older participants [30]. The *nature* of peer relationships, therefore, is crucial. Like childhood attachments, prosocial peer relationships act as a kind of safe haven or 'secure base' from which teenagers explore their world outside of the family home [31]. Such positive relationships may buffer or offer protection from the impact of adverse experiences and lack of parental closeness or support [32]. The converse is true when adolescents are involved in antisocial behaviours with peers who are doing the same thing [31].

While it is not possible to manufacture positive peer relationships, an awareness of their influence and an understanding of the potential effects of their absence is crucial in those being asked to consider mental and emotional health issues in young people. Senior clinicians asked to advise in such circumstances may be in a position to:

- ensure that such factors and the magnitude of their influence are taken into consideration in individual assessments and the process of formulation
- emphasise, when involved in teaching or training other practitioners in the children's workforce, with the primacy attributed to such relationships (and associated attitudes and behaviours) by young people in adolescence; such understanding is crucial in considering meaningful means of positive support and intervention

- promote local community and other initiatives which foster, model and provide acceptable adolescent-friendly settings which promote the possibility of prosocial and positive relationships

Family Relationships

Mental health difficulties and environmental stressors affecting parents have consistently been shown to have detrimental effects on children's well-being and development. Such effects were observed in both fathers and mothers. Phares et al [33] found that children's later emotional and behavioural needs were significantly determined by paternal mental health, even after controlling for maternal mental health. Parental mental health difficulties are linked to children having greater struggles with problem solving and with feelings of helplessness and hopelessness [34]. Furthermore, in social situations, children of parents with mental health difficulties display less active and exploratory play and have more generalised negative feelings towards peers [35].

The wider home context, beyond the effects of parental mental health and well-being, is a further family element which should be considered in terms of children's future health and development. Thus, homes where the atmosphere is characterised by high levels of conflict, difficulties with open communication, and lack of consistent responses are likely to have negative effects even beyond the impact of experience of early adversity or abuse [8]. Conversely and unsurprisingly, safe and nurturing familial attachment relationships, particularly parental/carer relationships, have been consistently found to promote mental and psychological well-being [36]. Relationships within the home that are emotionally attuned and offer clear and consistent boundaries provide the foundations for inter- and intra-personal qualities that build psychological resilience [37] as do a family's ability to solve problems together and to communicate openly [38]. Supportive relationships also buffer against the deleterious impact of adversity and abuse [39]. For example, children with mothers who are described as more supportive report feeling less affected by day-to-day stressors [40] and such characteristics have also been found to act to mitigate against the negative impact of crime and drug use [41].

There are some key underlying familial factors that underlie mental health prevention and the promotion of mental well-being and a range of parenting interventions that are offered to families to improve parent and child relationships (although this may vary across geographical areas). Again, such interventions can be considered to correspond to several of the formalised categories of prevention. Most of the well-established and evidence-based programmes (such as 'The Incredible Years' [42] and 'Triple P' [43]) are manualised and include focus on behaviour management, building strengths and relationship-building. There is a broad base of literature which emphasises the role of building attachments within families [44] and there are a number of psychotherapeutically informed approaches which focus on relationship building, such as Dyadic Developmental Psychotherapy (DDP) and 'video interactive guidance' (VIG) are popular and have a growing evidence-base. VIG is noted as an effective intervention within the NICE guidelines for adopted and cared for children [45]. Practical steps that can be taken include the following:

- ensuring a joined-up approach between children and adult services in terms of addressing children's emotional and mental health needs within a context of familial adversity; consider including 'Think Family' [46] or similar approaches as part of service design and remits

- establishing joint initiatives with other agencies and organisations to ensure coordinated provision for children, parents and families to avoid parallel process, gaps in provision and ensure access for professionals of appropriate advice supervision and support
- promoting a wider systems approach to addressing familial adversity based on accepted hierarchies of need [5,7] rather than individual psychopathology within families
- being clear about the role of family aspects in assessment
- considering whether flexible systemically-informed family work in such circumstances may be more acceptable, appropriate and effective than a more formal family therapy approach – i.e. favouring what is 'therapeutic' rather 'Therapy'
- supporting guided learning rather than mere provision of written or web-based or 'signposting' for struggling families

Individual Factors

Some individual qualities in children, which may have shaped by their experiences, can be fostered to promote well-being, prevent further deterioration if difficulties do arise, or to even act as an 'inoculation' in the face of adversity.

How a child views the future is important in considering future psychological well-being and prevention of later risk. A sense of hopelessness has been shown to predict future risk of self-harm and suicide in adolescents [47,48] and to predict other areas of risk including violence, substance use, sexual activity, and accidental injury in low-income inner city adolescents [49]. The most important aspect of hopelessness that seems to lead to increased risk appears not to be the expectation that a lot of negative events are likely to occur, but rather, the looking into the future and *not* feeling able to see anything positive [50]. In other words, seeing the future as empty rather than simply 'bad' is more likely to have a negative impact on mental health and increase future risk. Therefore, coping and ability to cope is something to be supported. Furthermore, the means whereby children learn to manage difficulties and conflict that will inevitably arise in life is clearly important. The ability to solve problems is linked to resilience in the face of adversity, with social problem-solving skills reducing the risk of suicide in females who have experienced abuse [51].

Consistently, having a hobby, skill or interest that is highly valued by the child is seen as a protective factor. This is true irrespective of whether a child is seen to come from a low or high-risk environment [28]. It seems that involvement in prosocial activities or in education/work are important protective factors, however, it is not the mere involvement in activities that is important. The key is for the child to feel that they are taking part in something that aligns with what they feel is personally important or valuable [52], which is what offers children and young people a sense of self-efficacy, self-esteem, and self-worth. Practical prevention in individual cases might therefore include:

- provision of the opportunity for all children and young people to explore what *they* are good at and what *they* feel is personally meaningful and, therefore, increasing hopefulness
- support for development of problem-solving skills
- approaches that support young people to cope following a specific difficult incident (e.g. psychological first aid or first line incident responses)

Safeguarding Children

The structures that exist within children's welfare practice also reflect the differing levels of preventative practice outlined earlier. Such structures exist in slightly different forms in most developed countries. In England and Wales such provision takes place within the statutory framework of The Children Act [53]. This is the most powerful statutory legislation governing the welfare of children and young people. The requirements of the act are largely coordinated by local authorities via social care departments of children's services in conjunction with the police and other agencies and organisations. The scope of intervention supported by the Children Act [53] reflects the degree to which a child's welfare is considered to be being placed at risk and varies from 'Early Help' (where a child and family are identified to be at risk of possible future harm and are in need of preventative care and support), through increasingly formalised and interventive statutory processes that respond to perceived levels of actual harm to the child ('Child in Need', 'Child Protection', entry into 'care of the local authority'). Remedial efforts within such situations are both child and family-orientated and there is a statutory duty for active health service participation in such endeavours. Such responsibilities and practice requirements are set out clearly in the overview document, 'Working Together to Safeguard Children' [54].

There are good reasons why safeguarding process should be seen as a key component of the remit of senior professionals working with children with emotional or mental health difficulties. Children subject to such process have frequently experienced disproportionate adversity and their families frequently experience a wide range of socio-economic difficulties or may be poorly equipped themselves to remedy maladaptive emotions and behaviours. Such situations are frequently complex and raise questions about mental health need and possible intervention at a juncture when children's emotional presentations give cause for considerable professional concern. Frequently children in such situations have not benefited from assessment, which has included informed and experienced mental health input (whether by advice, formal professional consultation or direct assessment) and if this is not available, questions and uncertainty prevail. In addition, children in such situations are recognised to have significant mental health needs [55]. Finally, referrals are frequently made to mental health services for children and families who, on assessment, are identified to have significant, hitherto unrecognised welfare needs. 'Escalation' of such needs in these circumstances can prove difficult and the involvement of a senior clinician can help facilitate this.

Active participation and understanding of the safeguarding process can thus represent important considerations in relation to identification and prevention of emotional/mental health difficulties and should not be seen as simply the remit of social work colleagues. For this aspect of their work clinicians will need:

- to understand relevant statutory safeguarding practice and expectations relating to it
- to be willing to participate in a collaborative way and advise about the extent to which formal mental health provision might be required
- to be willing to have a low threshold with regard to the need for initial assessment and cross-agency formulation of cases where high levels of emotional and behavioural difficulty are giving cause for professional concern
- to be willing to persist in situations where escalation of significant welfare needs is proving difficult

Strategic and Practice Considerations

Strategic Issues

In services working with children, good prevention approaches are likely to involve mutual understanding and cooperation between a range of agencies both at a strategic and at individual case-based levels. Such endeavours are likely to encompass the full range of primary, secondary and tertiary approaches and include some attention to concepts of health promotion. At a wider systemic level this is likely to require significant alignment not just at a day-to-day 'operational' level but also in terms of policy and political prioritisation; and the need for consensus in this is important. It is frequently the case that the impetus for new approaches is derived from a sudden and serious crisis event rather than a more considered and coordinated manner over time.

At a local level there exist early intervention or prevention strategies usually coordinated by public health clinicians in conjunction with a range of local providers, including local authorities, health, youth justice and the voluntary and community sector (also known as 'third sector' providers). It is important that senior clinicians and other senior professionals across agencies are aware of and able to contribute to such a strategy so that there is a clear bridge between strategic thinking and operational practice; only too frequently does such planning and strategy development take place separately from those involved in day-to-day practice. Accordingly, many senior clinicians remain unaware of the central tenets of local and wider systemic prevention policy, which in general is the remit at a local authority level of 'Health and Wellbeing Boards' [56]. This systems approach to prevention is essential and is likely to require longer-term strategic thinking rather than emphases on short-term projects and quick results. In line with the above it would seem important that senior clinicians within services focusing on child mental health:

- should be aware of local and wider prevention strategies, where they, along with the governance structure behind them, are agreed and overseen
- should be aware that prevention as a concept overlaps with, rather than is clearly separated from, day to day 'treatment' and 'intervention'
- should understand that much of their day-to-day work has or could have significant preventative benefits for children and young people
- should seek to emphasise and recognise the importance of the contribution made towards positive emotional and mental health made by services other than formal Children and Adolescent Mental Health Services (CAMHS) (such as schools, alternative educational provision, residential care, youth workers and the voluntary and community sector and others)
- should seek, wherever possible in practice, to develop good relationships and joint thinking across agencies to facilitate future collaborative endeavour

Practice Considerations

It is important to reiterate the degree to which, in clinical practice, it can be difficult for clinicians to appreciate the extent or nature of the contribution that they or their team may be making towards prevention. Formulation of a particular clinical situation is at the heart of good clinical practice and is instrumental in terms of formulating 'treatment' and ongoing care-planning. In the authors' experience, preventative aspects within formulation can be overlooked in favour of whatever immediate treatment and management of risk is considered necessary for the child under consideration.

Frequently, as with strategic policy at a governmental level, short-term needs and goals can be prioritised in favour of longer-term aspects and wider systemic considerations that could have particular preventative benefits. The development of a good formulation is a task requiring considerable clinical theoretical awareness and experience, particularly in complex situations where family and cross-agency professional consensus is required; the task is one which is frequently in the remit of the senior mental health clinician, and their ability to provide clarity about the necessary components of a formulation as well as support to others to contribute to it is likely to be instrumental. From a prevention perspective within the formulation process clinicians will need to give consideration to:

- longer-term considerations beyond the immediate need for 'treatment' and so a focus on longitudinal formulation alongside more immediate understandings
- consideration of issues relating to a child's particular vulnerabilities and strengths (and those of the family, community and professional system around them) and how these may be addressed beyond the immediate mental health 'problem'
- making use of accepted theoretical perspectives (traditionally associated with prevention): what has happened (e.g. ACEs); the wider context (e.g. social determinants of health); the coping capacity of the child, family or wider system (e.g. with reference to 'health harming behaviours')

Consideration of prevention of future emotional or mental health difficulties in the individual child can be complex. A dimensional approach when considering individual needs rather than an either/or linear conceptual framework is likely to be required. Such an approach is likely to require consideration of interactions between differing theoretical frameworks (for example, existing evidence about ACEs and theories of resilience), appreciation of the range of potential influences on the child or family in individual cases and some understanding of the concept of prevention in its various forms. It may also require flexibility of approach from the senior mental health clinician in terms of the types of roles that they may need to play in different circumstances. This flexibility of approach is perhaps the area of practice that is often overlooked as it demands less of the general clinical practice awareness but more on the positions or standpoints that need to be taken.

The key message for experienced and senior clinicians working with individual cases is that there is overlap between traditional treatment and prevention-informed practice and that the preventative component can best be sustained by the adoption of a flexible and systemically informed approach. Aspects of such an approach include:

- ability to support professional networks with key and frequently interconnecting theoretical concepts
- willingness to adapt involvement to include the wider systemic needs of the situation and to consider broadening definitions of 'treatment' and 'intervention' to include advisory and professional consultation and formulation skills as well as more traditional accepted forms of mental health input
- keeping the notions of treatment and prevention in mind in line with the acknowledged overlap between the respective theoretical concepts

In light of the above, the following practice considerations may be helpful to senior clinicians seeking to ensure better outcomes:

- identification of the child (often quite young) who is going to have long-term emotional difficulties and maintaining oversight to support professionals from other agencies.
- facilitation of accessibility to advice or consultative support and recognition of the importance of such input when direct involvement may not be appropriate or helpful.
- paying attention to language and ensuring mutual understanding in complex cross-agency situations and with families – avoiding descriptions of children with severe emotional or mental health difficulties as 'not having a mental health problem' or as having 'behavioural' (as opposed to complex emotional) problems.
- participating wherever necessary in key cross-agency processes such as 'child in need', 'child protection' or 'looked after children' core groups and meetings, special educational needs and youth justice processes.
- understanding the statutory landscape as it affects children, young people and their families beyond formal mental health or mental capacity legislation: being familiar with (or knowing who to ask about) welfare, educational or youth justice processes and statutory provision.
- understanding how key organisations function in local areas (familiarity with formal protocols) and also seeking to establish positive relationships with senior colleagues in other agencies (social care, education, youth justice, voluntary and community sector). This should be done where possible outside of crisis situations but in preparation for them on the basis that relationships are frequently more helpful than protocols in such circumstances.
- engagement with mental health and joint mental health/social care commissioners.
- understanding of the value of escalation of concern and safeguarding issues and realisation that this may require a senior experienced clinician in contentious or 'stuck' situations.
- awareness that professional disputes about complex cases frequently have a harmful effect on the child or family involved and that seeking to address these wherever possible in a courteous and respectful way may be particularly helpful.
- awareness of the value attached to senior clinical involvement in complex and risky situations (containing anxiety) and also of the value of supporting a situation being managed in a way that is proportionate or 'good enough' as opposed to ideal solutions being sought from elsewhere that may not be feasible or helpful.
- advocacy/facilitation of access when a young person or family with clear needs have apparently been denied access to a service without a clear reason or where there is evidence to suggest that they require such a service.

Conclusion

There is a tendency for prevention to be regarded as the business of professionals other than clinicians working in day-to-day clinical situations: these may include commissioners, public health practitioners and health and well-being teams. However, the theoretical perspectives that have been outlined in this chapter would seem to offer considerable opportunities for preventative thinking to inform and add interest to the role of the senior clinician in a way that is likely to benefit children, their families and other professionals. In many ways it could be seen as integral to the role of senior clinicians to be considering such matters and, should they do so, they will be well placed to be able to do this in the light of their professional experience and understanding not only of individual presentations but also of wider family and systemic factors that may influence outcomes for young people.

References

1. Marmot M. Health Equity in England: The Marmot Review 10 Years On. BMJ. 2020 Feb 25;368.
2. HM Government. *Government Response to Consultation on Transforming Children and Young People's Mental Health*. London: HM Government, 2018. Available from: https://assets.publishing.service.gov.uk/government/uploads/system/uploads/attachment_data/file/728892/government-response-to-consultation-on-transforming-children-and-young-peoples-mental-health.pdf.
3. Department of Health. *The NHS Long Term Plan*. Department of Health, 2019. Available from: https://www.longtermplan.nhs.uk/.
4. Creswell C. Editorial Perspective: Rapid responses to understand and address children and young people's mental health in the context of COVID-19. Journal of Child Psychology and Psychiatry. 2022 May 4;**64**(1):209–11.
5. Bronfenbrenner U. *Ecological Systems Theory*. London: Jessica Kingsley Publishers, 1992.
6. NHS Scotland. *Trauma Informed Practice : A Toolkit for Scotland*. NHS Scotland, 2021.
7. Maslow A. A Theory of Human Motivation. Psychological Review. 1943;**50**:371. Available at: https://psychclassics.yorku.ca/Maslow/motivation.htm.
8. Allen A, Donkin A. Adverse Childhood Experiences. In M Bush (ed.), *Addressing Adversity*. London: Young Minds and NHS Health Education England, 2018, 58–80.
9. Gerhardt S. *Why Love Matters – How Affection Shapes a Baby's Brain*. London: Routledge, 2004.
10. Petruccelli K, Davis J, Berman T. Adverse Childhood Experiences and Associated Health Outcomes: A Systematic Review and Meta-analysis. Child Abuse & Neglect. 2019 Nov 1;**97**:104127.
11. Felitti VJ, Anda RF, Nordenberg D, Et al. Relationship of Childhood Abuse and Household Dysfunction to Many of the Leading Causes of Death in Adults: The Adverse Childhood Experiences (ACE) Study. American Journal of Preventive Medicine. 1998 May 1;**14**(4):245–58.
12. Herzog JI, Schmahl C. Adverse Childhood Experiences and the Consequences on Neurobiological, Psychosocial, and Somatic Conditions Across the Lifespan. Front Psychiatry. 2018 Sep 4;**9**:420.
13. McCrory EJ, Viding E. The Theory of Latent Vulnerability: Reconceptualizing the Link Between Childhood Maltreatment and Psychiatric Disorder. Development and Psychopathology. 2015 May;**27**(2):493–505.
14. Department of Health. *Prevention Is Better than Cure: Our Vision to Help You Live Well for Longer*. Department of Health, 2018.
15. Siegel DJ. *The Developing Mind: Toward a Neurobiology of Interpersonal Experience*. New York: Guilford Press, 1999.
16. Ogden P, Minton K, Pain C. *Trauma and the Body: A sensorimotor Approach to Psychotherapy*. Norton Series on Interpersonal Neurobiology. New York: W. W. Norton & Company, 2006 Oct 17.
17. Neil L, Viding E, Armbruster-Genc D, et al. Trust and Childhood Maltreatment: Evidence of Bias in Appraisal of Unfamiliar Faces. Journal of Child Psychology and Psychiatry. 2022 Jun;**63**(6):655–62.
18. Matthews T, Danese A, Caspi A, et al. Lonely Young Adults in Modern Britain: Findings from an Epidemiological Cohort Study. Psychological Medicine. 2019 Jan;**49**(2):268–77.
19. Hanlon P, McCallum M, Jani BD, McQueenie R, Lee D, Mair FS. Association Between Childhood Maltreatment and the Prevalence and Complexity of Multimorbidity: A Cross-Sectional Analysis of 157,357 UK Biobank

Participants. Journal of Comorbidity. 2020 Jul 31;**10**:2235042X10944344.

20. Royal College of Psychiatrists. *No Health Without Mental Health: The Case for Action. Position Statement PS4*. London: Royal College of Psychiatrists, 2010.

21. NHS Digital. *Mental Health of Children and Young People in England 2021. Wave 2 Follow Up to the 2017 Survey*. London: NHS Digital, 2021. Available from: https://digital.nhs.uk/data-and-information/publications/statistical/mental-health-of-children-and-young-people-in-england/2021-follow-up-to-the-2017-survey.

22. NICE. *Public Health Guideline [PH40]. Social and Emotional Wellbeing: Early Years*. 2012.

23. HM Government. *Working Together to Safeguard Children. Statutory Framework: Legislation Relevant to Safeguarding and Promoting the Welfare of Children*. London: HM Government, 2018.

24. Thompson DR, Iachan R, Overpeck M, Ross JG, Gross LA. School Connectedness in the Health Behavior in School-Aged Children Study: The Role of Student, School, and School Neighborhood Characteristics. Journal of School Health. 2006 Sep;**76**(7):379–86.

25. Allen JP. The Attachment System in Adolescence. In J Cassidy, PR Shaver (eds.), *Handbook of Attachment: Theory, Research, and Clinical Applications*. New York: The Guilford Press, 2008, 419–35.

26. Blackmore S. *Inventing Ourselves – The Secret Life of the Teenage Brain*. London: Black Swan, 2018.

27. Laible D. Attachment with Parents and Peers in Late Adolescence: Links with Emotional Competence and Social Behavior. Personality and Individual Differences. 2007 Oct 1;**43**(5):1185–97.

28. Shelemy L, Knightsmith P. Building Resilient in the Face of Adversity. In: M Bush (ed.), *Addressing Adversity*. London: Young Minds and NHS Health Education England, 2018, 99–107.

29. Chester C, Jones DJ, Zalot A, Sterrett E. The Psychosocial Adjustment of African American Youth from Single Mother Homes: The Relative Contribution of Parents and Peers. Journal of Clinical Child and Adolescent Psychology. 2007 Jul 17;**36**(3):356–66.

30. Chein J, Albert D, O'Brien L, Uckert K, Steinberg L. Peers Increase Adolescent Risk Taking by Enhancing Activity in the Brain's Reward Circuitry. Developmental Science. 2011;**14**(2):F1–F10.

31. Zeifman D, Hazan C. Pair Bonds As Attachments: Reevaluating the Evidence. In J Cassidy, PR Shaver (eds.), *Handbook of Attachment: Theory, Research, and Clinical Applications*. New York: The Guildford Press, 2008, 436–55.

32. Bugental DB. Thriving in the Face of Early Adversity. Journal of Social Issues. 2004 Apr;**60**(1):219–35.

33. Phares V. Where's Poppa? The Relative Lack of Attention to the Role of Fathers in Child and Adolescent Psychopathology. American Psychologist. 1992 May;**47**(5):656.

34. Nolen-Hoeksema S, Wolfson A, Mumme D, Guskin K. Helplessness in Children of Depressed and Nondepressed Mothers. Developmental Psychology. 1995 May;**31**(3):377.

35. Lyons-Ruth K, Wolfe R, Lyubchik A. Depression and the Parenting of Young Children: Making the Case for Early Preventive Mental Health Services. Harvard Review of Psychiatry. 2000 Jan 1;**8**(3):148–53.

36. Greenberg MT. Attachment and Psychopathology in Childhood. In: J Cassidy, PR Shaver (eds.), *Handbook of Attachment: Theory, Research, and Clinical Applications*. New York: The Guilford Press, 1999, 469–96.

37. Seifer R, Clark GN, Sameroff AJ. Positive Effects of Interaction Coaching on Infants with Developmental Disabilities and Their Mothers. American Journal on Mental Retardation. 1991 Jul;**96**(1):1–11.

38. Walsh F. *Strengthening Family Resilience*. New York: The Guildford Press, 1998.
39. Gribble PA, Cowen EL, Wyman PA, Work WC, Wannon M, Raoof A. Parent and Child Views of Parent-Child Relationship Qualities and Resilient Outcomes Among Urban Children. Journal of Child Psychology and Psychiatry. 1993 May;**34**(4):507–19.
40. De Haan L, Hawley DR, Deal JE. Operationalizing Family Resilience: A Methodological Strategy. American Journal of Family Therapy. 2002 Jul 1;**30**(4):275–91.
41. Hawkins JD, Catalano RF, Kosterman R, Abbott R, Hill KG. Preventing Adolescent Health-Risk Behaviors by Strengthening Protection During Childhood. Archives of Pediatrics & Adolescent Medicine. 1999 Mar 1;**153**(3):226–34.
42. Webster-Stratton C. Bywater T. The Incredible Years® Series: An Internationally Evidenced Multi-modal Approach to Enhancing Child Outcomes. In B Fiese, M Whisman M Celano K Deater-Deckard E Jouriles (eds.), *APA Handbook of Contemporary Family Psychology*. Washington, DC: American Psychological Association, 2019, 343–59.
43. Sanders MR, Kirby JN, Tellegen CL, Day JJ. The Triple P-Positive Parenting Program: A Systematic Review and Meta-analysis of a Multi-level System of Parenting Support. Clinical Psychology Review, 2014;**34**(4):337–57.
44. Hughes DA. *Attachment Focused Parenting*. New York: W. W. Norton & Company, 2009.
45. NICE guideline NG26. *Children's Attachment: Attachment in Children and Young People Who Are Adopted from Care, in Care or at High Risk of Going into Care*. NICE, 2015. https://www.nice.org.uk/guidance/ng26.
46. Oxfordshire Safeguarding Children Partnership. *Think Family*. Oxford: Oxfordshire Safeguarding Children Partnership, 2025. Available from: https://www.oscp.org.uk/practitioners/multi-agency-procedures-and-resources/think-family/ (cited 28 April 2025).
47. McLaughlin JA, Miller P, Warwick H. Deliberate Self-Harm in Adolescents: Hopelessness, Depression, Problems and Problem-Solving. Journal of Adolescence. 1996 Dec 1;**19**(6):523–32.
48. Dori GA, Overholser JC. Depression, Hopelessness, and Self-Esteem: Accounting for Suicidality in Adolescent Psychiatric Inpatients. Suicide and Life-Threatening Behavior. 1999 Dec;**29**(4):309–18.
49. Bolland JM. Hopelessness and Risk Behaviour Among Adolescents Living in High-Poverty Inner-City Neighbourhoods. Journal of Adolescence. 2003 Apr 1;**26**(2):145–58.
50. MacLeod AK, Salaminiou E. Reduced Positive Future-Thinking in Depression: Cognitive and Affective Factors. Cognition & Emotion. 2001 Jan 1;**15**(1):99–107.
51. Kwok SY, Yeung JW, Low AY, Lo HH, Tam CH. The Roles of Emotional Competence and Social Problem-Solving in the Relationship Between Physical Abuse and Adolescent Suicidal Ideation in China. Child Abuse & Neglect. 2015 Jun 1;**44**:117–29.
52. Romans SE, Martin JL, Anderson JC, O'Shea ML, Mullen PE. Factors That Mediate Between Child Sexual Abuse and Adult Psychological Outcome. Psychological Medicine. 1995 Jan;**25**(1):127–42.
53. HM Government. *The Children Act*. London: HM Government, 2004. Available from: http://www.legislation.gov.uk/ukpga/2004/31/contents (cited 16 January 2023).
54. Department for Education. *Working Together to Safeguard Children 2023*. London: HM Government, February 2024. Available from: https://assets.publishing.service.gov.uk/media/669e7501ab418ab055592a7b/Working_together_to_safeguard_children_2023.pdf.
55. McCann JB, James A, Wilson S, Dunn G. Prevalence of Psychiatric Disorders in

Young People in the Care System. BMJ. 1996 Dec 14;**313**(7071):1529–30.

56. Department of Health and Social Care. *The Role of Health and Wellbeing Boards: Guidance*. Department of Health and Social Care, 2022. Available from: https://www.gov.uk/government/publications/health-and-wellbeing-boards-guidance/health-and-wellbeing-boards-guidance.

Chapter 22

Moving from Models of Liaison Psychiatry to Psychological Medicine: New Approaches

Isabel Paz, Kate Green, Harriet Stewart, Karen Steinhardt and Mina Fazel

Working in General Hospital environments can be an area of exciting innovation, often reflecting the advances and changes that are taking place in the patient population and problems that are being addressed. The term Liaison and Consultation Psychiatry has been used to describe the practice of working at the interface between somatic and mental health. Despite the term liaison meaning communication and cooperation, it can imply that mental health services are located elsewhere, potentially reinforcing a separation of mental and physical health that often, and especially from the perspective of the patient, can be arbitrary. Psychological Medicine, however, has a different connotation and implies an approach to care that places integration at the fore. Mental and physical health problems, if they can be easily separated, are still often comorbid, and therefore to provide good care for the patient as a whole, both aspects must be taken into consideration and treated simultaneously. The term Psychological Medicine is therefore used to describe the general hospital specialty working alongside other medical and surgical specialties; providing expert assessment and treatment of the mental health needs of patients admitted to acute hospitals, regardless of and alongside their other health needs. It is therefore not just a matter of semantics, but an understanding that psychology and psychiatry should play an integral role in the treatment of all patients in the general hospital.

Children's Psychological Medicine Team in General Hospitals

The Covid pandemic has had a profound impact on young people's mental health and the provision of services with an unprecedented subsequent demand for mental health services. NHS Digital prevalence data shows that 40% of young people report a deterioration in their mental health between 2017 and 2021 [1]. The data found an increase in rates of probable mental disorders of between 50% and 70% in under-19-year-olds. It also shows a 94% increase in the proportion of children and young people with possible eating problems [2].

One of the changing patterns in how young people present to mental health services is the observation that many arrive first at the emergency department of acute hospitals in crisis. This could be as a result of community Children and Adolescent Mental Health Services (CAMHS), as well as inpatient psychiatric provision for young people having been overwhelmed by the increase in demand. Furthermore, the proportion of admissions to pediatric wards in the UK with a primary diagnosis of a mental and behavioural disorder has increased substantially for the 5 years up to 2020/21 [2].

Even before the pandemic, the increase in demand for child and adolescent specialist psychiatric teams in the general hospital reflects the changing nature of paediatric services.

With the scientific advancements in care for some of the most complex patients, many children are surviving childhood – often with significant morbidity when they might not, previously, have survived. They are likely to have experienced multiple hospital admissions and medical investigations; all increasing the likelihood of comorbid mental health problems. Furthermore, there are increasing numbers of patients presenting with acute mental health presentations such as deliberate self-harm or eating disorders and those admitted to paediatric wards while waiting for inpatient psychiatric facilities. Children's Psychological Medicine (CPM) teams play a crucial role in the assessment and treatment of psychiatric comorbidities in children with the range of somatic health problems [3].

In 2016, Guthrie and colleagues published the results of a survey of 64 independent paediatric liaison psychiatry services in the USA. The most common reasons for consultation were suicide risk assessment, assistance in the diagnosis and management of medically unexplained symptoms, adjustment to medical illness, assessment for psychopharmacological intervention, delirium, treatment nonadherence and the management of children admitted to paediatric units to await psychiatric hospital placement [4].

In this chapter we will discuss a range of disorders where input from a psychological medicine team is needed in the general hospital setting. First, we will discuss disorders where psychological and medical care are closely interrelated and require fully integrated provision, such as for eating disorders and functional disorders. We will then discuss disorders involving the brain and neuropsychiatric presentations including neurodevelopmental disorders, traumatic brain injury and delirium. Following this we will describe psychiatric emergencies such as self-harm and also how to address the difficulties encountered in chronic illnesses and pain. We will then discuss some of the difficulties of managing psychiatrically unwell patients in the general hospital setting when their primary care needs are likely to be better managed in an inpatient psychiatric setting as well as some common presentations primarily seen in acute settings such as issues related to adherence to treatment, needle phobia, staff support following exposure to traumatic events and the implications of the Covid-19 pandemic.

Disorders Requiring Integrated Psychiatry and Paediatrics

Severe Eating Disorders

Eating disorders can be disabling and deadly. They are costly mental disorders that considerably impair somatic health and disrupt psychosocial functioning [5].

Between 1.25 and 3.4 million people have been estimated to have an eating disorder in the UK. The number of people being diagnosed and entering inpatient treatment for eating disorders in England alone has increased at an average rate of 7% year-on-year since 2009. This has been exacerbated further by the pandemic with an estimated 69% rise in hospital admissions for children and adolescents aged 17 and under, compared to data from the pre-pandemic year of 2019 [6]. A combination of social isolation, perceived lack of control, loss of routine, food insecurities and pressures to exercise have been identified as potential triggers. As a result, there has been a significant increase in referrals and wait times for specialist services particularly for anorexia nervosa, with increasing numbers presenting in either physical or emotional crisis to general hospitals – at times requiring naso-gastric (NG) feeding for their malnutrition.

The main aim of a medical admission is physical stabilisation, paying particular attention to the potentially life-threatening risk of re-feeding syndrome, however it is also a crucial period in the treatment process. In a likely long-term treatment trajectory, the CPM Team might be the first mental health professionals that are met. At times of crisis, young people and their families might be more receptive to engaging in psychoeducation about their condition, an essential preparation for the treatment journey ahead. It is also important to make sure that the care provided in hospital, from meal plans to supervision of meals and activity levels, as well as distress tolerance techniques, are in place as early as possible and consistent with those used by the receiving community team after discharge, so that there is continuity of approaches to care. In extreme situations when the young person is so unwell that they are unable to engage or lack capacity to do so, a Mental Health Act Assessment might be needed, particularly if the patient needs NG feeding against their will.

The input of the CPM team also involves the training of nursing and paediatric teams in the psychological and behavioural management of these patients, as without it the challenges these patients pose can be hard to manage in a busy acute hospital environment.

Medically Unexplained Symptoms/Functional Disorders

Medically unexplained symptoms (MUS) is a term used to describe a broad range of clinical presentations, where the symptoms the patient presents with cannot be fully explained by findings from somatic examinations and investigations. The experience of the symptoms for the patient is no different to the experience of those with identified organic pathology (such as a musculoskeletal injury), and in some cases both somatic and psychogenic symptoms co-exist. These disorders are more common in children (estimated prevalence of 10%), which can be understood from a developmental perspective as younger populations might not have the emotional repertoire or insight to explain and attribute their symptoms in light of their feelings. The severity of MUS can vary from mild and transient symptoms such as headaches to enduring and debilitating presentations such as functional neurological disorders. For some patients the symptoms will resolve spontaneously, but for others, the nature and severity of the condition will cause the patient and their family significant distress and disability, requiring specialist help.

Paediatric colleagues often find these 'complex presentations' challenging because regular symptomatic treatments are generally ineffective, which can then lead to multiple investigations and referrals across specialties. In the increasing litigious climate in which we work, it is understandable that health care professionals might want to ensure that more rare diagnoses are excluded, although some of these investigations might carry an iatrogenic risk. It can therefore often take some time and multiple attempts by various doctors to find a 'cause' before a functional diagnosis is even formally broached, although it might have been considered earlier in the diagnostic pathway.

Psychological Medicine specialists can play a significant role in the diagnosis and management of these presentations. Timely identification of recurrent presentations, discussions with the paediatricians to rationalise the need for investigations and interventions and containment of the health service anxiety generated by diagnostic uncertainty are all necessary steps towards successful management of the symptoms.

The next step is to discuss the diagnosis with the child and family. It is important that the explanation is given in a clear and non-judgemental manner, conveying that the lack of another medical explanation does not mean that the doctors do not know what the condition is or that the condition is not serious. Furthermore, it would be important to allay possible concerns about how patients might think we are interpreting their symptoms – for example, that the symptoms are all in the 'patient's head', or that the patient is consciously fabricating the symptoms. All of these are common miscommunications, which can cause iatrogenic harm by alienating the patient and their family, compromising future treatment. It is important to clarify that the symptoms remain significant, but the treatment focus is on symptom management rather than a quest to find a cause. Kozlowska et al have powerfully illustrated the iatrogenic stigma, erosion of empathy and compassion within the clinician–patient relationship and a lack of understanding about the disorder, through case examples of children and adolescents with functional neurological disorders [7].

Once a positive diagnosis has been made, the next step in the treatment process is psychoeducation about the condition, and a thorough assessment as early as possible to identify contributing factors and any psychiatric comorbidity, such as depression and anxiety, and also establishing healthy habits paying special attention to sleep. For complex cases the treatment should be multidisciplinary and include a programme of symptom rehabilitation, psychological management of the young person's anxiety, as well as a systemic approach with the family and school to identify and address maintaining factors.

Medically unexplained symptoms can be 'explained' and successfully treated, and the benefit to the child and the family, as well as the economic benefit in terms of reduction of unnecessary investigations and multiple medical appointments and hospital admissions is considerable. The expertise of CPM teams in these cases is particularly valuable, as they can contain the system, as well as the family, and by understanding the systemic factors at play, can create an environment of recovery [8].

Neuropsychiatric Presentations

The co-location of paediatric somatic and psychiatric services in the general hospital and the interdisciplinary discussions about patients that ensue from this, ensure that children and adolescents' needs are met [3]. Children with neurological disorders often present with comorbid psychiatric symptoms. These may be as a direct result of the pathological process in the brain or because of treatment side effects, stress, pain, adjustment to the diagnosis and/or prognosis. The complexity of these presentations is therefore best managed when CPM specialists and paediatric neurologists work together. Children presenting with psychosis for example, are tested for anti-NMDA encephalitis by paediatric neurologists but still need urgent psychiatric care. Children presenting to neurologists with Tourette's Syndrome may respond to psychological treatments such as Habit Reversal Training and psychiatric medication.

Delirium

Psychiatrists are often called to assess patients presenting with delirium as they can experience auditory and visual hallucinations and are in an acute confusional state. The cause is often due to a variety of factors including severe infections, responses to the addition and withdrawal of powerful sedative agents and whenever a patient is intubated. Delirium usually has a sudden onset and a fluctuating course [9]. The patient must be seen urgently for a mental state examination and a history from relatives obtained to establish the premorbid level of function. Ensuring that the patient is comfortable and that the environmental triggers for re-orientating the patient are prioritised (light during the daytime, a clock, reminders of which meal it is), reminding the patient that they are in hospital, and if needed, accessing visual aids, are simple but often overlooked interventions crucial in the management of delirium. The patient must be adequately supervised, to manage potential risk of self-harm. To reduce delirium in hospitalised children, health care providers should optimise the hospital environment (e.g. by reducing sleep disruption and keeping the child stimulated during the day), improve pain management, and decrease sedation (particularly use of benzodiazepines) [9]. In terms of treatment, the psychiatrist must exercise caution, as medication can worsen delirium, however, benzodiazepines and low-dose antipsychotic medication might be necessary to control agitation. These patients require frequent review and discussions with the treating team, so that treatment decisions are taken jointly. Delirium is often extremely distressing and traumatic for the patient and their family, with a moderate risk of subsequent PTSD [10].

Traumatic Brain Injury

PM psychiatrists are often called to see patients with acute traumatic brain injury whether accidental or due to deliberate self-harm. Tactful unravelling of the emotions and events prior to the head injury need to be determined, which can often be compromised if there is any retrograde amnesia. The effects of any coup or contra coup injury to the brain may require psychometric testing from a neuropsychologist alongside the multidisciplinary team needed to be able to address these complex presentations. Psychiatric follow-up for depression and PTSD are usually necessary, and this possibility should be discussed with the patient prior to discharge.

Functional Neurological Disorders

Functional neurological disorders are often the most extreme of functional presentations, and therefore given brief separate consideration, although the same principles apply as those in other medically unexplained symptoms. The added complexity in these cases derives from the level of disability that can ensue, and the subsequent anxiety that they can generate, not only in the patient and their family and school, but also for the treating clinicians. Particularly difficult are the cases where organic and functional pathology co-exist, such as non-epileptic seizures in a child with epilepsy. The two can be difficult to distinguish but both need treatment in their own right. As with other functional presentations it is best to treat in a multidisciplinary team involving education, CPM, Paediatrics and Social Care as appropriate.

Our case study below (see Beth) demonstrates how hospital paediatric neurologists and child psychiatrists worked with the CAMHS team. This enabled the team to better address the effect of comorbid conditions that might add to the difficulties experienced by the child and their parents.

Managing Comorbidities: Case Study

'Beth' is a 14-year-old who presented with severe 'tic attacks' and episodes of 'freezing' limbs, so that at times she could not walk or get into school. She had experienced some minor motor and vocal tics from around age 7 years. These had 'exploded' into episodes of anxiety and tic attacks within weeks of the Covid-19 lockdown. Parents described Beth as always having been very active but had great difficulty with peer relationships at primary school and she was seen by CAMHS for anxiety during this period.

Beth had not spent much time in secondary school, initially because of the lockdown but then stopped going altogether as a result of her symptoms. She reported that she had a few friends she talked to online. Beth was seen by the paediatric neurologist, who diagnosed a functional movement disorder and asked for her to be seen by a child psychiatrist.

CAMHS were also involved by this time and had commenced fluoxetine for her anxiety and clonidine for the tics. These medications were reported to be helping with the anxiety and the pre-existing tics, but the 'freezing' episodes worsened, restricting Beth in her activities.

In treatment, her parents were encouraged to pay selective attention to the symptoms by ignoring the tics and freezing, but to continue to be very responsive to Beth in all other activities. This was extremely difficult, especially, as expected, her symptoms worsened for the first few weeks, a period that typically extends from about 3–6 weeks. However, after this, Beth's functional symptoms, deprived of the reinforcement of her anxiety symptoms, started to subside. During this time, her parents were supported with weekly phone calls or appointments. Beth herself was involved in discussions throughout as it was crucial for her to understand why her parents were not responding to some of her symptoms, especially her tics.

After the tics/freezing episodes improved, Beth's anxiety symptoms became more prominent. She was treated with exposure and response prevention for her tics at CAMHS and returned to school, where she is reported to be managing well. She is currently awaiting ADHD and ASD assessments in the community.

Autism and Intellectual Impairment

A high proportion of young people presenting to services have difficulties related to anxiety and emotional dysregulation, both of which are common features presenting in individuals on the autism spectrum [11]. Many have autism without an intellectual impairment, but people with autism and/or intellectual impairment can share some presenting features. Both groups can struggle with change and the disruption to routine that admission to hospital involves, and both experience anxiety and find it difficult to identify their emotions and explain how they feel to others, particularly unfamiliar individuals. Patients do best where there is continuity of care, familiar people and objects, and when they understand what is about to happen and can plan for it. Being admitted to a paediatric ward involves repeated challenges to these young people and ways must be found of adapting the environment to make it less anxiety provoking. The needs will therefore be very different depending on whether an admission has been as an emergency or whether it is planned, and in complex presentations the CPM team can play an important role in assessment and planning, taking into account the developmental needs of the child or adolescent.

Complexity may lie in the multidisciplinary nature of the work that might need to be conducted, incorporating in variable degrees the following: genetic risk, disorders of early attachment, exposure to traumatic events, perceptions of pain, learning difficulties, communication difficulties and any possible safeguarding concerns. They may present with 'challenging behaviour', which the Royal College of Psychiatrists defines as: 'Behaviour of such an intensity, frequency or duration as to threaten the quality of life and/or physical safety of the individual or others, and is likely to lead to responses that are restrictive, aversive or result in exclusion' [12].

Fifty percent of children with ASD experience anxiety [11]. Common triggers are social judgements, performance pressures, school experience, sensory sensitivities being prevented from performing repetitive interests or activities or not having time to process experiences and overstimulation leading to feelings of being overwhelmed. Children and young people might have emotional outbursts at home where they feel safe, and behaviour can become challenging resulting in self-harm and admission to hospital. People with ASD often report suicidal thoughts and are at increased risk of death by suicide. Eighty percent of these individuals are likely to have a mental illness [13,14]. They are also more likely to develop schizophrenia, bipolar disorder, depressive disorder and ADHD. Perimenstrual disorders can also go unrecognised in this population. CPM clinicians also need to be aware of certain genetic conditions, which may present with particular behavioural phenotypes including self-injurious behaviour such as Lesch-Nyhan's and Smith-Magenis [15].

Placing, structure, routine and predictability are beneficial for many children and hospital passports are also helpful. These are personalised documents belonging to the patient listing their medical conditions and key information about the young person including likes and dislikes. It is compiled by parents and patients in partnership with hospital staff. The presence of staff with special interests and access to training on ASD and intellectual impairment might be a useful resource for the wards they work on as well as for other staff.

People with ASD and intellectual impairment can have greater sensitivity to medication at standard doses and therefore pharmacotherapy should be administered cautiously [16]. Useful prescribing principles are to start at a low dose and increase medication slowly; do not give more than one medication at a time and stop medications that have not been helpful. Plans involving the use of medication should be done early in the treatment process, taking into account the effects of any existing regular medication, as well as past experiences of other medications used, to avoid overmedication, and prevent potential errors when decisions are made in emergency situations by staff who might not know the patient well.

Psychiatric Emergencies

Deliberate Self-Harm

Children who present to the general hospital Emergency Department with signs of self-harm including overdose are usually first seen in A&E and then referred to the paediatric team to determine whether the child requires an admission to hospital [17]. This would usually be on medical grounds (need for treatment or observation for an overdose) but may also be on mental health or social grounds or both. NICE guidelines recommend that children presenting with self-harm should ideally be admitted overnight but presentations have increased disproportionately over time and due to capacity limitations, this is not routinely possible. In most settings only the physically compromised, those who have committed violent and potentially lethal acts, or those with safeguarding concerns, will result in admission to hospital. In any case, it is imperative to determine the child's intent to harm themselves by undertaking a full psychiatric assessment. Asking about suicidal ideation does not increase the risk of suicide [18]. Depending on local resources, patients may be seen first by a psychiatric nurse, psychologist or psychiatrist and a safety plan made for discharge home. They may be referred to the local CAMHS service for ongoing assessment and therapy or to the safeguarding team if the child is felt to have experienced maltreatment. In these cases, the CPM team have a crucial role to play in a multidisciplinary review where need for future input from community services will be determined.

It is very important to see the child on their own and without parents and carers to try to establish a relationship of trust, assess capacity and to understand the child's point of view.

Suicide is the third most common cause of death for adolescents. Completed suicide is more common in males and self-harming behaviour is more common in females. When

assessing a child or adolescent presenting with self-harm and suicidal ideation, asking about the factors associated with completed suicide is essential. These include:
- past history of suicidal thinking and behaviour with escalating intent
- high lethality of method (jumping from a height, hanging, researching lethal suicidal acts online) and access to such methods
- intention to die
- stressors (relationship problems, school or family difficulties)
- pre-existing mental illness (psychotic illness, depression, substance misuse, conduct disorder, anxiety, PTSD, eating disorder)
- isolation from support network (family, education, peers, homelessness)
- physical illness (cancer, diabetes)
- physical and sexual abuse
- family history of suicidal behaviour, suicide and parental mental illness
- hopelessness and worthlessness

Self-harm itself is a behaviour, but it may be related to a psychiatric diagnosis. Many young people who self-harm do so to reduce a feeling of high anxiety or emotional distress rather than to end their lives. This coping strategy works in the short-term but can become more severe over time if the underlying anxiety disorder is not treated. Some young people harm themselves as a way of self-punishment.

Carrying out a safety plan with the child and their parents and ensuring a transition to CAMHS with timely follow-up can be containing for families. It is often possible to identify certain activities that may reduce anxiety and ways of communicating the urge to self-harm. Mindfulness exercises and techniques to calm urges to self-harm (putting the hands in ice or snapping an elastic band for example) that avoid permanent harm and help to reduce distress are also helpful. The safety plan must include guiding the parents to ensure the home environment is safe, by removing sharps and ligatures. If parents feel unable to keep their child safe, then a multidisciplinary team (MDT) meeting with colleagues from Social Care, Education and CAMHS is often needed to enable a safer plan.

Chronic Health Conditions

There is broad consensus that children who have a chronic health condition are more susceptible to difficulties with their mental health, and a proportion of those may present with a psychiatric diagnosis that requires treatment [19,20,21]. The role of the CPM team may therefore include consideration of what preventative measures can be put in place – both by the medical team and by the young person and their family to facilitate positive mental health throughout the treatment journey as well as the management of more acute psychological distress where needed.

In the UK psychological input alongside medical teams was pioneered specifically for children and adolescents with diabetes and cystic fibrosis, primarily because of the impact that poor mental health could have on treatment adherence, as well as the heavy burden that both the condition and treatment could have on multiple areas of the patients' life [22]. The presence of a CPM team or a clinical psychologist within the team enhances holistic patient care and in several specialties is mandated within NICE guidance. Over time, the impact of this provision has been an increased appreciation of the assistance psychological approaches can bring to other chronic health conditions. The last 25 years has witnessed a significant increase in the number of clinical/paediatric psychologists employed to work with children and adolescents in acute hospital settings.

The role of the PM clinician will relate to the perceived long-term risks of the condition (Cancer, Duchennes Muscular Dystrophy), the burden of treatment (Juvenile Idiopathic Arthritis, Diabetes) as well as the potential life-changing impact of the condition (Differences of Sex Development). It will also be impacted by characteristics individual to the young person or family including gender identity, sexuality, ethnicity or culture (commonly described as the social graces) [23].

In all aspects of the role a 'formulation', identifying the key issues for the young person and the factors that exacerbate and maintain these, as well as background factors such as those above, are key to agreeing a psychological management plan. Communicating this formulation to the MDT can be crucial in ensuring a shared understanding of and a holistic approach to the issues.

At the time of writing, across the UK, all Children's Hospitals provide some level of psychology provision to paediatric patients in the hospital's out and inpatient services, with some employed directly by the acute service and others through CAMHS. Many will be embedded as a key member of the MDT working from neonates to young adults with a growing literature demonstrating the efficacy of psychological approaches within these populations. The role of the child and adolescent psychiatrist, however, is an emerging one within this field with only 50% of surveyed children's hospitals reporting direct access to psychiatry services within a liaison team and fewer than 20% offering an integrated service in the form of a psychological medicine team. However, with better awareness of the mental health needs as well as rising levels of psychiatric difficulty in the medical population the value of an integrated approach cannot be underestimated.

Psychiatrically Unwell Patients Stranded in the Hospital

Emergency departments are often the only place where young people and their families can literally walk in and access physical, as well as psychiatric care, particularly out of hours. There are a wide range of presentations, with deliberate self-harm and eating disorders being the most common, but also psychotic illnesses where a large potential differential might need to be ruled out, including autoimmune encephalitis. Many will therefore be discharged to the community, with a minority needing a specialist psychiatric facility. Unfortunately, some get stranded in Paediatric wards for long periods of time, while waiting for a psychiatric bed to become available; for example, there have been times where in the one of the general paediatric wards in the hospital in which the authors work, over one-third of patients were either waiting for a psychiatric inpatient bed or were under the care of Social Services needing a safe place to be discharged to. Often these patients suffer from complex trauma due to previous experiences of abuse or may have underlying undiagnosed neurodevelopmental difficulties such as autism, ADHD or intellectual impairment contributing to the presentation.

Young people in crisis require careful assessment and management in the Emergency department especially to determine if they pose a risk to themselves or others. Paediatric wards are usually not designed to care for these patients' needs, and there are often environmental factors to be addressed. Wards are often open (increased risk of absconding), have multiple ligature and oxygen points (self-harm and arson risk), and nursing staff not trained in managing acute psychiatric presentations.

The safe management of these patients require a prompt psychiatric evaluation to diagnose the acute psychiatric problem if there is diagnostic uncertainty. Treatment will be symptomatic and requires careful monitoring of mental state. Paediatric colleagues benefit from principles of behavioural de-escalation and rapid tranquilisation and often protocols assist these management complexities. Levels of nursing observation need to be determined, and at times specialist psychiatric nurses may be required. In the absence of more appropriate provision, security staff can become involved in the management of these young people when they display aggression, often leading to quite distressing situations. Chemical restraint might also be used in the absence of better environmental risk management. Protocols to plan for these eventualities are crucial and integrated services are often best placed to develop, audit and re-evaluate these in the context of a changing evidence base.

Finally, careful consideration must be given to the legal context, to ensure that the care and treatment provided is lawful. In children who are acutely mentally ill and are not consenting to treatment in the UK, a Mental Health Act assessment must take place, and detention to the acute hospital might be necessary in the absence of an appropriate psychiatric facility. In the case of children who do not meet criteria for detention under the Mental Health Act, but who are not safe to leave the hospital, and where the hospital is depriving them of their liberty, legal advice must be urgently sought, and a court authorisation might be required.

Other Areas Where Psychological Support Needed

Adherence and Needle Phobia

Children and adolescents, like adults, can struggle with procedures that they need to undergo. Difficulties typically referred to as 'needle phobia' can be very common with a systematic review highlighting how prevalent needle phobia is among the younger populations [24]. It can be helpful to identify the aetiology of the difficulties. In cases where the presenting anxiety is due to an underlying prior trauma (such as being held down for procedures, or being under considerable pain during, for example, a steroid injection into a joint) trauma therapy would be indicated; whereas fears about needles for a specific blood test often respond best to cognitive behaviour therapy including psychoeducation to address any catastrophic cognitions (e.g. I'll keep bleeding and then die) as well as timely exposure therapy.

Where treatment adherence is low the medical team are understandably concerned about the impact on disease management, and both the medical team and parents can find it frustrating when children are not adhering to treatment including medication, physiotherapy, occupational therapy or speech and language therapy. However, just giving more 'expert advice' at this point doesn't help – and indeed in some cases can generate even greater resistance in the young person. The CPM clinician can be invaluable in assessing which aspects may be getting in the way of adherence, including the child's understanding of their disease and treatment, the ease of taking the treatment, and how visible the treatment is to peers (adolescents with diabetes often talk about not wanting to test in front of their peers because it marks them out as different). By helping them to make sense of some of these dilemmas and giving them the psychological tools to make sense of what they want to achieve, this can in turn help individuals to adjust to their treatment and to their condition. Again, formulation with the family or even with the medical team can help the whole team to see the problem in a similar way and to act accordingly.

Adjustment

Contrary to what is often expected, children's mental health and emotional well-being are not directly related to the severity of their health condition. Instead, it is the *perceived* impact for the child on their life, including social, school, hobbies and activities and identity. Furthermore, how parents and other members of the family perceive the impact of the condition and its treatment on individual and family life contributes significantly to the overall picture. As such, involvement by the CPM clinician can focus on multiple people in the system as well as the young person.

As they get older, young people are increasingly expected to take an active role in the 'task' of starting to look after their condition and can end up feeling overwhelmed by the demands initially put on them if it is not done gently and carefully. Broadly speaking, it is useful to think about how the following aspects may impact on adjustment – both in the child and the parent/carer: pre-existing coping strategies and styles; health beliefs in the family culture and wider culture; health and treatment fears; religious beliefs; parental mental health difficulties and attachment styles in the family relationships.

Staff Support

The idea of enforced full-team 'debriefs' fell out of favour following the Cochrane review, which highlighted that psychological debriefing should not be assumed to be a beneficial approach to prevent PTSD after a potentially traumatic incident [25]. However, hospital personnel find some form of debriefing valuable and important after a significant event, and subsequently there is a variety of practices in place, not all of these helpful [26]. It is necessary therefore to have a system to assist staff members who have been exposed through their work to events that are particularly unexpected and distressing – which can include the surprise death of a patient on the ward or following accidents with multiple casualties. Hospitals benefit from staff who have received training and can access ongoing supervision to be available to support individuals and teams who need further support [27]. For example, some services utilise a narrative approach to ensure that everyone in the team (who would like to attend) has a shared understanding of all the events that have transpired, from the first contact with the hospital to the last. This in itself can address misunderstandings about what might have happened and feelings of guilt and anger that might have arisen in the confusion that often is present at these incidents. In parallel to this, individuals are able to seek specific personal support if needed following this so that they can be signposted accordingly.

Covid

The numerous and multiple impacts of the Covid-19 pandemic will only become truly evident as time progresses [28]. We will focus here on the impacts in the hospital system by discussing the impacts on children and adolescents who became unwell with Covid; the impacts of the pandemic on those with comorbidities and chronic health conditions and finally the impact of the pandemic on the hospital system. This is just a small area of the effect of the pandemic [29].

For those children and adolescents who had more severe consequences of Covid-19 infection, the most extreme of these consequences was paediatric multisystem inflammatory syndrome (PMIS) as well as the persistence of chronic 'long Covid' symptoms in the community. One study of PMIS showed that one-third of children had persistent symptoms after 8 weeks [30], and the psychological sequelae are important to ascertain in order to inform treatment approaches be that from traumatic memories to cognitive difficulties. In addition, there have been widespread reports of more child and adolescent presentations to the general hospital with severe eating disorders temporally associated with the periods of lockdown.

For those children who had pre-existing health vulnerabilities prior to the pandemic – either because of chronic illness or complex treatments that compromise the immune system, the pandemic has placed them in a precarious situation, where they might have had to miss hospital appointments and interventions, and they might have had to be even more isolated than their peers with impacts in health, education and social domains. The ongoing support of these children will likely benefit from integrated psychological medicine interventions. These changes for more vulnerable children are also evident for the most vulnerable children at home – for example those who live in situations of domestic abuse and violence with delayed hospital presentations.

In some reports the challenges described include heightened anxiety, disrupted routines, academic and social stresses associated with school closure, increased risk of domestic violence and abuse, and reduced access to physical and psychosocial support. However, this has not been a universally negative experience as, on the other hand, opportunities include reduced academic and social stress, increased time with families, reduced access to substances, easier access to health care using technology and opportunities to build resilience [31,32].

Finally, CPM teams can play an important role in helping a system under extreme stress. In the UK NHS staff have experienced significant challenges with redeployment, widespread staff sickness, loss of colleagues and exposure to the intense suffering of individuals unable to have in-person visits by their friends and relatives. These have all been areas where CPM teams can help with mitigating further difficulties.

Conclusions

In the broadest sense clinicians working in psychological medicine are involved in the assessment and treatment of mental health conditions, their impact on physical health conditions including adherence, and the reciprocal impact of the health condition on mental health. They have a key role within the MDT in keeping the psychological and mental health needs of the young person and their family at the forefront of their treatment and can act as a sounding board to the team, particularly where there may be concerns relating to unusual or unexpected presentations, changes in the condition over time, or changes in the engagement of the young person and family. It is perhaps intuitively obvious that any number of factors may impact on an individual's treatment course and that many of these factors may be external to the illness itself. The CPM clinician therefore has a valuable role to play in helping the young person, family and team to develop a formulation from which to understand changes and to plan and evaluate an appropriate intervention.

Psychological medicine teams are therefore likely to play a significant role in 21st-century medicine with better appreciation of how psychological well-being can impact on the presentation and treatment of every patient – no matter why they are in the hospital setting. It is not necessarily about seeing the most acutely unwell patients in the Emergency Department but instead focusing on the richness and range of psychological factors that impact on all aspects of medical care, and with the increasing sophistication of medicine rely more and more on specialists working together in teams.

References

1. Newlove-Delgado T, McManus S, Sadler K, et al. Child Mental Health in England Before and During the COVID-19 Lockdown. Lancet Psychiatry. 2021;8(5):353–54.
2. Vizard T, Sadler K, Ford T, et al. *Mental Health of Children and Young People in England, 2020: Wave 1 Follow Up to the 2017 Survey*. Surrey, United Kingdom: NHS, 2020. Available from: https://digital.nhs.uk/data-and-information/publications/statistical/mental-health-of-children-and-young-people-in-england/2020-wave-1-follow-up (accessed 8 May 2025).
3. Fazel M, Townsend A, Stewart H, et al. Integrated Care to Address Child and Adolescent Health in the 21st Century: A Clinical Review. JCPP Advances. 2021;1(4):e12045.
4. Guthrie E, McMeekin A, Thomasson R, et al. Opening the 'Black Box': Liaison Psychiatry Services and What They Actually Do. BJPsych Bulletin. 2016;40(4):175–80.
5. van Hoeken D, Hoek HW. Review of the Burden of Eating Disorders: Mortality, Disability, Costs, Quality of Life, and Family Burden. Current Opinion in Psychiatry. 2020;33(6):521.
6. NHS Digital. *Hospital Admitted Patient Care Activity 2020-21*. NHS Digital, 2021. Available from: https://www.gov.uk/government/statistics/hospital-admitted-patient-care-activity-2020-21 (accessed 8 May 2025).
7. Kozlowska K, Sawchuk T, Waugh JL, et al. Changing the Culture of Care for Children and Adolescents with Functional Neurological Disorder. Epilepsy & Behavior Reports. 2021;16:100486.
8. Blake L, Davies V, Conn R, Davie M. *Medically Unexplained Symptoms (MUS) in Children and Young People: A Guide to Assessing and Managing Patients under the Age of 18 Who Are Referred Top Secondary Care*. Royal College of Psychiatrists and Paediatric Mental Health Association (PMHA), 2018.
9. Dechnik A, Traube C. Delirium in Hospitalised children. The Lancet Child & Adolescent Health. 2020;4(4):312–21.
10. Norman S, Taha AA, Turner HN. Delirium in the Critically Ill Child. Clinical Nurse Specialist. 2017;31(5):276–84.
11. Adams D, Emerson L-M. The Impact of Anxiety in Children on the Autism Spectrum. Journal of Autism and Developmental Disorders. 2021;51(6):1909–20.
12. Barclay JE. *Challenging Behaviour: A Unified Approach College Report CR144*. Royal College of Psychiatrists, 2007.
13. Cassidy S, Bradley L, Shaw R, Baron-Cohen S. Risk Markers for Suicidality in Autistic Adults. Molecular Autism. 2018;9(1):1–14.
14. Cassidy S, Rodgers J. Understanding and Prevention of Suicide in Autism. The Lancet Psychiatry. 2017;4(6):e11.
15. Harris JC. Behavioral Phenotypes in Developmental Neuropsychiatric Disorders: Disrupted Epigenetics, Microdeletions, Sex Chromosome Aneuploidies, and Gestational Alcohol Toxicity. Current Opinion in Psychiatry. 2019;32(2):51–54.
16. Persico AM, Ricciardello A, Lamberti M, et al. The Pediatric Psychopharmacology of Autism Spectrum Disorder: A Systematic Review-Part I: The Past and the Present. Progress in Neuro-Psychopharmacology and Biological Psychiatry. 2021;110:110326.
17. Courtney DB, Duda S, Szatmari P, Henderson J, Bennett K. Systematic Review and Quality Appraisal of Practice Guidelines for Self-Harm in Children and Adolescents. Suicide and Life-Threatening Behavior. 2019;49(3):707–23.
18. Blades CA, Stritzke WGK, Page AC, Brown JD. The Benefits and Risks of Asking Research Participants About Suicide: A Meta-analysis of the Impact of Exposure to Suicide-Related Content. Clinical Psychology Review. 2018;64:1–12.
19. Garrett CJ, Ismail K, Fonagy P. Understanding Developmental Psychopathology in Type 1 Diabetes Through Attachment, Mentalisation and

Diabetes Distress. Clinical Child Psychology and Psychiatry. 2021;26(3):682–94.

20. Kyllönen MS, Ebeling H, Kautiainen H, Puolakka K, Vähäsalo P. Psychiatric Disorders in Incident Patients with Juvenile Idiopathic Arthritis-A Case-Control Cohort Study. Pediatric Rheumatology. 2021;19(1):1-7.

21. Maeda K, Hasegawa D, Urayama KY, et al. Risk Factors for Psychological and Psychosomatic Symptoms Among Children with Malignancies. Journal of Paediatrics and Child Health. 2018;54(4):411–15.

22. Allcock B, Stewart R, Jackson M. Psychosocial Factors Associated with Repeat Diabetic Ketoacidosis in People Living with Type 1 Diabetes: A Systematic Review. Diabetic Medicine. 2022;39(1):e14663.

23. Burnham J. Developments in Social GRRRAAACCEEESSS: Visible–Invisible and Voiced–Unvoiced 1. In Inga-Britt Krause (ed), *Culture and Reflexivity in Systemic Psychotherapy*. London: Routledge, 2018, 139–60.

24. Orenius T, LicPsych, Säilä H, Mikola K, Ristolainen L. Fear of Injections and Needle Phobia Among Children and Adolescents: An Overview of Psychological, Behavioral, and Contextual Factors. SAGE Open Nursing. 2018;4:2377960818759442.

25. Rose SC, Bisson J, Churchill R, Wessely S. Psychological Debriefing for Preventing Post Traumatic Stress Disorder (PTSD). Cochrane Database of Systematic Reviews. 2002(2):CD000560.

26. Twigg S. Clinical Event Debriefing: A Review of Approaches and Objectives. Current Opinion in Pediatrics. 2020;32(3):337–42.

27. Richins MT, Gauntlett L, Tehrani N, et al. Early Post-trauma Interventions in Organizations: A Scoping Review. Frontiers in Psychology. 2020;11:1176.

28. Howard-Jones AR, Bowen AC, Danchin M, et al. COVID-19 in Children: I. Epidemiology, Prevention and Indirect Impacts. Journal of Paediatrics and Child Health. 2022;58(1):39–45.

29. Lachman P. Where to Make a Difference: Research and the Social Determinants in Pediatrics and Child Health in the COVID-19 Era. Pediatric Research. 2021;89(2):259–62.

30. Kahn R, Berg S, Berntson L, et al. Population-Based Study of Multisystem Inflammatory Syndrome Associated with COVID-19 Found That 36% of Children Had Persistent Symptoms. Acta Paediatrica. 2022;111(2):354–62.

31. Serlachius A, Badawy SM, Thabrew H. Psychosocial Challenges and Opportunities for Youth with Chronic Health Conditions During the COVID-19 Pandemic. JMIR Pediatrics and Parenting. 2020;3(2):e23057.

32. Soneson E, Puntis S, Chapman N, Mansfield KL, Jones PB, Fazel M. Happier During Lockdown: A Descriptive Analysis of Self-Reported Wellbeing in 17,000 UK School Students During Covid-19 Lockdown. European Child & Adolescent Psychiatry. 2022:1–16.

Chapter 23

Forensic Mental Health Services for Young People

Oliver White

Introduction and Background

For the past two centuries, there have been concerns raised about the well-being of young people who have interactions with the criminal justice system [1] and/or who present with a risk of harm to others. The complexity of these young people arising from their risks and needs across multi-agency domains is such that conventional services are often not able to manage their mental health difficulties, including mainstream Children and Adolescent Mental Health Services [2,3]. There is, therefore, a clear role for specialist forensic Child and Adolescent Mental Health Services.

Forensic mental health services have developed considerably over the past 50 years. In the 1970s, there was no specialist forensic mental health provision for young people, and adult forensic mental health services primarily consisted of three special (high secure) hospitals as well as evidence to courts from a psychiatric expert witness. In the years since, there has been a significant expansion of secure adult forensic psychiatric inpatient provision (medium and low secure units) and, more recently, specialist community services today.

This is mirrored in the evolution of child and adolescent forensic mental health services, although with a slightly distinct focus. Adult forensic psychiatry has primarily focused on inpatient provision, with specialist community forensic mental health teams a relatively new development. Although secure forensic inpatient services for young people have existed since the 1980s, the development of specialist Community Forensic CAMHS has preceded such provision for adults. This mirrors the less restrictive approach for children and young people, including diversion away from custody.

Young People with Forensic Mental Health Needs

The number of first-time entrants to the youth justice system (aged 10 to 17) has consistently fallen over the past 10 years. In the period from 2012 to 2022, the number has fallen by 78% (from around 37,000 to just over 8,000) [4]. Reoffending rates have also reduced, but less consistently and more modestly; 31.2% in 2022, compared to over 40% prior to 2018. However, the frequency of reoffending (the number of offences committed by a young person) has increased during this period.

Although there are now fewer young offenders, there has always been concern about the complexity of the young people who present with concerns about their risk of harm to others and/or who may be in contact with the youth justice system. This complexity is increasing, with a high prevalence of adversity, instability, family conflict, deprivation and trauma. These young people are frequently victims of criminal activity themselves.

A significant number of them are under the care of local authorities or receive input from social services. A large portion have a history of low school attendance and poor academic attainment.

This group of young people experience frequent geographic and service transitions. They have historically been stigmatised and marginalised by services, which further complicates the establishment of trusting relationships with professionals and the overall system.

The high prevalence of mental illness in adolescent offender populations is well established. Rates of psychotic disorder, depressive disorder, anxiety disorder and PTSD are all increased compared to peers in the general population.

Adverse early life experiences frequently result in attachment difficulties and contribute to increased rates of conduct disorder and personality difficulties. Substance use disorders are also common.

The prevalence of learning difficulties and neurodevelopmental disorders (such as ASD and ADHD) among this cohort of young people is higher than that of the general population [5,6]. This aligns with the significantly elevated rates of individuals with learning disabilities or neurodevelopmental challenges who become involved in the criminal justice system and forensic services [7].

Young people who present with an increased risk of harm to others consequentially therefore have a wide range of forensic mental health needs [8,9,10,11,12].

Youth Justice Development

Policies concerning young people involved in the criminal justice system and/or present with a high risk of harm to others have evolved from a historical focus on punishment and deterrence to a greater emphasis on rehabilitation, education and welfare.

The establishment of the youth justice system in 1998 was a response to the increasing recognition that youth offending was not being addressed in a structured manner and that there was a lack of accountability at the local level for children involved in criminal behaviour. Youth Offending Teams (currently Youth Justice Services) were established via the Crime and Disorder Act 1998.

This is evidenced by the dramatic reduction in the number of young people in youth custody at any one time, from a steady level of approximately 3000 in the 10 years to 2009 to 450 in 2022. This is not solely driven by a reduction in offending by young people; there has been a recent focus on efforts to divert young people from custodial settings towards early intervention and community prevention [13,14].

Inpatient Forensic Mental Health Services for Young People

Inpatient care is required for a small cohort of young people who present with the most severe and complex mental disorders, including those associated with a high risk to self and/or others.

The increasing focus on community mental health treatment (including via enhanced community CAMHS teams such as crisis and home treatment services) has resulted in an increase in the overall complexity of young people who require inpatient admission. This has led to the expansion of specialist and secure inpatient services for young people, as the resources and environment within traditional Tier 4 General Adolescent Unit ('open') inpatient units is at times not sufficient to meet their needs.

Secure inpatient provision for young people consists of Adolescent Psychiatric Intensive Care Units (PICUs), Adolescent Low Secure Units, and Adolescent Medium Secure Units (MSU). Only the latter are forensic units; Adolescent PICUs and Adolescent Low Secure Units (LSUs) primarily focus on the assessment and treatment of young people who present with a significant risk of harm to self rather than others.

Adolescent Secure Forensic Psychiatric Hospitals (which operate according to medium secure standards) provide assessment and treatment for young people with mental and neurodevelopmental disorders who present with the highest levels of risk of harm to others, including those who have committed grave crimes. Young people who do not present with a high risk of harm to others (despite possible high risk of harm to themselves) should not be admitted to forensic units.

Scope of Adolescent Secure Forensic Psychiatric Hospital Provision

Provision of Adolescent Secure Forensic Psychiatric Hospitals increased from the first Adolescent MSU in 1985 [15] to over 100 beds across 7 units in 2008. This expansion included that it was increasingly common for young people in non-custodial settings to be referred to Adolescent Secure Forensic Psychiatric Hospitals; this includes girls in Adolescent LSU placements who also present with an increased risk of harm to others (often in the context of staff intervening to manage harm to self).

In the years since, the number of units and beds has gradually reduced to currently around 40 over 4 units. This is most notably due to fewer young people in custody and the expansion of Adolescent PICUs and Adolescent LSUs, which now primarily manage the predominantly female cohort of young people who present with a significant risk of harm to themselves, but only a moderate (if any) risk of harm to others. This contrasts with adult LSU provision, which has a clear referral criterion of risk of harm to others and therefore sit within broader adult forensic services.

There Adolescent Secure Forensic Psychiatric Hospitals in England operate as a national clinical management network. The network supports:

- A single national coordinated referral and admission pathway into individual service settings and across the network
- A coordinated national response that evidences equity of provision across services in England

The Adolescent Secure Forensic Psychiatric Hospital clinical network considers all inpatient referrals of young people from youth justice settings (courts and custodial units). In general, young people from these settings who require inpatient admission are likely to require medium security (there is no high secure inpatient mental health provision for young people; this need is met within medium security with enhanced care as required). The provision is particularly aimed at meeting the following needs:

- Where the young person with a mental disorder, including neurodevelopmental disorders such as learning disability and autism, presents a grave danger to the general public (including those who are high risk without an offending history and those charged with/convicted of specified violent or sexual offences under Schedule 15 of the Criminal Justice Act)

- Where the young person in custody (remand/sentenced) requires transfer to a psychiatric hospital and is directed to secure inpatient care by the Ministry of Justice (MoJ) via a Restriction Order under the Mental Health Act (S48/S49)
- Where the young person has been sentenced by a Crown Court to a Hospital Order (S37) that is accompanied by a Restriction Order (S41) under the Mental Health Act

Adolescent MSU Referral Criteria

- The young person is under 18 at the point of referral

and

- liable to be detained under Part II or Part III of the Mental Health Act

and

- presents significant risk to others with one or more of the following:
    - direct serious violence liable to result in injury to others
    - sexually aggressive behaviour
    - destructive and potentially life-threatening use of fire

and

- there is clear evidence prior to referral that serious consideration of less secure provision has been made and/or tested and discounted as the young person's needs/risk exceed the threshold for and ability of those services to manage.

Care Pathways into Adolescent Forensic Inpatient Provision

There are 4 recognised pathways into adolescent medium secure services:
- direct admission through a criminal court process or from youth justice custodial settings (majority)
- stepping up from low secure adolescent services
- admission from Adolescent PICU, a non-secure adolescent inpatient service, or (very rarely) directly from the community
- admissions from non-criminal justice and welfare settings including welfare secure units and specialist educational settings

Clinical Characteristics of Young People Admitted to Adolescent Secure Forensic Psychiatric Hospitals

The characteristics of 100 patients discharged from one of the Adolescent Secure Forensic Psychiatric Hospitals have been analysed [16]. Ages ranged from 12 to 18, with a mean age of 16.59. Sixty-one per cent were boys and 39% were girls. The group was predominantly White British, with 18% having different ethnic backgrounds (mixed race, Asian or Black British), of which one patient was a foreign national. Around 43% of female and 39% of male patients were subject to a full care order.

Twenty per cent of females and 8% of males were under Section 20 (Children Act 1989). The overall incident rate per occupied bed day was 0.55, meaning that each patient had an incident on average approximately once every 1.82 days. Females had an average incident rate of 0.99 per occupied bed day, which is nearly over four times higher than the male rate (0.26).

The length of stay ranged from one day (released by Tribunal) to 1364 days (3.75 years), with a mean of 276.40 days. The males had on average substantially shorter lengths of stay than the female patients. Forty-six patients (46%) were discharged to community settings, including parental homes, open residential care and residential schools. Thirty-eight (38%) were discharged to other hospitals, including 3 to adult open inpatient units, 13 (13%) to adult low secure, 12 (12%) to adult medium secure and 10 (10%) to Children and Adolescent Mental Health Service (CAMHS) units, both open and secure. Sixteen (16%) were returned to custody, following a clinical decision being made that they no longer required hospital treatment.

Thirty-two (32%) of the patients received a primary diagnosis of a psychotic disorder, including schizophrenia, schizoaffective disorder and substance-related psychotic episodes. These were predominantly male patients. Thirteen were diagnosed with mixed disorder of conduct and emotions with 19 (19%) predominantly female patients receiving the diagnosis of emerging emotionally unstable personality disorder. Nine patients (9%) were considered to have a conduct disorder as primary diagnosis, although most had comorbid diagnoses of childhood conduct disorder, although in other studies on adolescent forensic units this has not always been the case [17]. ASD was the primary diagnosis in (7%) of the young people. The remaining 14 patients (14%) had a variety of primary diagnoses.

The characteristics of the first 64 boys admitted to the same Adolescent Secure Forensic Psychiatric Hospital have been analysed in more detail [18]. They have increased unruliness, oppositionality, social insensitivity, family discord, substance abuse, delinquent predisposition, impulsive predisposition and depressive affect. Many of these strongly indicate emerging antisocial personality traits. Substance abuse correlated with overall incident rate during admission, and childhood abuse correlated with assault rate during admission. There was a high prevalence of risk factors for violence (as assessed via the SAVRY structured professional judgement tool [19]), particularly, 'history of violence', 'history of non-violent offending', 'past supervision and intervention failures', 'poor school achievement', 'stress and poor coping' and anger management problems. Several SAVRY risk factors had correlations with either the incident rate or the violence rate.

The characteristics of 30 consecutive females admitted to one of the Adolescent Secure Forensic Psychiatric Hospitals have also been analysed [20]. They presented with a range of significant and disabling difficulties across the three domains of Personality Patterns, Expressed Concerns and Clinical Syndromes. Cluster B and C personality difficulties in adult personality disorder diagnoses were prevalent. (Cluster B personality disorders are antisocial personality disorder, borderline personality disorder, histrionic personality disorder, and narcissistic personality disorder. Cluster C personality disorders are avoidant personality disorder, dependent personality disorder, and obsessive-compulsive personality disorder.) Clear evidence of PTSD was common, typically arising from past sexual abuse and exposure to violence. Many of the female patients have multiple risk factors for violence (as per the SAVRY), with a high prevalence of childhood history of maltreatment and problems with risk-taking and anger, as well as histories of self-harm and suicide attempts. Attachment difficulties exacerbated by a history of multiple placement breakdowns is highlighted, contributing to increased rates of impulsivity, anger and emotional dysregulation.

Community Forensic Children and Adolescent Mental Health Services

Development of Community Forensic CAMHS

Community Forensic Children and Adolescent Mental Health Services are focused on children and young people about whom there are concerns about their mental health and/or neurodiversity (including learning disability) who present high-risk towards others and/or are in contact with the criminal justice system.

In 2010, a needs assessment project [21] was carried out in London to examine the needs of young individuals who required assistance beyond the capabilities and resources of Tier 3 CAMHS clinicians and Youth Offending Team Health Workers. Findings include that the young people and their families and community were considered vulnerable and pose a risk to themselves and others. They faced multiple issues, with a significant portion (one-third) being female, and often come from unstable or fatherless households. Many were not engaged in education, training or employment and struggled with substance abuse or gang involvement. These individuals had the potential for, or were already exhibiting, severe violence and emotional or behavioural disorders. Due to their poor attendance and chaotic lifestyles, outreach services rather than clinic-based interventions were necessary, but there was a shortage of resources to meet the risk need. A comprehensive, multi-system approach was recommended to address the complex needs of these individuals, yet there was a lack of strategic planning and clarity of responsibility.

In 2013, a mapping of community provision for this group of high-risk young people about whom there are mental health concerns was undertaken [22]. This found that there was patchy geographical provision of dedicated specialist Community Forensic CAMHS provision across the UK, with significant areas of England and Scotland having no such service and were therefore reliant on spot-purchasing.

In the following years, policy development in child and adolescent mental health within NHS England [23,24] emphasised a need to improve mental health care and support for children and young people and created an opportunity to develop provision for the group who present with 'high risk' in terms of harm to self, harm to others and vulnerability. This included the recognition that conventional services may not meet their needs due to their complexity in various domains.

This resulted in the commissioning and provision, initially on a pilot basis but now as 'business as usual', of 13 regional Community Forensic CAMHS covering all of England. These services, some of which were evolutions of existing provisions, commenced between 2017 and 2019.

Despite a regional provision, Community Forensic CAMHS Teams are typically small and consist of clinicians with specialist awareness and experience of working with this cohort of high-risk young people, who due to their complexity of needs often have input from multiple agencies. Community Forensic CAMHS clinicians are from a range of professional backgrounds, including psychiatrists, clinical and forensic psychologists, nurses, social workers and other allied disciplines. Community Forensic CAMHS provide both indirect and direct interventions:

- 'Indirect' interventions refer to the advice and consultation aspects of the service. Such provision can involve (a) an initial short informal advisory discussion resulting in

a decision about whether further service involvement is required or (b) more formal professional consultation with a single professional or with a wider professional network.
- 'Direct' interventions involve the clinical face-to-face involvement of Community Forensic CAMHS: assessment of the young person, at times leading to treatment and other interventions when this is considered necessary and cannot be provided by existing services.

Community Forensic CAMHS Referral Criteria

The referral criteria for Community Forensic CAMHS are deliberately broad, to enable professionals who work with this cohort of complex, high-risk young people to access advice and consultation:
- the young person is under 18 years old

and
- there is concern regarding the young person's mental health (incorporating neurodevelopmental difficulties including learning disability and autism)

and
- the young person presents a high risk of harm towards others

and/or
- the young person is in contact with the youth justice system

Clinical Characteristics of Young People Who Receive Input from Community Forensic CAMHS

Small-scale evaluations of Community Forensic CAMHS provision prior to national commissioning provided some initial insights into the characteristics of young people accessing Community Forensic CAMHS and service activity. Out of a total of 278 referrals, the largest proportion of young people referred were male (82%), aged between 13 and 15 years (44%), White British (65%) and referred from mainstream CAMHS (52%) [25].

Analysis of the national Community Forensic CAMHS activity data [26] expands the understanding via analysis of 1311 advice cases and 1406 referrals. Key findings include:
- 84.7% were aged between 12 and 18 years, with some younger.
- 80% were referred due to violence or aggression.
- 35.5% had Social Care or Early Help Plans.
- 42.50% were known to have experienced inconsistent supervision or boundary setting.
- 22.6% had recent police contact.
- 46.7% had no youth justice input.
- 79.3% presented with at least one difficulty related to psychosis, anxiety, depression, post-traumatic features, ADHD, autism and longstanding behaviour and conduct difficulties. These were not mutually exclusive, with 58.4% having 2 presenting difficulties and 26.5% having 3 or more.
- 71.9% had accessed mainstream CAMHS before their referral.
- 50.9% had experienced/witnessed multiple traumatic events.
- 58.4% of young people presented with multiple difficulties.

The results of the study highlight the complexity of the young people referred to Community Forensic CAMHS and the need for specialist forensic mental health input to multi-agency networks that surround this cohort.

Community Forensic CAMHS Outcomes

The results of early regional evaluations suggested that Community Forensic CAMHS was highly valued in the professional community. They found a reduction in the potential for vulnerable young people to fall through the gaps between services [27] and referrals for out-of-area forensic assessments, avoiding displacement and additional costs [28].

As part of the pilot phase of national commissioning for Community Forensic CAMHS in England, a national evaluation of the provision was undertaken [29]. This identified the following key findings:

- There were significant improvements in the mental health and well-being (as measured by the Health of the Nation Outcome Scales for Children and Adolescents) and overall health and quality of life (as measured by the Health-Related Quality of Life Instrument for Children and Adolescents) for children and young people during the period in which they received input from Community Forensic CAMHS.
- Professionals in contact with this cohort of young people described that Community Forensic CAMHS input contained the network's anxiety, facilitated thinking around care and risk management, promoted interagency working, and provided direct intervention where needs were not met or identified.
- Several professionals noted that Community Forensic CAMHS involvement resulted in a lowering of risk presented by this group of young people and diverted them from admission to secure services.
- Children, young people and parents/carers who received input from Community Forensic CAMHS said that they were provided with high quality support, focused on good communication between and within involved parties and individualised to their needs.
- Parents/carers also discussed the importance of the knowledge and experience of Community Forensic CAMHS 'stepping in' to provide management and clarity in the situation.
- Children, young people, and parents/carers discussed a range of positive experiences and impacts following input from Community Forensic CAMHS, including improved mental health and well-being.
- Of children and young people for whom violence and aggression, sexually harmful behaviour or fire-setting was a concern at referral, between 39% and 52% were no longer a concern or had a suitable management plan in place at discharge.

Further thematic analysis of interviews with parents and carers across five regions [30] identified that Community Forensic CAMHS facilitated support via clear, joined-up communication, co-production of strategies and practical advice, facilitating understanding and 'holding' of anxiety. Further analysis of interviews with referring professionals [31] identified that Community Forensic CAMHS is an approachable and accessible service, provides good levels of communication, increases referrers' confidence, contains anxiety within the network via authority and expertise, facilitates thinking about risk and care and promotes interagency working.

References

1. Hagell A, Hazel N, Shaw C. *Evaluation of Medway Secure Training Centre.* London: Home Office, 2004.
2. NHS England. *The Five Year Forward View for Mental Health.* 2016. https://www.england.nhs.uk/wp-content/uploads/2016/02/Mental-Health-Taskforce-FYFV-final.pdf.
3. Griffin M, Hussain N, & Pittam G. *Evaluation of a Pilot Community Forensic Child and Adolescent Mental Health Service (FCAMHS) for Hampshire and the Isle of Wight (HIoW).* Oxford: Solutions for Public Health, 2010. Available from: https://www.sph.nhs.uk/wp-content/uploads/2017/07/HIoW-FCAMHS-Evaluation-Report-vfinal.pdf (accessed 26 January 2022).
4. *Youth Justice Statistics 2021/22: Youth Justice Annual Statistics for 2021 to 2022 for England and Wales.* England and Wales Youth Justice Board for England and Wales, 2023. https://www.gov.uk/government/statistics/youth-justice-statistics-2021-to-2022
5. Public Health England. *Learning Disabilities Observatory. People with Learning Disabilities in England 2015: Main Report.* Public Health England, 2016. Available from: https://assets.publishing.service.gov.uk/media/5a81e329ed915d74e3400976/PWLDIE_2015_main_report_NB090517.pdf.
6. Simonoff E, Pickles A, Charman T, Chandler S, Loucas T, Baird G. Psychiatric Disorders in Children with Autism Spectrum Disorders: Prevalence, Comorbidity, and Associated Factors in a Population-Derived Sample. J Am Acad Child Adolesc Psychiatry. 2008;47(8):921–29.
7. NHS England and NHS Improvement. *People with a Learning Disability, Autism or Both.* NHS England, 2019.
8. Department of Health. *Healthy Children, Safer Communities: A Strategy to Promote the Health and Well-Being of Children and Young People in Contact with the Youth Justice System.* Department of Health, 2009. https://lx.iriss.org.uk/sites/default/files/resources/dh_109772.pdf.
9. Harrington R, Bailey S, Chitsabesan P, et al. *Mental Health Needs and Effectiveness of Provision for Young Offenders in Custody and in the Community.* London: Youth Justice Board, 2005 https://data.parliament.uk/DepositedPapers/Files/DEP2013-2036/180493_-_YJB_-_Mental_Health_Needs.pdf.
10. Harrington R, Bailey S, Chitsabesan P, et al. *Mental Health Needs and Effectiveness of Provision for Young Offenders in Custody and in the Community.* London: Youth Justice Board, 2005.
11. Lane, R., D'Souza, S., Singleton, R., et al. Characteristics of Young People Accessing Recently Implemented Community Forensic Child and Adolescent Mental Health Services (F: CAMHS) in England: Insights from National Service Activity Data. Eur Child Adolesc Psychiatry. 2023;32:405–17.
12. Bailey S, Tarbuck P, Chitsabesan P, eds. *Forensic Child and Adolescent Mental Health.* Cambridge: Cambridge University Press, 2017.
13. Case S, Browning A. *The Child First Strategy Implementation Project: Realising the Guiding Principle for Youth Justice* [Report]. Loughborough University, 2021. Available from: https://hdl.handle.net/2134/16764124.v1.
14. Lightowler C, Orr D, Vaswani N. *Youth Justice in Scotland: Fixed in the Past or Fit for the Future?* Centre For Youth & Criminal Justice, 2014. Available from: https://www.cycj.org.uk/wp-content/uploads/2014/09/Youth-Justice-in-Scotland.pdf.
15. Bailey S, Thornton L, Weaver A. The First 100 Admissions to an Adolescent Secure Unit. Journal of Adolescence. 1994;17:207–20.
16. Hill SA, Ferreira J, Chamorro V, Hosking A. Characteristics and Personality Profiles of First 100 Patients Admitted to a Secure Forensic Adolescent Hospital. J Forensic Psychiatry Psychol. 2019;30(2):352–66.

17. Kaltiala-Heino R, Putkonen H, Eronen M. Why Do Girls Freak Out? Exploring Female Rage Among Adolescents Admitted to Adolescent Forensic Psychiatric Inpatient Care. J Forensic Psychiatry Psychol. 2013;24(1):83–110.

18. Hill SA, Argent SE, Lolley J, Wallington F. Characteristics of Male Patients Admitted to an Adolescent Secure Forensic Psychiatric Hospital. J Forensic Psychiatry Psychol. 2016;27(1):21–37.

19. Borum R, Lodewijks HP, Bartel PA, Forth AE. The Structured Assessment of Violence Risk in Youth (SAVRY). In RK Otto, KS Douglas (eds.), *Handbook of Violence Risk Assessment*. Routledge, 2011,438–61.

20. Hill SA, Brodrick P, Doherty A, Lolley J, Wallington F, White O. Characteristics of Female Patients Admitted to an Adolescent Secure Forensic Psychiatric Hospital. J Forensic Psychiatry Psychol. 2014;25(5):503–19.

21. Health in Justice LLP. *Health Needs Assessment of Young People in London with Complex Emotional, Behavioural and Mental Health Problems Who Are or May Be at Risk of Committing a Serious Crime*. London: Youth Justice Board and NHS Commissioning Support for London, 2010.

22. Peto LM, Dent M, Griffin M, Hindley N. Community-Based Forensic Child and Adolescent Mental Health Services in England, Scotland and Wales: A National Mapping Exercise. J Forensic Psychiatry Psychol. 2015;26(3):283–96.

23. NHS England. Future in Mind: Promoting, Protecting and Improving our Children and Young People's Mental Health and Wellbeing. London: Department of Health, 2015.

24. NHS England. *The Five Year Forward View for Mental Health*. London: NHS England, 2016.

25. Hindley N, Lengua C, White O. Forensic Mental Health Services for Children and Adolescents: Rationale and Development. BJPsych Advances. 2017;23(1):36–43.

26. Lane R, D'Souza S, Singleton R, et al. Characteristics of Young People Accessing Recently Implemented Community Forensic Child and Adolescent Mental Health Services (F: CAMHS) in England: Insights from National Service Activity Data. Eur Child Adolesc Psychiatry. 2017;23(1):36–43.

27. Griffin, M, Cleave N. *The Provision of Forensic Child and Adolescent Mental Health Services in the Thames Valley*. Oxford: Public Health Resource Unit, 2005.

28. Griffin M, Hussain N, Pittam, G. *Evaluation of a Pilot Community Forensic Child and Adolescent Mental Health Service (FCAMHS) for Hampshire and the Isle of Wight (HIoW)*. Oxford: Solutions for Public Health, 2010. https://www.sph.nhs.uk/wp-content/uploads/2017/07/HIoW-FCAMHS-Evaluation-Report-vfinal.pdf

29. Childs, J., Jacob, J., Labno, A., et al. *National Evaluation of Community Forensic Child and Adolescent Mental Health Services (Community F:CAMHS): Final Report*. Anna Freud Centre, 2021.

30. Jacob, J., Lane, R., D'Souza, S., Cracknell, L., White, O., & Edbrooke-Childs, J. 'If I Didn't Have Them, I'm Not Sure How I Would Have Coped with Everything Myself': Empowering and Supporting Parents/Carers of High-Risk Young People Assisted by Community Forensic CAMHS. Int J Forensic Ment Health. 2023;22(1):56–68.

31. Jacob J, Merrick H, Lane R, et al. 'Containing the Network': Referrers' Experiences of the Community Forensic CAMHS Consultation and Liaison Model. Int J Forensic Ment Health. 2024 Jul;23(3):264–76.

Index

13 Reasons Why (2019), 274

acceptance and commitment therapy (ACT), 289, 300
accommodation, assimilation and, 25
Acquarone, S., 60
action techniques, 302
activity scheduling, 300
adaptive behaviour assessment system (ABAS), 133
adaptive behaviours
  defined, 130–31
  measurement, 133–34
addictions, co-occurring with intellectual disabilities, 137
adherence to treatment, 348–49
adjustment to chronic conditions, 349
adolescence
  in normal childhood development, 30–31
  as risk factor for self-harm and suicide, 179
adolescent mentalization-based integrative therapy (AMBIT), 305
adolescent secure forensic psychiatric hospitals
  care pathways, 356
  characteristics of male and female patients, 357
  clinical characteristics of young people admitted to, 356–57
  referral criteria, 356
  scope of provision, 355–56
  standards of operation, 355
adverse childhood experiences (ACEs)
  assessment, 165
  biopsychosocial impact, 326
  cumulative effect, 326
  definition, 326
  examples, 52
  infant mental health and, 52
  and 'latent vulnerability', 326
  and neurodevelopmental conditions, 119
  potential physical impact, 41, 53
  as predisposing factors for BDD/DD, 284
  prevalence, 41
  and psychopathology in childhood, 41
  relationship with poverty, 41, 53
  relationship with 'social determinants of health', 326–27
  and the development of trauma-aware services and systems, 297
age of criminal responsibility, 88
  Northern Ireland, 94
  Scotland, 94
Ages and Stages Questionnaire, 58
Ainsworth, Mary, 22, 53
alcohol
  adolescence associated with initiation of alcohol use, 235
  alcohol use in pregnancy, 50, 133
    ASD, prenatal exposure as risk factor for, 120
    conduct disorder, prenatal exposure as risk factor for, 148
    foetal alcohol spectrum disorder, 37, 50, 133
    impact on foetal brain development, 37
  interventions for alcohol-using adolescents attending A&E, 237
  PTSD as predictor of alcohol use disorder, 234
  relationship with mood disorders, 233
  as risk factor for self-harm, 177
  trends in consumption, 234
alexithymia, 176
Amplified programme (Young Minds), 7
Angelman syndrome, 133, 138
'Angels in the Nursery' concept, 54
anorexia nervosa (AN), 245–47
  behavioural and psychological symptoms, 246
  diagnostic criteria, 245
  differential diagnoses, 246
  mortality rates, 11
  potentially irreversible long-term physical effects if left untreated, 245
  prevalence, 245
  severity ratings, 246
  temperament/personality factors and, 39
  treatment and management, 246–47
antidepressants, association with psychopathology, 37
anti-NMDA receptor encephalitis, association between psychiatric disorders and, 38
antisocial behaviours
  overview, 144
  genetic factors, 148, 149
  see also disruptive behaviour disorders.
antisocial personality disorder, 76
anxiety
  co-occurring with intellectual disabilities, 136
  role of tolerance of uncertainty, 309
  see also anxiety and depression; anxiety disorders.

363

Index

anxiety and depression
  association with excessive screen-time, 270
  autistic female children and, 119
  as differential diagnosis to BDD and DD, 282
  exposure to sexual trauma and, 233
  gender-diverse youth and, 315
  online CBT as treatment for, 172
  risk of for migrant and refugee children, 41
  social contact/peer relationships as mediating factor for, 309
  see also depression.
anxiety disorders
  age at onset, 169
  causes, 167
  continuity of disorders, 169–70
  course and outcomes, 169
  differentiating criteria, 168
  effectiveness of CBT for, 300
  interventions, 170–71
  normal childhood fears, 167
  prevalence, 168
  psychosocial interventions in CAMHS, 298
  as risk factors for self-harm, 176
  usefulness of diagnostic categories, 167
aripiprazole, 125, 205–6, 224
asenapine, 205, 224
assessments in child and adolescent psychiatry
  overview, 96, 111
  ADHD clinical evaluation, 105
  autism diagnostic interview, 105
  autism diagnostic observation schedule, 107
  case vignette, 97
  child and adolescent psychiatric assessment, 105
  cognitive functioning, 108
  confidentiality statement, 99
  development and well-being assessment, 105
  diagnostic interview for children, 105
  feedback, 110–11
  formulation and diagnosis, 108–10
  genogram, 104, 302
  history taking
    developmental history, 100
    educational history, 101
    parental health and education, 104
    principles, 99–101
    requesting external information, 101
    structure, 98
  information variability, 109
  introductions in assessment, 99
  managing expectations, 110
  Manchester child attachment story task, 107
  mental state examination, 101–3
    appearance and behaviour, 101–2
    insight, 103
    language and speech, 102
    mood, 102
    thought patterns, 102–3
  multidisciplinary approach, 98
  observational assessments, 107–8
  occupational therapy assessments, 108
  parents/carers and families, 103–4
    history taking, 104
    interview tools, 105
    observation of parent child interaction, 104
  physical examination, 105
  preparation for assessment in children and adolescents, 98–99
  the process of assessment in children and adolescents, 97–98
  purpose of assessment in children and adolescents, 96–98
  risk assessment, 103
  screening instruments, 106
  specialist assessments, 107
  speech and language assessments, 102, 108, 118
assimilation, 25
attachment disorders
  categorisation, 161
  disinhibited social engagement disorder, 161
  prevalence, 163
  reactive attachment disorder, 161
  relevance of attachment in child and adolescent psychiatry, 163
attachment styles, 161
attachment theory, 53–54
  ambivalent attachment, 22
  'Angels in the Nursery' concept, 54
  assessment tool, 107
  attachment styles overview, 162
  avoidant attachment, 22, 54
  disorganised attachment, 22–23
  'Ghosts in the Nursery' concept, 54
  insecure attachment, 53
  neurodivergent children and, 54
  normal childhood development and, 21–23
  relationship of insecure attachment and behaviour in later childhood, 23
  secure attachment, 22, 40
  'strange situation procedure', 22
  typical attachment behaviours, 53
  see also insecure attachment.
attention deficit hyperactivity disorder (ADHD), 121
  ADHD clinical evaluation, 105
  adverse outcomes associated with, 121
  ARFID associated with, 251

characterised in ICD-11, 121
childhood epilepsy
    associated with, 38
co-morbidities
    BDD, 279
    bipolar disorder, 204, 205
    disruptive behaviour
        disorders, 147
comparison of ICD
    and DSM
    classifications, 72
co-occurring with
    intellectual disability,
    134–35
differentiating from bipolar
    disorder, 203
efficacy of medications for,
    124–25
environmental risk
    factors, 121
genetic component, 52
heritability, 36, 121
non-pharmacological
    interventions, 125
obstetric complications
    associated with, 37
pharmacological treatment
    of resulting in
    reduction of SUD
    severity, 238
prevalence in males and
    females, 121
rating scales, 119
relationship with learning
    disability, 38
as risk factor for
    self-harm, 176
risk of substance misuse, 235
risperidone use, 153
traumatic brain injury
    associated with, 38
treatment approaches,
    124–25
Attwood, Tony, 309
autism
    comparison of ICD-10 and
        ICD-11 diagnoses, 70
    genetic component, 52
    and health inequality, 2
    as risk factor for self-
        harm, 176
autism diagnostic observation
    schedule
    (ADOS), 107
autism spectrum conditions
    (ASCs), co-morbidity

with destructive
    behaviour
    disorders, 148
autism spectrum disorder
    (ASD), 120
ARFID associated with, 251
and benefits of hospital
    passports, 345
characterised in ICD-11, 120
childhood epilepsy
    associated with, 38
common co-morbidities, 122
common triggers for
    anxiety, 344
co-morbid mental illness,
    prevalence of, 345
co-morbidity with BDD, 280
comparison of ICD and
    DSM
    classifications, 72
comparison with
    pathological demand
    avoidance, 120
co-occurring with
    intellectual
    disability, 134
diagnostic interview, 105
diagnostic observation
    schedule, 107
disordered eating behaviour
    and, 252
and early-onset psychosis,
    222–23
female vs male
    characteristics, 119
forensic in-patients,
    prevalence in, 357
'Good practice guide for
    professionals
    delivering talking
    therapies for autistic
    adults and children'
    (National Autistic
    Society), 305, 344
heritability, 120
obstetric complications
    associated with, 37
overlap with gender
    incongruence
    diagnoses, 315–16
perinatal environmental risk
    factors, 120
pharmacotherapy
    considerations, 345
potential associated genetic
    conditions, 345

prevalence, 76, 120
rating scales, 119
relationship with learning
    disability, 38
and risk of death by
    suicide, 344
role of tolerance of
    uncertainty, 309
treatment approaches, 124
Autism Strategy, 4
autoimmune/inflammatory
    conditions, association
    between psychiatric
    disorders and, 38
avoidant attachment, 22, 54
avoidant restrictive food intake
    disorder (ARFID), 11,
    71, 250–51
    associated with ASD, 251
    characteristics and possible
        signs of, 250–51
    classification, 250
    co-morbidities, 251
    prevalence, 250
    treatment and
        management, 251
Avon Longitudinal Study of
    Parents and Children
    (UK), 192

babies and young children,
    mental health of as
    neglected area of
    health care, see also
    infant mental
    health 49
Baker, L., 170
Bandura, A., 26
Beck depression inventory
    (BDI), 191
Beck's cognitive triad, 193
Beebe, B., 58
Beesdo-Baum, K., 170
behavioural activation, 193,
    298–99, 300
behavioural disorders
    co-occurring with
        intellectual
        disabilities, 137
    prevalence, 76
benzodiazepines, 137, 205,
    224, 343
Berens, A. E., 52
binge eating disorder
    (BED), 249
    characteristics, 249

binge eating disorder (cont.)
  physical consequences, 249
  prevalence, 249
  risk factors for development of, 249
  treatment and management, 249
bipolar affective disorder, co-occurring with intellectual disabilities, 136–37
bipolar disorder (BD), 201, 202–3
  aetiology, 148
  assessment, 203–4
  attempted suicide, prevalence of, 206
  classification, 202
  common co-morbidities, 204
  comparison of ICD-11 and DSM-5, 202
  controversy around the diagnosis, 201–2
  differential diagnoses, 203
  heritability, 203
  prognosis, 206–7
  treatment, 204–5
    co-morbid ADHD, 205
    depressive episodes, 205
    lithium, 206
    manic episodes, 205
    mixed episodes, 205
    relapse prevention, 205–6
    valproate, 206
Black, D., 54
bodily distress disorder (BDD)
  assessment, 285–87
    psychiatric assessment, 286
  bio-psycho-social explanatory model, 283–85
  case vignette, 280
  characteristics, 278, 279
  common co-morbidities, 280
  common symptoms, 279
  cultural aspects, 283
  diagnostic classification and clinical presentation, 278–79
  diagnostic overview, 279
  differential diagnoses, 282
  epidemiology, 282
  future perspectives, 292
  perpetuating factors, 284–85
  precipitating factors, 284

  predisposing factors, 284
  psychiatrists' role, 291–92
  as risk factor for self-harm, 176
  treatment, 291
    basic strategies, 287
    complementary techniques, 289
    education about symptoms, 287, 289
    general health promoting strategies, 289
    psychopharmacological interventions, 289
    specialised treatment, 289–91
borderline personality disorder (BPD)
  comparison with complex PTSD, 177
  hesitancy to diagnose, 177
  predictive validity of, 177
  as risk factor for self-harm and suicidality, 177
Bowlby, John, 21, 53, 61
brain development
  and infant mental health, 52
  optimal conditions for, 52
  role of early relationships in, 50–51, 52
  sensitivity of teenage brains to social input, 328
Brazelton, T. B., 58
Brazelton neonatal behavioural assessment scale (NBAS), 58
brief psychosocial intervention (BPI), 196
British Ability Scales (BAS) ©, 133
bulimia nervosa (BN), 247–49
  celebrity sufferers, 247
  common physical symptoms, 248
  co-morbidities, 248
  diabetes and, 248–49
  diagnostic criteria, 247–48
  novelty seeking behaviour and, 39
  treatment and management, 248
bullying, as risk factor for mental health problems in children, 40
Burnham, J., 301–2

cannabis, association with psychosis, 39, 223
Cantwell, D. P., 170
Carballo, J. J., 170
carbamazepine, 153
care system, mental health policy and, 12
case formulation
  definition, 296
  and psychosocial approaches, 296–97
  see also formulation.
'The Cass Review' (NHS England), 316
CBCL-Paediatric Bipolar Disorder (CBCL-PBD), 204
certificates, 301
challenging behaviour, RCPsych definition, 344
Chess, Stella, 23
child and adolescent mental health services (CAMHS)
  overview, 1
  assessment structure, 105
  benefits of early referral, 199
  combined categorical/dimensional approach, 69
  crisis teams and intensive home-based services, 183
  increased recognition of the importance of, 73
  inequalities in provision, 2
  psychosocial approaches. see psychosocial approaches
  role of classification in, 69
  specialist forensic services, see forensic mental health services.
  values-based practice training, 195
child and adolescent psychiatric assessment (CAPA), 105
child and adolescent psychotherapists (CAPTs), 303

child and family-focused cognitive-behavioural therapy, 206
Child Behaviour Checklist, 58, 204
child death overview panels (CDOPs), 2
child death review (CDR), 2
child development
  benefits of internet-based technology for, 265
  risks of internet-based technology for, 266
child interview, working model of, 58
child mania rating scale-parent version (CMRS-P), 204
Child Outcome Research Consortium (UK), 192
child parent psychotherapy, 61
Child Psychotherapy, 62
childhood development, normal, see normal childhood development.
The Children Act
  children's welfare practice and, 331
  scope of intervention supported by, 331
children and young people's mental health services (CYPMH), overview, 1, 13–14
Children and Young People's Mental Health Taskforce report (Scottish Government/COSLA), 3
chlamydia, association with mental health problems, 38
Chomsky, Noam, 26
Christchurch Health and Development Study (CHDS), 233
chronic fatigue, 278
chronic health conditions, 346–47
Circle of Security parenting programme, 61
citalopram, 197

classification of child and adolescent psychiatric disorders
  categorical vs dimensional, 67
  challenge to current systems, 67–68
  ICD and DSM classifications comparison between ICD 11 and DSM-5, 71–72
  efforts to harmonize, 67
  key updates, 70–71
  neurodevelopmental disorders, 72
  ICD-11 changes from ICD-10, 71
  most widely used systems, 67
  multiaxial classification and child and adolescent psychiatry, 69–70
  role in CAMHS, 69
climate change, potential role in depression, 194
clonidine, 125, 153
clozapine, 224
cognitive ability, and psychopathology in childhood, 38–39
cognitive behaviour therapy (CBT), 196, 299–300
  Cochrane review, 195
  combined treatment trials, 198
  effectiveness for eating disorders, 300
  as intervention for self-harm/suicide, 184
  interventions for antisocial behaviours, 154
  for OCD and body dysmorphic disorder, 171
  online CBT, 172–73
  potential benefits for reducing self-harm in adolescents, 184
  potentially beneficial components, 193
  for psychosis in children and adolescents, 225
  in psychosocial approaches, 299
  'third wave' approaches, 300
  trauma-focused (TF-CBT), 171, 173

  as treatment for bodily distress disorder/DD, 289
  as treatment for depression, 196
cognitive development
  four stages, 25
  in normal childhood development, 25
cognitive functioning, assessing, 108
cognitive remediation therapy (CRT), 225
community forensic CAMHS
  clinical characteristics of young people admitted to, 359–60
  development of, 353, 358–59
  interventions provided by, 358
  outcomes, 360
  referral criteria, 359
community-based treatments, clinical outcomes, 12
compassion-focused therapy (CFT), 300
complex PTSD (C-PTSD)
  attachment styles overview, 162
  the concept of complex trauma, 164
  diagnostic criteria, 165, 166, 177
  differential diagnosis, 166–67
  ICD-11 categorisation, 164
  interventions, 172
  RAD and DSED seen as potential pre-cursor to, 161
  see also post-traumatic stress disorder (PTSD).
compulsive sexual behaviour disorders, 72
conduct disorder/conduct-dissocial disorder, 23, 71–72, 145–46, 233, 354
  adverse childhood experiences and, 354
  associated factors, 144
  characteristics, 76, 137, 144–45, 147, 148
  diagnostic criteria, 73
  differentiation of ODD from, 144

conduct disorder (cont.)
    IED and, 147
    insecure attachment and, 23
    learning disability as risk factor for, 38
    multimodal interventions, 154
    neurobehavioural disinhibition and, 233
    NICE recommendations for young people at risk of, 154
    pharmacotherapy, 153
    prenatal risk factors, 148
    sexual trauma and, 233
    undesirable outcomes associated with a diagnosis of, 147
consanguinity, and risk of autosomal recessive genetic conditions, 119
cortisol
    potential impact on brain and body, 52
    potential role in depression, 192
Costa, Paul, 24
Costello, E. J., 169
Council for Child Internet Safety, 264
Covid-19 pandemic, 78, 194
    and health inequalities, 2, 323
    impact on CYP, 1, 10, 254, 271, 339, 340, 343, 349–50
    impact on data collection, 231
    and increased online gambling, 271
    and increased prevalence of eating disorders, 1, 10, 194, 254, 271, 340
    and increased use of digital therapies, 255
    lockdowns, 255, 271, 343
    and PMIS, 349
    and psychopathology in childhood, 42
    and the transformation of the digital landscape, 264
Crime and Disorder Act 1998, 354

criminal justice pathway, psychiatrist's role in. *see under* legal perspectives.
criminal justice system
    concerns raised about well-being of young people who have interactions with, 353
    EMCDDA guidance on substance misuse, 239–39
    prevalence of youth contact with, 78
    see also adolescent secure forensic psychiatric hospitals; community forensic CAMHS; forensic mental health services.
criminal responsibility, age of, *see* age of criminal responsibility.
crisis services and home treatment teams, 12
Crowell Play Procedure, 58
cyberbullying, 272–73
    case vignette, 282
    comparison with traditional in-person bullying, 272
    definition, 272
    mental health impact, 272–73
cyclothymic disorder, ICD-11 and DSM-5, 202
CYP-IAPT (improving access to psychological therapy for children and young people) programme, 8, 13
cystic fibrosis, 346
cytomegalovirus, association with mental health problems, 38

Dadds, M., 167
debriefing of hospital personnel, value of, 349
delirium, 340, 342–43
demographics and correlates of mental disorder, 74–75
depression

aetiology, 192–94
attachment-informed theories, 193
case vignette, 42
clinical features, 190
cognitive theories, 193
common co-morbidities in adolescent depression, 191
diagnosis, 190
diagnostic criteria, 191
epidemiology, 190
heritability, 36
inpatient admission, 200–1
prevalence in preschool age children, 190
prevalence in the perinatal period, 50
prognosis, 200–1
protective factors, 192
psychosocial interventions in CAMHS, 298
and rates of substance use disorder, 233
rating scales, 191–92
as risk factor for self-harm and suicide, 177
risk factors
    biological, 192–93
    developmental and psychological, 193
    environmental, 193, 194
    familial, 192
    and the role of serotonin in neuroplasticity, 192
treatment
    brief psychosocial intervention (BPI), 196
    CBT, 196
    combined treatment trials, 198
    digital health interventions, 196
    ECT, 200
    evidence-based treatment options, 195
    exercise programmes, 198
    family-focussed treatment, 196
    iatrogenic effects, 197
    interpersonal psychotherapy (IPT), 196
    medication, 197–98

citalopram, 197
common side effects of
    SSRIs, 197
fluoxetine, 197–98
combined treatment
    trials, 198
ketamine, 200
sertraline, 197
venlafaxine, 200
music therapy, 198
nature-based, 198
options, 195
outcomes, 201
predictors of outcome, 199
preventative
    interventions, 194
psychological therapy,
    196–97
    adverse effects, 197
school-based
    interventions, 195–96
stepped care model, 195
transcranial magnetic
    stimulation, 200
treatment resistant
    depression (TRD),
    199–200
    see also anxiety and
    depression.
Deprivation of Liberty
    Safeguards
    (DoLS), 82
development and well-being
    assessment
    (DAWBA), 1,
    105, 192
developmental coordination
    disorder (DCD), co-
    occurring with
    intellectual
    disabilities, 135
developmental language
    disorder, comparison
    of ICD and DSM
    classifications, 72
developmental learning
    disorders, 122
developmental milestones,
    normal childhood
    development, 19–21
developmental motor
    coordination disorder
    (dyspraxia), 122
developmental speech or
    language
    disorders, 121

diabetes mellitus (DM)
    association between
    psychiatric disorders
    and, 38
    disordered eating in the
    context of, 248–49
    and treatment
    adherence, 346
diagnosis, formulation and,
    108–10
Diagnostic and Statistical
    Manual of Mental
    Disorders (DSM), 67
Diagnostic Classification of
    Mental Health and
    Developmental
    Disorders Infancy
    and Early
    Childhood, 49
diagnostic interview for
    children (DISC), 105
diagnostic overshadowing, 138,
    153, 305
dialectical behaviour therapy
    (DBT), 304
    as intervention for self-
    harm/suicide, 184
    as therapy for eating
    disorders, 252–53
Digital Bodies (Bell et al), 255
digitization and health
    information
    technology, 7–9
disability, parent–infant
    psychotherapy in the
    context of, 60
disinhibited social engagement
    disorder (DSED), 71
    comparison with RAD, 161
disorders
    classification by ICD and
        DSM, 67
    potential for overlap, 68
disorganised attachment,
    22–23
disruptive behaviour disorders
    overview, 144
    aetiology, 148–49
    assessment, 149–52
    biological factors, 148
    co-morbid developmental
        and mental health
        issues, 147
    comparison of ICD and
        DSM
        classifications, 72

conduct-dissocial disorder,
    145–46
    diagnostic criteria, 146
    definition and
        categorisation,
        144–47
    epidemiology, 147–48
    estimated cost to society, 144
    functional imaging
        studies, 148
    heritability, 148
    impulse control disorders,
        146–47
    interaction between genetic
        and environmental
        factors, 149–53
    oppositional defiant
        disorder, 144
    personality disorder, 147
    prevalence, 147
    psychopharmacology, 153
    psychosocial approaches,
        153–55
    psychosocial factors, 148
disruptive mood dysregulation
    disorder (DMDD),
    72, 202, 203
disruptive/dissocial
    disorders, 71
dissociative disorders (DD)
    assessment, 285–87
    psychiatric
        assessment, 286
    biopsychosocial explanatory
        model, 283–85
    case vignette, 281
    characteristics, 278
    common co-morbidities, 280
    common symptoms, 280
    cultural aspects, 283
    diagnostic classification and
        clinical presentation,
        278–79
    diagnostic overview, 281
    differential diagnoses, 282
    dissociative neurological
        symptom disorder
        (DNSD), 280
    epidemiology, 283
    future perspectives, 292
    perpetuating factors, 284–85
    precipitating factors, 284
    predisposing factors, 284
    psychiatrists' role, 291–92
    and risk of medication
        errors, 280

dissociative disorders (cont.)
    treatment, 291
        basic strategies, 287
        complementary
            techniques, 289
        education about
            symptoms, 287, 289
        general health promoting
            strategies, 289
        psychopharmacological
            interventions, 289
        specialised treatment,
            289–91
dopamine
    dysfunction of implicated in
        pathophysiology of
        tics, 122
    increased levels of during
        self-injury, 182
    risk-taking behaviours
        and, 30
Down syndrome
    (trisomy 21), 132
dyadic developmental
    psychotherapy
    (DDP), 329
dynamic developmental
    psychotherapy
    (DDP), 304
dyslexia, 136, 148
dyspraxia, 122

early adversity
    awareness of long-term
        physical and mental
        health impact,
        323
    mitigating role of positive
        social
        determinants, 326
'early experiences', and infant
    mental health, 51
early intervention in psychosis
    services, 11–12,
    225–26
early puberty, potential role in
    depression, 193,
early relationships
    effects on structure and
        function of the
        brain, 52
    examples of challenges
        for, 50
    role in brain development,
        50–51, 52
    and temperament, 50

Early Years Healthy
    Development Review
    Report (HM
    Government,
    2021), 10
early-onset psychosis (EOP)
    overview, 219
    aetiology, 220
    antipsychotic medication,
        224–25
        common side effects,
            224–25
    ASD and, 222–23
    clinical symptomatology,
        221–22
    common co-morbidities, 223
    course and prognosis, 221
    diagnostic assessment/
        differential diagnosis,
        222–23
    early intervention services,
        11–12, 225–26
    environmental factors, 220
    epidemiology, 219–20
    genetic factors, 220
    medical causes of psychotic
        symptoms, 222
    neurodevelopmental
        origins, 220
    prevalence of psychotic
        symptoms in
        childhood, 220
    psychosocial
        interventions, 225
    risk factors, 220
    treatment, 223–26
eating disorders (ED), 340–41
    overview, 244–45
    anorexia nervosa, 245–47
    avoidant restrictive food
        intake disorder,
        250–51
    binge eating disorder, 249
    bulimia nervosa, 247–49
    case vignette, 43
    clinical implications and
        future directions,
        256–57
    common co-morbidities, 253
    complex presentations,
        251–53
    Covid-19 pandemic and,
        42, 350
    diagnostic criteria
        changes, 244
    digital therapies, 255–56

eating disorder services, 11
effectiveness of CBT for, 300
impact of social media, 244,
    253–55
main aim of medical
    admission, 340–41
medical emergencies
    guidance, 246
as method of self-harm,
    180–81
NHSE Guidance, 11
other specified feeding and
    eating disorders, 250
prevalence, 340
    CYP, 256
    gender diverse youth, 315
    male/female differences,
        11, 76
research limitations, 256
role of the CPM team, 341
social media/the internet
    and, 40, 255, 274
temperament and
    personality
    influences, 39
education
    benefits of internet-based
        technology for, 266
    risks of internet-based
        technology for, 266
electroconvulsive therapy
    (ECT), as treatment
    for difficult-to-treat
    depression, 200
elimination disorders, 71
emotional development,
    normal childhood
    development, 24–25
emotional disorders,
    prevalence, 75, 190
emotional literacy, 25
emotional regulation, 24
    role of temperament, 24
    self-harm as strategy for, 181
encopresis, 71
Engel, George, 34, 109
enuresis, 71
epidemiology of child and
    adolescent
    psychiatric disorders,
    73–78
    behavioural disorders, 76
    demographics and correlates
        of disorder, 74–75
    effects of Covid-19
        pandemic, 78

emotional disorders, 75
hyperactivity disorders, 76
mental health in CYP, 1–2
other disorders, 76–77
self-harm and suicide, 77
substance misuse and
criminal justice
contacts, 77–78
in the UK, 73–74
epigenetics, definition, 52
epilepsy
associated with psychiatric
disorders in
childhood and in later
life, 38
co-occurring with
intellectual
disabilities, 138
ethnic minority communities,
access to services, 2
ethnicity
as correlate of disorder, 75
and risk of depression, 194
Euphoria (2019), 274
European Monitoring Centre
for Drugs and Drug
Addiction, 239
exposure therapy, 298, 300
externalisation, 301
eye movement desensitisation
and reprocessing
(EMDR), 171, 304

factitious disorder, as
differential diagnosis
to bodily distress
disorder and DD, 282
family focused treatment for
early onset and
youth, 206
family life cycle, 302
family nurse partnership
programme, 10
family risk factors, for
psychopathology in
childhood, 40
family therapists, 302
family-based therapies, as
intervention for self-
harm/suicide, 184
Faraone, S. V., 121
febrile seizures, 38
Felitti, V. J., 52
fibromyalgia, juvenile,
278
'fitspiration', 253, 274

Five Year Forward View for
Mental Health
(FYFVMH), 4, 5,
11, 13
fluoxetine, 153, 197–98, 205
combined treatment
trials, 198
foetal alcohol spectrum
disorder (FASD), 37,
50, 133
foetal valproate syndrome,
118
Foley, D. L., 170
forensic mental health
services, 353
historical perspective, 353
inpatient care, 354
prevalence of mental illness
in adolescent offender
populations, 354
secure inpatient provision
for young people, 355
young people with forensic
mental health needs,
353–54
youth justice development,
354
see also adolescent
secure forensic
psychiatric hospitals;
community forensic
CAMHS.
formulation
4 Ps approach, 109
bio psycho social
approach, 109
commonly used methods,
109–10
the concept of, 181, 296
developmental
approach, 110
and diagnosis, 108–10
requirements of the task,
333
Fragile X syndrome, 118, 132
Fraiberg, Selma, 54, 61
Frank, J., 53
Fraser Guidelines, 83,
Freud, Sigmund, 24, 53
Fukuyama, Francis, 235
functional family therapy
(FFT), 305
functional gastrointestinal
disorders, 278
functional neurological
(symptom) disorder

(conversion
disorder), 278
functional neurological
disorders, 343
functional somatic syndromes
(FSS), 278
Future in Mind (Department of
Health & NHS
England 2015), 3, 11

Galloway, S., 50
gaming
brain changes associated
with, 272
and compulsive/addictive
behaviours, 270
encouraging a balance of
gaming
behaviours, 271
questions to ask about, 268
gaming disorder, 270–72
definition, 270
link with online
gambling, 271
research on, 271–72
gender diverse youth
co-morbid mental health
problems,
315–16, 319
considerations in assessment
and treatment of, 317
and 'de-transition', 319
differential diagnosis,
314–15
distal or proximal stressors
experienced by, 316
domains of health care
overlap, 318
epidemiology, 314
gender incongruence
defined, 314
gender-affirming model of
care, 316–17
controversy around, 316
lack of long-term follow-
up, 318
post-treatment mental
health outcomes, 318
impact of the increasing
trend, 314
male/female patterns, 314
prevalence, 313, 314, 318
research on mental health
in, 318
sexual and gender minorities
terminology, 313

gender diverse youth (cont.)
  suicide prevention as focus of treatment, 317
  and 'The Cass Review' (NHS England), 316
  unique stressors faced by, 313
gender identity, normal childhood development, 31–32
general data protection regulation (GDPR), 8,
general hospitals
  benefits of working in, 339
  increase in demand for child and adolescent specialist psychiatric teams, 339
generalised anxiety disorder, prevalence, 169
genetic syndromes, case vignette, 43
genetics
  association with neurodevelopmental disorders, 118, 120
  and risk factors for psychopathology in childhood, 36–37
  role in infant mental health, 52
  role in intellectual disabilities, 132
genogram, 104, 302
Getting It Right First Time (GIRFT), 8
'Ghosts in the Nursery' concept, 54
Gillick Competence, 83,
Gin, K., 220
global developmental delay, 132
Gosling, C. J., 124
'The Great Disruption' (Fukuyama), 235
Green, J., 124
grooming
  definition, 273
  online grooming and sexual exploitation, 273
guanfacine, 125
Guthrie, E., 340

habit reversal training, 342

Harold, G., 104
Health and Care Act (2022), 5
Health and Social Care Act (2012), 1
Health and Wellbeing Boards, 323, 332
health care access
  benefits of internet-based technology for, 266
  risks of internet-based technology for, 267
health inequalities, likely impact on mental health, 2
health promotion, strategies for, 324
Heckman, J. J., 54
heritability of psychiatric disorders
  ADHD, 36, 121
  ASD, 120
  bipolar disorder, 201, 203
  depression, 36
  disruptive behaviour disorders, 148
  neurodevelopmental disorders, 119
  schizophrenia, 37, 220
Herman, J., 164
herpes simplex, association with mental health problems, 38
history taking
  developmental history, 100
  educational history, 101
  parental health and education, 104
  principles, 99–101
  requesting external information, 101
  structure, 98
holistic models of care, 9
home treatment teams, crisis services and, 12
hopelessness, potential consequences of a sense of, 330
hospital passports, benefits of, 345
human immunodeficiency virus (HIV), association with mental health problems, 38
Human Rights Act 1998, 81–82

hyperactivity disorders, prevalence, 76

The Identification of an Intellectual Disability, an A to H Framework (IDIDA2H©), 133–34
impulse control disorders, 72, 146–47
  CBT as treatment for, 154
  intermittent explosive disorder, 147
  prevalence, 147
  pharmacotherapy, 153
  pyromania, 146–47
Incredible Years Programme, 62, 299, 329
infants
  definition, 49
  development of peer relationships, 28
  etymology, 55
  language development, 26
  process of bonding between parents and, 21
  see also attachment theory
infant mental health
  adverse childhood experiences and, 52
  assessment
    observation of infants and their relationships, 58
    tools and measures, 58–59
  behaviourism and cognitive theory, 54
  brain development and, 52
  coining of the phrase, 54
  definition of infants, 49
  diagnosis and formulation of mental health problems, 59
  dissociation, avoidance and miscuing strategies, 55
  'early experiences' and, 51
  early relationships and, 50–51, 52
  epigenetics and, 52
  fathers' mental health and, 51
  genetic factors, 52
  impact of parental functioning on, 51

importance of good mental health in infancy, 49
importance of support for parents and other primary caregivers, 51
infant mental health services
the case for, 54–55
composition of specialist IMH teams, 56
Northern Irish provision, 3
psychiatrists' role, 56–57
Scottish provision, 3
Scottish provision, Perinatal Mental Health Care Pathway, 57
service design and provision, 55, 56
stepped care model, 56
interventions, 59–62
child parent psychotherapy, 61
Circle of Security parenting programme, 61
family nurse partnership, 62
infant-parent psychotherapy and parent–infant psychotherapy, 60
narrative, 60
neonatal behavioural assessment scale, 60
newborn behavioural observation, 60
other commonly used interventions, 62
video interaction guidance, 61, 299
key ingredients for a healthy and safe start in life, 50–51
maternal mental health problems and, 50
nurturing factors, 49
pathology, psychoanalysis and attachment theory, 53–54
pregnancy and, 50
prevalence of problems with, 49
RCPsych report, 49

role of a safe and stimulating environment, 51
infectious agents, association with mental health problems, 38
inpatient treatment
comparison with community-based treatments, 12
drive to reduce reliance on in England, 4
insecure attachment, 53
association with adolescent depression, 193
as 'general vulnerability' to mental health problems, 163
inconsistent caregiving associated with, 40
key role in child and adolescent psychopathology, 173
and later diagnosis of behavioural disorders, 23
linked to anxiety, 163
and PTSD, 23
integrated care boards (ICBs), 5
integrated care models, 9
requirements for development of, 13
value of for children with chronic health conditions, 347
see also psychological medicine.
integrated care partnerships (ICPs), 5
integrated care systems (ICSs), 5,
key aims, 5
and provider collaboratives, 5
Integration and Innovation: working together to improve health and social care outcomes for all (White Paper, 2021), 9
intellectual disabilities
overview, 19, 130
defining, 130–32
assessment

adaptive behaviours measurement, 133–34
IDIDA2H© framework, 133–34
IQ measurement, 133
association of ARFID with, 251
causes
environmental, 133
genetic, 132
co-occurring conditions, 136–37, 138
ADHD, 134–35
assessment of, 138–39
autism, 134
behavioural disorders, 76
borderline intellectual functioning, 136
comparison of ICD-10 and ICD-11 criteria, 138
developmental coordination disorder, 135
developmental learning disorders, 136
developmental speech and language disorders, 135
'diagnostic overshadowing' and, 138
mental health disorders, 140
treatment of, 139–40
differential diagnoses, 134–37
interventions
biological interventions, 140
capacity and consent, 140
psychological interventions, 139
social interventions, 139
mild, 131
moderate, 131
normal distribution at 2 standard deviations below mean, 131
and physical health, 138
prevalence of mental disorders by ICD-10 category, 135
profound, 132

intellectual disabilities (cont.)
　provisional disorder of
　　intellectual
　　development, 132
　relationship with mental
　　health, 2
　research recommendations,
　　140–41
　severe, 132
　　see also learning
　　disabilities.
intelligence quotient (IQ)
　defined, 130
　measurement of, 133
　as predictor of adult-onset
　　schizophrenia, 38
intermittent explosive disorder
　　(IED), 147
　prevalence, 147
International Classification of
　　Diseases (ICD), 67
International Consortium for
　　Health Outcomes
　　Measurement, 192
internet-based
　　technology (IBT)
　overview, 264, 275
　benefits, 265–66
　clinical role, 267
　compulsive use and
　　addiction, 270
　and copycat behaviour,
　　273–74
　cyberbullying, 272–73
　digital history screening
　　questions, 267–68
　　additional assessment, 268
　　advice for parents/
　　　guardians, 268
　gaming disorder, 270–72
　importance of
　　understanding for
　　clinicians, 265, 267
　increasing use of by children
　　and young
　　people, 264
　online grooming and sexual
　　exploitation, 273
　potential for a 'digital
　　divide', 264
　risks, 266–67
　social media, see social media.
interpersonal psychotherapy
　　(IPT), 196
　short-term benefits for
　　depression, 195

interpersonal psychotherapy
　　for depressed
　　adolescents
　　(IPT-A), 304
intersex, 31, 313, 315
invisible friends, 301

juvenile fibromyalgia, 278
Juvenile Offenders Act 1847, 93

Kaufman Brief Intelligence
　　Test, 133
ketamine
　misuse of, 223
　as treatment for difficult-to-
　　treat depression, 200
Kiddie Schedule for Affective
　　Disorders and
　　Schizophrenia
　　(K-SADS), 191, 204
Klein, Melanie, 53
kleptomania, 146, 153
Kohlberg, L., 27
Koot, H. M., 169
Kozlowska, K., 342

lamotrigine, 206
Lanarkshire IMH
　　Observational
　　Indicator Set, 59
language and speech,
　　assessment of,
　　102, 108
language development
　developmental speech or
　　language
　　disorders, 121
　in infancy, 26
　learning theory, 26
　nativist theory, 26
　newborn babies, 26
　normal childhood
　　development, 26
　social learning theory, 26
Larsson, H., 121
Leach, P., 52
learning disabilities
　challenges for families caring
　　for children with, 39
　co-morbidity with bodily
　　distress disorder, 280
　and concerns around staff
　　knowledge and
　　training, 4
　genetic risk factors, 39
　impact on parents, 39

　and patterns of self-harm, 180
　prevalence in adolescent
　　offender
　　populations, 354
　relationship with
　　psychiatric/
　　neurodevelopmental
　　disorders, 38
learning theory of language
　　development, 26
legal perspectives
　overview, 81
　'Bournewood gap', 82
　Children Act 1989, 84, 85
　consent and competency, 83
　court system
　　Crown court, 93
　　family courts, 93
　　secure custodial estate for
　　　young people, 93–94
　　sentencing options, 93
　　youth courts, 93
　Deprivation of Liberty
　　Safeguards
　　(DoLS), 82
　devolved nations, 94
　Gillick Competence and
　　Fraser Guidelines, 83
　Human Rights Act 1998,
　　81–82
　intellectual disabilities and
　　consent to
　　interventions, 140
　Juvenile Offenders Act
　　1847, 93
　Liberty Protection
　　Safeguards (LPS), 83
　Mental Capacity Act 2005
　　(MCA), 82
　Mental Capacity
　　Amendment Act
　　2019, 83
　Mental Health Act 1983
　　(amended 2007)
　　(MHA), 84, 85–88
　　Section 37 Guardianship
　　　order, 88
　　treatment under, 84
　parental responsibility, scope
　　of, 83–84
　psychiatrist's role in criminal
　　justice pathway,
　　88–92
　　assisting the young person
　　　through the Court
　　　process, 90

dangerousness, 91–92
disposals, 91
diversion to hospital, 89
fitness to be interviewed, 88–89
Part III MHA provisions, 91
psychiatric defences, 92
transfer from custodial settings, 89–90
leptospirosis, association with mental health problems, 38
Lesch–Nyhan syndrome, 345
LGBTQ youth, relationship with mental health, 2, 194
Liaison and Consultation Psychiatry, *see also* psychological medicine 339
Liberty Protection Safeguards (LPS), 83
Lieberman, Alicia, 54, 61
lifespan diagnostic approach, 70
lithium, 205
lockdown restrictions, impact on mental health, 194
long term plan, *see* NHS Long Term Plan (LTP).
looked after children, and mental health policy, 12
lurasidone, 224

major depressive disorder (MDD)
characterisation as treatment resistant depression, 199
Covid-19 pandemic and increase in prevalence of, 194
overlap with common co-morbid mental disorders, 199
prevalence in adolescence, 190
malaria, association with mental health problems, 38
Manchester child attachment story task (MCAST), 107
Manoli, D. S., 120

Marryat, L., 53
Maslow's Hierarchy of Needs, 325
maternal depression, potential role in depression, 192, 193
maternal infections in pregnancy, potential impact on the infant, 120, 133
maternal mental health
and infant mental health, 50
as predictor of child mental health, 40
McCrae, Robert, 24
McCrory, E. J., 326
McFadyen, A., 56
Mead, M., 53
measles, 133
association with mental health problems, 38
median nerve stimulation, as possible treatment for tics, 125
medical emergencies in eating disorders (MEED) guidance, 246
medically unexplained symptoms (MUS)
common miscommunications, 341
diagnosis and management, 341–42
meaning of, 341
melatonin
potential role in depression, 193
as treatment for sleep disturbance, 124
Mellow Programme, 62
meningitis, 133
Mental Capacity Act 2005 (MCA), *see also under* legal perspectives, 82–83
Mental Capacity Amendment Act 2019, 83
Mental Health and Wellbeing Strategy (Scottish government), 3
Mental Health Bill, 4
mental health conditions co-occurring with intellectual disabilities, 136–37

global pre-Covid-19 pandemic prevalence, 190
prevalence in the UK, 1–2
adolescent girls, 1
comparison of ethnic groups, 1
as risk factors for self-harm, 176
Mental Health of Children and Young People in England Survey 2017 (NHS Digital, 2018), 190
Mental Health of Children and Young People in England Survey 2020 (NHS Digital, 2022), 34, 194
mental health policy
England, 3–5
integrated care systems, 5
primary care networks, 5
provider collaboratives, 5
referral and access, 5–6
service delivery, 12
overview, 6, 7
approaches to, 7–10
service delivery framework
crisis services and home treatment teams, 12
data and quality improvement, 7–9
early intervention psychosis services, 11–12
early years support, 10
eating disorder services, 11
integrated and holistic models, 9
looked after children, 12
THRIVE framework, 10
transition and support for adolescents and young adults, 10–12
trauma-informed approaches (TIAs), 9
workforce development, 13, 27
Northern Ireland, 3
Scotland, 3
Wales, 2–3
mental health promotion, 324

mental health support teams (MHSTs), 4, 327
mental illness
　childhood origins, 327
　prevalence in children, 34
mental state examination, 101–3
　appearance and behaviour, 101–2
　insight, 103
　language and speech, 102
　mood, 102
　thought patterns, 102–3
mentalisation-based treatment adapted for adolescence (MBT-A), 184
Mesman, J., 169
Mian, N. D., 169
migration, as risk factor for psychopathology in childhood, 41
Mindfulness-Based Therapies (MBT), 289
minority groups, prevalence of self-harm in, 180
minority stress theory, 313
Missed Opportunities (Centre for Mental Health), 10
mood, assessment of, 102
mood disorders
　co-occurring with intellectual disabilities, 136
　as risk factors for self-harm, 176
moral development
　'Heinz dilemma', 27
　normal childhood development, 27
　stages of, 27
mothers object relations scales, 58
multi-systemic therapy (MST), 154, 305
Muris, P., 167
music therapy, as treatment for depression, 198

naltrexone, 153
narrative therapy, 171, 301
National Autistic Society, 'Good practice guide for professionals delivering talking therapies for autistic adults and children', 305
National Child Mortality Database (NCMD), 2
nativist theory of language development, 26
nature-based interventions for depression, 198
needle phobia, 348
Nelson, C. A., 52
neonatal abstinence syndrome, 50
neonatal behavioural assessment scale (NBAS), 60
neurobehavioural disinhibition in childhood, relationship with substance misuse, 233
neurodevelopmental disorders (NDD), 2, 71
　overview, 113, 125
　ADHD, 121
　ASD, 120
　assessment, 117–20
　　developmental history, 118
　　exposure to alcohol or drugs in utero, 118
　　family history, 119
　　hearing and visual impairments, 118
　　importance of enquiring about tics, 118
　　multidisciplinary approach, 117
　　observation of the child, 119
　　psychometric assessment, 118
　　psychosocial, 118–19
　　rating scales and assessments, 119–20
　　speech and language therapy, 118
　case examples, 113–17
　case vignette, 42
　classification
　　comparison of ICD-10 and ICD-11, 114–16, 123
　　problems with, 113
　developmental learning disorders, 122
　developmental motor coordination disorder, 122
　developmental speech or language disorders, 121
　genetic associations, 118, 120
　health inequalities and, 323
　heritability, 119
　ICD and DSM classifications, 72
　pathological demand avoidance, 120–21
　as predisposing factors for bodily distress disorder/DD, 284
　prevalence in adolescent offender populations, 354
　sleep disturbance, prevalence, 118
　tic disorders, 122–23
　treatment approaches
　　ADHD, 124–25
　　ASD, 124
　　general principles, 123–24
　　specific disorders of development and language, 125
　　tic disorders, 125
　see also individual disorders.
Neurofibromatosis Type 1, 118
neuroplasticity, depression and the role of serotonin in, 192
New York Longitudinal Study, 23
newborn behavioural observation (NBO), 60
NHS Benchmarking, 8
NHS Long Term Plan (LTP), 2, 4, 6
　aims for crisis services, 12
　aims for young people, 10
　commitments, 4,
　funding, 4
　integrated and holistic service provision commitment, 6
　investment plans, 6
　post-Winterbourne View commitments, 4
　prevention support, 323
　publication and funding, 4

recruitment and training goals, 309
waiting times commitment, 2
NICE guidance
ADHD treatment, 124, 238
antipsychotic treatment, 204, 223
anxiety disorders, 170
assessment in CAMHS, 149
bipolar depression, 205
bipolar disorder, 204, 205
depression rating scales, 191
depression treatment, 197, 199
disorder-based nature, 68
eating disorders, 246, 247, 248, 249, 251, 253
interventions for adopted and cared for children, 329
nursery education, 327
patient/carer training, 154
psychoeducation for ADHD and autism, 299
on psychological approaches for neurodivergent CYP, 305
psychological approaches to chronic health conditions, 346
on psychosocial interventions, 298
PTSD, 171
self-harm, 182, 183, 345
stepped care model, 195
on systemic approaches, 300
trauma-focused CBT (TF-CBT), 173
non-binary, 31
non-epileptic seizures, 278, 280, 282, 283
non-violent resistance (NVR), psychosocial interventions in CAMHS, 302–3
normal childhood development, 19
overview, 6
adolescence, 30–31
attachment theory, 21–23
cognitive development, 25
developmental milestones, 19–21
emotional development, 24–25

gender identity, 31–32
language development, 26
peer relationships, 28
personality, 24
play, 28
puberty, 30–31
sexual orientation, 31–32
sleep, 28
social competence and morals, 27
temperament, 23
vulnerability and resilience, 24
Northern Ireland, mental health policy, 3

obesity, potential role in depression, 193
obsessive-compulsive disorder (OCD)
association of ARFID with, 251
psychosocial interventions in CAMHS, 298
as risk factors for self-harm, 176
obstetric complications associated with psychiatric disorders, 37
olanzapine, 205, 224,
Oliver McGowan Mandatory Training on Learning Disability and Autism, 4
online gambling, mental health implications, 272
opiates, use of in pregnancy, 50
oppositional defiant disorder (ODD), 23, 71, 72, 144
characteristics, 76
differential diagnoses, 71
ICD-11 categories and definitions, 145
insecure attachment and, 23
other specified feeding and eating disorders (OSFED), 250

paediatric autoimmune neuropsychiatric disorders (PANDAS), 123

paediatric liaison psychiatry services, survey of, 340
paliperidone, 225
paracetamol, association with psychopathology, 37
parenting
dysfunctional parenting as risk factor for antisocial behaviours, 149
impact of unrealistic parental expectations, 23
understanding the impact of on a child's development, 22
parents
associations between mental health of child and, 40
impact of parental functioning on infants' development, 51
mental health, relationship with children's well-being and development, 329
parents/carers and families
assessment principles, 103–4
history taking, 104
interview tools, 105
observation of parent child interaction, 104
parity of esteem, meaning of, 1
pathological demand avoidance (PDA), 120–21
patient-reported experience measures (PREMs), 8
patient-reported outcome measures (PROMs), 8
peer relationships
characteristics of positive relationships, 328
development of in infancy, 28
as mediating factor for anxiety and depression, 309
preventative role, 328–29
and psychosocial approaches to neurodivergent CYP, 309

peer relationships (cont.)
　role in normal childhood
　　development, 28
　role of play in development
　　of, 28
perinatal mental health
　　services,
　　transformation
　　proposals in
　　England, 4
persistent physical symptoms
　　(PPS), 278
personality
　'Big Five' theory, 24
　normal childhood
　　development, 24
　and psychopathology in
　　childhood, 39
　role of temperament in
　　formation of, 24
personality disorder, 147
　co-occurring with
　　intellectual
　　disabilities, 137
　differentiating from
　　C-PTSD, 166
　differentiating from
　　PTSD, 166
　disordered eating behaviour
　　and, 252,
Phares, V., 329
phenylketonuria, 133
phthalates, 121
physical examination, 105,
physical health, and
　　psychopathology in
　　childhood, 37–38
Piaget, Jean, 25
pica, 250
play
　and development of peer
　　relationships, 28
　importance for brain
　　development and
　　communication,
　　51
　and language
　　development, 26
　normal childhood
　　development, 28
　structured assessment
　　around, 107
Play Therapy, 62
pleiotropy, 36
positive parenting
　　programmes, 10

postpartum psychosis,
　　prevalence, 50
posttraumatic stress disorder
　　(PTSD), 163,
　　171–72, 273
　attachment styles
　　overview, 162
　cyberbullying and, 273
　diagnostic criteria, 163,
　　165, 166
　differential diagnosis, 166
　effectiveness of CBT for,
　　300
　EMDR as treatment for, 304
　evidence of in female forensic
　　in-patients, 357
　ICD-11 categorisation, 164
　insecure attachment and, 23
　interventions, 280
　as predictor of alcohol use
　　disorder, 234
　prevalence and causes,
　　163–64
　secure attachment as
　　protective factor, 163
　see also complex
　　PTSD.
poverty
　mental health impact, 193
　relationship between health
　　and, 53
Powell, B., 61
Prader-Willi Syndrome, 133
pre-frontal cortex, 30
pregnancy
　alcohol use in, 50, 133
　and infant mental health, 50
　maternal infections in,
　　potential impact on
　　the infant, 120, 133
　and substance use, 37
preschool autism
　　communication
　　treatment
　　(PACT), 124
prescribed medications,
　　association with
　　psychopathology,
　　37
prevention and early
　　intervention
　overview, 323, 334
　aspects of a flexible and
　　systemically
　　informed approach,
　　333–34

　clinical practice
　　considerations,
　　332–34
　defining prevention, 324
　distinction between
　　prevention and
　　promotion, 324–25
　in education settings, 327–28
　evidence-based
　　programmes, 329
　family relationships and,
　　329–30
　impact of early adversity,
　　325–27
　see also adverse
　　childhood
　　experiences (ACEs).
　individual factors, 330
　Maslow's Hierarchy of
　　Needs, 325
　peer relationships and,
　　328–29
　practical strategies, 330
　primary prevention, 324
　renewed attention to, 323
　role of 'social determinants
　　of health', 326–27
　safeguarding
　　perspectives, 331
　secondary prevention, 324
　strategic issues, 332
　tertiary prevention, 324
prolactin, potential role in
　　depression, 193
psychiatric co-morbidity, use
　　of in ICD-11, 70
psychiatry, focus on the concept
　　of disorder, 67
psychological medicine
　overview, 339, 350
　autism and/or intellectual
　　impairment, 344–45
　chronic health conditions,
　　346–47
　co-morbidity management
　　case study, 343–44
　CPM teams in general
　　hospitals, 339–40
　delirium, 342–43
　disorders requiring
　　integrated psychiatry
　　and paediatrics,
　　340–44
　eating disorders, 340–41
　functional neurological
　　disorders, 343

impacts of the Covid-19
  pandemic, 349–50
integrative focus, 339
medical unexplained
  symptoms/functional
  disorders, 341–42
needle phobia, 348
neuropsychiatric
  presentations, 342–43
psychiatric emergencies,
  self-harm, 345–46
psychiatrically unwell
  patients stranded in
  hospital, 347–48
staff support, 349
support for adjustment to
  chronic
  conditions, 349
traumatic brain injury, 343
treatment adherence
  support, 348–49
psychological therapy, 196–97
adverse effects, 197
psychopathology in childhood
ACEs and, 41
case vignettes, 42–43
cognitive ability and, 38–39
Covid-19 pandemic and, 42
environmental risk factors,
  37–42
family risk factors, 40
genetic risk factors, 36–37
migration risk factors, 41
physical health and, 37–38
prenatal/perinatal risk
  factors, 37
relationships between
  variables, 34
risk and protective
  factors, 34
risk factor levels, 36
school and community risk
  factors, 40
socio-economic inequalities
  and, 41
substance use and, 39
symptomatic approach, 69
technology and social media
  risk factors, 40–41
temperament and
  personality risk
  factors, 39
terminology used in
  epidemiological
  research, 35
psychosis

overview, 219
CBT as treatment for, 225
early intervention services,
  11–12, 225–26
psychological medicine
  perspective, 342
psychotic illnesses as risk
  factor for self-harm,
  176
see also early-onset
  psychosis (EOP).
psychosis/schizophrenia,
  co-occurring with
  intellectual
  disabilities, 137
psychosocial approaches, 153,
  296, 305, 306
ACT, 300
anxiety disorders,
  298
behavioural approaches
child focused, 298–99
parent focused, 299–305
case formulation and,
  296–97
CBT, 299–300
common elements and core
  principles, 297–98
compassion-focused
  therapy, 300
depression, 298
disruptive behaviour
  disorders, 153–55
evidence-based practice
  and, 298
examples of influencing
  psychosocial factors,
  296–97
future perspectives, 309–10
intervention types, 296
meaning of, 296
neurodivergent CYP, 305–9
capacity to consent, 306
direct individual therapy
  elements of, 309
indicators for, 305–7
environmental
  adaptations, 308
eye contact, 307
indicators for direct
  individual therapy,
  305–7
language and
  communication, 307
masking, 307
peer relationships, 309

special interests, 308
value of concrete
  strategies, 308
visual supports, 307–8
non-violent resistance,
  302–3
OCD, 298
other psychosocial
  interventions, 304
parent/carer training
  approaches, 299
psychodynamic approaches,
  303–4
psychoeducation, 299
systemic approaches, 300–1
therapy/change techniques,
  301–2
psychotic disorders, prevalence
  in forensic
  in-patients, 357
puberty
behavioural impact on
  adolescents, 30
the process, 30
Tanner stages, 31
pyromania, 146–47

quetiapine, 205
The Quick Test (QT)©, 133

randomised controlled trials,
  exclusion of young
  people from, 195
reactive attachment disorder
  (RAD), 71
comparison with DSED, 161
re-authoring, 301
refeeding syndrome, 340
reflexivity, 301
relational reflexivity, 302
self-reflexivity, 301
relationships, sex and health
  education (RSHE), 6
repressed memories, 303
research domain criteria
  (RDoC), 68
resilience
normal childhood
  development, 24
relationship with
  temperament, 24
revised children's anxiety and
  depression scale,
  192
Riding the Rapids, 299
risk assessment, 103

at risk mental states
(ARMS), 12
risperidone, 123, 125, 153, 205, 224–25
routine outcome measures (ROMs), 8, 298
Royal College of Psychiatrists Practice Standards, 236
rubella, 120, 133
rumination disorder, 250
Rutter, M., 167

schedule for affective disorders and schizophrenia mania rating scale, 204
schizophrenia
  association with obstetric complications, 37
  childhood onset schizophrenia, 219
  heritability, 37, 220
  schizophrenia spectrum disorders, 219
school-based interventions for depression, 195–96
school-based mindfulness training (SBMT), 196
schools
  RSHE curriculum, 6
  setting up of mental health support teams in, 4, 327
Schore, A., 51
Scotland, mental health policy, 3
screening instruments, 105–6
Secondary Impulse Control Syndrome, 72
secure attachment, 22, 40
  parent/carer training approaches, 299
  as protective factor against PTSD, 163
Segal, L., 55
seizures
  febrile, 38
  prevalence in childhood, 38
selective mutism, 71
selective serotonin reuptake inhibitors (SSRIs)
  combination treatment, 198
  common side-effects, 197
  and disruptive behaviour disorders, 153

FDA 'Black Box' warning on suicidality, 198
and treatment resistant depression, 199, 200
self-esteem, acceptance as important source of, 28
self-harm, 304
  addictive component, 182
  ADHD as risk factor for, 176
  autism as risk factor for, 176
  body dysmorphic disorder as risk factor for, 176
  co-morbidity with bulimia, 248
  cyberbullying and, 273
  DBT as treatment for, 304
  disordered eating as method of, 180–81
  function of, 178, 181
  mindfulness exercises, 346
  NICE guidelines, 182
  as psychiatric emergency, 345–46
  as risk factor for future suicidality, 179
self-harm/suicide, 330
  aetiology and association with mental health conditions, 176–78
  depression as risk factor for, 177
  epidemiology, 178–80
  family adversity and, 178
  formulation of, 181–82
  gendered differences, 178, 180
  importance of asking about factors associated with, 346
  interventions, 183–85
  CBT, 184
  crisis teams and intensive home-based services, 183
  DBT, 184
  family-based therapies, 184
  hospital admissions, 184–85
  MBT-A, 184
  NICE recommendations, 183

  pharmacological treatment, 184
  psychological, 183
  secure units, 185
  methods used, 180–81
  population-based study, 177
  prevalence, 77, 178
  pre-pandemic prevalence, 2
  prevention strategies, 178
  public health concerns, 176, 178
  risk assessment, 182–83
    collaborative and therapeutic approaches, 183
    NICE guidelines, 182
    personalised approach, 182–83
    utility of risk assessment tools, 103, 182
  risk factors, 177–78, 179
  role of social media, 178
  safety plan, 346
  terminology and definitions, 176
SEND and alternative provision improvement plan (UK Gov, 2023), 4
separation anxiety disorder, 71
serotonin, role of in neuroplasticity, 192
sertraline, 197
sexual exploitation, online grooming and, 273
sexual orientation/gender identity
  as correlate of disorder, 74
  normal childhood development, 32
  as risk factor for self-harm/suicide, 180
Skinner, B. F., 26
sleep, normal childhood development, 28
sleep disorders, co-occurring with intellectual disabilities, 138
sleep disturbance
  managing, 124
  relationship with depression, 193
Smith-Magenis syndrome, 133, 345

social competence and morals, normal childhood development, 27
social learning theory of language development, 26
social media, 268–70
 benefits, 269
 challenges and clinical risks, 269
 compulsion or addiction to, 270
 and copycat behaviour, 274
 and cyberbullying, 272
 definition, 268
 mental health impact, 194, 244, 253–55, 274
 positive and negative influences/impacts, 40–41, 297
 and psychopathology in childhood, 40–41
 questions to ask about usage of, 267–68
 role of in self-harm/suicide, 178, 194
 use of by CYP, 269
 used by online groomers, 273
social prescribing, 296
socialisation
 benefits of internet-based technology for, 265
 risks of internet-based technology for, 266
socio-economic status
 as correlate of disorder, 75
 and psychopathology in childhood, 41
 as risk factor for mental health problems, 40
 and risk of ADHD, 121
sodium valproate, association with psychopathology, 37
Solihull programme, 62
somatic symptom disorder, 278
speech and language assessments (SAL), 102, 108, 118
staff recruitment and retention, 13, 27
State, M. W., 120
Stein, A., 51, 104
Steiner, Claude, 25
stepped care model
 depression treatment, 195

infant mental health services, 56
Stepping Forward to 2020/2021 (2017), 13
'strange situation procedure', 22
Strengths and Difficulties Questionnaire (SDQ), 1
streptococcal infection
 association with acute onset of tics or OCD, 123
 association with mental health problems, 38
substance misuse
 overview, 231, 240–40
 ADHD as risk factor for, 235
 assessment of, 236–37
 and brain myelination, 235
 co-morbidities, 231–33, 248
 European Monitoring Centre for Drugs and Drug Abuse Quality Standards, 239
 interventions
  atomoxetine, 238
  Cannabis Youth Treatment Study, 237
  complex interventions, 238
  fluoxetine and CBT, 238
  interagency coordination, 240
  multidimensional family therapy, 237
  multisystemic therapy, 238
  secondary prevention, 237
  single modality intervention, 237–38
  substances and complex psychopathology, 238–40
 origins of substance use disorders
  deviant peers, 234
  early behaviour problems, 233
  family environment, 232
  mood and other mental disorders, 233–34
  trauma, 233–34
  trends, 234–35

presence of in completed adolescent suicides, 236
prevalence, 77–78, 231–32
and psychopathology in childhood, 39
psychosocial harms, 235–36
rates among adoptees, 233
relationship with economic growth and development, 232
as risk factor for self-harm, 177
substance use disorder
 DSM-5, 232
 ICD-11, 231
substance-related avoidable deaths, 236
US national co-morbidity study – adolescent supplement, 231, 233
suicidal thoughts, cyberbullying and, 273
suicide
 NCMD report, 2
 presence of substance misuse in completed adolescent suicides, 236
 prevalence as cause of death for adolescents, 345
 prevalence of attempts in adolescent onset bipolar disorder, 206
 rates of in the UK, 179
 risk of in adolescents with PTSD, 163
 social media as risk factor for, 194
sustainability and transformation partnerships (STPs), 5
synaptic pruning, 52
syphilis, association with mental health problems, 38
systemic lupus erythematosus (SLE), association between psychiatric disorders and, 38
systemic thinking, 302

Tanner stages of puberty, 31

technology, impact of rapid growth in, 297
temperament
  the concept of, 39
  early relationships and, 50
  'easy' characteristics *vs* 'difficult', 23
  and psychopathology in childhood, 39
  relationship with vulnerability and resilience, 24
  role of in emotional regulation, 24
  role of in personality formation, 24
  'slow-to-warm-up' children, 23
tension type headache, 278
theory of mind, childhood development, 26
therapeutic letters, 301
'thinspiration', 253, 274
Thomas, Alexander, 23
thought patterns, assessment of, 102–3
threat processing, 327
THRIVE Framework, 10, 309
thyroid stimulating hormone, potential role in depression, 193
tic disorders, 122–23
  characterised in ICD-11, 122
  treatment approaches, 125
tics, importance of enquiring about, 118
Timid to Tiger, 299
Tourette's Syndrome, psychological medicine perspective, 342
toxoplasmosis, 38, 133
  association with mental health problems, 38
training, CYP-IAPT programme, 13
transcranial magnetic stimulation, as treatment for difficult-to-treat depression, 200
Transforming Care (2012), 4

Transforming CYP Mental Health Provision Green Paper (2017), 4, 6
transgender, 32, 180, 313
trauma
  assessment of in children and adolescents
    asking difficult questions, 165
    very young children, 165–66
  cyberbullying and, 273
  debriefing of staff after traumatic incident, 349
  EMDR as treatment for, 304
  impact of exposure to in childhood, 24
  interventions, 173
  potential role in depression, 194
  as precipitating factor for bodily distress disorder/DD, 284
  prevalence of exposure to, 164, 173
  principles of trauma informed care, 165
  relationship with bipolar disorder, 201, 207
  relationship with self-harm, 182
  trauma-focused (TF-CBT), 171, 173
  trauma-informed approaches to mental health policy, 9
  see also complex PTSD (C-PTSD); post-traumatic stress disorder (PTSD).
traumatic brain injury, 343
  potential role in depression, 193
  as risk factor for ADHD, 38
  as risk factor for neuropsychiatric problems, 38
treatment adherence, support for, 348
Treatment for Adolescents with Depression Study (TADS) (JAMA, 2004), 198, 200
Treatment of Resistant Depression In Adolescents (TORDIA) study (Emslie *et al.*), 200
Triple P-Positive Parenting Program, 62, 299, 329
tuberous sclerosis, 118, 133, 138
type 1 diabetes mellitus, disordered eating in the context of, 248–49

valproate, 37, 113, 118, 153, 205, 206
Vasey, M. W., 167
venlafaxine, 200
video interactive guidance (VIG), 61, 299, 329
Viding, E., 326
Vineland adaptive behaviour scales, 133
The Voice of the Infant Best Practice Guidelines and Infant Pledge, 56
vulnerability and resilience, normal childhood development, 24

Wales, mental health policy, 2–3
Watch, Wait & Wonder, 62
Watch Me Play, 62
Wechsler adult intelligence scale, 133
Wechsler intelligence scale for children (WISC) ©, 133
Wechsler nonverbal scale of ability, 133
Wechsler preschool and primary scale of intelligence, 133
Wechsler individual attainment test, 108
White, Michael, 301
'window of tolerance', 326, 327

Winnicott, Donald, 53
Winterbourne View Hospital, 4
workforce development, 13, 27
WPATH (World Professional Association for Transgender Health), 316

young mania rating scale, 204
Youngstrom, E. A., 203
youth justice system
   development of, 354
   numbers of first-time entrants, 353

ziprasidone, 205, 224

For EU product safety concerns, contact us at Calle de José Abascal, 56–1°,
28003 Madrid, Spain or eugpsr@cambridge.org.

www.ingramcontent.com/pod-product-compliance
Ingram Content Group UK Ltd.
Pitfield, Milton Keynes, MK11 3LW, UK
UKHW022107150326
469019UK00019B/1498